CLINICAL LABORATORY INSTRUMENTATION AND AUTOMATION

Principles, Applications, and Selection

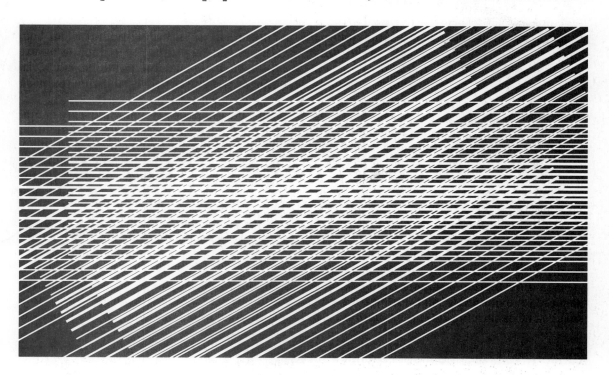

KORY M. WARD, PhD, MT(ASCP)

Assistant Professor
Medical Technology Division
School of Allied Medical Professions
The Ohio State University
Columbus, Ohio

CRAIG A. LEHMANN, PhD, CC(NRCC)

Associate Professor and Chair,
Division of Diagnostic and Therapeutic Sciences
School of Allied Health Professions
State University of New York at Stony Brook
Stony Brook, New York

ALAN M. LEIKEN, PhD

Associate Professor
Health Science and Management
Department of Allied Health Resources
School of Allied Health Professions
State University of New York at Stony Brook
Stony Brook, New York

W.B. SAUNDERS COMPANY

A Division of Harcourt Brace & Company
Philadelphia
London   Toronto   Montreal   Sydney   Tokyo

CLINICAL LABORATORY INSTRUMENTATION AND AUTOMATION

Principles, Applications, and Selection

Library of Congress Cataloging-in-Publication Data

Clinical laboratory instrumentation and automation: principles, applications, and selection / [edited by] Kory M. Ward, Craig A. Lehmann, Alan M. Leiken.—1st ed.

p. cm.

ISBN 0–7216–4218–7

1. Pathological laboratories—Automation.   I. Ward, Kory M.
   II. Lehmann, Craig A.   III. Leiken, Alan M.
   [DNLM: 1. Equipment and Supplies.   2. Laboratories.
   3. Technology, Medical—instrumentation.   QY 26 C6409 1994]

RB38.C58 1994   616.07'028—dc20

DNLM/DLC   92–48469

W.B. SAUNDERS COMPANY
A Division of
Harcourt Brace & Company

The Curtis Center
Independence Square West
Philadelphia, Pennsylvania 19106

Clinical Laboratory Instrumentation and Automation:
Principles, Applications, and Selection

ISBN 0–7216–4218–7

Last digit is the print number: 9   8   7   6   5   4   3   2   1

W.B. SAUNDERS COMPANY
A Division of
Harcourt Brace & Company

The Curtis Center
Independence Square West
Philadelphia, Pennsylvania 19106

Library of Congress Cataloging-in-Publication Data

Clinical laboratory instrumentation and automation: principles, applications, and selection / [edited by] Kory M. Ward, Craig A. Lehmann, Alan M. Leiken.—1st ed.

p. cm.

ISBN 0–7216–4218–7

1. Pathological laboratories—Automation.   I. Ward, Kory M.
II. Lehmann, Craig A.   III. Leiken, Alan M.
[DNLM: 1. Equipment and Supplies.   2. Laboratories.
3. Technology, Medical—instrumentation.   QY 26 C6409 1994]

RB38.C58 1994   616.07′028—dc20

DNLM/DLC   92–48469

Clinical Laboratory Instrumentation and Automation: ISBN 0–7216–4218–7
Principles, Applications, and Selection

Printed in the United States of America

Last digit is the print number: 9   8   7   6   5   4   3   2   1

Contributors

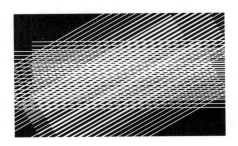

BARBARA J. CLEVELAND, MPH, MT(ASCP)
Graduate Teaching Assistant, The Ohio State University School of Allied Medical Professions; Medical Technologist—Toxicology; University Reference Laboratories, Columbus, Ohio
Fundamental Principles of Electronics Instrumentation for the Measurement of Blood Gases and Electrolytes

ROBERT P. DeCRESCE, MD, MPH, MBA
Assistant Professor of Pathology, Rush Medical College; Director of Clinical Laboratories, Rush–Presbyterian–St. Luke's Hospital, Chicago, Illinois
Clinical Chemistry Automation

KAREN M. ESCOLAS, MS, MT(ASCP)
Clinical Assistant Professor, School of Allied Health Professions, Department of Medical Technology, Health Sciences Center, State University of New York at Stony Brook, Stony Brook, New York
Laboratory Information Systems

JOSEPH G. FINK, MD
Clinical Associate Professor of Pathology, New York Medical College–Metropolitan Hospital Center, New York, New York
Preventive Maintenance and Troubleshooting

DEBORAH T. FIRESTONE, MA, MT(ASCP) SBB
Clinical Assistant Professor, School of Allied Health Professions; Department of Medical Technology, Health Sciences Center, State University of New York at Stony Brook, Stony Brook, New York
Particle Counters

DONALD J. GARTNER, MS, MT(ASCP)SH
Associate Professor, School of Allied Health Sciences, Clinical Laboratory Sciences; Indiana University School of Medicine; Administrative Supervisor, Hematopathology, Department of Pathology, Indiana University Hospital, Indianapolis, Indiana
Automated Hematology Analyzers

EDWARD HARRIS, BS
Regional Sales Manager, Spectrophotometer
Products, Milton Roy Corporation, Rochester,
New York
Spectrophotometry

LINDA M. KASPER, MS, MT(ASCP)SC
Program Director, Medical Technologist Program,
Indiana University Medical Center, Indianapolis,
Indiana
Automated Instrumentation (Generic)

DAVID D. KOCH, PhD
Associate Professor, Department of Pathology and
Laboratory Medicine, University of Wisconsin;
Director, Clinical Chemistry Laboratory,
University of Wisconsin Hospital and Clinics,
Madison, Wisconsin
*Instrumentation for the Measurement of
Blood Gases and Electrolytes*

YUN-SIK KWAK, MD, PhD
Assistant Professor of Pathology, Case Western
Reserve University School of Medicine; Chief,
Pathology and Laboratory Medicine Service, VA
Medical Center, Cleveland, Ohio
*Chemistry Instrumentation for the Small Office
Laboratory*

CRAIG A. LEHMANN, PhD, CC (NRCC)
Associate Professor and Chair, Division of
Diagnostic and Therapeutic Sciences, School of
Allied Health Professions; Program Director,
Medical Technology, State University of New
York at Stony Brook, Stony Brook, New York
*Improving Laboratory Efficiency Through
Workflow Analysis*
*The Impact of Instrumentation on Laboratory
Costs*
A Word From the Manufacturer

ALAN LEIKEN, PhD
Associate Professor of Health Sciences and
Management, School of Allied Health
Professions, State University of New York at
Stony Brook, Stony Brook, New York

*Improving Laboratory Efficiency Through
Workflow Analysis*
*The Impact of Instrumentation on Laboratory
Costs*

MARK S. LIFSHITZ, MD
Clinical Associate Professor of Pathology;
Director of Clinical Laboratories, New York
University School of Medicine, New York, New
York
Clinical Chemistry Automation

JAMES E. LOVE, Jr, PhD, MBA
Senior Development Engineer, Clinical
Diagnostics Division, Eastman Kodak Company,
Rochester, New York
Electrophoretic Instrumentation Systems

**TIMOTHY G. McMANAMON, PhD,
DABCC**
Instructor, Clinical Laboratory Science, Mercy
School of Health Sciences; Clinical Chemist,
Mercy Hospital Medical Center, Department of
Pathology, Des Moines, Iowa
Chromatography Instrumentation Systems

HERBERT K. NAITO, PhD, MBA
Chief, Clinical Chemistry, Pathology and
Laboratory Medicine Service; Associate Director,
National Center for Laboratory Accuracy and
Standardization, VA Medical Center, Cleveland,
Ohio
*Chemistry Instrumentation for the Small Office
Laboratory*

SHESHADRI NARAYANAN, PhD
Clinical Professor of Pathology, New York
Medical College; Attending, Department of
Pathology, New York Medical College–
Metropolitan Hospital Center, New York,
New York
Preventive Maintenance and Troubleshooting

RICHARD O. PFAU, PhD, MT(ASCP)
Assistant Professor, Adjunct Faculty, School of
Allied Medical Professions, College of Medicine;

Assistant Professor, Adjunct Faculty, Department of Anthropology, The Ohio State University, Columbus, Ohio
Forensic Instrumental Applications

JOHN R. SNYDER, PhD, MT(ASCP)SH
Dean and Professor, School of Allied Health Sciences, Associate Dean, Indiana University School of Medicine, Indianapolis, Indiana
Automated Hematology Analyzers

VIVIEN A. SOO, MS, MT(ASCP)
Section Supervisor, Special Chemistry/Toxicology, University Hospital, State University of New York at Stony Brook, Stony Brook, New York
Immunochemistry Analyzers

BERNADETTE L. THORNTON, MT(ASCP)
Senior Technologist, Quality Control, The Ohio State University Hospital, Columbus, Ohio
Instrumentation Systems: Reliability and Validity Issues

DAVID J. THORNTON, PhD, C(ASCP)
Director, Clinical Chemistry Laboratory, Children's Hospital, Columbus, Ohio
Instrumentation Systems: Reliability and Validity Issues

GEORGE T. TORTORA, PhD
Associate Professor, School of Allied Health Professions, Health Sciences Center, State University of New York at Stony Brook; Head of Clinical Microbiology, University Hospital, Stony Brook, New York
Automation in Clinical Microbiology

KORY M. WARD, PhD, MT(ASCP)
Assistant Professor, Medical Technology Division, School of Allied Medical Professions, The Ohio State University, Columbus, Ohio
Spectrophotometry
Electrophoretic Instrumentation Systems

F o r e w o r d

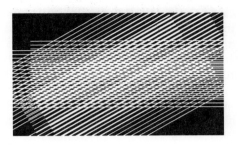

AUTOMATION AND INSTRUMENTATION: FIVE DECADES OF APPLIED TECHNOLOGY

The growth of automation in the clinical laboratory is the result of two key factors: the clinician's need for increasing amounts of diagnostic information and the rapid availability of new technology for the development of laboratory instrumentation. In this book, *Clinical Laboratory Instrumentation and Automation: Principles, Applications, and Selection,* a variety of core technologies are described. Many of these technologies have been applied to clinical laboratory automation. Their success is based on three factors that have stood the test of time: reliability in producing consistent analytical data with a minimum of downtime, ease of training to ensure technology transfer, and cost effectiveness. These factors have been a constant challenge to the teams of chemists, engineers, physicists, and programmers who have developed automated systems over the last five decades.

The growth of laboratory automation began in the early 1950s to meet the demands of clinicians for diagnostic information. The periods can be viewed by decade and give us valuable insight into the development cycle of which we are all a part.

1950–1959
Trial and Error: The First Steps

These years represent the initial growth phase of clinical laboratory instrumentation. The decade began with emphasis on the classic techniques of quantitative analytical biochemistry and manual cell counting. Training emphasized the skills of pipetting and rigid conformance to protocol. Simple photometers reading percent transmission often represented the only instrumentation in the chemistry laboratory with the exception of pH meters. The latter were essential, since many laboratories still made their own reagents. The analysis of sodium and potassium using bulky flame photometers was just beginning. Much more common in the clinical laboratory were electrophoresis systems for protein fractionation. All these systems required manual pipetting of sample and were labor-intensive. Physicians usually received reports from individual laboratory sections with little interpretive background information.

Throughout the decade, automation became more evident in the laboratory. The commercial development of the Technicon AutoAnalyzer system in 1957 established continuous flow as a viable technology for routine clinical chemistry analysis. Simulation of manual techniques on an automated system was the basis of the Robot Chemist developed by Warner-Chilcott Instruments Division. These original chemistry analyzers were single-channel systems performing tests in a sequential manner. On the completion of a single test they could be switched to a new method and samples rerun for new parameters. Availability of these new analytical tools encouraged laboratorians to develop adaptations of traditional assays to the new instrumentation.

By the end of the decade, several companies were offering flame photometers for the routine analysis of sodium and potassium. The new units were compact and were available on a 24-hour basis for "STAT" reporting. The use of temperature-controlled spectrophotometers enabled the laboratory to perform kinetic assays for many clinical enzyme assays. The Coulter and Sanborn companies were developing particle counters that enabled the automation of the routine manual cell counting procedures used in the standard complete blood count (CBC).

1960–1969
Automation for Every Laboratory

The variety of developments during this period was fueled by the wide acceptance of automated analysis in the clinical laboratory. The decade began with the rapid expansion of single-channel analyzers into a wide variety of laboratory settings. By 1965, multichannel analyzers that generated chemistry and hematology profiles were available. In 1968 the first Oak Ridge Conference was held, announcing the concept of centrifugal analysis. The availability of solid-state electronics utilizing transistors allowed the instrument designer to switch from analog to digital systems. Vacuum tubes were replaced by solid-state devices and printed circuit boards combining multiple functions. Servicing of complex systems was resolved by replacing boards instead of troubleshooting at the individual component level. The first laboratory computer systems began to appear. The rapid growth of new systems in this decade paralleled the growth of laboratory medicine and its increasing consumption of laboratory data. In retrospect, this was the first decade in which there was unlimited access to laboratory data because of the impact of laboratory automation.

As automated workstations came to be routinely used in the laboratory, it soon was apparent that their efficiency could be increased by simultaneous operation of several modules to obtain multiple results from a common sample. A single operator could then produce subsets of patient results that were usually ordered as panels. Examples of this ordering pattern were calcium and phosphorus; albumin and total protein; and sodium, potassium, chloride, and bicarbonate. The laboratory could now produce results faster than they could be calculated and collated into a completed patient report. Out of this dilemma evolved the concept of multiple analysis. The first successful application was the Technicon SMA 12 system. This continuous-flow system processed 30 samples per hour for 12 parameters commonly ordered in acute-care hospitals. It was followed by a second model, the SMA

12-Survey, which focused on tests used on outpatients to produce a biochemical profile on an ambulatory population. By the end of the decade, the SMA 12/60 and 6/60 systems were available from Technicon. These systems could be run simultaneously, producing an 18-test profile. There was a similar development from manufacturers of discrete analyzers. The Hycel Mark X utilized their manual kit reagents to produce a ten-channel analyzer by duplicating these manual assays on an automated system. By the end of the decade, large-scale discrete analyzers were available from AGA, Vickers, Coulter, and Damon, and a 17-test analyzer was being developed by Hycel. The chemistry profile became an integral part of admission testing for hospitalized patients as well as part of the routine testing done on outpatients.

Multiple analysis was not restricted to clinical chemistry. One of the early applications of the original AutoAnalyzers was the determination of hemoglobin on whole blood samples. This was coupled to a particle counter and led to the development of multiple analyzers for hematology. The SMA 4 generated results for hemoglobin, white and red blood cell counts, and hematocrit value, while the SMA 7 included calculated indexes. This was followed by the introduction of the Coulter S system, which measured red and white cells, mean cell volume (MCV), and hemoglobin directly from a whole blood sample and calculated the hematocrit value, mean cell hemoglobin concentration (MCHC), and mean cell hemoglobin (MCH) automatically.

1970–1979
Technology Expansion: The Computer-Driven Analyzer

In this decade, computers were designed into many of the analytical systems that came into common use. It is reflected in the design approach utilized on the Technicon SMAC (Sequential Multiple Analyzer Plus Computer) system and in the design of the three centrifugal analyzers that came on the market in the early 1970s. These analyzers, based on the GEMSAEC concept, were the Electro-Nucleonics GEMSAEC, the Union Carbide CentrifiChem, and the American Instruments Company RotoChem. These systems all depend on the use of onboard computers and microprocessors to capture changes in absorbance and convert them to calculated concentrations. They also controlled the repetitive operation of the systems, replacing the mechanical cams and timing devices previously utilized in system design. The use of onboard computers also made possible the development and routine use of a single unit dose chemistry analyzer, the Du Pont ACA. This system incorporated the reagents into subsections of a single unit dose reagent pack. This pack was identified to the system by the use of a bar code reader. An onboard computer then initiated the appropriate analytical steps.

Another development that came to the forefront in the beginning of the 1970s was the successful utilization of ion-selective electrodes (ISEs) for the routine analysis of sodium and potassium. This technology was first applied to the Photovolt Stat Ion and the SMAC systems. By the middle of the decade, it was in widespread use on the ASTRA systems developed by the Beckman Corporation. It also was applied to STAT systems by the Nova and Orion companies. The utilization of ISEs for sodium and potassium analysis is now taken for granted, but in the early 1970s it was a new technology.

By the end of the decade, most manufacturers were routinely developing instruments around available computer systems. IL and Roche developed second-generation centrifugal analyzers with increased rates of analysis, automatic sample handling, and adaptability to laboratory information systems (LIS). In fact, by the end of the decade, most manufacturers were routinely designing LIS interfaces into their systems to interact with a wide variety of second-generation laboratory information systems that had become available.

Progress was made in automated white cell differential counts using two distinct approaches—pattern recognition and cytochemical continuous flow-analysis. The pattern recognition systems were developed at the LARC analyzer by Corning Scientific Instruments and Hematrak by the Geometric Data Corporation. These systems were automated microscopes that used digital imaging processing techniques to identify the morphologic features of the different types of white cells. The continuous-flow Hemalog-D system from the Technicon Instruments Corporation used cytochemical staining to differentiate the populations in conjunction with light scattering. Instead of a count of 100 cells on a slide, 30,000 leukocytes were viewed per sample. Regardless of technology, automation now made it possible for differentials to be routinely run by general laboratory technologists with the same accuracy previously obtained only by experienced senior technologists.

1980–1989
Random Access Comes of Age

A new type of automated system, the random access analyzer, became generally available in this decade. Random access analyzers offered the capability of a broad test menu on a single system. They generally had the capability of onboard reagent storage for up to 30 different assays, and the operator could choose any number of tests on a given sample depending upon on-system reagent availability and the appropriate software to perform and calculate the tests ordered. These systems generally had

sampling rates from 120 to 480 tests per hour. Throughput of patient samples was determined by the number of tests ordered for each sample. The major advantage of these systems was the reduction in number of workstations, relative ease of operation, and 24-hour availability to cover off-peak workloads. These systems were generally more complex and expensive than the batch analyzers but offered cost-effective processing of the laboratory workload.

Developers of these systems took advantage of a variety of technologies to offer random access capability to the laboratory. One of the most interesting approaches was that developed for use on the Kodak Ektachem systems, which utilized a multilayer film slide technology for a variety of assays. Operators would choose the tests required through a keyboard CRT display, and the system would automatically aliquot samples and select the appropriate slides in the analyzer module. The reaction of samples was accomplished by the diffusion of the specimen through a series of film layers, and the final results were read in a reflectometer or ion-selective electrode detection system. Random access also was accomplished for more conventional systems using liquid reagents by the development of metering systems that used as little as 3 μL of sample and reagent volumes of 300 μL or less. These systems were usually based on positive displacement devices (Hamilton syringes) controlled by computer command. Reactions took place either in disposable cuvettes mounted on a rotor or on systems that contained onboard cuvette washing systems that allowed recycling of the permanent cuvettes.

The Coulter DACOS, the Cooper DEMAND, and the Hitachi 705 were examples of random access analyzers that became available in this decade. The Technicon RA-1000 and CHEM 1 systems utilized an inert fluorocarbon to maintain the integrity of samples and reagents in their analytical pathways, permitting simplified medical design. The American Dade PARAMAX incorporated reagents in a "pill" form that were reconstituted as needed, thereby simplifying reagent handling. Regardless of the technological approach, the laboratory now had a variety of random access systems to choose from, simplifying workflow patterns and decreasing the need for batch analyzers dedicated to single tasks.

1990–1999
The Era of Consolidation

The development of new instrumentation in the 1990s reflects a period of consolidation and retrenching by both the developers and the users of laboratory automation. Many of the companies involved in instrument development have become part of larger organizations through the merger process. Major changes in applied technology require significant investment and long years of development before they produce profits. The financial impact of development is now carefully assessed before projects are launched. The increased regulatory requirements imposed on the manufacturer also add to the costs of development.

The users of laboratory automation have their own concerns. In a health system going through a period of cost review, how much will be allocated to the laboratory? Will it be perceived as a provider of useful clinical information or an area of excessive costs? Will local laboratories be forced to consolidate and share services, increasing the turnaround time now offered? What will be the impact of new technology on lowering operating costs while providing timely information to physicians?

One cannot predict the future, but this brief review of the history of automation conveys a central message: *change*. This has been the only constant in the utilization of instrumentation in the clinical laboratory. We, as users of this equipment, have had the opportunity to be on the leading edge of the changes in the clinical laboratory. Our knowledge of instrumentation will secure our future.

Jacob B. Levine, M.B.A., C.C. (NRCC)
Director
Clinical Evaluations and Product Labeling
  Diagnostics Division
Miles Inc.
Tarrytown, New York

P r e f a c e

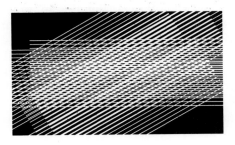

Although designed primarily for the clinical laboratory science student, this textbook will be a valuable resource to many individuals, from those who work with clinical laboratory instrumentation to those who support clinical laboratory instrumentation, such as the manufacturers. The intended audience for *Clinical Laboratory Instrumentation and Automation: Principles, Applications, and Selection* includes associate and baccalaureate degree students of clinical laboratory science programs, graduate students in clinical laboratory science, pathology residents, medical students, and practitioners. This textbook is designed to be used in conjunction with other courses or textbooks within formal clinical laboratory science–related educational programs, to serve as the "stand-alone" textbook for a comprehensive clinical laboratory instrumentation course, or to be a reference book for clinical laboratory practitioners, researchers, and industry personnel. Written to provide the reader with a broad-based understanding of clinical laboratory instrumentation principles, it offers specific applications of these principles by the manufacturers and describes the processes of instrument selection.

The clinical laboratory practitioner must not only possess the skills necessary to understand the basic operation of clinical laboratory instruments but also be able to make intelligent decisions about the acquisition of instrumentation to meet the needs of the specific laboratory. Further, the practitioner is now challenged to verify the reliability of all instruments brought into the laboratory, according to federal regulations. Accordingly core chapters describing analytical theory and principles of basic electronics, spectrophotometry, electrochemistry, chromatography, electrophoresis, particle counting, and immunochemical methodologies are included, in addition to chapters on the use of computers and laboratory information systems for automation, operation management, interfacing, and quality assurance verification. Individual chapters are devoted to instrument reliability issues, laboratory information systems, and troubleshooting. To enhance the student's or practitioner's knowledge about selection of laboratory instruments, chapters on workflow analysis and economic issues related to instrument selection are included. One chapter deals comprehensively with chemistry instrumentation for the small office laboratory.

This book incorporates contributions from experts in various fields of clinical laboratory instrumentation. Each chapter was written with the intent to provide the reader with the most current technological information while presenting the material in an enjoyable and readable style. In keeping with the principles of good educational practice, each chapter commences with learning objectives and key words, which are boldfaced when they first appear in the discussions. All chapters conclude with multiple-choice test questions that test the reader's comprehension of major concepts. A glossary offers assistance with vocabulary related to instrumentation and automation.

Some unique features of this textbook include a general discussion of automation followed by specific chapters addressing automation in hematology, clinical chemistry, and microbiology. Readers will also find a special chapter devoted to forensics instrumentation. Because of the diversity and complexity of the major automated systems in the marketplace today, this book also of-

fers an appendix entitled "A Word From the Manufacturer." This provides a direct link to information supplied by the manufacturers, the aim of which is to provide the reader with a comparative summary of the current major automated chemistry systems. Additionally, in an effort to equip the student to deal with government regulations, the chapter entitled "Instrumentation Systems: Reliability and Validity Issues" is offered. This chapter provides a practical approach to instrument reliability verification, and ongoing quality assurance measures that must be in place in order to meet federal regulatory requirements.

We, as the editors, hope that this textbook will meet the needs of individuals who work with clinical laboratory instruments or are involved with their acquisition. It is our goal to cover the spectrum of laboratory instrumentation and automation by describing the principles of operation; by introducing the systems currently on the market; and by helping to enable operators of laboratory instruments to make proper judgments on selection, maintenance, troubleshooting, and quality assurance issues. Finally, to foster the understanding of the principles of computerization and laboratory information systems that enhance delivery of accurate laboratory results in a timely fashion.

Kory M. Ward
Craig A. Lehmann
Alan M. Leiken

Acknowledgments

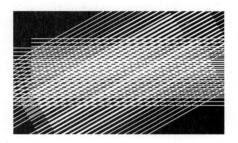

We would like to thank all the manufacturers who have worked with us over the last two years. Their commitment to the education of laboratorians has been highly commendable.

We would also like to thank our families for their support and sacrifices: Tim Bibler; Trevor and Brendan Ward; Susan, Jason, and Aaron Lehmann; and Nancy, Tracy, and Amy Leiken.

Many thanks to Peg Monigold and Janet Polak for their manuscript preparation and all the detailed activities relevant to it.

Last, but not least, we give special thanks to the following individuals at the W.B. Saunders Company: Selma Ozmat, Editor, for inviting us to do this project, and to Scott Weaver, Developmental Editor, for his ability to keep us on track. We also wish to recognize the work of Ellen B. Zanolle, Designer; Megan Guenthardt, Production Manager; and Peg Shaw, Illustration Specialist.

Contents

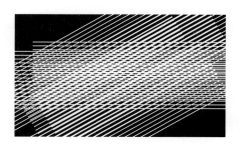

Chapter 15

DAVID J. THORNTON, PhD C (ASCP), and BERNADETTE L. THORNTON, MT (ASCP)

Chapter 16

JOSEPH G. FINK, MD, and SHESHADRI NARAYANAN, PhD

Chapter 17

CRAIG A. LEHMANN, PhD, CC (NRCC), and ALAN LEIKEN, PhD

Chapter 18

ALAN LEIKEN, PhD, and CRAIG A. LEHMANN, PhD, CC (NRCC)

CLINICAL LABORATORY INSTRUMENTATION AND AUTOMATION

Principles, Applications, and Selection

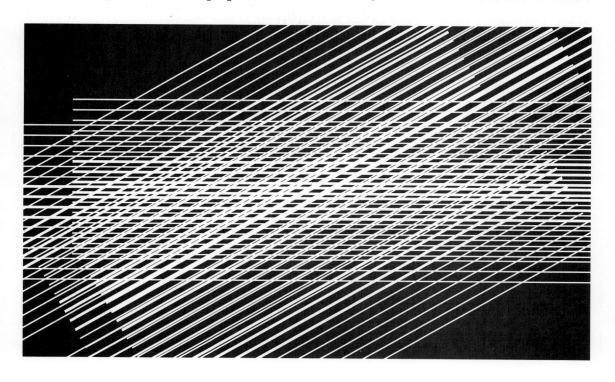

Chapter 1

FUNDAMENTAL PRINCIPLES OF ELECTRONICS

BARBARA J. CLEVELAND, MPH, MT (ASCP)

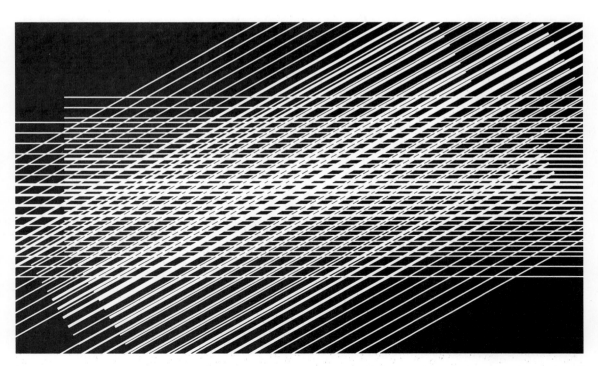

LEARNING OBJECTIVES

After studying this chapter, the student should be able to:

- Define terms essential to a basic understanding of laboratory electronics.
- Properly perform basic electronic calculations.
- List the electrical properties of insulators and conductors.
- Define Ohm's law and characterize its relationship to the control of light from excitor lamps and its influence on electrophoretic migration.
- List the major sources of electricity. Describe the construction and operation of basic electronic components.
- Explain the principle associated with the use of the Wheatstone bridge and list examples of laboratory instruments that employ this configuration.
- Summarize the construction, function, and proper replacement of electrical fuses.
- Describe the characteristics and generation of direct current and alternating current.
- Differentiate between series and parallel circuits.
- Outline the rectification process.
- Describe the operation of commonly used laboratory readout devices.
- List examples of:
  a. clinical applications of the principles of electronics.
  b. instrument uses of the components of electronics.

KEY WORDS

Alternating current. An electrical circuit in which the flow of electrons is bidirectional, moving first in one direction and then in the other.

Capacitor. An electrical circuit element with the ability to store an electrical charge.

Diode. A solid-state device (or electron tube) having only two active elements or electrodes that allow current flow in only one direction.

Direct current. An electrical current in which the electrons flow in only one direction.

Emitter. One of the elements of a transistor; comparable to the cathode of the electron tube.

Gain. The amount of amplification of input voltage to output voltage.

Integrated circuit. A major electrical device containing several electrical components such as to allow the device to perform multiple electronic functions.

Semiconductor. A material with a resistivity between that of conductors and insulators; a solid-state electrical device, called a diode, made of silicon (or germanium) ``doped'' crystal.

Solid-state circuit. An electrical circuit that uses semiconductor diodes and transistors instead of vacuum tubes.

Transducer. A device that changes physical energy, such as pressure, light, and heat, into electrical energy.

Transformer. A device containing a primary and a secondary coil, linked by magnetic lines of force, used to transfer and increase or decrease electrical energy from one circuit to another.

Transistor. A solid-state, three-electrode semiconductor device that functionally replaced the vacuum tube.

Wheatstone bridge. An electrical configuration using four resistors that act in pairs to compare some unknown parameter to a known parameter according to Ohm's law.

INTRODUCTION

Instruments are major tools in the modern clinical laboratory. Many of them require very little maintenance and are compact and easy to operate; still these instruments need to be properly maintained to assure precision in their operation. Although laboratorians are not electricians, they need to have a basic knowledge of what is actually happening electronically when a laboratory instrument is being used. Covers may need to be removed; bulbs, fuses, and even circuit boards may need to be replaced. Switches, needles, digital readouts, recorders, and computers all may require some level of electrical understanding. In a sense there is continual communication between the user and the electronic instrument. This communication is certainly improved when one has a better knowledge of the operation and electronics of the instrument.

Although most of the instrument troubleshooting problems are related to basic maintenance, or to the lack of it, some are electronic. Something as simple as proper fuse replacement can be a critical issue: a very expensive instrument can be damaged by replacement of a fuse with one that allows more current to be pulled by the instrument.

The purpose of this chapter is to present basic and understandable electronics by providing explanations and examples of major electronic events.

ELECTRICITY

The word *electric* is rooted in the Greek word "amber," which stands for a yellow-brown fossil resin. The rubbing of amber with a cloth or fur produces forces of attraction and repulsion. This force, termed *electric attraction* and *electric force* by the English physicist William Gilbert, is that property which moves electrons; it is a fundamental property of all charged particles.

The electric charge that is generated by the rubbing of amber is due to friction, to be discussed later with sources of electricity. For now, the basics of electricity will be reviewed by looking at the structure of atoms and molecules.

Atomic Structure

A general knowledge of atomic structure is essential for understanding chemical combination reactions, ionization processes, the properties of insulators and conductors, the mechanisms of current flow, and all electrochemical applications used in the clinical laboratory.

The atom is the basic component of all matter. It is composed of orbital negative electrons surrounding an electrically positive nucleus of protons and, except for hydrogen, neutral neutrons (Fig. 1-1). The negative charge of the electrons is equal to the positive charge of the protons; therefore, the atom is an electronically balanced structure.

Most materials exist as compounds of various elements. Thus, a molecule is the smallest combination of atoms. When the molecules of a substance are altered to form

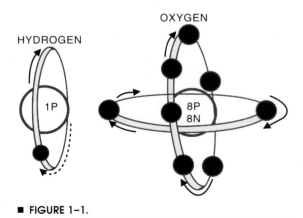

■ FIGURE 1-1.

Hydrogen and oxygen atoms.

a new molecule, a "chemical" change has occurred. When molecular changes involve reactions between charged particles, they are electrical changes.

Periodic elements are arranged according to their ascending atomic number, atomic weight, or mass number (number of protons and neutrons in the nucleus) period and group. From the atomic number (Z), one can tell the charge on the nucleus and the number of protons (and electrons) in the structure. Hydrogen has an atomic number of 1, which means that it has one proton and one electron. The mass number of hydrogen is 1.0080, which may be considered as 1.01 for our purposes. Oxygen, with its atomic number of 8 and mass number of 16, has 8 electrons, 8 protons, and 8 neutrons.

Orbital electrons are arranged in successive shells (and subshells) designated K, L, M, and so on (Fig. 1–2). Shell electron capacities are 2, 8, 18, and 32 from the nucleus to the outermost shell. The electrons in the outer shells are responsible for the chemical properties of the element. These electrons are not tightly bound to the nucleus and are therefore capable of participating in chemi-

cal and physical reactions. Examples are those that are involved in visual, ultraviolet, and fluorescence spectrophotometry; flame excitation and atomic absorption methods; and electrochemical applications. The inner shell electrons are tightly bound to the nucleus; therefore, alteration of the inner shell structure is best facilitated by high-energy particles, gamma rays, and x-rays. Applications in nuclear medicine, procedures using radioisotopes, and x-ray technology employ many of the principles associated with nuclear neutron–proton ratios and alterations of the inner shell structure.

Ionization

Aqueous solutions of acids, bases, and salts are called *electrolytes* because they conduct electricity. Electrolytes also show rapid chemical reactions and cause greater changes in the colligative properties of a solvent than an equimolar concentration of a nonelectrolyte, nondissociated solute. For example, an electrolyte solution of sodium chloride (NaCl) or calcium chloride (CaCl$_2$) will be highly dissociated; the effect on the colligative property, respectively, is two and three times that of an equimolar solution of a nondissociated compound. In short, a compound that has the ability to carry a charge is called an electrolyte. Such compounds are also able to dissociate partially or completely. According to the "Arrhenius theory of electrolytic dissociation," molecules of electrolytes give rise to charged particles called ions when dissolved in an aqueous solution. The charge carried on the ion is equal to the valence on the ion.

Consider a covalent compound with two shared electrons, such as hydrogen chloride (HCl) (Fig. 1–3A). The shared electrons are oriented so as to be nearer the chlorine atom than the hydrogen atom; therefore, the chlorine is negative with respect to hydrogen. If HCl is placed in an electrical field, the negatively charged chlorine will be ori-

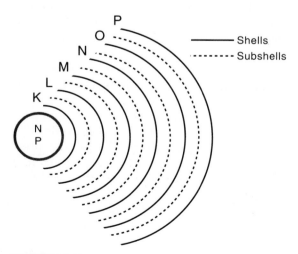

■ FIGURE 1–2.

Shells and subshells.

(A)

H $\overset{..}{\underset{..}{Cl}}$:

Electrons are shared
closer to the chlorine;
therefore, the chlorine
is negatively charged.

(B)

$HCl + H_2O \quad >> \quad H_3O^+ + Cl^-$

$HNO^3 + H_2O \quad >> \quad H_3O^+ + NO_3^-$

Covalent polar

(C)

: $\overset{..}{\underset{..}{Cl}}$: $\overset{..}{\underset{..}{Cl}}$:

Covalent nonpolar

■ **FIGURE 1–3.**

A, Covalent arrangement for HCl. *B,* Polar orientation. *C,* Arrangement for covalent nonpolar Cl₂.

ented to the positive plate; the hydrogen, with its positive charge, will be oriented to the negative plate. As illustrated in Figure 1–3*B,* the ionization of HCl (and other covalent compounds) involves a reaction with the solvent. The ability to develop a polar orientation in an aqueous solution is an important factor supporting ionization of covalent compounds. This condition of polarity is not seen with the chlorine molecule, Cl₂, because the shared pair of electrons are midway between the two chlorine atoms (Fig. 1–3*C*).

An electrovalent compound, such as potassium chloride (KCl), illustrated in Figure 1–4, will exist in the crystalline state as ions. This compound is formed from the original elements by the transfer of electrons from one atom to another. Many salts and bases are electrovalent and exist as ions both in the solid state and in solution; there-

fore, ionization is the process of separation of ions are that already present.

We can now summarize that the process of ionization creates charged particles from atoms or molecules. An atom (or molecule) is said to be excited when its internal energy is raised above its normal state. This excess energy can force loosely bound electrons out of orbit. A positive ion can result from the loss of electrons, and a negative ion can result from electron gain. Redox reactions, such as those seen with a galvanic cell, are reactions in which electrons are lost and gained. The oxidation potential of an element is the tendency for that element to act as an oxidizing or reducing agent. Consider Figure 1–5(a). One chemical element acts as an oxidizing agent by having an affinity for electrons of other elements; these other elements are, therefore, oxidized in the presence of this agent. In Figure 1–5*B,* the chemical element acts as a reducing agent because of the ease with which it gives up electrons. Other elements are reduced in the presence of this element.

Applications in the clinical laboratory utilize this phenomenon of ionization. Redox reactions are essential components of elec-

(+) (-)
K   Cl   >>> K⁺   +   Cl⁻
Solid/crystal   Ionization

■ **FIGURE 1–4.**

Electrovalent KCl.

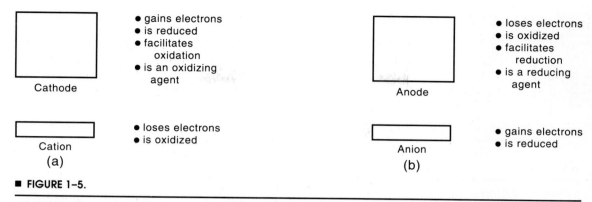

■ FIGURE 1–5.

Redox activity.

trochemical cells. One example of an electrochemical cell is the basic battery, which has two poles, the anode and the cathode, which serve as an electron donor and acceptor, respectively.

When organic compounds are burned in a hydrogen-air flame, they ionize. The flame-ionization detector, used with gas chromatography, burns the effluent sample presented to it in a hydrogen-air gas mixture to produce ionized organic compounds. Each sample is detected by creating changes in flame conductivity as the solutes elute from the column and are burned; the ions produced are detected by a pair of electrodes. The sample may be quantified for the chemical in question by comparing the conductivity and ionization properties of the sample with those of standards.

Ionization of covalent compounds produces a hydronium ion (a positively charged water molecule). Endosmosis, also called electro-osmotic force, produced when an acetate substrate is used for electrophoresis, is due to the production of a hydronium molecule. When a serum sample for electrophoretic separation of albumin and globulins α-1, α-2, β, and γ is placed in an alkaline buffer of pH 8.6 to 8.8, all of these proteins take on a negative charge. It is expected that these proteins would migrate, according to the magnitude of their individual charges, toward the positive pole of the electrophoretic system. This is true for the most part. However, some fractions migrate in the opposite direction when endosmosis is present. This is the case when the γ-globulin, with its negative charge, migrates toward the negative pole.

Conductors and Insulators

Substances like silver and copper permit the free motion of a large number of electrons. This is because these substances contain excess electrons that have been dislodged from the outer shell and can exist outside the atom. These "free" electrons are responsible for carrying the current in a conductor. The more free electrons in a substance, the better the substance acts as a conductor. Silver is a very good conductor of electricity and is the metal used to establish certain electrical parameters, e.g., amperes and the coulomb.

A conductor becomes an active conducting system when supplied with a direct current source (generator or battery); the charge is carried as electrons are forced to move through the system by being repelled from the negative ($-$) pole toward the positive ($+$) pole of the source (Fig. 1–6). Electrons

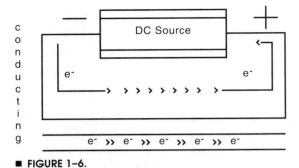

■ FIGURE 1-6.

Active conducting system.

are forced out of orbit as electrons move toward neighbor atoms. This process is repeated throughout the length of the conductor.

Conductance is the movement of electrons through the conducting material. Most chemical changes take place in the material with the passage of these electrons, and the current is maintained by the moving electrons.

With electricity and ionization, electrolytes also conduct electric current through the movement of ions toward positive and negative poles (Fig. 1-7).

Conductivity is defined as the ability to carry current when a voltage source is applied. When the current is being carried by electrolytes, the concentration of the ions determines the amount of current that can be carried. There is a direct proportionality relationship between current carried and ion concentration.

When a metal is used, conductivity is influenced by the resistance that the conductor offers to the flow of electrons. This resistance (to be discussed later as resistivity) varies with the make-up of the conductor, the length and cross-sectional area of the conductor, and the reaction temperature. In fact, conductivity is the reciprocal of resistivity, and conductance, abbreviated mho (which is ohm spelled backward), is the reciprocal of resistance.

The principle of the Coulter counter, which is used to count red blood cells (RBC) and white blood cells (WBC), is based on conductivity and resistance. The instrument is equipped with a constant voltage and two salt-filled electrodes, one inside a glass vessel and the other outside. The glass vessel contains a small orifice (hole) of a specified diameter, depending on which blood cells are being counted. The salt solution serves as a current conductor. When a cell moves through the orifice, it acts as a resistor to current flow by displacing the conducting solution. The size of the particle determines the magnitude of the change in resistance. The magnitude and number of current spikes in a sample are used to determine the size and number of cells present per volume of solution.

We know that atoms have orbital electrons existing in shells and in subshells, and that the electrons in the outer shell reflect the valence of the atom as well as the number of electrons that must be gained or lost to obtain a full shell. How is this important in conduction and insulation?

Certain atomic interactions lead to the formation of molecules with an orbital called the valence band, a band of electrons that occupy a minimum energy level. These molecules also have an adjacent conduction band, which is an orbital of a higher energy level that is normally not filled (Fig. 1-8). Electrons in the valence band can move to

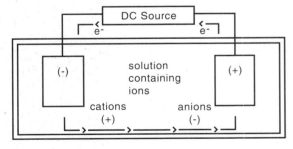

■ FIGURE 1-7.

Movement of electrolytes.

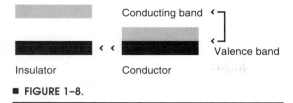

FIGURE 1–8.

Valence and conducting bands of insulators and conductors.

the conducting band with the addition of energy. While in the conducting band they are free to move around. This transition to the conducting band leaves a hole in the molecular structure. In a conductive metal this hole is easily filled by an electron from somewhere else in the material. When an electrical field is applied to the conducting material, the electrons move.

The conducting band of an insulator is not as close to the valence band; therefore, there are large energy gaps that make it difficult for electrons to make the transition to the conducting band. Insulators have very few free electrons and require very large amounts of energy to break the influence of the nucleus on the electron (Table 1–1).

The conducting ability of semiconductors is somewhere between that of a conductor and an insulator. The construction and function of semiconductors will be discussed later with diodes and transistors.

Electromotive Force

Current

Now we have seen that a charge moves in an orderly fashion through a conductor when a direct current source is supplied. Early investigators believed that the charge moved from positive to negative (conventional current flow), but we now know that the flow of electrons in a metal conducting

system is from negative to positive (electron current flow). This orderly flow of electrons is the electric current (I), and it is measured as the ampere (A), named after a French physicist, André Ampère. The energy of each electron is due to the charge (Q) and is measured in coulombs (C), named after another French physicist, Charles Coulomb. One coulomb is 6.24×10^{18} electron charges, and one ampere is 1 coulomb/second. Other units of current measurement include the milliampere (mA) and the microampere (μA). The ease with which the current flows depends on the material through which the current is flowing, or the resistance (R) to current flow. The force that moves the electrons through the conducting material is the voltage (V). The rate of current flow is influenced by both the resistance and the voltage.

A current can be generated so as to flow in one direction and maintain a constant value. This is called **direct current** (DC). We have seen that the battery can serve as a DC source. Such a current can also be generated by a DC generator.

Alternating current (AC) can be considered to be an entire sine wave. It is generated commercially. We know it as the electricity that comes from wall outlets. The current flows first in one direction and then in the other; therefore, its current flow is characterized by frequency, amplitude, a constant change in direction, and an accompanied variation in voltage.

TABLE 1–1. EXAMPLES OF CONDUCTORS AND INSULATORS

CONDUCTORS	INSULATORS
Silver	Dry air
Copper	Glass
Aluminum	Mica
Zinc	Rubber
Brass	Asbestos
Iron	Bakelite

Resistance

Resistance is a useful component of electricity; it generates heat, allows for control of electron flow, and regulates voltage.

We have noted that the conducting ability of a material depends on the number of free electrons; likewise, some materials are more resistive than others. Conductivity and resistivity are related as reciprocal functions of each other, meaning that a good conductor will have low resistivity. The resistivity of a wire is influenced by the length of the wire and the cross-sectional area. The resistance relationship to resistivity is expressed as

$$R = \rho\ L/A,$$

where R is the resistance (Ω), rho (ρ) is the resistivity of the wire (specific for the type of material) in ohm cm, L is the length of the wire in cm, and A is the cross-sectional area in cm^2. See Table 1–2 for examples of resistivity.

A resistor (see Fig. 1–16 for the symbol for a resistor) is a poor conductor of electricity that is introduced to "resist" the flow of current. It is an essential component of the production of an electromotive force. As we will discover later with our discussion of Ohm's law (E = IR), altering the resistance will cause a change in the current (I) or the voltage (E, EMF, or V). Resistance is measured in ohms (Ω) and is defined as a voltage drop of 1 volt when a current of 1 ampere flows through it.

TABLE 1–2. EXAMPLES OF RESISTIVITY

MATERIAL	RESISTIVITY IN 10^{-6} ohm cm
Aluminum	2.6
Brass	6.0
Carbon	350.0
Copper	1.7
Mercury	94.1

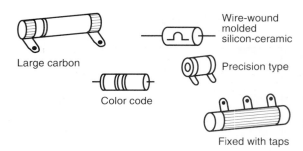

■ **FIGURE 1–9.**

Fixed resistors.

There are several different types of resistors. Most often displayed are the various types of fixed and variable resistors (see Fig. 1–16 for the symbol for a resistor). As their names imply, fixed resistors have set values, and variable resistors are adjustable or can change with some specified function. Many fixed resistors are made of carbon. This is understandable, because carbon has a resistivity of 350 microhm cm, meaning that it is a highly resistive element. Figure 1–9 presents examples of the various types of fixed resistors.

The resistance value of the carbon-rod type of resistor is indicated by a standard color code. As illustrated in Figure 1–10, the first and second significant figures are indicated by the first and second bands, respectively. The third band is the multiple and tells the number of zeros to add, or the

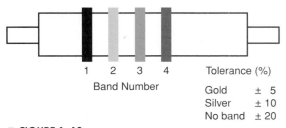

■ **FIGURE 1–10.**

Resistor color code.

TABLE 1–3. VALUES FOR
COLOR-CODED RESISTORS

COLOR	SIGNIFICANT FIGURE	MULTIPLIER
Black	0	1
Brown	1	10
Red	2	100
Orange	3	1000
Yellow	4	10000
Green	5	100000
Blue	6	1000000
Violet	7	10000000
Gray	8	100000000
White	9	1000000000

placement of the decimal point. The fourth band tells the tolerance of the resistor. If the fourth band is absent, the tolerance is considered to be 20 percent. See Table 1–3 for code values.

Some fixed resistors are popular for electronic uses when precision is not a major factor. When greater precision is required, say ± 1 percent, the wire-wound types of resistors are used.

Variable resistors are used extensively in clinical laboratory instruments. These uses will be expanded upon later in the section on resistor functions. For now, we will briefly describe them and mention some of their functions. There are two major types: the two-terminal rheostat and the three-terminal potentiometer. They function as zero and offset voltage knobs, as major components of the **Wheatstone bridge,** and as the slidewire configuration of the null-balancing potentiometric recorder. Several types of variable resistors are illustrated in Figure 1–11.

Sources of Electricity

Physical energy is converted to electrical energy (electricity) by a device called a transducer. There are five major sources of electricity. A mechanical source is (1) static electricity and that which comes from induction generators. Other sources include (2) photoelectric, (3) thermoelectric, (4) chemical, and (5) piezoelectric.

Voltage production by magnetic induction (generating a magnetic field around a current-carrying coil or wire) is widely employed for production of vast quantities of electrical power, as is seen in commercial electricity. Induction is also the basis for the construction and operation of inductive devices, e.g., coils (the d'Arsonval meter), transformers, relays, and solenoids.

No doubt we have all experienced static electricity, in which electrons are transferred, owing to friction, through the rubbing of certain materials. This type of electricity can pose a problem with laboratory instruments, especially if they are not properly grounded. There is usually not a prob-

Potentiometer

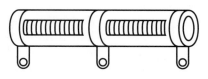

Enamel
adjustable
resistor

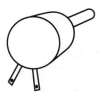

Rheostat

■ **FIGURE 1–11.**

Variable resistors.

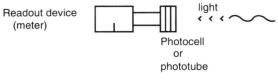

■ **FIGURE 1–12.**

Photoelectric voltage production.

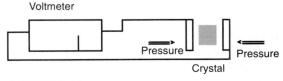

■ **FIGURE 1–14.**

Piezoelectric voltage production.

lem with instruments today because they are equipped with the three-pronged electrical plug, which allows for the flow of unwanted electricity, including static electricity, from the chassis of the instrument to the earth.

With photoelectric sources, an electrical charge develops when light strikes certain types of photosensitive (light-sensitive) materials, e.g., selenium alloy, and causes electrons to be emitted from the surface of the material. A current is detected as light energy is converted to electrical energy (Fig. 1–12).

Thermoelectric voltage production uses the thermocouple, a heat-sensing device illustrated in Figure 1–13, in which two dissimilar metals are pressed together to form hot and cold junctions. The voltage developed depends on the difference in temperature between these junctions.

Electrochemical reactions are examples of chemical reactions that are sources of electricity. As previously illustrated (refer to the earlier discussions on ionizations and electrolytes and to Fig. 1–7), when two dissimi-

lar metals are connected to a DC source and placed in a conducting solution, an electromotive force develops between them.

Piezoelectric electromotive force is an example of electricity that develops from pressure to crystals, such as quartz (Fig. 1–14). When the pressure to the crystal is constant, the electrons flow in one direction (dictated by the laws of physics and chemistry) until the crystal is neutrally charged. Decompression of the crystal causes the pressure to flow in the opposite direction. The EMF produced by this method is very low. Such crystals, however, are sensitive to changes in temperature and changes in mechanical force; use is limited to special applications.

Voltage

The force that causes electrons to move through a conductor is termed *electromotive force* (EMF). The volt (V), used to measure this quantity, is defined as that force required to move 1 coulomb per second (1 amp) through a resistance (R) of 1 ohm (Ω). The volt is also equal to 1 joule per coulomb. The terms *electromotive force* and *volt* are synonymous. *Potential* and *potential difference* are two other terms that are often used instead of voltage or EMF. In general, potential can be defined as the power or ability to do something that has not yet come into being. The force required to move electrons has the ability to move electrons, and therefore has the potential to move electrons. The electrons are moved between two points;

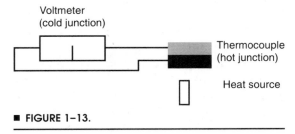

■ **FIGURE 1–13.**

Thermoelectric voltage production.

therefore, the potential difference is the ability to move the electron from point 1 to point 2.

A battery (see Fig. 1–16 for the symbol for a battery) is a device (a cell or system of cells in a common container) that converts chemical energy into electrical energy. It contains two poles, is capable of being a spontaneous conductor of electricity, and serves as a DC source.

Ohm's Law

The ohm (Ω), as mentioned, is the amount of resistance offered to current flow in a circuit. As a matter of fact, the definitions for resistance (R), current (I), and voltage (EMF or E) are related. This relationship was described by George Ohm, a 19th century German physicist, as Ohm's law:

$$E = IR$$

For precision in photometric measurements, it is essential that the current supplied to the excitor lamp be constant, thereby assuring that the output from the lamp is constant. Some spectrophotometric instruments use a ballast lamp to regulate the current to the lamp through resistance. When the current to the lamp starts to increase, the resistance supplied by the ballast also increases. When the current decreases, the ballast resistance also decreases. This function of holding the current constant can also be performed by a voltage regulator. Both the ballast lamp and the voltage regulator employ the principles related to Ohm's law.

It is important to understand Ohm's law also in its association with the buffer and substrate (migration medium) used for electrophoretic separations. The migration solution is a conductor because the buffer ionizes. The substrate is saturated in the buffer, and therefore it is also a conductor.

TABLE 1–4. IR DROP

RESISTOR (Ω)	IR DROP (V)	DIVISION POINT	VOLTAGE
25	0.375	b	1.125
50	0.750	c	0.375
25	0.375	d	0.000

However, the substrate also offers resistance. When the voltage source (E) is applied to the electrophoretic system, the buffer and substrate supply the other necessary constituents (I and R), according to Ohm's law.

We now know that voltage is the force required to push current through resistance (Fig. 1–15 and Table 1–4). We might summarize that the voltage "drops" from the initial value to zero as the current is pushed through the resistor.

For the sake of illustration, let's say that a 1.5-volt battery is used to push a current of 0.015 amp through a 100-ohm resistor. In Figure 1–15A, the voltage at point a is 1.5. The voltage drops by a magnitude of I $\times$ R as the current is pushed through the resistor. Thus the terms *voltage drop* and *IR drop* are synonymous. The voltage at point b is 0.

In Figure 1–15B, the total resistance of 100 Ω is shared between three resistors, 25, 50, and 25. The voltage will drop between points a and d from 1.5 volts to 0.0 volt but will be "divided" based on the value of the resistor.

Power

The watt (W) is a measure of power (P); it is the work done when 1 volt moves 1 ampere, which is, by definition, 1 joule per second. The volt equals 1 joule per coulomb; therefore, the definition for power must include voltage, current, and Ohm's law:

$$P = VI = RI^2 = V^2/R$$

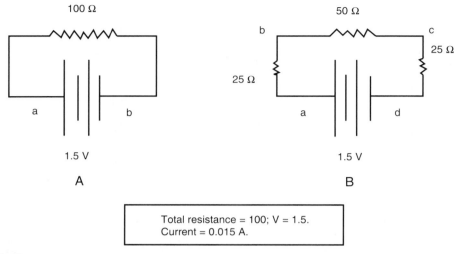

Total resistance = 100; V = 1.5.
Current = 0.015 A.

■ **FIGURE 1–15.**

Voltage drop or IR drop.

What does the power rating (wattage) on an electrical component tell us? In short, it tells us the amount of electrical power required to operate the device, or whether the component can handle the amount of electricity to be passed through it. We will see how this applies when we discuss fuses and fuse replacement.

CURRENT FLOW AND CIRCUIT CONFIGURATIONS

Electrical Components

Many of the laws and principles of electronics are exemplified in the construction and function of electronic devices. (See Fig. 1–16 for a key to the component symbols used to diagram electronic devices.)

Capacitors

Capacitors (see Fig. 1–16 for the symbol for a capacitor) have several functions, all of which are related to the ability of the capac-

itor to store charge and release an electrical charge. The amount of charge stored is directly proportional to the voltage across the capacitor. This may be expressed as $Q = CV$, where Q represents the stored charge, C is the capacitance, and V is the applied voltage. The capacitor is constructed of two thin, chargeable metal plates separated by an insulating material called the dielectric. The value of the capacitance is influenced by

1. The size of the capacitor plate; therefore, the capacitance is directly proportional to the plate area.
2. The distance between the two plates; the capacitance is inversely proportional to the distance.
3. The permittivity (related to the insulating ability) of the dielectric medium. Air, mica, Mylar, and Teflon are some materials that have been used as the dielectric.

How does a capacitor store charge? Figure 1–17 is a simple illustration of a capacitor in three phases of storing charge.

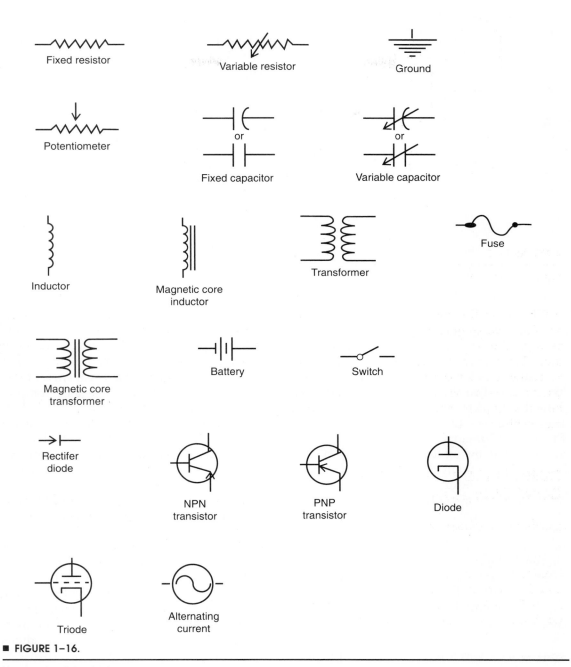

■ **FIGURE 1–16.**

Key to circuit symbols.

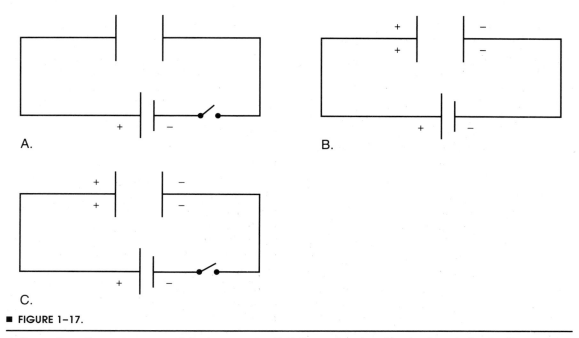

■ **FIGURE 1–17.**

A, Capacitor with no charge on plates in open circuit. *B,* Capacitor charging due to polarity of voltage source in closed circuit. *C,* Charged capacitor in an open circuit.

Figure 1–17*A* represents the initial stage of charging. The effect of the applied voltage is not realized by the plate because the circuit is open. When the circuit is closed, as in Figure 1–17*B,* current flows and the plates are charged owing to the polarity of the source. The current does not pass through the dielectric because of its insulating ability. When the potential of the plates and that of the source are equal, the current will stop flowing. Figure 1–17*C* illustrates that the capacitor is capable of holding the charge even when the circuit is opened. A resistor may be used with a capacitor in a special configuration to control the rate of charging and discharging of the capacitor. A capacitor–resistor configuration can be used as a part of the rectification and filtering system to convert alternating current to pulsating direct current, and finally to direct current.

Capacitors also can be used as current flow regulators that block direct current and allow the passage of alternating current.

Resistor Functions

Earlier, we discussed the resistor and how it might be used to control current and voltage. The type of resistor most often used for these functions is the variable resistor—the rheostat and primarily the potentiometer, or the "pot" as it is sometimes called.

A rheostat is a variable resistor with two terminals, say A and B, that represent the total resistance (Figs. 1–9 and 1–18*A*). The rheostat can be adjusted so that the resistance between these two points is any intermediate value within the range of variation. An example of the rheostat in use is the light-dimming device. The use of rheostats in the clinical laboratory is limited.

The potentiometer, illustrated in Figures 1–11 and 1–18*B,* is a device with three ter-

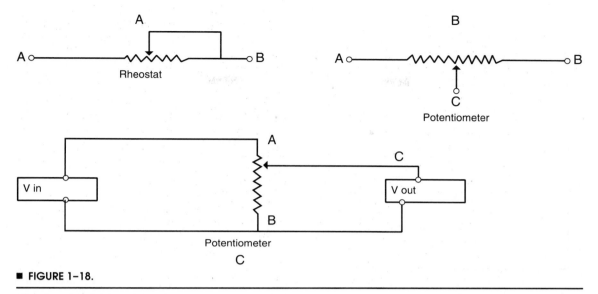

■ **FIGURE 1–18.**

Circuitry of variable resistors.

minals, points A, B, and C. Point C is the variable point between the fixed points A and B. This means the total resistance is represented by AB, or AC plus CB. The potentiometer differs from the rheostat in that when the wiper arm is moved the total resistance does not change, but the total effective resistance does change the current and the voltage. In Figure 1–18C, any situation that causes the wiper arm C to move will cause the output voltage to vary according to Ohm's law. When the wiper arm is at point A, the output voltage will be equal to the input voltage. When the wiper arm is at point B, the output voltage will be 0.

The Wheatstone bridge configuration, illustrated in Figure 1–19, may at first seem complex. The truth is that its operation can be explained by simple ratio and proportion, because there are three knowns and one unknown in a proportional set-up. The variable resistors R_1, R_2, and R_3 are considered as having known values. The value of the R_x resistor is to be determined. A galvanometer is placed between points b and d to deter-

mine the voltage of the system. Initially the bridge is balanced so that there is no difference (null point) in the potential across the bd terminal; the galvanometer will read 0. The sum effect of R_1 and R_2 determines the value for I_1. The resistors R_3 and R_x are responsible for determining the value of I_2. Changes in the balance of the system, through changes in R_x, will be reflected by a change in the galvanometer reading. As we shall see later in the section on measurement and readout devices, R_x can serve as many different things—for example, as the thermocouple of a freezing point osmometer or the indicating wire in a thermal conductivity gas chromatographic detector.

Induction and Inducers

As you may remember from academic courses such as physical science or physics, a magnetic field is induced around a current-carrying wire. If you grasp this wire with your right hand, your fingers will indicate the direction of the magnetic lines of

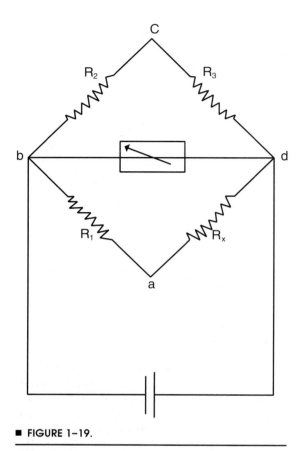

■ **FIGURE 1–19.**

Wheatstone bridge.

force when your thumb is pointing in the direction of current flow. This is called the right-hand rule. The left-hand rule is used to determine the direction of the force lines when electron flow is used and the thumb is pointing in the direction of electron flow.

The magnetic field of a straight current-carrying conductor is weak. If we shape the wire into a loop, the magnetic field cuts the plane of the loop because the lines of force are now perpendicular to the plane of the loop. In short, the magnetic field intensity at the center of the loop is increased by coiling the wire. A coiled wire acts like a magnet when current is passed through it, and

coiling the wire to form a solenoid is the basis for the formation of electromagnets. If the solenoid is wrapped around an iron core, the number of force lines is greatly increased and a stronger electromagnet is created. Coiled configurations are a key part of devices like servomotors. Electromagnets are essential components of buzzers, relays, and electric meters.

An EMF is created in a conductor that is cutting across magnetic lines of force. This EMF is proportional to the rate at which the lines are being cut. If the conductor is moving at a continuous rate, the EMF induced is also continuous. One way to do this is to rotate the coil between the poles of a magnet. Induction is used in the construction of electric generators for the production of direct current (DC) and alternating current (AC).

Figure 1–20 illustrates the circuit symbols for common inductors.

Transformers

How can you get enough voltage to operate a piece of equipment that requires 200 volts from a line source (amount of voltage supplied from the wall plug) of 110 volts? Before we answer this question, let's pose another. What would happen if two conduct-

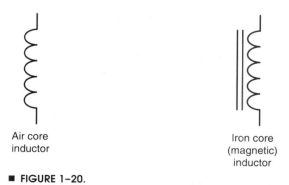

Air core inductor

Iron core (magnetic) inductor

■ **FIGURE 1–20.**

Circuit symbols for common inductors.

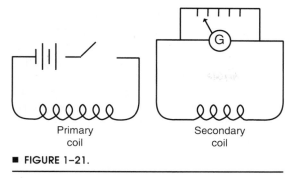

■ FIGURE 1–21.

Faraday's induction experiment.

ing coils were brought into close proximity with each other? Faraday performed such an experiment (Fig. 1–21). Using two coils carefully insulated from each other, he connected one coil, called the primary coil, to a battery, and another coil, the secondary coil, to a galvanometer. He noted that when he closed the switch on the primary coil, there was a momentary current in the secondary coil. We know that when an alternating current is induced in a primary coil, a changing magnetic field is created that results in the generation of a back EMF in the primary coil. A current can also be measured in the secondary coil. The concentration of the magnetic field can be increased by winding the insulated wires around a central core, such as iron.

Figure 1–22 illustrates the simple construction of a **transformer.** Electrical energy is transferred from the primary coil to the secondary coil with no direct connection between the coils. Voltage is the electrical factor most often used to describe transformer action.

The voltage induced in the secondary coil is opposite that of the primary coil. This means that when the AC voltage is in the positive half of the cycle, the induced voltage in the secondary coil is in the negative half of the cycle; when the AC voltage is in the negative half of the cycle, the induced voltage in the secondary coil is in the posi-

tive half of the cycle. When the number of turns in the primary coil is less than the number in the secondary coil, the voltage induced in the secondary coil will be greater than that of the primary coil. This is called a *step-up transformer.* Likewise, a *step-down transformer* has fewer turns in the secondary coil than are found in the primary coil. The voltage induced is directly related to the number of turns in the coils and is related through the following equation:

$$V_s/V_p = N_s/N_p$$

where V_s is the voltage in the secondary coil
V_p is the voltage in the primary coil
N_s is the number of turns in the secondary coil
N_p is the number of turns in the primary coil

Now to work a problem. Let's say that the primary coil has 50 turns. We are interested in "stepping up" our voltage from 110 V to 200 V. By simple ratio and proportion we can calculate that the secondary coil would need approximately 91 turns to achieve the voltage desired.

Vacuum Tubes and Semiconductor Diodes

It is unlikely to find vacuum tubes in laboratory instruments unless the instrument

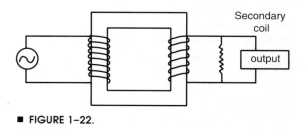

■ FIGURE 1–22.

Transformer construction.

was constructed in "those good old days" of black and white television. Therefore, we discuss the vacuum tube because of its mode of action and its relationship to rectification, amplification, and the operation principle of the semiconductor diode.

The vacuum tubes are illustrated in Figure 1–23. The most common types are the diode, triode, and pentode.

The basic vacuum tube has a heater and two electrode elements, one being the cathode and the other the anode. The heater, usually a tungsten filament, supplies heat to the cathode from which electrons are emitted. The cathode functions as the electron **emitter** and the anode serves as the collection plate (Fig. 1–24). The tube functions on the principles of thermonic emission, attraction of unlike charges, and repulsion of like charges. When a direct current source is connected to the tube, with negative lead to the heater/cathode and positive lead to the plate/anode, the vacuum tube is said to be *forward-biased*, as illustrated in Figure 1–25A. When the filament is heated, electrons are emitted from the negatively charged cathode. These electrons are attracted toward the positively charged anode, forming an electron cloud. This forward-biased diode is now a key device in conducting current through the system. When the leads of the source are connected in reverse, the negative charges on the plate and the cathode repel each other; there is no current flow and the diode is said to be *reverse-biased*, as in Figure 1–25B.

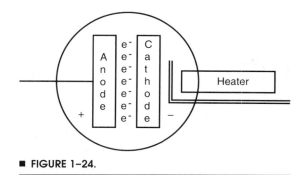

■ **FIGURE 1–24.**

Schematic of a vacuum tube.

What happens when the source is alternating current? This source can be thought of as both negative and positive. When the negative part of the cycle is in connection with the cathode, the positive part of the cycle can be thought of as in connection with the anode. This is the same forward-biased, current-conducting situation that was mentioned previously. The current flows in one direction. When the negative part of the cycle is in connection with the anode and the positive part of the cycle is in connection with the cathode, the current does not flow; the system is reverse-biased. We now see how a diode facilitates the conversion of alternating current to direct current. This initial step converts alternating current to pulsating direct current. It is pulsating because there are gaps in the cycle caused by the time associated with the reverse-biased phase. We will see how pulsating direct current is converted to direct current when we discuss rectification.

The triode, illustrated in Figure 1–23, is a vacuum tube that contains an additional element, the grid, which is positioned between the emitter and the plate. The grid voltage can be varied from zero to increasing negative voltage. Fewer electrons flow to the plate when the grid voltage is more negative than the cathode. Also, there is a corresponding increase in plate resistance and a

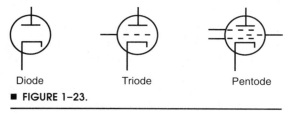

| Diode | Triode | Pentode |

■ **FIGURE 1–23.**

Circuit symbols for vacuum tubes.

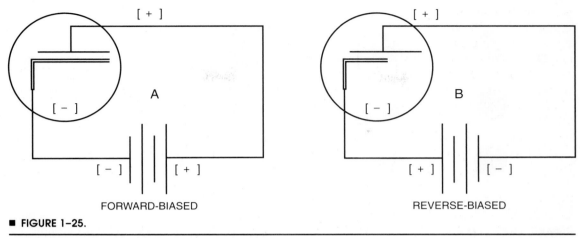

■ FIGURE 1–25.

Forward-biased and reverse-biased vacuum tubes.

decrease in conventional current flow. Electron flow virtually ceases when the grid voltage is at its maximum. The reverse is true when the grid voltage is at 0; the plate resistance is decreased and electron flow is at its maximum. This action allows the triode to function as an amplifier. The grid controls the increase in amplification, which is also expressed as the gain (G), or ratio of voltage output to input voltage:

$$G = V_0/V_I$$

Consider a triode controlled so that its plate is more positive and its grid more negative than the cathode emitter. Such a tube would be able to operate at grid values between 0 and maximum; it would also be able to handle waveforms (alternating current) with values that are ± the 0 mean. When an AC signal is applied to the triode, the positive portion of the sine wave produces an amplified negative output; the negative portion of the sine wave produces an amplified positive output. Therefore, a small input voltage can be amplified to a larger output voltage. This amplification process is very similar to that of the transistor, as we shall see.

A semiconductor electronic component is a **solid-state circuit** with applications similar to that of the vacuum tube. Zener diodes, junction diodes, amplifiers, detectors, oscillators, rectifiers, switching elements, transistors, and integrated circuits are all examples of semiconductor applications.

Key to the operation of the **semiconductor** are the crystalline structure, with its covalent bonding, and the composition of the semiconductor. Silicon and germanium, each having the property of being tetravalent, are materials commonly used for the construction of this device. The tetravalent property facilitates the formation of the crystalline structure in that the four valence electrons covalently bond with four electrons from adjacent atoms (Fig. 1–26).

Pure forms of silicon or germanium are of no use as semiconductors because there are no free electrons. We have seen that electrons are the carriers of negative charge. To explain current flow in a semiconductor, we must introduce a positive charge carrier, the "hole."

The conducting property is given to the crystal when it is "doped" with an impurity that creates extra negative or positive

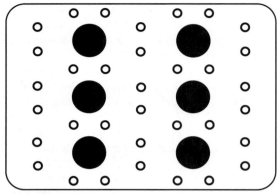

■ **FIGURE 1–26.**

Crystal of silicon or germanium.

charge carriers. The impurity element is considered a donor or acceptor based on whether it has an excess or deficiency of loosely bound electrons. Examples of donor impurities are pentavalent elements such as arsenic, antimony, or phosphorus, each being able to increase the number of negative charge carriers by introducing an extra electron to the crystal. The semiconductor formed is called the N-type (Fig. 1–27A). When the pure crystal is "doped" with a trivalent element such as aluminum, gallium, or boron, an electron deficiency called a "hole" is created. This "hole" is considered to be the positive charge carrier. The trivalent elements are examples of acceptor impurities, and the semiconductor formed is called the P-type (Fig. 1–27B).

A P-N junction diode, illustrated by Figure 1–28, is created when P- and N-type semiconductors are joined and the negative and positive charges migrate to form a junction. Free electrons move across the junction to fill the holes near the P-region while holes move across the junction to capture free electrons near the N-region. Ionization is created in the P and N regions, creating ionized acceptors in the P-region, which have a negative charge, and ionized donors in the N region, which have a positive charge. Also, there are holes in the P-region with a

positive charge and free electrons in the N-region with a negative charge. The net charge in each region is a function of the positive and negative charges in that region. The created junction potential has a sign opposite to that of the designated material and, therefore, serves as a barrier potential to prevent further migration of holes and electrons. Barrier potential is important in conducting current in a semiconductor because it acts like the plate and cathode in the vacuum tube diode.

As mentioned earlier, in a forward-biased, current-conducting diode the plate is positive with respect to the heated cathode. An

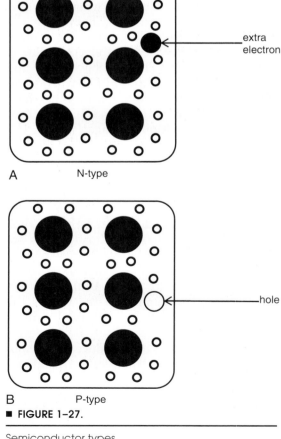

A   N-type

B   P-type

■ **FIGURE 1–27.**

Semiconductor types.

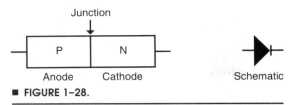

■ FIGURE 1–28.

P-N junction diode.

external voltage source will facilitate current flow across a P-N junction if the leads are connected so that the external potential is greater than the barrier potential, in a forward-biased direction. This causes a reduction in barrier potential and allows more electrons to flow from the N-type material across the junction; likewise, more holes travel across the junction from the P-type material. Electrons are also moving from the negative terminal of the external source and from the P-type terminal in the external circuit to the positive terminal of the external source. Therefore, current is conducted through the diode. Examine Figure 1–29A. Current will not flow when the leads of the external source are reversed in relationship to those of the diode terminal, and the diode is called reverse-biased, illustrated in Figure 1–29B.

Let's expand our discussion of diode functions by looking at rectification and filtration. Consider that when the voltage source is alternating current, such as that supplied by the wall outlet, the waveform produced is the sine wave. As mentioned earlier, a transformer is used to obtain the desired voltage by varying the number of turns in the primary and secondary coils. However, another problem exists. Electronic devices work on direct current; therefore, the alternating current sine wave must be converted to direct current. This is accomplished by rectifying and filtering the alternating current line voltage.

Rectification is the process of converting the alternating current sine wave to direct current by using a diode, which allows current to flow in only one direction; one half of the sine wave is detected and a pulsating direct current is produced.

Filtration involves capacitors and resistors (or inductors). By impeding the current flow and storing charge and releasing it, unwanted portions of the pulsating direct current can be eliminated. The pulsating direct current is converted to a constant-output direct current. Figure 1–30 illustrates the half-wave rectifier and the full-wave rectifier. The full-wave rectifier differs from the half-wave rectifier in that it can accommodate the entire sine wave.

A special diode application is that of the Zener diode. The term *Zener breakdown* re-

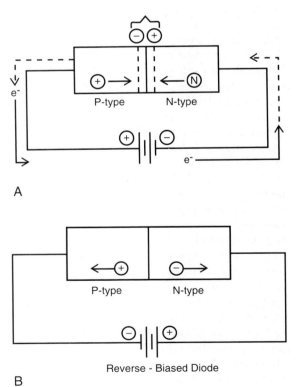

A

B

■ FIGURE 1–29.

A, Forward-biased and *B,* reverse-biased diodes.

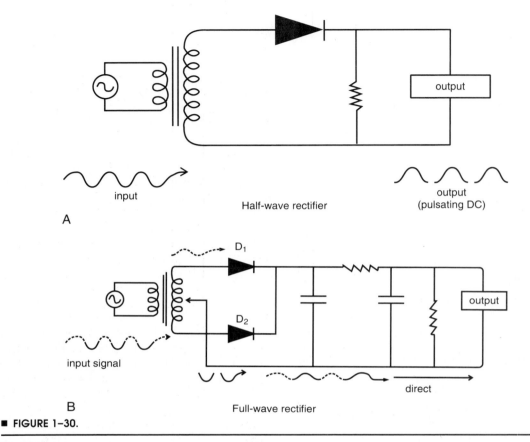

input

Half-wave rectifier

output
(pulsating DC)

A

D₁

D₂

input signal

output

direct

B

Full-wave rectifier

■ **FIGURE 1–30.**

Rectifiers.

fers to an excess increase in current (also termed *avalanche current*), applied in the reverse direction over a diode so as to exceed the ability of the diode to resist current flow. This phenomenon led to the construction of the Zener diode, a diode that can withstand Zener breakdown. Zener diodes function at the reverse breakdown point by conducting the current through it. If strategically placed in a circuit, at a point where a voltage level must not be exceeded, it may be used as a voltage regulator.

Transistors

The vacuum tube, for the most part, has been replaced by a three-electrode semicon-ductor, solid-state electronic device called a **transistor.** They are smaller, require little or no warm-up time, can be operated at lower voltages, and have a much longer life span than do vacuum tubes. The basic transistor is constructed of the same types of semiconducting materials as previously discussed with the P-N junction diode; thus, they are referred to as NPN and PNP transistors. Other transistor structures use P and N materials, but only the NPN and PNP types are discussed here.

The NPN transistor consists of N-type material for the emitter, thin P-type material for the base, and N-type material for the collector. The reverse is true for the PNP transistor (Fig. 1–31).

■ **FIGURE 1–31.**

Transistors.

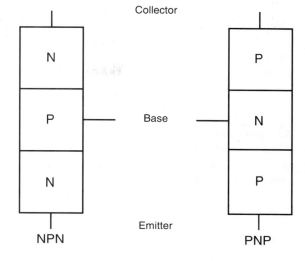

The functions of the emitter, base, and collector can be compared with the function of the vacuum tube: with the NPN transistor, electrons flow from the emitter into the base and then to the collector. With the PNP transistor, holes are emitted from the emitter. Current flow is controlled by the base, much like that of the vacuum tube grid.

Both NPN and PNP transistors, like vacuum tubes, can amplify an input signal. As an alternating current input voltage is introduced at the base of the transistor, the emitter-base bias is changed; therefore, current flow through the transistor is changed. As the base becomes more positive, more electrons are attracted by the base of an NPN transistor; fewer holes are attracted by the base of a PNP transistor. The reverse is true as the base becomes more negative. In any case, a small alternating current input signal is amplified as a larger output signal.

Circuit

Series and Parallel Circuits

A *series circuit* is one in which current consecutively flows through several different loads and returns to the source. For the sake of illustration, let's compare this to a series of wall outlets in, say, a mobile home. Think of this as the current flowing from the source in the back bedroom, along one wall toward the front of the home, and returning to the source along the other wall. What happens to the circuit if one of the wall outlets burns out? The circuit will be broken and current flow will stop.

With the *parallel circuit* configuration, the current divides into branches. If one branch fails to operate, the current flow is rerouted; the entire circuit is not halted.

Most often an electrical configuration is a combination of series and parallel circuits, and the resultant current flow is a function of both types.

How are electronic components influenced by series, parallel, and series-parallel circuits? The simplest of these is illustrated by the resistor in series, where R_{total} is the sum of the R values in the series circuit. This is calculated as:

$$R_T = R_1 + R_2 + \ldots R_N$$

The resultant current and voltage are functions of the circuit configuration and Ohm's law. Refer to the earlier discussion on voltage drop and voltage division.

The total resistance for a parallel circuit configuration is less than the resistance of the resistor in the smallest branch because the current flow is divided. This is calculated as:

$$1/R_T = 1/R_1 + 1/R_2 + \ldots 1/R_N$$

In contrast, the calculations for capacitors in series and in parallel are opposite to the calculations for resistors; the calculation for capacitors in series is:

$$1/C_T = 1/C_1 + 1/C_2 + \ldots 1/C_N$$

and the calculation for capacitors in parallel is:

$$C_T = C_1 + C_2 + \ldots C_N$$

Since laboratory instruments consist of series, parallel, and series-parallel configurations, the calculations will involve a combination of all relative equations.

There are two other possible circuits, both of which are not planned. The first is the short circuit, a path of low resistance to the flow of electrons, caused by wires touching. This causes the instrument to draw an excess of current. There is a possible short in an instrument when it continues to blow a fuse. The second type of circuit is the open circuit. This is an incomplete circuit. Consider a hypothetical situation in which an instrument function, say a sample probe operation, is controlled by a series configuration; the sampling process does not work. The problem may be due to a break in the circuit. It may be something as simple as a loose connection.

Integrated Circuits

An **integrated circuit** (IC), illustrated in Figure 1–32, is an electronic device that incorporates many other electronic components, so that the IC can perform several functions. Resistors, capacitors, diodes, and transistors are all examples of components that are incorporated into a silicon "chip"; thus, the IC may be thought of as a complete circuit. It is small and complex, is made of semiconductor material, and may be designed to serve many functions, one of which is in computer technology. One application of the IC is in large-scale integration (LSI), which facilitates reduction of major electronic systems to a few chips.

Circuit Boards

With the advent of IC and LSI came the ability to place major operational functions together on a chassis, the printed circuit board (Fig. 1–33). One board can contain several integrated circuits and additional

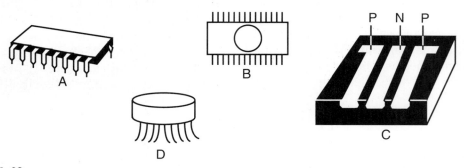

■ FIGURE 1–32.

Integrated circuit structure and function.

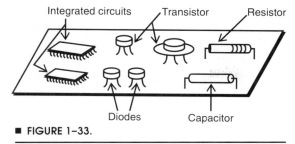

■ **FIGURE 1–33.**

''Simple'' circuit board.

resistors, capacitors, and transistors. These are all soldered according to some specific circuit diagram. The advantage of this is that the board can be quickly and easily maintained or changed should the prescribed function fail. Also, boards are generally changed by the technologist troubleshooting the instrument or a technologist assigned to instrument maintenance. This facilitates in-house repair of the instrument.

MEASUREMENT AND READOUT DEVICES

Electrical and Light Meters

An electromagnet is a wire-wound magnet, a coil, that behaves according to the laws of induction; a magnetic field is established when an electric current is passed through a wire. This field increases and decreases with the current. Consider two magnets: one is a small electromagnet with a voltage source, a pointer (or light suspension with a mirror set-up), and the ability to rotate in the field of the other, which is a larger, fixed horseshoe-type magnet. What happens to the coil when an electric current is passed through it? It will rotate to align itself in the magnetic field. The stronger the current passed through it and the greater the generated magnetic field, then the greater the rotation of the coil-pointer. If such a meter, supplied with a scale, is

placed in a measuring instrument, it can be used to equate change in current to some desired parameter; the current flowing through the coil will be directly proportional to the angular rotation of the coil. The scale can be calibrated to indicate amps, volts, or ohms, as with the multimeter, or it may be set to indicate concentration of an analyte. This device represents the basic structure and operation of the d'Arsonval galvanometer, illustrated in Figure 1–34.

Applications of the Wheatstone Bridge

Null-Point Systems

Many laboratory instruments use the principle of null point in some form or another. The *null point* is that point at which the voltage in an indicating line is equal to that in a reference line—hence no difference.

Figure 1–35 is a much-abbreviated illustration of the events in a null-point system. First we must note that V(error) = V(in) − V(ref). We must also note that V(ref) is equipped with a variable resistor. Assume that an analysis has been performed that involves a sample blank solution and test samples (a standard, a control, and an unknown). Each of these samples will elicit a different response because of their varied concentrations. We must know a start point, so the sample blank solution is used to set the zero. When the sample blank solution is introduced to the sample line, the zero knob is used to set the scale to 0. Though it may not be, V(error) is assumed to be 0. Next we introduce a test sample, the standard, to the sample line. This causes a change in V(error). The servomotor moves to set the system to null-point balance. The offset knob is used to indicate the corresponding concentration on the scale. Now we introduce the control to the sample line. Once again V(error) is changed. The servomotor

■ **FIGURE 1–34.**

D'Arsonval galvanometer.

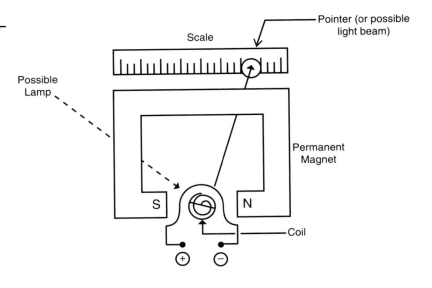

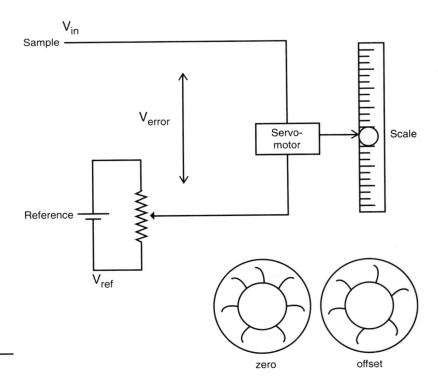

■ **FIGURE 1–35.**

Basic null-balancing system.

moves to balance the system as the scale indicates the concentration of the control. If it is in range, we can continue with our analysis.

Freezing Point Osmometry

Earlier, under the section on the Wheatstone bridge, we saw how several resistors could be used to establish the null-point condition. Suppose that we have a temperature-sensing thermistor and three variable resistors, as is illustrated in Figure 1–36. As the thermistor detects the released heat of fusion (see principle of freezing point osmometry) the galvanometer of the Wheatstone bridge moves, re-establishing balance. Some form of a scale-offset mechanism can be used to indicate the osmolality of the sample.

Thermal Conductivity Detector

The thermal conductivity detector, a detector used in gas chromatography, is illustrated in Figure 1–37. It consists of a reference cell resistor (R_{ref}) through which the carrier gas passes, a sample cell resistor (R_{sample}) through which the carrier gas and vaporized sample mixture pass, and two variable resistors that serve as detectors.

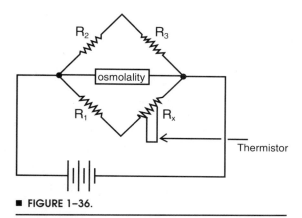

■ **FIGURE 1–36.**

Osmolality and Wheatstone bridge.

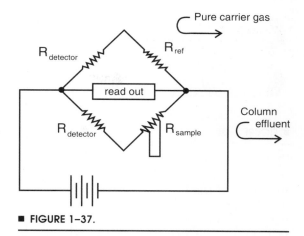

■ **FIGURE 1–37.**

Thermal conductivity detector.

The temperature of a heated filament in the sample stream is changed if the gas from the column contains eluted materials. This change in the temperature is measured by a change in the resistance. With the balancing of the Wheatstone bridge, there is an indication of the concentration of the sample that caused the change in conductivity.

FUSES AND PROPER FUSE REPLACEMENT

A fuse is a protective device, inserted in series, between the line voltage and the instrument. Most fuses found in laboratory instruments are like one of those illustrated in Figure 1–38. They are generally small, glass-covered cylinders, with metal-capped ends. Inside the fuse is a wire filament with a wattage rating; this filament serves as a resistive element. This element is designed to melt at a certain temperature, thereby creating a gap in the circuit and stopping the flow of current. The melting of the element is controlled by the equation heat = I^2R; as mentioned earlier, any condition that causes the instrument's circuit to draw too much current will cause the fuse to blow.

The wattage rating indicates the operat-

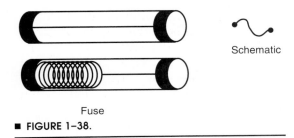

Schematic

Fuse

■ **FIGURE 1–38.**

Fuses.

ing limits of the fuse and is designed to have a value that protects the instrument. It is very important to understand that the fuse is a protective device, and that the same type of fuse, with the same ratings, should be used in replacement.

Let's say that an instrument continues to blow a fuse. What happens if the fuse is replaced by another with a larger capacity? If the reason for the blown fuse was a short or liquid in the instrument, the problem has not been solved; in fact, another has been created. The instrument can now draw more current, possibly causing damage to electrical components.

DIGITAL ELECTRONICS

Just as the vacuum tube was replaced by transistors, many basic laboratory components have been replaced by digital electronics. To understand "from whence we've come," let's first look at analog electronics. As the name implies, analog operations use numbers to represent physical quantity data; circuit properties can have real number values with analog electronics. Think of a scale, or better yet, a number line; a real number can be any number, with a continuum of values on that number line.

An example of an analog application is that of a mechanical integrator, one that determines the area under the curve. Another example is a device that determines watts by applying Ohm's law.

How does digital electronics differ from analog electronics? The exact mechanisms of digital electronics will not be emphasized because of the complexity of the subject; however, basic concepts will be discussed. Digital electronics uses Boolean algebra to apply two-state logic; this generally means "ON" and "OFF" and employs the two-digit binary numbering system. Binary numbers are used to represent logic statements. For example, true may be represented by "1" and false may be represented by "0." The instrument works through a series of switches, known as gates, which either block or pass electrical current; thus the "ON/OFF" situation is established. Since we are talking about complex circuit designs, many paths need to be controlled; thus there are many types of gates. And yes, it is the integrated circuit that allows for these complex functions.

What are gates and how do they function? Gates are essential components of digital electronics: they admit or reject signals. Consider the following examples of Truth Tables for switches; closed/on is represented by "1," and open/off is represented by "0" (Table 1–5).

One type of gate is the "AND" gate, as

TABLE 1–5. TRUTH TABLES

"AND" GATE		
SWITCH A	SWITCH B	LAMP
Open (0)	Open (0)	Off (0)
Closed (1)	Open (0)	Off (0)
Open (0)	Closed (1)	Off (0)
Closed (1)	Closed (1)	On (1)

"OR" GATE			
SWITCH A	SWITCH B	SWITCH C	LAMP
0	0	0	0
1	0	0	1
0	1	0	1
0	0	1	1
1	0	1	1
1	1	0	1
0	1	1	1
1	1	1	1

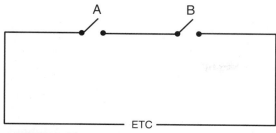

■ FIGURE 1–39.

AND gate.

shown in Figure 1–39. Here there are two switches in series. As can be seen, the only time the lamp is lit is when both switches are closed. Another type of gate is the "OR" gate. Consider that there are three switches in parallel, as illustrated in Figure 1–40. Review the previous discussions on parallel circuits. As expected, the only time the lamp is off is when all three switches are open.

There are other circuit gate configurations; however, they will not be discussed here.

It is important to understand digital electronics because the instruments have changed, some more drastically than others. There may be servomotors on some recorders, but more likely there are digital readout devices. Microprocessors and microcomputers are an integral part of laboratory in-

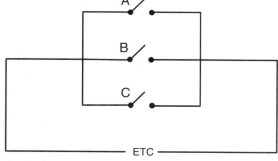

■ FIGURE 1–40.

OR gate.

struments. On some instruments, baseline adjustment is not performed by simply turning the zero knob; it might be through the use of a computer. A sample blank is placed into the system and the instrument is instructed to perform a scan. The information from the scan sets the blank.

ELECTRONIC APPLICATIONS IN THE CLINICAL LABORATORY

How might the clinical laboratory scientist use basic electronic information? Where in the clinical laboratory are electronic principles applied? Let's review some of what has been discussed and point out specific places where certain electronic principles apply. Table 1–6 summarizes electronic principles and illustrates their application in the clinical laboratory.

Electrolyte solutions may be considered as

TABLE 1–6. ELECTRONIC APPLICATIONS IN THE CLINICAL LABORATORY

ELECTRONIC PRINCIPLE	APPLICATION EXAMPLES
Conductivity	Particle counters
	Sample probes
	Thermal conductivity detector
	Urea nitrogen electrode
Ionization	Flame ionization detector
Polarography	Glucose detection electrode
Potentiometry	Ion-selective electrodes
	Variable resistor functions
	Readout devices
	Zero/offset knobs
Ohm's law	Electrophoresis
	All forms of current conduction
Rectification/ filtration	Power supplies to instrument
Resistance/wattage	Fuse replacement
Wheatstone bridge	Double-beam analyzers
	Flame photometry/internal standard
	Freezing point osmometry/ thermistor
	Thermal conductivity detector

electrical conductors. A serum sample, as well as other biologic fluids, can also conduct electricity, thereby completing a circuit. Many sample probes are equipped with sample indicator electrodes that attempt to complete a simple circuit. If a nonconducting situation exists, such as "NO SAMPLE," an open circuit is detected. Certain particle counters use conductivity as well as resistance.

Electrochemical reactions, such as in potentiometry, coulometry, and polarography, have replaced many of the titration and colorimetric procedures. Ion-selective electrodes are employed for the detection and quantification of electrolytes; special conductivity electrodes are used to detect concentrations of urea nitrogen.

Other applications include gas chromatography, flame ionization, thermal conductivity, and electron capture (not discussed in this chapter).

Discriminator circuits allow for selection of a particular size of radioisotope, based on the pulse produced.

Since a fuse is an important part of the most sophisticated laboratory instrument, the importance of proper fuse replacement cannot be overemphasized.

Last, but not least, by having an understanding of the laboratory instrument and the science associated with its operation the role of the laboratory scientist is much more than simply pushing buttons and following instructions.

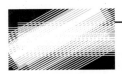

REVIEW QUESTIONS

Choose the one correct answer.

1. Many laboratory components work on direct current, yet the power source is alternating current. The _____ of the instrument converts AC to DC.

   a. transducer
   b. transformer
   c. rectifier
   d. voltage regulator

2. The generalized resistance to flow of an alternating electrical current, applied to capacitors and inductors as well as resistors, is

   a. impedance
   b. semiconductance
   c. inductance
   d. potential energy

3. The transistor is the major component of the

   a. resistor
   b. transducer
   c. amplifier
   d. rectifier

4. Static electricity is removed from an instrument via

   a. capacitor
   b. ground
   c. rectifier
   d. transducer

5. The main difference between a conductor and an insulator is

a. the Z number of the material
b. the element configuration
c. the number of positive charges
d. the number of free electrons

6. An electromotive force is induced in any conductor that is moving across

a. a transformer
b. voltage potential
c. an insulator
d. magnetic lines of force

7. Given the following schematic, the total capacitance is

a. 1.9×10^{-6} F
b. 5.1×10^{-1} μF
c. 20 F
d. 2.0×10^{-5} F

8. The bands on a carbon resistor are painted red-green-yellow-silver, in order. Its ohmic resistance is

a. 25,000 Ω, 5% tolerance
b. 25,000 Ω, 10% tolerance
c. 250,000 Ω, 10% tolerance
d. 2500 Ω, 5% tolerance

9. Which resistor must be placed in parallel with a 2.5 K and a 1.5 K to equal R_T of 431.6 Ω?

a. 400 Ω
b. 6.8 K
c. 800 Ω
d. 5.2 K

10. Given the following schematic, the calculated total resistance is

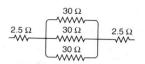

a. 1.23 Ω
b. 15 Ω
c. 7.55 Ω
d. 6.6×10^{-2} Ω

11. What is the voltage required to send a total current of 6 amps through three series-connected resistors of 4, 8, and 10 ohms?

a. 128 V
b. 132 V
c. 24 V
d. 60 V

BIBLIOGRAPHY

Ackerman PG: *Electronic Instrumentation in the Clinical Laboratory.* Boston, Little, Brown, 1972.
Bender GT: *Principles of Clinical Instrumentation.* Philadelphia, WB Saunders, 1987.
Bureau of Naval Personnel: *Basic Electricity.* New York, Dover, 1962.
Bureau of Naval Personnel: *Basic Electronics.* New York, Dover, 1968.
Diefenderfer AJ: *Principles of Electronic Instrumentation,* 2nd edition. Philadelphia, WB Saunders, 1979.
Eggert AA: *Electronics and Instrumentation for the Clinical Laboratory.* New York, John Wiley, 1983.
Ferris CD: *Guide to Medical Laboratory Instruments.* Boston, Little, Brown, 1980.
Hicks R, Schenken JR, Steinfauf MA: *Laboratory Instrumentation,* 2nd edition. New York, Harper and Row, 1980.
Jacobowitz H: *Electricity Made Simple.* Garden City, New York, Doubleday and Company, 1959.
Kaplan LA, Pesce AJ: *Clinical Chemistry: Theory, Analysis and Correlation,* 2nd edition. St. Louis, CV Mosby, 1989.
Lee LW, Schmidt LM: *Elementary Principles of Laboratory Instruments,* 5th edition. St. Louis, CV Mosby, 1983.
Miller R: *Electronics the Easy Way,* 2nd edition. Hauppauge, NY, Barron's Educational Series, 1988.
Zbar PB: *Basic Electricity: A Test-lab Manual,* 4th edition. New York, McGraw-Hill, 1974.
Zbar PB, Sloop JG: *Electricity-Electronics Fundamentals: A Text-lab Manual,* 2nd edition. New York, McGraw-Hill, 1977.

Chapter 2

SPECTROPHOTOMETRY

KORY M. WARD, PhD, MT (ASCP)
EDWARD HARRIS, BS

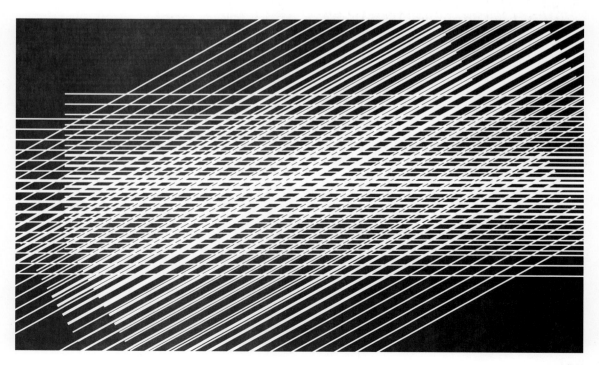

LEARNING OBJECTIVES

After studying this chapter, the student should be able to:

- State the Beer-Lambert law and apply this law in the calculation of the concentration of an analyte in an unknown solution.
- Describe the mathematical relationship between percent transmittance (% T) and absorbance (A).
- Identify the major components of a spectrophotometer, explain their functions, and differentiate between single-beam, double-beam, and split-beam configurations.
- Define bandpass and describe its relationship to instrument performance.
- Describe how to monitor the performance of a spectrophotometer with respect to wavelength accuracy, stray light, linearity, and photometric accuracy.
- Given a manufacturer's "spec sheet," define the terminology and rate the performance features as good, fair, or poor.
- List ten priorities to be considered when selecting a spectrophotometer.

KEY WORDS

Absorption. Light that will not pass through a solution. It is the process by which energy in the form of electromagnetic radiation is transferred to a substance when the radiation interacts with the substance.

Bandpass. The range of wavelengths between which the peak absorption is half the transmittance. This range represents the distribution of wavelengths that pass through the exit slit of the monochromator. This term corresponds to the slitwidth of the spectrophotometer.

Beer's law. An equation that shows the linear relationship existing between absorption and the concentration of the absorbing species. The law states that the absorbance of a homogeneous sample of an absorbing substance is directly proportional to the concentration of the absorbing substance: $A = abc$, where A = absorbance, a = absorption coefficient, b = distance the light travels through the sample, and c = concentration.

Cuvette (cuvet). The receptacle in which the sample is placed, allowing light bands exiting the monochromator to pass through before striking the detector. There is a wide variety of cuvettes. The choice depends on the type of analysis and the sample volume.

Detector. A device designed to convert the energy of incident radiation into an electric output that is a useful measure of the radiation that is incident on the device.

Diffraction grating device. A monochromatic wavelength selector (monochromator) that consists of a series of parallel grooves, equally spaced, allowing a light beam that strikes it to be dispersed into several linear spectra.

Drift. A slow, unidirectional change in the output of an instrument that occurs over several days or weeks in a system, representative of long-term instability. Drift occurs because of temperature changes and/or aging of the light source and electronic components.

Filter. A device that selectively passes certain wavelengths of light and will absorb others. A glass (Wratten) filter has one or two layers of colored glass.

Flow cell. A type of sample holder that is designed as a flow-through cuvette. Sample is introduced via tubing.

Linearity. The extent to which a range over a response (e.g., absorbance) is directly proportional to the concentration; also, the relationship between two variables that yields a straight line when plotted on a graph.

Noise. Random fluctuations in a system that occur abruptly, representative of short-term stability.

Quality control checks. Performance tests run daily, weekly, or monthly to verify photometric accuracy, photometric linearity, and wavelength accuracy, and to determine whether stray light is entering the system.

Resolution. In spectrophotometry, this term can be substituted for bandwidth.

Scanning. The collection of data (e.g., absorbance) over an entire wavelength range. This feature on a spectrophotometer allows one to determine the maximal absorbance wavelength of an absorbing solution.

Specification sheets (spec sheets). A manufacturer's list of performance and special features provided for a particular instrument.

Spectrophotometer. An instrument that measures the amount of monochromatic light passing through a solution by means of an adjustable monochromator such as a prism or a diffraction grating.

Stray radiant energy (stray light). Light (wavelengths) other than those exiting from the sample which strike the detector. Usually this is room light that has entered the instrument.

INTRODUCTION

Before the end of the 19th century, gravimetric and volumetric analyses were performed exclusively as quantitative measurements. By the beginning of the 20th century, an analytical instrument, the spectroscope, was introduced. This invention, along with the rapid development of photoelectric tubes, transistors, integrated circuits, and semiconductors, allowed for a more sophisticated method of quantitation. Today, in the contemporary clinical laboratory, many analytical procedures utilize the principles of spectrophotometric instrumentation. In fact, most automated systems incorporate spectrophotometric techniques within the body of the analyzers.

Spectrophotometry utilizes the principle of light absorption, at specific wavelengths, by the analyte. This physical property is characteristic for the substance being measured and is the basis of this analytic method. Specific patterns of electromagnetic radiation absorption are characteristic for biochemical substances. The electromagnetic wavelength absorption pattern of a substance can therefore be the basis for its identification. Once the spectral absorption pattern is known, the wavelength of maximal absorbance can be selected for quantitative purposes. Furthermore, the relative amount of light absorbed by the analyte is directly proportional to the concentration of the analyte. To determine the exact concentration of an *unknown* in solution, the unknown is evaluated relative to a *standard* and referenced against a *blank* solution.

Just as organic molecules may be quantified by their absorption of ultraviolet, visible, or infrared radiation, elements such as sodium may also be quantified based on their ability to absorb or emit light of a particular wavelength selectively. These observations form the basis for three additional spectral analyses: emission spectrophotometry, atomic absorption spectrophotometry, and fluorometry.

This chapter presents the principles, components, and quality control checks for visible and ultraviolet spectrophotometry. Flame emission photometry, fluorometry, and atomic absorption spectrophotometry will be discussed in Chapter 4, Instrumentation for the Measurement of Blood Gases and Electrolytes. Infrared spectrophotometry and mass spectrophotometry will be discussed in Chapter 12, Forensics Instrumentation. The spectral techniques of nephelometry and turbidity will be presented in Chapter 3, Particle Counters.

SPECTROPHOTOMETRIC PRINCIPLES

Theory of Light Waves

To understand how spectrophotometric measurements are made, a discussion of light and wave theory is necessary. Newton discovered that white light is actually a composite of all the wavelengths of visible light, and that the human eye can see these colors if white light is directed onto a prism. Later, after Newton's discovery, it was discovered that light traveled in waves, and the actual color perceived by the eye is a function of wavelength. For example, green light has a wavelength of 540 nm, and red light has a wavelength of 760 nm. The entire visible spectrum ranges from 380 nm (violet) to 760 nm (red). Electromagnetic radiation above and below the visible spectrum is in the infrared and ultraviolet regions, respectively. The following discussion involves wave theory and the mathematical relationship between the amount of light transmitted through a solution and the concentration of the absorbing species in the solution.

Light travels in waves. A single wave consists of *wavelength* and *amplitude*. The wavelength (λ) is the distance from the crest of one wave to the crest of the next wave. The amplitude is the peak height of a wave, which also determines its intensity. Based on the preceding information, the speed of light (which can be measured in photons) is equal to the wavelength times the *frequency* (γ). The number of waves per second is the frequency. Because the speed of light is constant (3×10^9 meters per second), there is a relationship between wavelength and frequency; that is, as the wavelength of light increases, the frequency decreases. The wavelength, measured in nanometers (1 nm = 10^{-9} meter), is thus inversely proportional to frequency. The shorter the wavelength, the higher the frequency, i.e., energy.

Actually, visible light and ultraviolet light are only a small portion of the entire family of radiation known as the *electromagnetic spectrum*. The entire electromagnetic spectrum consists of gamma rays, x-rays, ultraviolet (UV), visible (VIS), infrared (IR), microwaves, and radio waves. Figure 2–1 illustrates the relationships of wavelength (λ), frequency (υ), and energy (E) in the electromagnetic spectrum. The energy of light can be measured by the formula $E = h\upsilon$, where h = Planck's constant* and υ is derived by the formula $\upsilon = [\{c/n\}]/\lambda]$ (c = the speed of light in a vacuum,† n = the refractive index of the medium, and λ = wavelength).

Since matter consists of protons, neutrons, and electrons, the electrons exist in a number of energy states. The transition from the ground state to an excited state requires a specific amount of energy depending on an atom's unique electronic configuration. The electrons are held in orbit by electrostatic forces. Matter interacts with specific energies (wavelengths) based on the

---

*Planck's constant is equal to 6.626×10^{-34} joule/second.

†The speed of light in a vacuum = 3×10^{10} m/second.

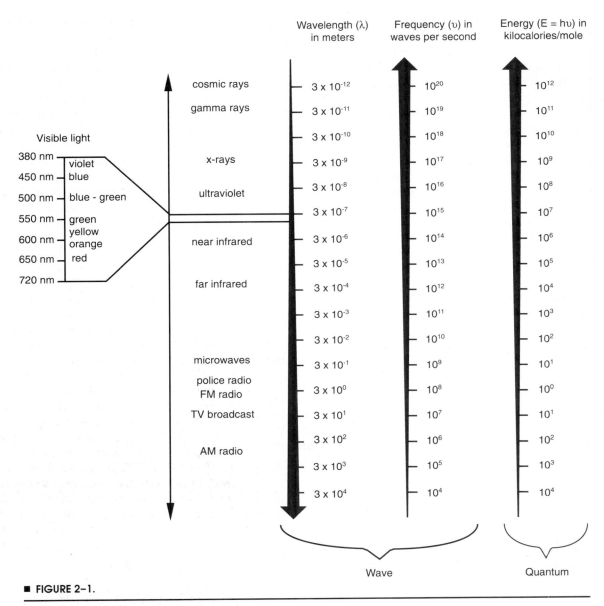

■ **FIGURE 2–1.**

The electromagnetic spectrum.

molecule's electronic structure. The energy generated by the UV and VIS light of the electromagnetic spectrum has sufficient energy to excite electrons from the ground state to the first energy level (an excited state). This interaction in UV/VIS spectro-

photometry is called **absorption.** The measurement of the interaction of radiant energy with matter in the UV and VIS portion of the electromagnetic spectrum is called *spectrophotometry*. A *spectrophotometer* is an analytical instrument that measures the fraction of radiant energy (light) transmitted through a sample. *Transmittance* (T) varies logarithmically with the concentration of the absorbing species, as follows: $T - 10^{-abc}$. Rearranging the equation gives the following:

$$Log (1/T) = 2 - log T = abc$$

where a = molar absorptivity, b = pathlength of sample, and c = concentration of absorbing species. By substituting absorbance (A) for the transmittance term, absorption and concentration become directly proportional.

$$A = 2 - log T \quad or \quad A = abc$$

This equation is referred to as the Beer-Lambert law (also known as the Beer-Bougher law), or **Beer's law,** and is very important in the measurement of samples in a spectrophotometer. This equation shows a linear relationship existing between the absorbance and concentration of the absorbing species. That is, as the concentration of an absorbing species *(sample)* in-creases, more light is absorbed by the sample. Specifically, this law states that the amount of light absorbed (A) by a solution is proportional to its absorbing index, i.e., a, molar absorptivity, which will vary with wavelength; b, the pathlength through which the light travels; and c, the concentration of the solution.

By comparing the amount of radiant energy absorbed at a specific wavelength in a sample solution to the energy absorbed of a known concentration of that sample at the same wavelength, one can quantify the amount of that analyte in solution. By plotting absorbance values obtained at a wavelength versus the known concentration, a standard curve can be constructed. If this plot is directly proportional, then it follows Beer's law. Figure 2–2 shows the relationship between absorbance and concentration.

Various instruments have evolved that use the absorbance of light to determine concentration. The earliest application was the color comparator, followed by the filter photometer and the spectrophotometer. The color comparator was a device that allowed light to travel through both a solution of

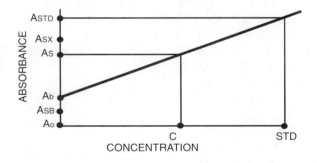

Ao = 000A = distilled water

Ab = absorbance of the reagent blank

ASTD = absorbance of STD (reaction mixture)

ASB = absorbance of sample blank

ASX = absorbance of sample (reaction mixture)

ASX − ASB = AS = absorbance due to constituent being measured in the sample (sample blank correction)

Read AS on standard curve. Concentration of constituent being measured = C.

Note: Reagent blank = reagent + distilled water as sample.
Sample blank = sample + distilled water as reagent.
Water blank = distilled water.

■ **FIGURE 2–2.**

Relationship of absorbance to concentration.

known concentration (a standard solution) and one of unknown concentration (sample solution). The user visually compared the transmitted light and adjusted the pathlength until the light transmitted from both solutions appeared to be of the same intensity.[1] Knowing the pathlength (b) and the molar absorptivity coefficient (a), the unknown concentration could be computed using the Beer-Lambert law. The major drawback to this method of spectrophotometry was that it was only as good as the user's ability to match the intensity of the light transmitted.

With the addition of a photodetector, a new generation of spectrophotometric analysis developed. The *filter photometer* uses glass filters to isolate a band of wavelengths to be passed through the solutions, and it employs the photodetector to detect the amount of light transmitted through the solution. The *photodetector* converts the radiant energy of the light transmitted through the solution to electrical energy. The electrical signal is then relayed to a meter calibrated in percent transmittance (% T) units and/or absorbance [i.e., optical density (OD)]. The Beer-Lambert law (A = abc) is employed with the photometer when the pathlength (b) is constant and the wavelength is constant. The absorbance (A) derived from % T is detected, and the concentration (c) can be calculated using a standard curve and semilog graph paper. The user of this instrument must prepare a series of *standard solutions* of known concentration, measure % T or absorbance (OD), and prepare a plot of absorbance readings (y-axis) versus the concentration (x-axis). Refer to Figure 2–2 (graph of absorbance vs. concentration). A straight line will result in the range of concentrations that follows Beer's law. Thus, any unknown concentration with an absorbance that falls in the linear region of the graph can be determined.

In the 1930s, another instrument that applied the principles of light absorption and photodetection was developed. This instrument, known as a *colorimeter,* or *spectrometer,* differed from the filter photometer in that the method of isolating specific wavelengths from white light was by means of a *prism* or **diffraction grating device.** Figure 2–3 illustrates the isolation of wavelength from white light via a filter, a prism, and a diffraction grating device. This type of

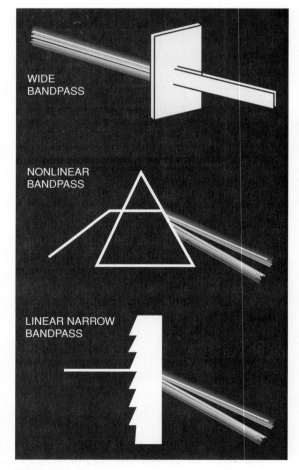

WIDE BANDPASS

NONLINEAR BANDPASS

LINEAR NARROW BANDPASS

■ **FIGURE 2–3.**

Comparison of wavelength isolation from white light by a filter, prism, and a diffraction grating device.

instrument allowed one to select a narrower bandpass. In other words, accuracy was improved because specific wavelengths of light could be selected, thus allowing for improved absorbance detection.

COMPONENTS OF THE SPECTROPHOTOMETER

The major components of a *single-beam* spectrophotometer are the light source, the wavelength isolator, the sample compartment, the detector, and the readout device. Figure 2–4 shows these components. This instrument differs from *double-beam* and *split-beam* spectrophotometers, which have beam splitters that are used to separate the light source into two beams. We will now

discuss each component of the single-beam spectrophotometer and how it works.

Light Source

A UV/VIS spectrophotometer contains two types of energy sources, one for the visible portion, usually defined as 320 to 1000 nm, and another for the ultraviolet portion of the spectrum, usually defined as 100 to 390 nm. An incandescent *tungsten light source* is used for the visible portion, and a hydrogen *deuterium lamp* is used for the UV portion. The tungsten lamp is usually of tungsten halogen origin and gives off a continuous emission of light of 340 to 950 nm, offering a stable and long-lasting (500+ hours or more) energy supply. The UV lamp contains a gas, usually of hydrogen origin such as

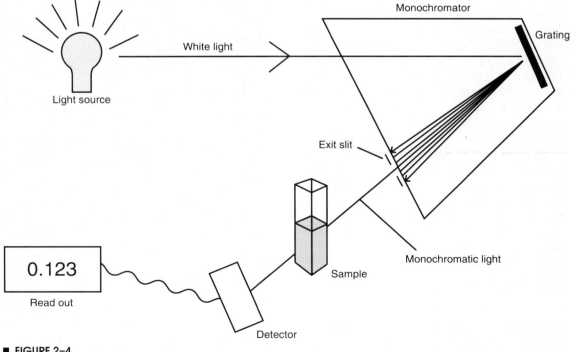

■ **FIGURE 2–4.**

Conventional components of a single-beam spectrophotometer. (Courtesy of Milton-Roy Corporation, Rochester, NY.)

deuterium, in a quartz envelope, which allows for easy penetration of the UV light rays and gives off a *continuous spectrum* of 200 to 360 nm. Deuterium discharge lamps have three to five times greater spectral intensity than hydrogen lamps.

The interchange from the visible and UV lamps occurs usually in the 340 to 360 nm range and is accomplished with a lamp interchange mirror, which toggles between the two lamps (Fig. 2–5). Actually, light from the deuterium lamp is directly focused on a relay lens, enters a condenser lens, and then goes onto a series of concave mirrors that cause the light to strike the monochromator. Light from the tungsten lamp is first reflected off a mirror and then follows the same course as the deuterium-generated

light. Improvements in the light sources have been made recently. A tungsten-halogen visible source lamp has the advantage of providing more energy and a longer life than a plain tungsten lamp. In the latter, the tungsten that evaporates from the filament will coat the glass envelope, thereby decreasing the energy output. The incorporation of low-pressure halogen vapor, such as iodine or bromide, and the presence of a lamp envelope of fused silica increase the lifetime of the tungsten filament used in the more recently introduced quartz-halogen lamp.[2]

Because lamps age with use, it is prudent to schedule periodic lamp inspections and to replace lamps as necessary after a certain number of hours of operation. Lens paper

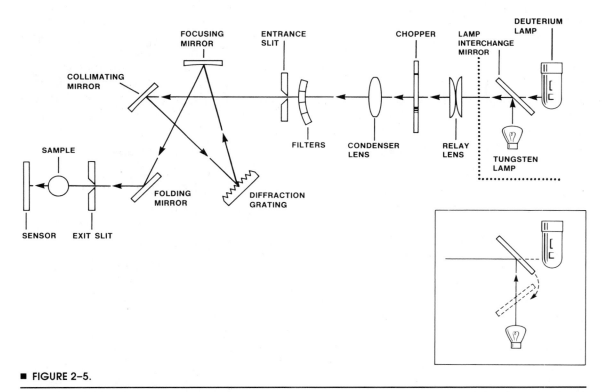

■ FIGURE 2–5.

Tungsten and deuterium lamps with an interchange mirror. (Courtesy of Milton-Roy Corporation, Rochester, NY.)

should be used to hold and position the lamp during replacement, because smudges and fingerprints will cause uneven light emissions. To complement the light source contained in the spectrophotometer, an optical system consisting of lenses and slits modifies the light beam before and after it strikes the monochromator. The latest light source available for spectrophotometers is tunable laser beams. These are capable of providing monochromatic light, and thus discrete wavelengths can be emitted.

Wavelength Isolator (Monochromator)

The purpose of the wavelength isolator or *monochromator* is to isolate the light into individual bands. Although we cannot separate a single wavelength of light, a group or band can be isolated and sent from the monochromator into the sample compartment.

The monochromator is made up of an entrance slit, a dispersion device, and an exit slit. The entrance slit focuses the light (VIS or UV) onto the dispersion device in the monochromator to be isolated into individual bands that are then passed through an exit slit into the sample compartment.

Three devices are used to separate white light into a specific band: the *filter,* the *prism,* and the *grating.* The simplest way to isolate light transmitted by the energy source is to use the **filter.** Two types of filter are commonly employed, an *interference filter* and a glass or *Wratten (absorption) filter.* In the glass filter, one or more layers of colored glass are placed in the path of the light beam, thus allowing only those wavelengths of light that are not absorbed by that particular color to be transmitted through the sample. In a Wratten filter, a colored gelatin is placed between two clear glass pieces, thus allowing only certain wavelengths of light to be transmitted through the glass and to the sample. The other wavelength bands are absorbed in the gelatin. The advantages of utilizing a filter for separation are its low cost and minimal maintenance requirement. The major disadvantage is that it sends a broad band of wavelengths through the sample and does not allow for a continuous spectrum.

The interference filter works on a principle similar to that of the glass filter previously described. Generally, when these types of wavelength isolators are used the instrument is called a photometer. It should be noted that with a filter photometer, only discrete wavelength ranges are available. Instruments that utilize a fixed wavelength have interference filters (Fig. 2–6).

A *prism* works on the principle that light will be refracted at specific angles, depending on the wavelength of the light entering and exiting the transparent material. A prism can be made from either glass or quartz, depending on the wavelength ranges of choice (VIS or UV). A focusing lens is usually employed in order to condense the light on the prism. The advantages of utilizing a prism in a monochromator are that the prism is inexpensive and offers a good

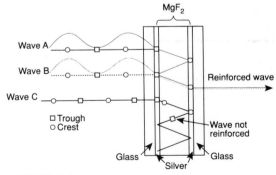

■ **FIGURE 2–6.**

An interference filter. Wave A reinforced by wave B breaks through. Wave C is not reinforced by any wave and does not break through. (From Khazanie P: Spectrophotometry. *In* Anderson SC, Cockayne S (eds): *Clinical Chemistry: Concepts and Applications.* Philadelphia, WB Saunders, 1993, p 79.)

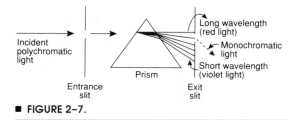

■ FIGURE 2–7.

Diffraction of white light with a prism. (From Khazanie P: Spectrophotometry. *In* Anderson SC, Cockayne S (eds): *Clinical Chemistry: Concepts and Applications.* Philadelphia, WB Saunders, 1993, p 79.)

means of separating out the light into its bands. The major disadvantage is that it gives a nonlinear separation of the bands, in which the lower bands, such as violet, bend more upon exiting the prism than does the red band at the other end of the spectrum (Fig. 2–7). To perform a proper wavelength calibration on a prism instrument, several wavelengths must be measured because of this nonlinear refraction of light.

A *diffraction grating* consists of a series of parallel grooves that are equally etched on a glass surface, allowing the light beam that strikes it to be dispersed into several linear spectra (Fig. 2–8). The surface is usually a piece of glass that has been coated with aluminum, which is an excellent reflector of UV and visible energy. The spacing, which is

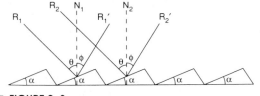

■ FIGURE 2–8.

The principle of reflectance grating. Two incident rays, R_1 and R_2, are in phase, emerging as R_1' and R_2'. Those rays not in phase will be destroyed by interference. α = blade angle; θ = angle of light striking; ϕ = reflectance angle. (From Khazanie P: Spectrophotometry. *In* Anderson SC, Cockayne S (eds): *Clinical Chemistry: Concepts and Applications.* Philadelphia, WB Saunders, 1993, p 79.)

numerous, can be planar-etched, which is quite expensive and tedious. Most gratings used in spectrophotometers today are blazed and holographically replicated. That is, they are copied directly from a master grating. These gratings are usually a criss-cross design that greatly reduces second-order radiation, thereby minimizing **stray radiant energy** (SRE), that is, wavelengths other than the intended, that strike the detector. A grating operates on the principle that light waves will bend around a corner upon striking material set at specific angles. By controlling the angle of deflection, we can get the proper wavelength of the light beam at a different angle.

The advantage of a diffraction grating is that it offers linear dispersion of the light over the entire UV and visible range. For this reason, only two wavelengths are needed to calibrate this type of instrument. As the incident light strikes the grooves on the reflectance grating, many tiny spectra are formed, one from each groove. Spectra that are in phase reinforce one another, and those out of phase cancel one another. The final result is a linear line spectrum that is parallel.[3] The disadvantage of a grating instrument is that it is usually more expensive than filter or prism-based units.

Effect of Monochromator on Bandpass

The movement of the grating or prism, which is mounted in the monochromator, allows the specific bands of light to strike the exit slit and enter the sample compartment. This movement is accomplished either manually by turning a knob or by way of a motor controlled by a microprocessor or computer. In the monochromator system, two types of slits are encountered. There is a slit at the entrance, which focuses the light on the grating or prisms, where it can be dispersed with a minimum of stray light. The second slit is the exit slit, which isolates the se-

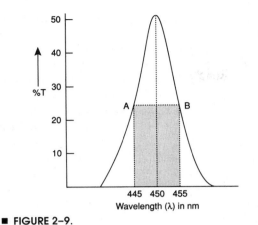

■ **FIGURE 2–9.**

Bandpass of a spectrophotometer (isolated by a filter). (From Khazanie P: Spectrophotometry. *In* Anderson SC, Cockayne S (eds): *Clinical Chemistry: Concepts and Applications.* Philadelphia, WB Saunders, 1993, p 80.)

lected narrow band of wavelengths. By increasing the width of the exit slit, the band of emerging light is broadened, thus increasing intensity but decreasing spectral purity. The range of wavelengths exiting the slit is called the **bandpass,** or **bandwidth.** The bandwidth is the measure of the distribution of wavelengths that are passed through the exit slit of the monochromator and corresponds to 75 percent of the energy that is passed through the sample. The point at which bandpass is measured is at one half the peak transmittance. In Figure 2–9, the peak transmittance is 50 percent T at 450 nm. One half of the peak transmittance is 25 percent T, which is represented by points A and B at 445 and 455 nm, respectively. The bandpass in this example is 10 nm. Typically, interference filters produce bandpass widths of 10 to 20 nm; prisms and gratings produce narrower bandpass widths of less than 5 nm.[3]

As the bandwidth of the spectrophotometer increases, the sharpness of the peaks decreases, owing to less resolution. The absorbance maximum may shift owing to side peaks being incorporated in the primary peak, and the absorptivity decreases. Bandpass is one of the most important specifications of the monochromator. Bandpass, indicated in nanometers (nm) (20, 5, or 2), describes the purity of the light passing through the sample. Specifically, bandpass is defined as the spectral transmittance, equal to one-half the peak transmittance. In other words, bandpass is that range of wavelengths passing through the exit slit of the wavelength-selecting device.

Three factors determine the bandpass of an instrument: (1) the light intensity output of the source, (2) the efficiency of the system to isolate wavelength bands, and (3) the sensitivity of the detector. Although narrow bandwidths offer greater resolution and sensitivity, there is a decrease in intensity.

Figure 2–10 illustrates the effect of bandpass on spectral **resolution**. The spectral peaks at wavelengths 400, 410, 415, 420, and 425 nm are not resolved by the 30-nm bandpass instrument; instead, there is a broad peak in the 410- to 425-nm region. In

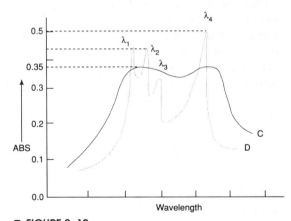

■ **FIGURE 2–10.**

Effect of bandpass on spectral resolution. Comparison of the spectral scan using a wide bandpass width (curve C) and a narrow bandpass width (curve D). (From Khazanie P: Spectrophotometry. *In* Anderson SC, Cockayne S (eds): *Clinical Chemistry: Concepts and Applications.* Philadelphia: WB Saunders, 1993, p 80.)

contrast, the 8-nm bandpass instrument not only is able to isolate the five spectral peaks shown but also yields a greater absolute absorbance at 625 nm.

Sample Holders

The vessel in which the sample is placed, allowing light bands exiting the monochromator to pass through before striking the detector, is called the **cuvette.** Cuvettes may be round, square, cylindrical, or rectangular. Generally, the sample compartment is designed to accommodate a variety of cell shapes and sizes. A square cuvette, because of the parallel sides, provides the greater accuracy. The round sides cause more light scatter of the incident light beam. Furthermore, striations in the round cuvettes can cause reflection of some of the incident light.

Glass is suitable for measurements in the visible region of the spectrum; however, whenever analyses are performed in the ultraviolet region of the spectrum, *quartz* cuvettes are required. The lime in glass cuvettes absorbs the ultraviolet radiation. Some specially manufactured plastic disposable cuvettes, which allow ultraviolet light to be transmitted through them, may also be utilized. Most cuvettes used routinely in the clinical laboratory have pathlengths of 1 cm. Although longer pathlength diameters are sometimes required when a sample is very dilute, the 1-cm pathlength is considered to be the reference. To measure samples with low volumes, microcells can be used. Microcells are cuvettes that hold volumes of 100 μL or less. With microcuvettes, it is important that the cell be aligned so that maximal light passes through the sample.

Significant errors may be introduced because of stray light during the detection of the light transmitted through the cuvette. Whenever readings are being made, the light shield should cover the cuvette well. Extraneous light will result in loss of accuracy. Additional error also can be introduced if the cuvettes have fingerprints, smudges, scratches, or cloudiness. To minimize these effects, cuvettes should be carefully cleaned and wiped with a lint-free cloth or lens paper. To maximize precision, cuvettes should always be placed into the cuvette holder in the same direction. For analyses requiring no loss in precision due to the cuvette, optically matched cuvettes are desirable.

Another type of sample holder is the **flow cell.** With these types of cuvettes, the sample is introduced into the cell via tubing (usually Teflon) that is connected to inlet and outlet ports on the cell. A peristaltic pump is generally employed to "draw" the sample through the tubing and into the cell. These flow-through cuvettes provide a constant light path and have the advantages of speed and ease of measurement. The flow cell, however, must be rinsed with distilled water between measurements to minimize carry-over from one sample to the next. In some instances with flow cells, it is necessary to regulate the temperature. Temperature regulation is a requirement in certain kinetic assays.

Detectors

Detectors utilized within the spectrophotometer are usually one of three types: *photomultiplier tube, photocell,* or *photodiode.* A detector converts the electromagnetic radiation into an electrical signal. There is a direct relationship between the intensity of the electromagnetic radiation and the electrical signal produced.

Photomultiplier Tube

A photomultiplier tube works on the principle of converting light energy into electri-

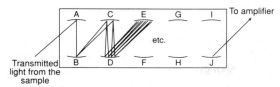

■ **FIGURE 2–11.**

Schematic of a photomultiplier tube. A = cathode; B–J = dynodes represented by crescent shape. (From Khazanie P: Spectrophotometry. *In* Anderson SC, Cockayne S (eds): *Clinical Chemistry: Concepts and Applications.* Philadelphia, WB Saunders, 1993, p 81.)

cal impulses that are amplified and directed to a readout device. The photomultiplier tube is made of a photosensitive metal that absorbs light energy and emits electrons in proportion to the radiant energy that strikes the surface. These electrons are transmitted to a secondary stage where they are amplified, producing more electrons, and then transmitted to a third stage for another amplification that is four- to six-fold. This process continues until the amplified signal is sent to the readout device as an electric current. Some of today's photomultiplier tubes have as many as 15 stages (dynodes).[3] (Refer to Fig. 2–11). Photomultiplier tubes have rapid response times, show little fatigue, and offer good sensitivity in both the ultraviolet and visible ranges. Photomultiplier tubes can be found in both visible and UV/VIS spectrophotometers.

Photocell (Phototube)

A photocell (phototube) consists of a curved, light-sensitive cathode and a narrow, cylindrical anode (Fig. 2–12). A photocell is coated with a photosensitive material at the cathode, such as cesium, that emits electrons when radiant energy strikes it. The emitted electrons are then collected at the anode. An electric current results, which is detected externally as a voltage change across a resistor. The electric current flows to the detector, where it is measured.

Photodiodes (Light-Sensing Diodes)

Photodiodes, or light-detecting diodes (LDDs), differ from phototubes in that they are usually made of a silicon material. More recent designs employ silicon chips that convert light energy to an electrical signal for detection. The silicon chip results in greater accuracy and speed and offers an expanded bandpass range.[3]

Readout Devices

Readout devices include the analog (meter), the digital, the recorder (X-Y or Y-T), and the RS232 for computer interfacing. An *analog* output represents a transmittance reading from the amount of light. In the digital output, analog signals are converted to digital values for processing by a central processing unit (CPU).

Spectrophotometer Designs

Based on the optical geometry, conventional spectrophotometers can be categorized into three different types: single-beam,

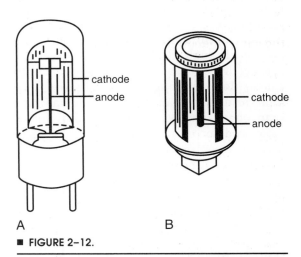

A   B

■ **FIGURE 2–12.**

Phototube configurations. *A,* Conventional type; *B,* cartridge type.

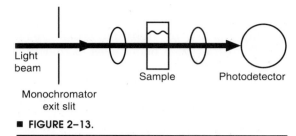

Single-beam spectrophotometer optics design. (Courtesy of Milton-Roy Corporation, Rochester, NY.)

double-beam, and split-beam (sometimes referred to as dual-beam). There is also the photodiode array.

In a *single-beam spectrophotometer* (Fig. 2–13), a reference solution is placed in the sample compartment and % T is adjusted to 100 percent (or 0 absorbance). The sample is then placed in the compartment and measured. This type of spectrophotometer offers excellent energy efficiency and low design cost but is subject to drift and poor stability. For this reason, a constant check of the solution (the "blank") versus the sample is necessary. Single-beam spectrophotometers generally are not suitable for scanning applications.

Scanning is the ability of the spectrophotometer to make continuous photometric readings (usually in absorbance units) over a wavelength range. This feature is accomplished through mechanical rotation of the grating device over a continuous wavelength range. Most scanning instruments are of the dual- or double-beam type. Before making a scan on a sample, a blank or baseline is measured to compensate for differences in the energy output over that range. The purpose of scanning a sample is to find where the absorbance peak(s) are and to determine any interferences that may cause false readings. Figure 2–14 shows a printout of a wavelength scan.

In the *double-beam spectrophotometer* (Fig. 2–15), the light beam is split into separate beams by a chopper motor. Each

beam, approximately of equal energy, is directed to two cell holders, one containing a reference cell and the other a sample to be measured. A ratio between the two is obtained. This type of spectrophotometer offers excellent stability and low drift but a higher design cost. Additionally, since only 50 percent of the energy is diverted to the sample, highly absorbing species cannot be directly measured. This type of spectrophotometer is used for scanning applications when a sample absorbance is changing rapidly over time (in a nonkinetics application).

The third type of spectrophotometer is the *split* or *dual beam* (Fig. 2–16). In this system the light beam is split in two by a beam splitter. But instead of 50 percent of the light beam being sent through a reference and sample cell holder, a small fraction, 15 to 20 percent, is sent through air as a reference beam. A reference cell is placed in a sample compartment and % T is adjusted to 100 percent T or 0 absorbance. The sample is then placed into the sample compartment

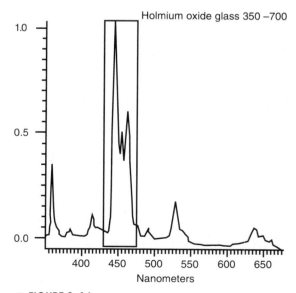

■ **FIGURE 2-14.**

Spectral scan of holmium oxide glass, from 350 to 700 nm. (Courtesy of Milton-Roy Corporation, Rochester, NY.)

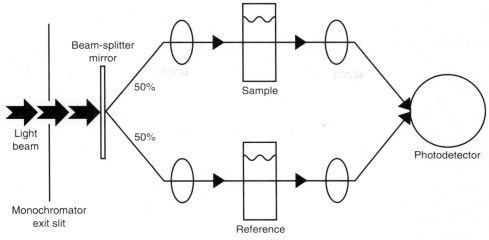

■ **FIGURE 2–15.**

Double-beam spectrophotometer optics design. (Courtesy of Milton-Roy Corporation, Rochester, NY.)

to be measured. In the dual-beam spectrophotometer the energy directed through the sample compartment is much higher than that in the double-beam; excellent stability is achieved with low drift, and the cost is moderate. This spectrophotometer is also designed for scanning applications. Samples in which absorbance values change rapidly over time are unsuitable for this type of instrument.

Photodiode Array

Another type of spectrophotometer is the *photodiode array* (PDA) (Fig. 2–17). Unlike a conventional spectrophotometer, in which

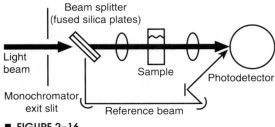

■ **FIGURE 2–16.**

Split-beam (or dual-beam) spectrophotometer. (Courtesy of Milton-Roy Corporation, Rochester, NY.)

light is separated into individual bands and transmitted through a sample, a PDA passes all bands of light through the sample. After passing through the sample the light is then separated, in a spectrograph compartment, by means of a fixed grating that projects the individual bands onto an array. This array contains a series of diodes (detectors) that convert the light energy into electrical impulses. Since there are multidetectors in this type of system, a range of wavelengths can be detected simultaneously, rather than sequentially as with a conventional spectrophotometer. Generally the electrical impulses are passed onto a computer for rapid data analysis and display. Depending on the wavelength range to be measured, a PDA can contain a deuterium and a tungsten lamp for analysis over a 190 to 950 nm range. The number of diodes on the array determines the resolution; that is, the greater the number of diodes over a given wavelength range, the better the resolution.

PDA is an important tool in the analysis of kinetic assays in which one can measure both substrate and product formation at different wavelengths simultaneously. It is

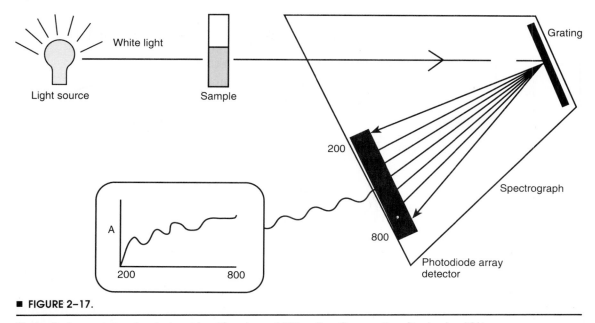

■ **FIGURE 2–17.**

Photodiode array spectrophotometer. (Courtesy of Milton-Roy Corporation, Rochester, NY.)

also utilized in applications that require continuous scanning, because of its speed—commonly less than 1 second over the wavelength range.

Power Supply

The power supply in any UV/VIS spectrophotometer must provide stable and continuous power to the circuits. Batteries are used in some spectrophotometers. The advantage is that batteries provide direct current and portability. This is important in some applications that may require field testing.

QUALITY CONTROL AND THE SPECTROPHOTOMETER

As with all instruments, performance evaluation is important in ruling out one of the three sources of error in testing procedures: faulty test chemistry, operator error, and instrument performance. To assure the accuracy of the data being generated, periodic inspection of the spectrophotometer used in the clinical chemistry laboratory is an absolute necessity. **Quality control checking** of the spectrophotometer performance is achieved by regular inspections of wavelength accuracy, detector linearity, and stray light. These are the minimum checks recommended by the American Association for Clinical Chemistry.[4] Fluctuations in the meter readout and the line voltage should also be noted and corrected. Automated instruments should be checked for **noise** and **drift.** The random fluctuations in absorbance readings seen on strip-chart recorders are indicative of noise. Noise refers to the quality of short-term stability. Drift can be seen as a slow, unidirectional change that occurs over several days. Figure 2–18 illustrates instrument noise and drift.

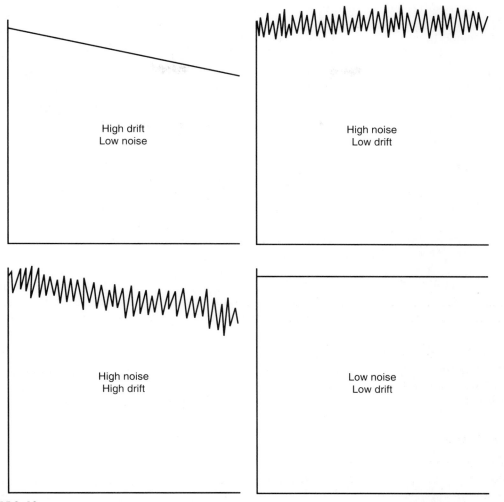

High drift
Low noise

High noise
Low drift

High noise
High drift

Low noise
Low drift

■ **FIGURE 2–18.**

Spectrophotometer noise and drift.

Wavelength Accuracy

Wavelength accuracy implies that the radiation striking the sample is that of the wavelength indicated on the dial or display. One assumes that the light exiting the monochromator is the bandpass selected by the operator. By definition, wavelength accuracy is the agreement between the wavelength reading of the spectrophotometer and the actual wavelength. The monochromator alignment and its bandwidth are the factors responsible for wavelength accuracy. If a spectrophotometer exhibits wavelength inaccuracies, the absorbance readings will be erroneous. For example, if the bandwidth of the light coming from the monochromator is wider than the solution's spectral absorbance peak, these "extra" wavelengths will be transmitted and reach the detector, causing falsely low results. These readings will actually show the slope of a peak absorbance, not the peak height. Verification of wavelength accuracy can be accomplished by using special rare earth filters or solutions that have sharp absorption peaks at specified wavelengths. Alternately, light sources that have sharp emission lines may also be used.

The most accurate method to determine the wavelength accuracy of the spectrophotometer is to select a light source such as a deuterium or mercury lamp and fit it into the instrument, if possible. Deuterium lamps emit prominent line spectra at 486 and 656 nm and a less prominent line at 380 nm.[6] To check the wavelength accuracy with either of these light sources, the wavelength dial is set 5 to 10 nm below the expected wavelength, and then the dial is turned toward the wavelength chosen. The point of maximal absorbance is the actual wavelength being detected. The process is repeated in the reverse direction. The two observed wavelengths should agree with each other and the true wavelength $\pm$ 0.25 nm. If these determinations do not agree, the wavelength-dial linkage must be adjusted.[7] Wavelength checks must be made at a minimum of three wavelengths for prism instruments, since they are nonlinear, and at a minimum of two wavelengths for grating instruments.

The most frequently used method to check wavelength accuracy is with holmium oxide or didymium glass filters. Didymium has characteristic absorbance peaks in the visible region of the spectrum at 573, 586, 685, 741, and 803 nm, whereas holmium oxide filters have absorbance peaks in both the visible and ultraviolet regions of the spectrum.

Since didymium shows characteristic broad peaks at several wavelengths, it is the filter of choice for the calibration of wide-bandpass instruments; holmium oxide is

often used for calibration of narrow-bandpass instruments. These filters may be purchased from the National Bureau of Standards.

Stable chromogenic solutions also can be used as a secondary wavelength calibration standard. To verify calibration after a filter has been employed, solutions such as cobalt ammonium sulfate, cobalt chloride, potassium chromate, or nickel sulfate may be utilized. For example, potassium chromate (40 mg/L) has absorbance peaks at 340, 375, 400, and 450 nm. Although chromogenic solutions are inexpensive, they have the disadvantages of being subject to preparation errors, contamination, and aging.

Although the most accurate method to check for wavelength accuracy is to replace the light source with a deuterium or mercury lamp, which has distinct, sharp spectral lines, this method is rarely used because it is a more cumbersome technique.

Photometric Linearity and Accuracy

Photometric **linearity** is the ability of the detector to respond properly in the conversion of light impulses to electrical signal over the entire detector range. If a photocell is able to produce an output that is proportional to the light intensity from the cuvette, varying concentrations of a solution should result in a straight line. The cause of nonlinear photometric readings can be traced to the detector, the amplifier, or the readout device. Nonlinear or inaccurate photometric readings will result in nonlinearity of absorbance values.

The most common method of measuring photometric linearity is with neutral glass filters. These filters are placed in the light path at various wavelengths, and the transmittance values (versus air) are obtained and compared with filter certified values. As an alternative, any solution used for absorbance checks, e.g., ammonium sulfate, can be diluted and used for linearity studies.

Stray Radiant Energy

As defined earlier, stray radiant energy (SRE) is energy of other than the intended wavelengths that strikes the detector without passing through the sample. This energy may come from light leaks within the sample compartment (e.g., scratches on the cuvette) or energy leaks may be due to misaligned cells (particularly with microcells), improper light source (improper replacement), and misaligned optics.

Stray radiant energy causes a lower absorbance reading for the sample being analyzed. This will result in a nonlinear relationship between absorbance and concentration (i.e., one that does not follow Beer's law). The most reliable method for testing stray light is with glass cutoff filters. These filters are placed in the light path, and the transmittance values obtained are compared with certified values of that filter for that wavelength. Stray light is a greater problem at either end of the visible region of the spectrum.

AUTOMATION OF SPECTROPHOTOMETERS

Instrument Control

First-generation spectrophotometers were manually operated. Dials of the instrument were turned to control the functions of wavelength selection, "zeroing" (0 absorbance or 100 percent transmittance), and "blanking." All these adjustments were made by turning knobs on the outside of the instrument. Figure 2–20 shows an early spectrophotometer with knob controls.

Now, through the use of a microprocessor, functions previously performed manually can be controlled through a key pad and data displayed on a screen (Fig. 2–19).

Data Output

The meter was the earliest and simplest form of data display on the spectrophotometers. A galvanometer translated the electrical signal from the photodetector to a needle deflection on the meter display. The values of absorbance and percent transmittance

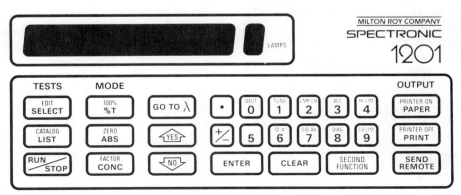

■ **FIGURE 2–19.**

Keyboard functions on a spectrophotometer. (Courtesy of Milton-Roy Corporation, Rochester, NY.)

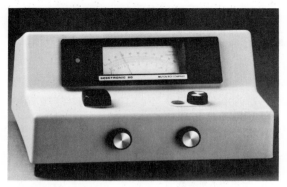

■ **FIGURE 2–20.**

An early spectrophotometer with a meter display. (Courtesy of Milton-Roy Corporation, Rochester, NY.)

were read by the operator. Figure 2–20 illustrates an early spectrophotometer with a meter display.

The next advancement for data output was the digital display (Fig. 2–21). With digital display, the readings were made quickly and accurately. Today one typically finds light-emitting diodes (LEDs), liquid crystal displays (LCDs), vacuum fluorescent displays, and cathode ray tubes (CRTs) used for display of the readings.[8] Now, with addi-

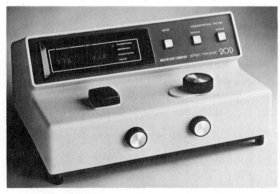

■ **FIGURE 2–21.**

A spectrophotometer with a digital display. (Courtesy of Milton-Roy Corporation, Rochester, NY.)

tional circuitry, a calculation factor can be introduced so that the absorbance data can be converted to concentration.

More recent spectrophotometers have the capability to send digital signals across serial or parallel ports to communicate with a printer or a computer interfaced to the instrument. In addition to supplying the absorbance/transmittance readings and the concentration, newer spectrophotometers have built-in microprocessors that are capable of graphics display. An entire spectral scan may be viewed via the CRT and downloaded to a printer or plotter for a hard copy (Fig. 2–22).

Data Manipulation

As technology advanced, spectrophotometers with early microprocessors could be set for both end-point and kinetic analysis. For the kinetic assays, a change in absorbance over time (ΔA) could be monitored and enzyme activity calculated. Figure 2–23 is a data printout for the kinetics mode from a modern microprocessor-controlled spectrophotometer. Now, many data manipulations are possible. Table 2–1 summarizes the data manipulation features of the state-of-the-art spectrophotometers.

Some future trends in data handling include the use of "flash memory cards." Measuring 2 by 4 inches in size and containing up to 40 megabytes of memory, these cards utilize integrated circuits to store and retrieve data rapidly. The advantage of these cards over current computer-driven systems is that data are stored electronically. The data can also be transferred to desktop or notebook computers for further data manipulation. These cards allow the user to set up test parameters easily and collect data from the instrument rapidly.

■ **FIGURE 2–22.**

A CRT hardcopy printout of a spectrophotometer scan with menu options. (Courtesy of Milton-Roy Corporation, Rochester, NY.)

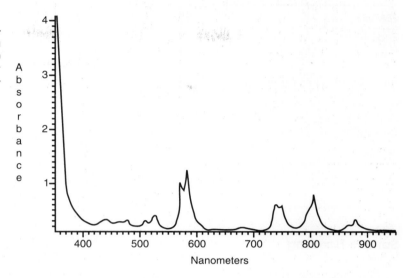

■ **FIGURE 2–23.**

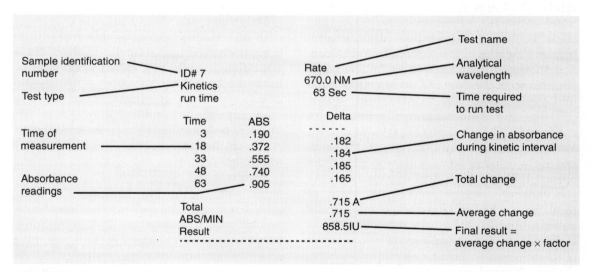

Data printout for the kinetics mode from a modern spectrophotometer. (From Altemose IR, et al: Evolution of instrumentation for UV/VIS spectrophotometry. *Journal of Chemical Education* 63(11):A263, Nov 1986.)

TABLE 2-1. DATA MANIPULATION FEATURES USED FOR CLINICAL LABORATORY APPLICATIONS

FEATURE	DESCRIPTION
End-point	Measures A, % T, or concentration of a sample after an initial time
Linear standard curve	Measures concentration of a sample relative to a known set of standards, from which a linear regression curve has been generated
Nonlinear standard curve	Measures the concentration of a sample relative to a set of standards that have a nonlinear response. Various curve fits used to fit the points are point-to-point, cubic, spline, quadratic, and linear equations
Kinetics	Measures the change in absorbance over time (rate analysis); generally used in the measurement of enzymatic activity
Multiple wavelengths	Measures absorbance of an unknown at various wavelengths Examples: *Absorbance ratio* of two wavelengths to test for purity of DNA; *Three-Point Net* (Allen's Correction)—three wavelengths are used to correct for interferences

Sample Handling

The first generation of spectrophotometers relied on the operator to insert the cuvettes containing the sample one at a time. Later, flow cells were introduced. Flow cells allow for rapid, discrete sampling, emptying, and rinsing of the sample from the cell. Automation of multiple samples is made possible with the flow cell design. One of the first clinical analyzers to incorporate a flow cell was the Autoanalyzer (Technicon Instruments Corporation, Tarrytown, NY). Multiple samples could be read by the process of continuous flow. A debubbled stream passed through the narrow glass flow cell, the ends of which were optically clear, so that light from the monochromator could pass through it. Flow cells are also used in the detector systems of high-pressure liquid chromatography (HPLC), a clinical laboratory technique described in Chapter 5, Chromatography Instrumentation Systems. Many spectrophotometers can be interfaced with a shuttle tray that holds the test tubes containing the samples; a probe delivers the sample to the flow cell.

INTERPRETATION OF MANUFACTURER'S SPECIFICATION SHEETS

Manufacturers always provide customers with advertising brochures describing their company's spectrophotometer models. These **specification sheets,** called **spec sheets,** present a capsulized summary of the instrument's performance limits, data management capabilities, and any special features. Many details are listed on these spec sheets. A typical list of specifications is presented in Table 2–2.

Performance specifications generally include wavelength range accuracy and precision, bandpass (slit width), photometric detection range, and stray light minimums. Other instrument options include scanning speed (if applicable), data management capabilities, host computer compatibility, and instrument sampling features. Generally the light source will not be specifically identified; instead, the wavelength range will be given. As mentioned earlier, a tungsten lamp is used for the visible region of the

TABLE 2–2. INTERPRETATION OF MANUFACTURERS' SPECIFICATION SHEETS

SPECIFICATION	COMMENTS	EXAMPLE
Wavelength range	Indicates what wavelength ranges are covered for that instrument	325–1000 nm (visible) 190–1000 nm (UV/VIS)
Wavelength accuracy	The agreement of the wavelength displayed and those passed through the monochromator	±2 nm
Wavelength repeatability	Sometimes referred to as *reproducibility*, how well the instrument can go back to the same desired wavelength	±0.3 nm
Spectral slit width	Sometimes referred to as *bandwidth*, the band of wavelengths exiting the monochromator	2 nm
Photometric accuracy	Indicates the ability of the detector to respond correctly to various intensities of light	±0.005 A at 1.00 A
Photometric range	Indicates the range the instrument can respond in transmittance (% T), absorbance (A), and concentration (C)	To 200% T − 3.000 to 3.000 A −9999 to 9999 C
Photometric stability	Sometimes referred to as *drift*, indicates how the photometric readings in absorbance will change over time, usually at the baseline (0.00 A)	±0.002 A/hr at 0.00 A
Stray light	Sometimes referred to as *stray radiant energy* (SRE), the amount of energy other than the intended wavelength striking the detector	Less than 0.05% at 220 nm and 340 nm
Slewing speed	Refers to the speed with which the instrument can go from one wavelength to another	6000 nm per minute
Scanning speed	For a scanning spectrophotometer, refers to the speed at which the instrument can collect data over a wavelength range	5–3000 nm per minute
Stability	Noise and drift limits	Noise: ±0.005 A/15 minutes Drift: ±0.010 A/hour
Data processing	The software or microprocessor control functions, e.g., data management capabilities	Kinetic rate calculations; standard curve calculations; standard curve calculations at multiple wavelengths
Special features	Readout options	CRT display; printer
	Data storage	20 tests with a battery backup
	Accessories	Flow cell (sipper); multicell holder; automatic sample handler

electromagnetic spectrum, and a vapor lamp such as deuterium is used for the UV range. Both lamps will be present in the instruments that have both UV and visible range capability. As illustrated earlier in Figure 2–5, if the operator must switch from the visible to the UV range, a mirror in the spectrophotometer is repositioned so that the vapor lamp light now passes through the entrance slit onto the rest of the optical system, including the monochromator. Also listed in the spec sheets are the wavelength reliability limits.

Technical details, such as grating rulings per inch, agreement of wavelength setting and actual reading, and the the wavelength precision limits are detailed. A quality spectrophotometer will have a wavelength accuracy of $\pm$ 2 nm and a precision of $\leq$ 0.5 nm. Bandwidth (bandpass) is usually listed as *slit width*. High-performance spectrophotometers used in the clinical laboratory should have slit widths of $\leq$ 2 nm. *Resolution* is another term substituted for bandwidth. Photometric accuracy and range also are listed. In addition, the absorbance, transmittance, and concentration display ranges will be noted. The amount of stray light reflected onto the detector will be given as the amount of SRE, defined earlier. Normally, the SRE is less than 0.1 percent T. The stability features of *noise* and *drift* are other performance features noted.

The spec sheet also includes other instrument features and control options. If a wavelength driver is present, the *scanning* and *slewing speeds* are listed. (These terms are defined in Table 2–2.) Generally, the manufacturer summarizes any special options available with the particular model. These options, unrelated to the instrument performance, may include sample handling, data calculations and storage, time and temperature control, display and printer options, and computer interface options.

CONSIDERATIONS IN SELECTING A SPECTROPHOTOMETER

Most of the clinical laboratory tests performed in today's laboratory are run on automated systems, discussed in forthcoming chapters; however, in many situations stand-alone spectrophotometers are still used. Although criteria for selection of a spectrophotometer are similar to those applied to the large automated systems, some thought should be given to defining specific considerations for spectrophotometers in more detail.

Table 2–3 gives a priority list of questions the laboratorian should address before the purchase of an instrument. The first question to be answered is "What tests will be performed on the instrument now and in the future?" If the tests will require both UV and visible region analyses, then a UV/VIS spectrophotometer is necessary. This feature cannot be altered at a later date. Another related question is "Is scanning a requirement?" If the laboratory staff intend to establish new methods for research or other purposes, this feature may be necessary in order to identify the wavelength best suited for the particular determination. Additionally, spectral scanning to identify drugs of abuse may be desired. Likewise, spectral scanning of hemoglobin to differentiate oxyhemoglobin from methemoglobin will require this feature. The other related feature is whether a single-, split-, or double-beam optical configuration is desired. Remember, only split- and double-beam spectrophotometers are appropriate for scanning.

Another important question is "What degree of accuracy is required?" If scanning is being performed, the best resolution possible is required. If only routine quantitations

TABLE 2–3. PRIORITY CONSIDERATIONS FOR SELECTION OF A SPECTROPHOTOMETER

1. What test(s) will be performed?
2. Is scanning required?
3. What degree of accuracy is required?
4. What type of sample holder(s) is (are) required?
5. Is automation of sampling required?
6. What type of data manipulations is required?
7. What is the ability of the instrument to be interfaced?
8. Can the instrument be upgraded for possible future needs?
9. What are the warranty and service considerations?
10. What are the budgetary considerations?

will be performed on the instrument, a more moderately priced spectrophotometer with a larger, but adequate, bandpass may be considered.

Next, the sample considerations need to be addressed. "What type of sample holders will be required?" If very little sample volume will be available, microcuvettes are necessary. If the concentration of the analyte is very low, as in parts/million, then a spectrophotometer capable of handling a longer pathlength cell will be a must. Another sample consideration is the need for automation. A large number of samples per run or multiple operations per run (e.g., kinetic assays) will obviate the need for a flow cell.

The next consideration relates to data manipulations. "Is interfacing to a laboratory computer a need?" "Is storage of data desired?" "What type of calculations are necessary (e.g., multiple wavelength comparisons)?" "How should the data be displayed—hard copy, video display?"

After all the performance and special features options have been identified, the technologist should now address the warranty and instrument purchase cost. When considering the warranty agreement, the laboratorian needs to determine whether the instrument will be repaired on-site or off-site. Once the instrument is purchased, proper maintenance will be necessary. In fact, laboratory staff need to document maintenance and quality control checks for these instruments to comply with the Clinical Laboratory Improvement Act (CLIA)[9] guidelines for all licensed laboratories.

Whenever a new spectrophotometer is being considered for purchase, all the preceding considerations need to be identified. After the questions have been answered, the final consideration is the reputation of the manufacturer. A more detailed presentation of instrument selection is given in Chapters 17 and 18.

SUMMARY

Spectrophotometry has a wide range of both industrial and clinical applications. Any compound that will react with a chemical to produce a color or transmit light can be measured by this technique. In the clinical market, spectrophotometry is performed predominately in the visible and UV regions of the electromagnetic spectrum. In addition, both *end-point* and *kinetic reactions* are used.

An understanding of the spectrophotometer's components—light source, monochromator, sample holder, detector, and readout device—is necessary to perform the appropriate quality control checks, maintain and troubleshoot the instrument, and interpret the manufacturer's spec sheets.

Today, advances in microprocessors and computers have increased the spectrophotometer's capabilities in data manipulation, test storage, and retrieval, which has led to advances in automation. Many of the modern spectrophotometers are now microprocessor-controlled, which allows for automatic functions such as movement of the grating motor, automatic blanking for the reference cell, and automatic conversion from % T to absorbance (A) values. Additionally, a microprocessor offers automatic calculation of standard curves and curve-fitting. Overall, modern spectrophotometers offer improved sensitivity, reliability, and ease of operation.

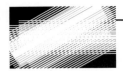

REVIEW QUESTIONS

Choose all the responses that are true.

1. If a blue sample is placed in a spectro-photometer, which of the following statements are true?

   a. The sample absorbs energy at the 630–650 nm range.
   b. The sample absorbs energy at the 430–450 nm range.
   c. The sample transmits energy at the 630–650 nm range.
   d. The sample transmits energy at the 430–450 nm range.

2. As the bandwidth of a spectropho-tometer goes from 10 nm to 2 nm, the spectral resolution

   a. increases.
   b. decreases.
   c. remains the same.

3. A typical spectrophotometer contains which of the following components?

   a. photocell, light source, detector, readout device, cell
   b. detector, dispersion device, light source, sample compartment, readout device
   c. monochromator, light source, readout device, detector, photo-diode
   d. sample compartment, cell holder, light source, detector, readout de-vice

4. Which of the following statements is/are true?

   a. A split-beam spectrophotometer has three beams.
   b. A double-beam spectrophotom-eter has a reference cell and sam-ple cell.
   c. Split-beam and double-beam spectrophotometers generally pro-vide more stable readings than sin-gle-beam spectrophotometers.
   d. All scanning spectrophotometers are double-beam.

5. When measuring a sample in a 10-mm cell with low absorbance readings, one can increase the sensitivity by

   a. diluting the sample.
   b. placing the sample in a 5-mm cell.
   c. placing the sample in a 50-mm cell.
   d. placing the sample in a 5-cm cell.

REFERENCES

1. Altemose IR: Evolution of instrumentation for UV-visible spectrophotometry: Part I. *J Chem Educ* 63:A216–A223, 1986.
2. Narayanan S: *Principles and Applications of Labo-ratory Instrumentation.* Chicago, ASCP Press, 1989, pp 8–17.

3. Khazanie P: Spectrophotometry. *In* Anderson SC, Cockagne S (eds): *Clinical Chemistry: Concepts and Applications.* Philadelphia, WB Saunders, 1993, pp 72–91.

4. Frings CS: Spectral techniques. *In* Kaplan LA, Pesce AJ (eds): *Clinical Chemistry: Theory, Analysis and Correlation.* St. Louis, CV Mosby, 1984, pp 51–73.

5. *Laboratory Instrumentation Evaluation, Verification, and Maintenance Manual.* Northfield, IL, College of American Pathologists, 1989, pp 61–72.

6. Rand RN: Practical spectrophotometric standards. *Clin Chem* 15:839–863, 1969.

7. Edisbury J: Practical hints on absorption. *In Spectrophotometry.* New York, Plenum Press, 1967, p 176.

8. Lott JA: Practical problems in clinical enzymology. *Crit Rev Clin Lab Sci* Dec:277–301, 1977.

9. Altemose IR: Evolution of instrumentation for UV-visible spectrophotometry: Part II. *J Chem Educ* 63:262–266, 1986.

10. *The Federal Register* 57(4):7164–7165, 1992.

C h a p t e r   3

PARTICLE COUNTERS

DEBORAH T. FIRESTONE, MA, MT (ASCP) SBB

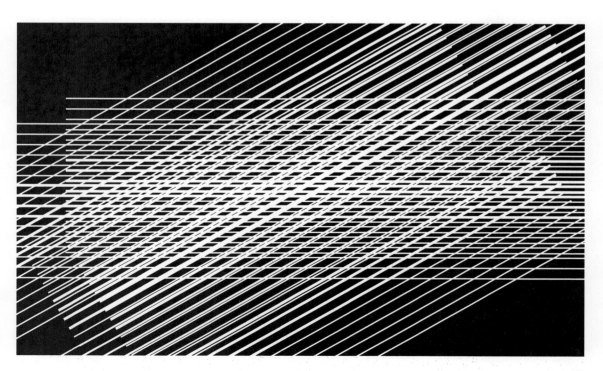

LEARNING OBJECTIVES

After studying this chapter, the student will be able to:

■ Describe the principle of electrical impedance and explain how this principle is applied to enumeration of blood cells.

■ Compare and contrast the principles of flow cytometry with nephelometry and turbidimetry.

■ Diagram and label the components of a laser-based flow cytometer and cell sorter.

■ Discuss the incorporation of various types of filters and dichroic mirrors in a flow cytometer system to achieve analyses on different cells.

■ List at least three clinical applications for flow cytometry.

■ Compare and contrast nephelometry and turbidimetry in terms of instrumentation, principles, and sensitivity.

■ Explain the term *microparticle-enhanced nephelometric immunoassay.*

■ List at least three clinical applications for nephelometry and turbidimetry.

■ Write the principle of osmometry.

■ Compare and contrast measurement of colligative properties based on principle, limitations, and clinical applications of the following: freezing point, vapor pressure, colloidal pressure, and boiling point.

■ Calculate osmolality given the patient's serum sodium, blood glucose, and blood urea nitrogen values.

■ Calculate and give the purpose of the osmolal gap.

KEY WORDS

Coincidence correction. Electronic circuitry that corrects for the possibility that two cells will pass through an aperture at one time.

Colligative properties. The four physical properties of a solution: boiling point, freezing point, vapor pressure, and osmotic pressure, that are related to the number of particles in solution and can, in turn, be measured to determine the osmolality of a solution.

Dichroic mirror. A mirror that splits a beam of energy and directs specific portions of it in two different directions.

Fluorochrome. A molecule, used to tag an antigen or an antibody, that is capable of absorbing light and re-emitting it as fluorescence.

Histogram. A computer-generated, single-dimensional display of cellular analyses, such as volume. Analysis or measured values are shown on the X-axis, and the concentration is shown on the Y-axis.

Impedance. Opposition to the flow of alternating current, which is a result of the combined effect of resistance and reactance; an application of this principle is applied in cell-sorting instrumentation.

Laser. An acronym for Light Amplification by Stimulated Emission Radiation; this beam of light is very intense, highly collimated, and often used in nephelometers.

Light scatter. The interaction of light directed on particles suspended in solution, resulting in the bending of light, at various angles, away from its original path.

Microparticle-enhanced nephelometric immunoassay. A technique that utilizes submicron-sized particles as carriers of antibodies, so that the reaction of the coated antibody with the antigen will result in a suspended particle large enough to scatter light and thus be detected by a nephelometer.

Nephelometry. The technique of employing a specially designed spectrophotometer to detect light scatter, produced by particles suspended in solution, at an angle different from that of the incident light source.

Refraction. The bending of incident light after it passes from one medium to another of different density. Light scatter at right angles is strongly influenced by this phenomenon.

"Sort logic." A computerized logic that is applied to a cell-sorter instrument in which cells are identified electronically as they pass a laser beam; this results in certain cells being charged and redirected for further analyses.

Turbidimetry. The measurement of a decrease in percent transmittance of an incident beam of light as it passes through a solution containing suspended particles.

HISTORY

Some of the earliest laboratory techniques used for counting particles involved the time-consuming, laborious, and somewhat inaccurate method of counting cells one at a time. Counting chambers, invented in the 1800s, were carefully filled with a fixed amount of diluted blood, and red and white blood cells were painstakingly counted. Price-Jones, in 1933, developed a method for sizing cells that involved projecting a stained blood film on a piece of paper, outlining the cells and measuring their diameter. A simpler and less accurate method of red blood cell sizing involved inserting a micrometer disk in the eyepiece of a microscope.[1]

One of the earliest methods for automatically counting cells in suspension was described by Moldavan in 1934. A suspension of cells (red blood cells or stained yeast) was forced through capillary glass tubes onto a microscope stage and then counted by a photoelectric apparatus attached to the ocular. Problems surrounding this technique included maintaining an adequate flow rate and obstruction of the ocular by large cells. The incorporation of the laminar sheath flow principle into subsequent photoelectric counters alleviated these problems. The sheath flow principle is the basis for almost all flow cytometer instruments in use today.

The light-scattering properties of particles were first recognized by Pope and Healy in 1938. They observed that when antibody and antigen were mixed in the proper proportions and intersected by a light source, light was scattered. The clinical usefulness of these findings was demonstrated by Schultze and Schwick when they observed that the intensity of light scattered was proportional to the amount of precipitate formed between some plasma proteins and their specific antibody. This was the basic principle of the nephelometer, which was not in practical use in the clinical laboratory until the 1970s. Automated nephelometers are routinely used in the laboratory today for the analysis of proteins.[2]

In 1949, Wallace Coulter filed for a patent entitled "Means for Counting Particles Suspended in a Fluid." This led to the development of the "Model A" Coulter Counter, which had the capacity to perform cell sizing automatically. This methodology sizes cells using the electrical impedance principle, which relates the volume of the particles to the amplitude of the signal. Subsequent refinements in the initial instrumentation have produced an automated, computerized, sophisticated photoelectric device capable of performing simultaneous multiparameter measurements on red and white blood cells and platelets.

Fulwyler, in 1965, developed the first cell sorter, which had the capacity to separate cells based on their Coulter volume. At the same time, Kamentsky independently developed a flow cytometer that had the ability to measure the nucleic acid content and **light scatter** of cells using spectrophotometry. In addition, he used electrostatic techniques to separate cells in flow, and today the electrostatic cell sorter is the most common instrument of its type in the laboratory.

Subsequent discoveries concerning (1) the relationship between light scatter and cell size and internal complexity, (2) the properties of fluorochromes, and (3) staining and subsequent detection of cancer cells, coupled with the introduction of the laser as a light source, have had a tremendous impact on state-of-the-art instrumentation in the clinical laboratory today. Current flow cytometers have the ability to rapidly quantify and analyze multiple chemical and physical properties of cells or cellular constituents.[3]

The purpose of this chapter is to provide an overview of the methodologies used for measuring the number and properties of particles and their applications in the clinical laboratory. These particles may be individual cells (B-lymphocyte, red blood cell, platelet), cellular structures (chromosomes), or antigen-antibody complexes. In addition, the **colligative properties** of a solution, which are a function of the number rather than of the individual properties of particles, can be measured.

This chapter is divided into three sections: electrical impedance, light scattering techniques, and osmometry.

Electrical impedance and light-scattering techniques provide quantitative and descriptive information about particles. Electrical impedance is a change in electrical resistance as cells in a conductive liquid pass through an orifice. Light-scattering techniques refer to the ability of individual cells to scatter light (flow cytometry) and antigen-antibody complexes to scatter (nephelometry) or transmit (turbidimetry) light.

Osmometry measures the colligative properties (freezing point depression, vapor pressure reduction, osmotic pressure) of a solution, which in turn relates to the number of particles in solution.

ELECTRICAL IMPEDANCE

Principle

W. H. Coulter is responsible for developing the principle of electrical **impedance.** Coulter, in 1956, described this principle:[4]

The instrument employs a non-optical scanning system providing a counting rate in excess of 6,000 individual cells per second with a counting interval of 15 seconds. A suspension of blood cells is passed through a small orifice simultaneously with an electric current. The individual blood cells passing through the orifice introduce an impedance change in the orifice determined by the size of the cell. The system counts the individual cells and provides cell size distribution. The number of cells counted per sample is approximately 100 times greater than the usual microscope count to reduce the statistical error by a factor of approximately 10 times.

The Coulter method performs measurements on cells through electrical impedance, which is defined as a change in electrical resistance when a cell that is in a conductive liquid passes through an orifice. This method is based on the fact that cells are relatively poor conductors of electricity. Figure 3–1 illustrates the electrical impedance method of counting and sizing cells. Cells are suspended in a conductive liquid that serves to insulate the cells as they pass through the aperture. The center of the aperture is the optimal sensing zone. One electrode is submerged in the cell suspension, and the other is placed within the aperture tube. As the cells pass through the aperture, the resistance of the electrical path between the electrodes is increased. This, in turn, generates an electrical pulse that can be counted and sized. Electronic circuitry corrects for the possibility that two cells may pass through the aperture at one time (**coincidence correction**).

In the Coulter instrumentation, blood aspirated into the blood-sampling valve is divided into two separate volumes. One volume is mixed with diluent and delivered to the red blood cell (RBC) bath where red blood cell and platelet counting are performed as the cells pass through the red blood cell aperture. As the blood sample passes through the aperture, the current between the internal and external electrodes changes each time a cell passes through. This produces a voltage pulse, the magnitude of which is proportional to the size of the cell, and the number of pulses is directly proportional to the cell count. Particles that measure between 2 and 20 fL are counted as platelets while all particles above 36 fL are counted as red blood cells. The mean corpuscular volume (MCV) is also calculated as cells measuring between 36 and 360 fL pass through the aperture. The red blood cell aperture size is 50 × 60 microns. Cells are channeled into 256 channels that are each 1.3 fL wide.

In a separate bath, a volume of blood is mixed with diluent and a cytochemical-lytic reagent. A white blood cell (WBC) count is performed as cells pass through an aperture, and a difference in electrical resistance is recorded. Cells greater than 35 fL are recorded as white blood cells. The white blood cell aperture size is 100 × 75 microns, and cells are channeled into 256 channels of 1.64 fL width. Hemoglobin determinations are done using a photometric procedure.[4] White blood cell differential counts are performed by first mixing the blood sample with a lysing reagent that removes the red blood cells and preserves the membranes of the white blood cells. The cells are then introduced to a flow cell where they are evaluated for volume (as measured by impedance), conductivity (using high-frequency radio waves), and light scatter (measured as the cells pass through a laser light beam). Using these three criteria, cells are then isolated and identified.[5]

The RBC, WBC, platelet, and hemoglobin data are transmitted to a computer for the

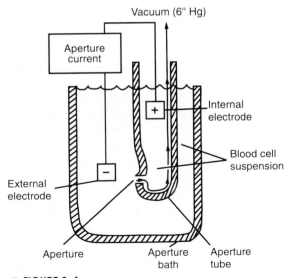

■ **FIGURE 3–1.**

Coulter method of counting and sizing.

generation of test results and **histograms.** The computer corrects for the presence of statistical outliers and aperture obstructions. The counting baths of some instruments have three apertures that function as independent systems, whereas others have only one aperture and the sample is counted three times. The data from the three countings are analyzed to verify that at least two of them are within statistical range of each other. If not, the data are not included.

The computer derives the MCV and red cell (erythrocyte volume) distribution width (RDW) from the RBC histogram and the mean platelet (thrombocyte) volume (MPV) and platelet count from the platelet histogram. The hematocrit, mean corpuscular (erythrocyte) hemoglobin (MCH), and mean corpuscular (erythrocyte) hemoglobin concentration (MCHC) are computed.[4]

Although the Coulter method of counting cells by electrical resistance has been on the market for the longest period of time, it is not the only instrumentation available that counts cells in this manner. Interested readers are referred to Chapter 9 on hematology automation in this book for a more detailed discussion of additional instrumentation.

Clinical Applications

Electrical impedance instrumentation is used primarily in the hematology laboratory for the enumeration of white and red blood cells and platelets. Additional parameters (hemoglobin, MCV, RDW, white blood cell differential) are available depending on the sophistication of the analyzer.

LIGHT-SCATTERING TECHNIQUES

Laser-Based Flow Cytometry

Principle

Flow cytometers measure the properties of cells and cell organelles that are suspended in a moving liquid medium. Cells pass single file through a sensing area during which time they are illuminated by a **laser** beam. The cell intersects the laser beam, and the light that is transmitted consists of both scattered (forward and 90 degree) and fluorescent light, which is directed by lenses and focused onto photomultiplier detectors. Computers then collect and analyze the data.

Modern flow cytometers have progressed to such an advanced state of sophistication that they are capable of analyzing up to 70,000 events/second[6] from a variety of sources and analyzing and storing multiparameter information that includes number of cells, presence/absence of surface markers, and intricate analysis of intracellular constituents. The use of **fluorochromes** with a diversity of excitation and emission wavelengths and their conjugation to monoclonal antibodies have contributed to the sophistication of present instrumentation.

Components of a Flow Cytometer/Sorter

The major components of a flow cytometer include a cell transportation system, light source, flow chamber, filters, lenses, mirrors, photodetectors, and computers for data analysis.

Cells to be analyzed by flow cytometry come from a variety of sources: lymph nodes, peripheral blood, bone marrow, tumors, and various other tissues. The preparation of cells will depend on their source, since some cell suspensions (lymph nodes, fibroblasts for chromosome analysis) require more preparation than others (peripheral blood or bone marrow).

Following preparation, cells are placed in a suspending medium and introduced to the system using pressurized gas (usually nitrogen), which transports them from the sample cup to the flow cell. Most modern flow cytometers use a quartz flow cell, which offers the advantage of eliminating light scatter due to the liquid stream itself. This in turn improves the resolution of the system. The alternative to the quartz flow cell is the "jet-in-air" excitation mode, which means that the cells exit the flow cell before being illuminated by the laser beam. In this method, light is scattered by both the cells and surrounding medium.

Figure 3–2 diagrams the components of a laser-based flow cytometer and cell sorter.

As cells enter the flow cell, they are surrounded by a low-pressure fluid known as the sheath fluid. This outer stream of fluid creates a laminar flow that forces the inner sample stream to the center of the total stream and results in the single file alignment of the cells. This process, known as hydrodynamic focusing, prevents cells from sticking and subsequently adhering to the sides of the flow cell, thereby disrupting the laminar flow.[7]

Cells are then intersected by a light source. Laser beams and high-pressure mercury and xenon arc lamps are examples of light sources used. Laser beams are advantageous to use as light sources because they provide a source of monochromatic light of a single wavelength that is highly concentrated into a single beam.[8] A narrow metal bar, known as an obscuration bar, prevents the laser beam from striking the photomultiplier tube.[7] Lasers, however, are costly and

larger than other light sources. Examples of laser beams include argon, krypton, xenon, helium-neon ion, and dye. High-pressure mercury and xenon arc lamps are less expensive to purchase and maintain; they are smaller and therefore easier to incorporate into instruments. However, they produce a lower light output at all wavelengths, and filters used in conjunction with the light source are not capable of producing monochromatic beams.[9] The light that is transmitted by the cells as they intersect the light source consists of fluorescent and scattered light.

Fluorescent signals can be measured when cells are labeled with an appropriate fluorochrome. Fluorochromes are available over the entire ultraviolet and visible spectrum. Table 3–1 lists fluorochromes that are used in flow cytometry.

Electrons of a fluorescent material that absorb wavelengths of light can be raised to a higher energy level. Once raised to these higher energy levels, these excited electrons emit energy in the form of fluorescence before they then fall back to a lower energy state. The emitted energy describes the emission spectrum and is of a higher wavelength (lower energy level) than the energy absorbed. As can be seen from Table 3–2, each fluorescent compound has its own unique set of excitation and emission spectra.

The utility of a fluorochrome for incorpo-

TABLE 3–1. FLUORESCENT DYES COMMONLY USED IN FLOW CYTOMETRY

DNA CONTENT	RNA CONTENT	ANTIBODY CONJUGATION	BASE COMPOSITION

Propidium iodide
Acridine orange
	Acridine orange
	Pyronin Y
	Thioflavin T
		Fluorescein
		  isothiocyanate
		Phycoerythrin
		Fluorescein
		  isothiocyanate avidin
		Rhodamine
		  isothiocyanate
			Hoechst 33258
			  (adenine and
			  thymine)
			Chromomycin A3
			  (guanine and
			  cytosine)

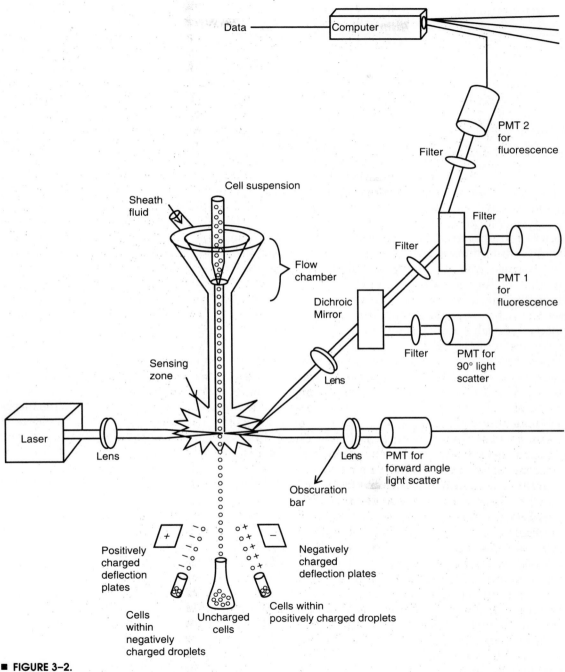

■ **FIGURE 3–2.**

Diagram of flow cytometer and cell sorter.

TABLE 3–2. EXCITATION AND EMISSION SPECTRA FOR COMMON FLUOROCHROMES AVAILABLE FOR ANTIBODY CONJUGATION

	SPECTRAL RANGE >50% OF PEAK	
	EXCITATION (nm)	EMISSION (nm)
Fluorescein isothiocyanate	480–505	510–540
Rhodamine isothiocyanate	560–600	585–625
Texas red	580–605	600–635
Phycoerythrin	490–570	565–590
Phycocyanin	580–640	630–665
Allophycocyanin	620–660	645–675

ration into a flow cytometer is dependent on the ease with which it can be conjugated to a monoclonal antibody, the spectral region in which it absorbs and emits light, and the brightness of fluorescence.[9] The intensity of fluorescence will be proportional to the amount of fluorochrome present when the fluorochrome is excited by light of a fixed wavelength.[6] The excitation and emission spectra of each fluorochrome, as well as the wavelength of the exciting light (i.e., laser) needs to be carefully evaluated before incorporation into a system, as it is important to be able to differentiate between the excitation and emission wavelengths when making measurements.

Consider the fluorochromes FITC (fluorescein isothiocyanate) and PE (phycoerythrin). As can be seen from Table 3–2, the excitation ranges for FITC and PE are 480 to 505 nm and 490 to 570 nm, respectively. If both these fluorochromes are excited by an argon laser (488 nm), they would absorb light, be raised to a higher energy level, and emit light of a higher wavelength (emission spectrum) than the wavelength of light that was originally absorbed. This then allows for the distinct separation of the fluorescent emissions (Figure 3–3).

Filters possessing unique properties are strategically placed to reflect/pass certain wavelengths of light. Three types of filters are available for incorporation into a flow cytometer. Long pass filters allow light with a wavelength longer than a specified value to pass through and block light with a wavelength below this value. Short-pass filters do the opposite (allow light of a lower wavelength to pass while blocking the higher wavelength), and bandpass filters allow light between specified values to pass through.[6]

Dichroic mirrors split a beam of energy and direct specific portions of it in two different directions. For instance, a dichroic mirror may allow shorter wavelengths to pass through but reflect wavelengths longer than a certain value.[6]

Figure 3–4 illustrates how multiple filters

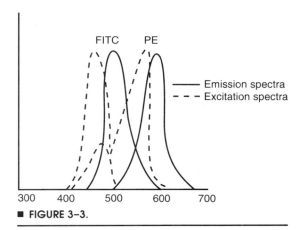

■ FIGURE 3–3.

Separation of excitation and emission spectra of fluorescein isothiocyanate (FITC) and phycoerythrin (PE).

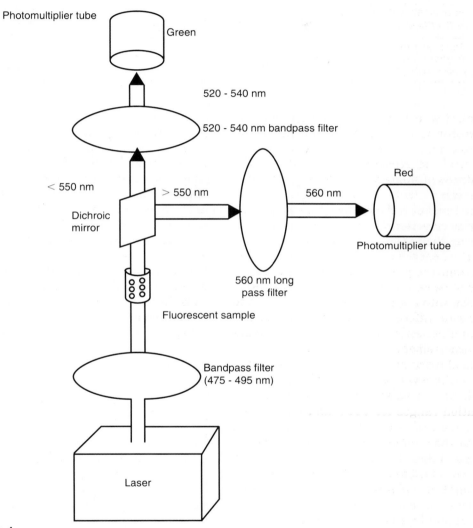

Photomultiplier tube

Green

520 - 540 nm

520 - 540 nm bandpass filter

Red

< 550 nm

> 550 nm

560 nm

Dichroic
mirror

Photomultiplier tube

560 nm long
pass filter

Fluorescent sample

Bandpass filter
(475 - 495 nm)

Laser

■ **FIGURE 3–4.**

Optical path of a flow cytometer.

and dichroic mirrors can be used to perform simultaneous analyses of cells labeled with two fluorescent dyes excited by one light source. An argon laser passes through a bandpass filter (475 to 495 nm) and illuminates a fluorescent sample. The emitted light (which is of a higher wavelength than the excitation wavelength) reaches a dichroic mirror, which directs light with a wavelength greater than 550 nm (red area of the spectral range) through a long-pass filter to a photomultiplier tube. Light emitted with a wavelength of less than 550 nm passes through the dichroic mirror. The bandpass filter selects light between the wavelengths of 520 and 540 nm (green area of the spectral range) to reach the photomultiplier tube.

Light is scattered in either a forward or a 90-degree direction. The forward angle light scatter is proportional to cell size, and the 90-degree or right angle light scatter is proportional to the granularity of the cell. Light scatter at right angles is influenced strongly by **refraction,** which allows for cells of equal size to be differentiated by their internal structure. For instance, cells possessing more internal complexity (e.g., granulocytes) will scatter more light than cells with less internal complexity (lymphocytes).[8]

Forward angle light scatter travels to the appropriate light detector. At 90 degrees to the laser beam are beam splitters that divide the light among the remaining photomultiplier tubes (90-degree light scatter and fluorescence). The photomultiplier tubes amplify the signals and either display them on a screen or store them for later use.[10]

The sophistication of modern flow cytometers allows for the selective analysis of certain portions of the parameters being displayed. Simultaneous analysis of forward and 90-degree light scatter allows for the separation of granulocytes, monocytes, and lymphocytes based on their size and granularity. Electronic gates can be used to delineate which populations of cells are to be studied further. For example, when analyzing cell surface markers on peripheral blood lymphocytes, it is important to "gate out" red blood cells, platelets, and other cellular debris so that only the population of interest is left. Once the population to be studied has been identified (in this case lymphocytes), it is possible to differentiate these cells further through the use of monoclonal antibodies and fluorochromes. The conjugation of FITC to anti-CD4 and PE to anti-CD8 will allow for the separation of T_{helper} (CD4) and $T_{suppressor}$ (CD8) cells. Other combinations of parameters and gating can be used, since the analytical capabilities of the instrumentation are extensive.

Flow cytometers can be equipped with either one or two laser beams. Instrumentation with a single laser beam can generate two scatter (forward and 90-degree) and from one to three fluorescent signals, whereas a second laser beam has the ability to generate one or two additional fluorescent signals.

Flow cytometers have the additional capability of physically sorting objects (cells) from the liquid suspension. The separation of cells can be based on one or a combination of parameters for further analysis. Although this is primarily a research tool, it also has been used clinically in bone marrow transplants either to rid the marrow of an unwanted cell population or to enrich for a needed one. In cell sorters (see Figure 3–2), a fluid stream carrying cells is passed through a small orifice, forming a fluid jet. The chamber (also known as the nozzle) is vibrated, and the jet breaks up into tiny uniform drops. Cells of interest are identified with electronic gating, as described earlier, and a **"sort logic"** is set up that tells the instrument via the computer when to initiate a pulse. Prior to a cell being pinched off into a droplet, a voltage pulse is applied to the stream when a cell of interest (i.e., satisfies the sort logic) intersects the laser beam. This results in only certain droplets being charged. The desired droplets (which contain the desired cells) carry a charge while the uncharged droplets do not. The droplets pass through an electrical field generated by electrical deflection plates, and the charged droplets are deflected into suitable collection containers for further analysis while the uncharged droplets pass through.[3]

Clinical Applications

Applications of flow cytometry in the clinical and research laboratory are extensive. The availability of monoclonal antibodies has allowed for the rapid quantification of populations of T and B cells. This has proved to be beneficial in evaluating the status of the immune system, diagnosing and following patients with leukemias and lymphomas, autoimmune or immune deficiency diseases, and monitoring a patient's response to drug therapy. The division of T and B cells into subpopulations through the use of monoclonal antibodies has allowed for the immune status of patients with certain diseases (e.g., human immunodeficiency virus) to be monitored by following CD4 (T_{helper}) and CD8 ($T_{suppressor}$) cells. In addition, the classification scheme of lymphomas and leukemias has been remarkably expanded by using monoclonal antibodies to phenotype subpopulations of cells.

Flow cytometry can be used in cell cycle analysis by staining the cells with a fluorescent dye such as propidium iodide and quantifying the number of cells in any one cycle. The amount of fluorescence bound is proportional to the amount of DNA present. This is clinically important because some malignant cells contain more DNA than normal cells, and these generally have a poorer prognosis (with the exception of some pediatric malignancies). DNA analysis has been used in the diagnosis and management of breast and bladder cancer and in the diagnosis and classification of leukemias and lymphomas.

In addition, flow cytometry can be used to perform chromosomal karyotyping by staining cells in metaphase, lysing, and evaluating them. A histogram is generated that represents the different groups of chromosomes, and interpretations with regard to translocation and trisomy can be made.

White blood cell differential counts can be performed on a flow cytometer. The light scattering pattern of unstained cells allows for the cells to be identified as neutrophils, monocytes, or lymphocytes. Once stained, it is possible, depending on the stain used, to differentiate the cells further into basophils, eosinophils, and metamyelocytes. Fluorescent dyes such as acridine orange, thioflavin T, or pyronin Y can be used to stain for RNA content and allow for the elucidation of reticulocytes.[11]

In the future, flow cytometry will undoubtedly play a major role in all areas of the clinical laboratory:

- In identifying the DNA composition of microorganisms
- Expanding genetic screening through the use of selective gene probes
- Following the pathogenesis of infectious diseases by monitoring the presence of new antigens in host cells
- Monitoring the effectiveness of therapeutic agents against specific cell populations by following the ability of the drug to bind to a cell and subsequent metabolic alterations[12]

Nephelometry and Turbidimetry

Principle

The basic principle of antigen-antibody reactions is that an antigen [Ag], when reacted with its specific antibody [Ab], will form a complex [AgAb].

As seen in Figure 3–5, increasing amounts of antigen are added to a constant amount of antibody. In the initial stages of the reaction, when small amounts of antigen are present in proportion to the amount of antibody present, the reaction is said to be in antibody excess, or prozone. As increasing amounts of antigen are added, a zone of equivalence is reached in which optimal conditions are present for the reaction of antibody and antigen and the resultant formation of precipitate. As the amount of antibody stays constant and more antigen is added, the region of antigen excess, or post-zone, is reached. The initial reaction of antibody with antigen occurs within minutes, whereas the formation of lattice networks that lead to visible precipitation may take place over a few hours.

Light of an appropriate wavelength that strikes the antigen-antibody complex can be transmitted, absorbed, reflected, or scattered. **Turbidimetric and nephelometric immunoassays** detect the presence of particles in solution by their ability to transmit and scatter light, respectively.

Light-Scattering Properties of Particles

The light-scattering properties of particles were first described by Lord Rayleigh over

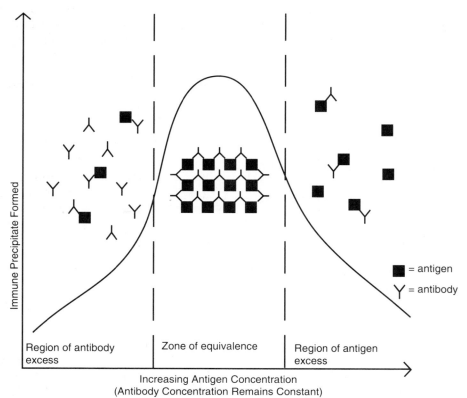

■ **FIGURE 3–5.**

Antigen-antibody precipitin curve.

100 years ago. Light scattered by a homogeneous population of particles is dependent on the relationship between the wavelength of the light and the size of the particle. Figure 3–6 illustrates the three different types of light scatter that may occur: Rayleigh, Mie, and Rayleigh-Debye. Rayleigh describes a phenomenon in which light is scattered symmetrically about the particle when the wavelength of the light is greater than the size of the particle (d < 0.1 lambda). Mie scatter occurs when the wavelength of the light is much smaller than the size of the particle (d > 10 lambda), and most of the light is scattered in a forward direction due to out-of-phase backscatter. When the wavelength of the light is approximately equal to the size of the particle, the scatter seen is Rayleigh-Debye, and more light is scattered in a forward as opposed to a backward direction.[13]

Components of Nephelometers and Turbidimeters

The basic components of the instrumentation used to measure the turbidimetric and nephelometric properties of particles (Fig. 3–7) are similar and include a light source, filter and collimating system, lens, sample cuvette, and detector. Turbidimetric determinations can be performed on most automated clinical chemistry analyzers and spectrophotometers, whereas dedicated instrumentation (i.e., a nephelometer) is required for nephelometric assays.

Light sources most commonly used are mercury arc lamps, tungsten/iodide lamps, and helium-neon lasers. Lasers provide a monochromatic light of a single wavelength, which is highly concentrated into a thin, intense beam. However, they are costly and provide only a limited selection of fixed

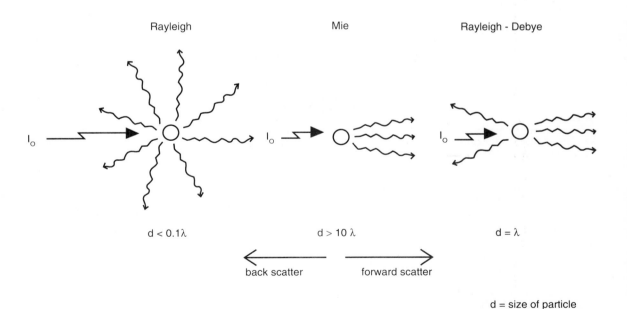

■ **FIGURE 3–6.**

Light-scattering properties of particles.

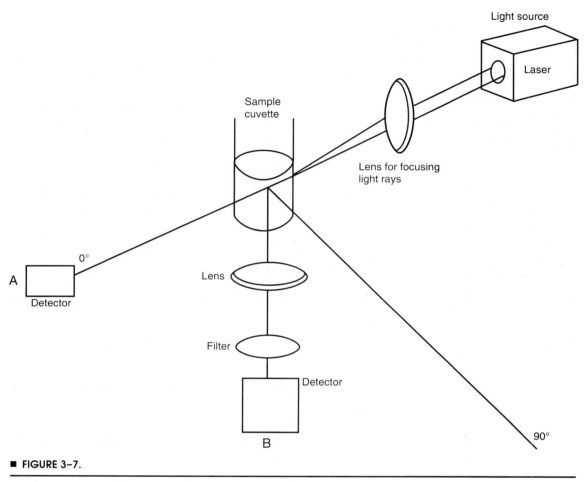

■ FIGURE 3–7.

Schematic of light-scattering instrumentation. *A,* Light-scattering measurements for turbidimetry; *B,* forward scatter nephelometer.

wavelengths, in contrast to other light sources that provide a variety of wavelengths that can be selected through the use of a filter.[2]

A collimating system and wavelength selector (such as a filter) are used only for light sources other than lasers. When a laser is used as a light source, a lens focuses the light source onto the sample cuvette.

A fixed amount of a high-titer, high-affinity antibody is added to varying amounts of antigen. The resultant antibody-antigen reactants are placed in the sample cuvette and intersected by the beam of light. Measurement of the light scattered by the particles in solution is made by the detector.

A filter is introduced near the detection device to ensure a high "signal-to-noise" ratio and a relatively high degree of sensitivity. Detectors must be matched to the wavelength of the incident light, and their placement depends on whether transmitted or scattered light is being measured. Turbidimetric measurements are made at 180 de-

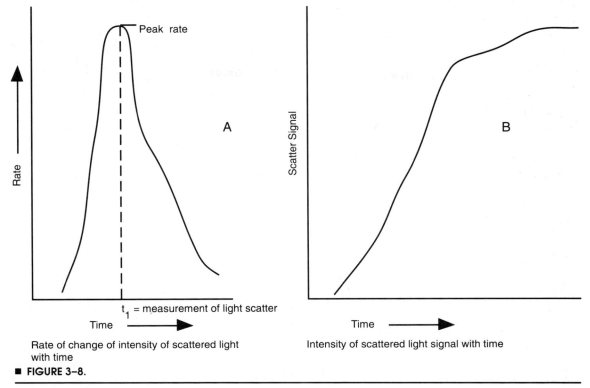

Peak rate

A

Rate

t_1 = measurement of light scatter

Time

Rate of change of intensity of scattered light
with time

Scatter Signal

B

Time

Intensity of scattered light signal with time

■ **FIGURE 3–8.**

Kinetic analysis of light scattering.

grees to the incident beam. The placement
of the detector in nephelometers is dependent on the light-scattering properties of the
particles in suspension.[2]

Antigen-antibody systems contain a heterogeneous population of particles with dimensions of between 250 and 1500 nm. The
wavelengths of the light sources used in
most commercial nephelometers are between 340 and 650 nm. Since the wavelength of the light is equal to the average
size of the particles being measured, the majority of the light scatter will be in the forward (as described by Rayleigh-Debye) as
opposed to the 90-degree angle. Detectors
can be placed anywhere from 5 to 90 degrees
to measure light scatter. However, for
nephelometers to achieve the greatest degree of sensitivity, they should be equipped

to measure light in a forward as opposed to
a 90-degree angle.[2]

Rate Versus End-Point Determinations

The reaction of antibody with antigen
may be measured in one of two ways: rate
(kinetic) or end-point (equilibrium) determinations. In rate determinations (Fig. 3–8A),
measurements are made within the first few
minutes, when the largest change in the intensity of scattered light with respect to
time takes place. Rate determinations have
several distinct advantages: (1) they do not
require that a separate reagent blank be
run (the instrument electronically subtracts
the background signal from that of an unreacted sample), (2) more samples can be
assayed in a fixed amount of time, and (3)

there is no interference by turbidity. The value of the maximum rate of light scattering is directly proportional to the antigen concentration.[2]

In an end-point assay, reaction times vary, and the change in intensity of scattered light with respect to time is small (Fig. 3–8B). A separate reagent blank is required in an end-point assay, and a reasonable amount of time (anywhere from 10 minutes to 1 hour) must elapse before readings are taken.[2] Rate nephelometric assays have been shown to correlate well with end-point determinations,[14] and both can be applied to nephelometric and turbidimetric assays.

Carrier Particles in Nephelometric Assays

In some instances, antigen-antibody reactions do not result in complexes that are sufficiently large to scatter light. For example, rheumatoid factors (RF), which display antibody characteristics against the immunoglobulin IgG, are not capable of forming a visible agglutinate when complexed with IgG. In these instances, the antigen (i.e., IgG) is bound to a carrier particle (i.e., latex). The interaction of the IgG-coated latex particle with its specific antibody (RF) causes agglutination of the latex particles and a resultant scattering of the incident light.

Another example of carrier particles being used is in the **microparticle-enhanced nephelometric immunoassays** used for the quantitation of immunoglobulins. In this assay, immunoglobulins are bound to microspheres, which will then agglutinate with their specific antisera. When free immunoglobulins (IgG, IgM, IgA) are present, agglutination between the immunoglobulin-coated microsphere and its specific antisera will be inhibited.[15]

Nephelometric Inhibition Assay

A nephelometric inhibition assay (NIA), which is a competitive binding assay, has been developed for the indirect measurement of small molecules (e.g., haptens). Previously, the method of choice for measuring small-molecular-weight compounds was radioimmunoassay, which is time consuming and laborious. Haptens typically have a small molecular weight and cannot induce an immunologic response without help, but they can react with antibodies that are specific to themselves. Antibody specific for the hapten is produced by immunizing an animal with a hapten complexed to a carrier molecule.

In the nephelometric inhibition assay, haptens are coupled to a different molecule (i.e., large protein molecule), which is now known as the "developer antigen." This developer antigen competes with free hapten (the unknown component being measured) for combining sites on a fixed amount of antibody. The amount of light scatter is inversely related to the concentration of free hapten. This assay is more sensitive than conventional nephelometric assays[16] and has been found to correlate well with radioimmunoassay (RIA).[17]

Sensitivity of Nephelometric and Turbidimetric Immunoassays

The sensitivity of automated nephelometric methods has been much improved over manual counterparts. This is due, in part, to the incorporation of polymers into the sample mixture, the detection of antigen excess, and discriminating between background scatter and scatter intrinsic to the antigen-antibody complex. The addition of polymers such as polyethylene glycol (PEG) to the antigen-antibody mixture in the sample cuvette increases the speed of complex formation (thereby decreasing the reaction time) and the intensity of light scattered. The ability of an instrument to compensate for antigen excess is critical, because accurate measurements of antigen can be made only in the ascending limb of the precipitation curve. Most modern instrumentation has the ability to detect and monitor antigen excess automatically.[18] The detection of background scatter is diminished by measuring light scatter at a forward rather than a 90-degree angle and by electronically subtracting background signals (rate nephelometry) or taking a blank reading (endpoint nephelometry).

The sensitivity of turbidimetric assays is dependent on the ability of the detector to measure small changes in light intensity. The use of spectrophotometers with high-quality detection systems and light sources with low wavelengths results in adequate sensitivities for most turbidimetric assays.

A comparative study of turbidimetric and light-scattering techniques on a centrifugal analyzer equipped with a multipurpose optics system found that nephelometry was more sensitive than turbidimetry in the measurement of immunoglobulins.[18] Other studies have found that while nephelometry and turbidimetry are generally comparable in sensitivity, nephelometry may be more sensitive when low levels of antigen-antibody reactions are being measured.

Clinical Applications

The most frequently measured biologic fluids include serum, cerebrospinal fluid, and urine. The clinical applications of nephelometry and turbidimetry include the measurement of plasma proteins (immunoglobulins A, G, and M, complement components C3 and C4, albumin and acute phase reactants), hormones, drugs (gentamicin, phenobarbital, phenytoin, and theophylline), rheumatoid factor, circulating immune complex, and antistreptolysin O. In addition, turbidimetry has clinical applications in the bacteriology laboratory in the measurement of antibiotic sensitivities.

OSMOMETRY

Principle

Osmometry determines the osmolality of a solution by measuring the colligative properties of that solution. The colligative property of a solution relates to the number of particles in solution rather than their mass, charge, size, or chemical composition. When a solute is dissolved in a solvent, the colligative properties of the solution will change in a linear relationship as the number of particles in solution increases. The changes in the colligative properties include an increase in the boiling point and osmotic pressure and a decrease in the freezing point and vapor pressure.

Solution molality, or the number of moles (gram molecular weight) of solute per kilogram of solvent, provides a measure of the amount of dissolved solute. The osmolality of a solution is a measure of the total number of moles of particles in 1 kilogram of solvent. When 1 mole of any non-ionic solute is dissolved in 1 kilogram of solvent, the colligative properties of the solution change by a uniform amount because a mole contains a uniform number of particles (Avogadro's number is 6.02×10^{23} particles). For non-ionic solutes, the changes in the colligative properties of this 1-molar solution are that the boiling point is increased by 0.52 C°, the vapor pressure drops by 0.3 mm Hg and the freezing point drops by 1.86 C°. The osmotic pressure also increases.[19]

One osmol is defined as Avogadro's number of particles. In solution, 1 molecule of glucose does not ionize and hence, 1 osmol is present. One molecule of sodium chloride (NaCl) and one molecule of calcium chloride

(CaCl) will dissociate into 2 and 3 osmols of particles, respectively, if complete ionization occurs.[20]

Measurement of Colligative Properties

The colligative properties that are most commonly measured in the laboratory are the freezing point and vapor-pressure depression. The osmotic pressure may be measured by colloid osmotic pressure.

Freezing Point Depression

Freezing point depression involves supercooling a sample, agitating the sample until it freezes and subsequently crystallizes, and then measuring the heat of fusion. The heat of fusion is measured by a thermistor, which is a variable resistance heat sensor. The thermistor is connected to a Wheatstone bridge, which can detect the change in resistance caused by the heat of fusion of the sample.

The sample, into which a thermistor probe and stirring wire have been inserted, is lowered into a cooling bath and supercooled to several degrees below its freezing point. The temperature of the bath is maintained at -6 to -9 C° through the use of a cooling liquid such as ethylene glycol into which refrigerator coils are immersed. The sample is gently stirred during this cooling step. When sufficient cooling has occurred, as indicated by the galvanometer, crystallization (formation of ice crystals) of the sample is initiated by a vigorous agitation of the wire. The heat of fusion is liberated, causing the temperature of the solution to increase, as recorded by the galvanometer, toward its true freezing point, where ice and water are in equilibrium with one another. During this period of time, the galvanometer indicates that the Wheatstone bridge is balanced with the measuring potentiometer,

and the temperature is measured. The solution remains at the freezing point until all the solvent (water) is frozen. The galvanometer then begins changing direction as the sample cools down again to bath temperature. Readings are usually in milliosmoles (10^{-3} osmols); however, conversions can be performed if the instrument reading is in degrees. The temperature read during the equilibrium process is the freezing point of the solution and is inversely related to the osmolality. Figure 3–9 illustrates the freezing point thermodynamics of a sample.

In some osmometers that measure freezing point depression, a light beam galvanometer is used as a visual display, and the operator watches the spot of light in order to record the equilibrium point. In other instruments, the entire process is automated and the osmolality reading is displayed digitally.[19, 20]

Vapor Pressure Depression

The vapor pressure depression of a sample is determined thermometrically through the use of a fine wire thermocouple. The thermocouple determines the dew point temperature, which is the temperature at which dew forms on a cold surface at a fixed humidity level in a closed chamber.

A small amount of sample placed on a filter paper disk is inserted into the sample chamber through the use of a sample slide, and the chamber is sealed. The sample and chamber equilibrate, and the temperature (reference) is recorded. The thermocouple, which is suspended above the sample, is then Peltier-cooled below the dew point temperature, and water begins to condense on its surface. The electrical current is turned off, and the heat of condensation causes the thermocouple temperature to rise to the temperature at which condensation ceases. When this plateau is reached (equilibrium between condensation and evaporation), the

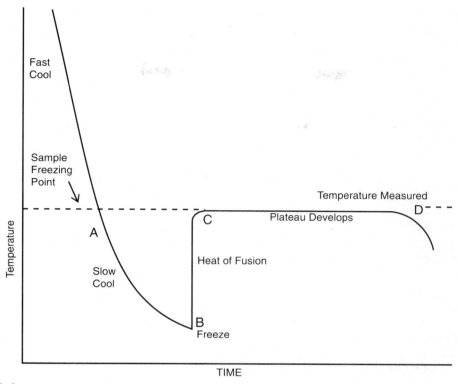

■ FIGURE 3–9.

Freezing point thermodynamics. The sample is supercooled (A) to several degrees below its freezing point (B). Heat of fusion is released; the ice-water mixture is in equilibrium (C), and the freezing point is measured (D).

dew point temperature is recorded. This final temperature, which can be reported in units of osmolality, is proportional to the dew point temperature depression, which in turn, is a function of the vapor pressure. Manual and automated instruments are available to determine the dew point temperature depression.

The advantages of this particular methodology are that a small sample size is required, and no special sample tubes are necessary because the paper disks serve as specimen carriers. Particular attention must be paid to the handling of the sample to avoid contamination.[19, 20]

Colloid Osmotic Pressure

This particular methodology is dependent on the osmotic properties of molecules. A two-chamber pressure system is separated by a semipermeable membrane (permeable to small molecules, impermeable to large molecules). One chamber is filled with the sample to be analyzed, and the other chamber (reference) is filled with isotonic saline. Saline moves to the sample chamber until the back pressure prevents further flow. This back or negative pressure equals the colloid osmotic pressure of the unknown sample. A sensitive pressure transducer detects this negative pressure, and the oncotic pressure is recorded in mm Hg.[20]

Boiling Point Elevation

This methodology is not useful for the measurement of clinical samples because the proteins will coagulate and grossly change the composition of the sample.

Formula for Calculation of Osmolality

The osmolality of a sample can be determined mathematically. The formulas that follow contain only those constituents that significantly affect osmolality.

SI Units (Système International d'Unités)

Calculated osmolality (mOsm/kg) =
$$2 \times Na \ (mmol/L) + glucose \ (mmol/L) + BUN \ (mmol/L)$$

Historical Units

Caluated osmolality (mOsm/kg) =
$$2 \times Na \ (mEq/L) + \left[\frac{Glucose \ (mg/dL)}{18} + \frac{BUN \ (mg/dL)}{2.8} \right]$$

These formulas use molarity rather than molality, as this compensates for the presence of other serum components and accounts for theoretic corrections that were not included. The factor 2 includes the presence of the sodium cation and chloride anion. Glucose and BUN molecules do not dissociate and therefore are counted only once. The factors 18 and 2.8 in the historical units formula represent the molecular weights of glucose and BUN, respectively, and allow for the conversion from deciliters to liters.

The calculated osmolality can be compared with the measured osmolality—the difference is known as the osmolal gap.

Osmolal Gap

Osm/kg =
$$measured \ Osm/kg - calculated \ Osm/kg$$

The average osmolal gap is near 0. An abnormal osmolal gap indicates the presence of abnormal concentrations of substances in the blood that have not been measured.[13]

Sample Collection

Blood serum and urine samples are most commonly measured, but other body fluids (peritoneal, pleural, spinal) may be used. The blood sample should be collected with a minimum of stasis. Blood and urine samples should be centrifuged in a timely manner and stored in a sealed container. Serum and urine samples are stable for several days when kept in stored vials at -5 C° and for several months when frozen at -20 C° or less. If a test cannot be performed in a timely manner, the specimen should be frozen and then warmed to room temperature before analysis.

Sera to be analyzed should be free of particulate matter as they could act as seeding agents in the freezing point depression methodology. Volatile agents (e.g., ethanol) will not be detected by vapor pressure but can be measured by freezing-point depression. Anticoagulants other than heparin can increase the osmolality.

Normal serum osmolality is 285 to 310 mOsm/kg. The normal levels for urine osmolality depend on the hydration of the patient and can range from 50 to 1400 mOsm/kg.[13]

Clinical Applications

The most common uses of osmometry are to detect unmeasured substances in the plasma, monitor electrolyte fluid therapy, and assess the concentrating ability of the kidneys.

Only a few substances are present in plasma in sufficient amounts to affect the plasma osmolality. The most common substances that can be ingested in sufficient amounts to affect the measurements are alcohols.

The ratio of urinary to serum osmolality can sometimes be used to study kidney function and to monitor burn patients, critically ill patients, and those with kidney disorders. If a random urine sample is dilute, no conclusion can be made about the concentrating ability of the kidneys; the test must be repeated on a specimen obtained the next morning following a night of fluid restriction.[13]

Freezing-point depression is the most common technique in the clinical laboratory. Vapor pressure osmometers are a relatively new technique. They have been used in cystic fibrosis screening because of the small amount of sample needed for a measurement.

The major use of the colloid osmotic pressure is to monitor the water-plasma protein balance in the detection and treatment of conditions leading to pulmonary edema.[13]

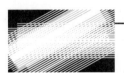

REVIEW QUESTIONS

Choose the best answer.

1. All the following statements are true, concerning electrical impedance measurements, EXCEPT:

   a. As cells pass through the the aperture, the resistance of the electrical path between the electrodes is decreased.
   b. Electronic circuitry that corrects for the possibility that two cells may pass through the aperture at one time is called coincidence loss.
   c. As blood passes through the aperture, the current between the internal and external electrodes changes each time a cell passes.
   d. The voltage produced as the cell passes through the aperture is directly proportional to the size of the cell.

2. The light-scattering technique in which light scattered by an individual cell is detected is known as

   a. microparticle-enhanced nephelometry.
   b. rate nephelometry.
   c. turbidimetry.
   d. flow cytometry.

3. Turbidimetry differs from nephelometry in that

a. it is a more sensitive analytical technique.
b. it measures light scattered at a 90° angle.
c. it measures a decrease in the transmittance of light from the incident beam after it exits the solution of suspended particles.
d. it requires a dedicated instrument with a laser beam.

4. A device used in flow cytometers to split a beam of energy and direct specific portions of it into two different directions is known as a

a. short bandpass filter.
b. long bandpass filter.
c. specified bandpass filter.
d. dichroic mirror.

5. Clinical applications for nephelometry include all the following, EXCEPT:

a. plasma proteins.
b. urine proteins.
c. serum lipids.
d. drugs.

6. All the following statements are true concerning rate nephelometry, EXCEPT:

a. A reagent blank does not have to be run.
b. There is no interference from turbidity.
c. Fewer samples can be assayed in a fixed period of time than in endpoint nephelometry.
d. The value of the maximum rate of light scattering is directly proportional to the antigen concentration.

7. Omolality can be measured in the clinical laboratory by instrumentation that detects:

a. freezing-point depression.
b. vapor pressure depression.
c. boiling-point depression.
d. A and B.

8. Given Na^+ = 154 mEq/L; glucose = 120 mg/dL; and BUN = 35 mg/dL, the serum osmolality is

a. 387 mOsm/kg.
b. 327 mOsm/kg.
c. 312 mOsm/kg.
d. 233 mOsm/kg.

REFERENCES

1. Wintrobe MM: *Clinical Hematology.* Philadelphia, Lea and Febiger, 1961.
2. Kaplan LA, Pesce AJ (eds): *Nonisotopic Alternatives to Radioimmunoassay; Principles and Applications.* New York, Marcel Dekker, 1981.
3. Melamed M, Lindmo T, Mendelsohn M: *Flow Cytometry and Sorting,* 2nd edition. New York, Wiley-Liss, 1990.
4. *Coulter Stks Manual.* Hialeah, Florida, Coulter Electronics, 1990.
5. Poulsen KB, Bell CA: Automated hematology: Comparing and contrasting three systems. *Clin Lab Sci* 4:16–17, 1991.
6. *Fluorescent Microbead Standards.* North Carolina, Flow Cytometry Standards Corporation, 1988.
7. Patrick CW, et al: Flow cytometry and cell sorting. *Lab Med* 15:740–745, 1984.
8. Haynes JL: Principles of flow cytometry. *Cytometry Suppl* 3:7–17, 1988.
9. Owens MA: Role of the laboratory in clinical flow cytometry: Present and future. Cytometry Suppl 3:101–103, 1988.
10. Hoffman RA: Approaches to multicolor immunofluorescence. *Cytometry Suppl* 3:18–22, 1988.
11. Grogan WM, Collins JM: *Guide to Flow Cytometry Methods.* New York, Marcel Dekker, 1990.
12. Waller KV, Bruzzese DB: Flow cytometry in the clinical laboratory. *Lab Med* 16:480–484, 1985.
13. Kaplan LA, Pesce AJ: *Clinical Chemistry; Theory, Analysis and Correlation.* St. Louis, CV Mosby, 1984.
14. Sternberg JC: A rate nephelometer for measuring specific proteins by immunoprecipitin reactions. *Clin Chem* 23(8):1456–1464, 1977.
15. Cuillier ML, Montagne P, Bessou TH, et al: Microparticle-enhanced nephelometric immunoassay

(nephelia R) for immunoglobulins G, A, and M. *Clin Chem* 37(1):20–25, 1991.

16. Finley PR: Nephelometry: Principles and clinical laboratory applications. *Lab Management* 20:34–45, 1982.
17. Cheng A, Bray K, Polito A: Nephelometric inhibition assay for gentamicin. *Clin Chem* 25(6):1078, 1979.
18. Hills LP, Tiffany TO: Comparison of turbidimetric and light-scattering measurements of immunoglobulins by use of a centrifugal analyzer with absorbance and fluorescence/light-scattering optics. *Clin Chem* 26(10):1459–1466, 1980.
19. Ferris CD: *Guide to Medical Laboratory Instruments*. Boston, Little, Brown, 1980.
20. Hicks MR, Haven MC, Schenken JR, McWhorter CA: Laboratory Instrumentation. Philadelphia, JB Lippincott, 1987.

BIBLIOGRAPHY

Bender GT: *Principles of Chemical Instrumentation.* Philadelphia, WB Saunders, 1987.

Brown BA: *Hematology: Principles and Procedures.* Philadelphia, Lea and Febiger, 1988.

Narayanan S: *Principles and Applications of Laboratory Instrumentation.* Chicago, American Society of Clinical Pathologists Press, 1989.

Tietz NW: *Textbook of Clinical Chemistry.* Philadelphia, WB Saunders, 1986.

Turgeon ML: *Clinical Hematology; Theory and Procedures.* Boston, Little, Brown, 1988.

Van Dilla M, Dean P, Laerum O, Melamed M: *Flow Cytometry: Instrumentation and Data Analysis.* New York, Academic Press, 1985.

Part I Electrochemistry

INTRODUCTION

POTENTIOMETRIC METHODS

AMPEROMETRIC METHODS

COULOMETRIC METHODS

**PRACTICAL APPLICATIONS AND ISSUES IN CLINICAL LABORATORY
ELECTROCHEMICAL ANALYSIS**

RECENT AND FUTURE TRENDS

Part II Emission and Absorption Spectroscopy

ELECTROMAGNETIC RADIATION

FLAME TECHNIQUES

Flame Characteristics

Burners

Flame Temperature

ATOMIC ABSORPTION

Instrumentation

Interference

Flameless Atomic Absorption

FLAME PHOTOMETRY

Internal Standard

Instrumentation

INDUCTIVELY COUPLED PLASMA EMISSION SPECTROSCOPY

CHEMILUMINESCENCE

FLUORESCENCE

Instrumentation

Fluorescence Polarization

Chapter 4

INSTRUMENTATION FOR THE MEASUREMENT OF BLOOD GASES AND ELECTROLYTES

DAVID D. KOCH, PhD
BARBARA CLEVELAND, MPH, MT (ASCP)

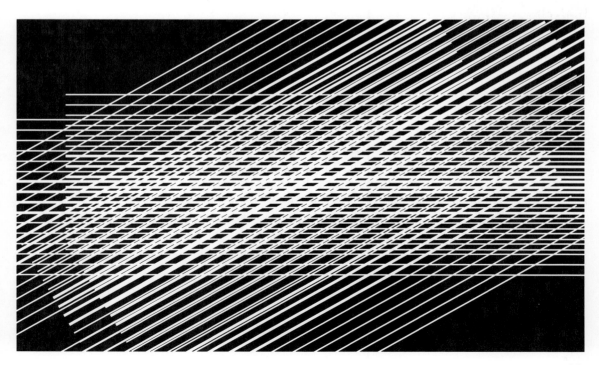

LEARNING OBJECTIVES

After studying this chapter, the student should be able to:

- Differentiate between the following principles: potentiometry, amperometry, voltammetry, coulometry, and polarography.
- Describe the construction of the following indicator electrodes: glass, liquid membrane, precipitate-impregnated, solid-state, gas-sensing, and enzyme.
- Give the principle of measurement for pH, pCO_2 and pO_2.
- Explain the ionophore systems used to measure K^+ and Cl^-.
- Give the principle of coulometric analysis and name the general term for an instrument that applies this technique in the clinical laboratory.
- Give the relative merits of direct potentiometry.
- Describe by illustration and explain the principle of operation for flame emission photometry and atomic absorption.
- List basic instrumental components and describe the function of each component.
- Characterize the burner assembly and flame profiles for flame photometry and atomic absorption; describe the processes taking place in each part of the flame; explain how these processes and burner assembly are related to flame optics.
- Describe the circumstances leading to the selection of emission and absorption analytical approaches as well as the advantages and limitations associated with each.
- Describe the purpose for and the technique of internal standardization as related to flame techniques; list the criteria for a chemical to serve as the internal standard.
- List interferences associated with flame techniques and suggest ways of eliminating these interferences.
- Describe the principle of and the instrumentation associated with inductively coupled plasma emission spectroscopy.
- Explain the principle of fluorometry and the significance of differences in the optics path as related to those in the basic spectrophotometer; draw a block diagram of the essential components of the basic fluorometer and describe the function of each.

- Explain the relationship between fluorescence, phosphorescence, and chemiluminescence.
- Summarize analytical problems and interferences associated with fluorescence techniques and describe ways of eliminating them.
- Explain the principle of fluorescence polarization and describe application of this principle in the clinical laboratory.

KEY WORDS

Amperometry. The branch of electrochemistry that utilizes information gained from applying a fixed potential to an electrochemical cell and then measuring current produced because of an oxidation or reduction reaction.

Atomic absorption. A spectrophotometric method to determine the concentration of elements in a solution by vaporizing them in a flame and measuring their absorption of characteristic wavelengths.

Chemiluminescence. A chemical reaction that produces light.

Chopper. A component that interrupts an electrical current or light beam, converting it from direct current to alternating current through mechanical or electrical means.

Coulometry. An analytical technique similar to amperometry. The main difference is that the current needed to convert a substance completely is measured and used to determine the concentration.

Electrochemistry. The study of chemical reactions occurring because of the flow or presence of electrons between two dissimilar substances.

Electrode. An electrochemical interface or half-cell that can be used with another interface to make useful measurements.

Flame photometry. A photometric method to determine the concentration of an element in a flame-vaporized sample by measuring the intensity of its emission spectra.

Fluorescence. That property of some substances that allows them to absorb light energy at one wavelength and re-emit some of it at a longer wavelength; the immediate emission (10^{-8} sec) of light after it has absorbed radiation.

Hollow cathode lamp. A lamp containing an inert gas and a metal cathode that emits wavelengths, characteristic of the cathode.

Indicator electrode. The electrochemical half-cell with a potential that varies in response to some analyte.

Inductively coupled plasma. A photometric method to determine the concentrations of elements in an electrically heated argon gas ''plasma'' source by measuring the intensity of their emission spectra.

Internal standard. A known concentration of a substance (element or compound) added to a sample to correct for certain characteristics of a procedures, e.g., flame instability.

Ion-selective electrode (ISE). An indicator electrode used in potentiometry that responds to a specific ion in the sample.

Junction potential. A potential arising at the interface between the inner electrode fluid of the reference electrode and the sample.

Line spectra. Discontinuous emission of essentially monochromatic light.

Liquid membrane electrode. A porous polymer membrane indicator electrode in which a nonpolar liquid is soaked. A hydrophobic ion-exchanger or neutral carrier ionophore that selectively reacts with the ion of interest is dissolved into the nonpolar liquid.

Phosphorescence. The delayed release (10^{-2} to 100 sec) of absorbed radiation.

Potentiometry. An analytic technique making use of the information gained from determining a potential difference (volts) between two interfaces (e.g., electrodes) measured at equilibrium and with no current.

Reference electrode. An electrode that has a known, constant half-cell potential and against which the relative potential of the working or indicator electrode is measured.

Saturated calomel electrode (SCE). A practical reference electrode containing an inert wire (e.g., platinum) in contact with elemental mercury, mercurous chloride (calomel), and a saturated solution of potassium chloride.

Silver-silver chloride electrode (Ag/AgCl). A popular reference electrode constructed of a silver wire, or platinum wire coated with silver, for which some of the silver is converted to silver chloride by electrolysis in hydrochloric acid.

Voltammetry. An analytic technique similar to amperometry, in which the potential is varied in some way and the current-potential relationship is monitored.

Working electrode. The electrode that consumes or produces electrons, which can be measured as current and related to the amount of analyte.

Part 1

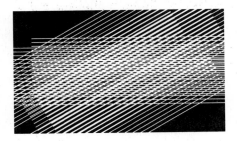

Electrochemistry

DAVID KOCH, PhD

INTRODUCTION

Clinical laboratory science faces profound challenges in the 1990s. Some of these demands originate from the technologic capabilities available today, as mentioned in the Preface to this book. Physicians now expect a level of service that only a decade or so ago would have been impossible for most laboratories to deliver. On the other hand, perhaps the fact that technology has preceded the demand is fortunate—clinical laboratory scientists can find the tools with which they may meet the challenge. But what requirements should analyzers fulfill?

The preferred characteristics of a device intended for determining the concentration of analytes in human body fluids are:

- precision
- accuracy
- true biologic concentration

- low cost
- short dwell time
- no warm-up time
- large throughput
- small sample volume
- wide linear range
- no carryover
- easy maintenance

Several other characteristics that need to be assessed when deciding whether to accept an instrument might be suggested; the subject of selecting methods is discussed in detail in Chapters 13 and 15. Certainly clinical laboratory methods must be precise, so physicians can assume that a noticeable shift in the values means something real is happening with their patients. And these methods must be accurate—in acceptable agreement with the "right answer" (whenever that value is knowable). Related to accuracy, the measurement ideally should be of the true biologically active entity. Cost pressures demand that these determinations be performed with as little reagent and consumable cost as possible. Speed and convenience are very important practical considerations for clinical laboratories today, meaning emphasis should be placed on response time, warm-up time, ability to handle all types of workload, avoidance of dilutions, ease of maintenance, and other issues. Does any analyzer match these characteristics? It may seem impossible; however, a good pH electrode/pH meter combination comes as close as any instrument to meeting all these demands.

The pH electrode is an example of an **ion-selective electrode (ISE)**. Other ISEs serve as the means by which several measurements in laboratory medicine, particularly clinical chemistry, are now made. Most of these methods also come close to satisfying the requirements listed earlier. ISEs are based on the technique known as **potentiometry**. To understand how ISEs fulfill the characteristics sought in an ideal body fluid analyzer (or when these characteristics are not fulfilled, how to deal with that situation), we must study potentiometry. But potentiometry is one branch of the field of **electrochemistry**, so we first need to consider electrochemistry in general—some terms, fundamentals, and applications.

Electrochemistry may be defined as chemical reactions occurring because of the flow or presence of electrons. It is thus governed by the transfer of energy from electrons to chemicals, or the potential for such transfer. The chemicals are in contact with the electrons at surfaces or *interfaces*. Hence, electrochemistry could be described as the study of charged interfaces, the delineation of forces governing the transfer of electrons across them, and the harnessing of these electrochemical interfaces and forces for useful applications.

Current and potential are key elements of electrochemistry. *Current* (i) is the flow of electrons through a substance such as a solution or a wire, and it is measured in coulombs of charge (essentially numbers of electrons) per second, or *amperes. Resistance* (R) is the term describing the opposition of a substance to current flow, and it is measured in *ohms*. For current to flow, the *potential* (E, or ability to do work) applied to the system must be greater than the resistance exhibited by that system. When current exists, such a potential energy must also exist. The opposite is not always true, however; a potential may be present without current flow. The branch of electrochemistry that makes use of the information gained from determining this potential at zero current is potentiometry which, as mentioned, is the technique important to ion-selective electrodes. The potential is computed in *volts* (V). Actually, measuring the potential of any one electrochemical interface is impossible; only the potential difference between two such interfaces can be measured. These interfaces are generally termed **electrodes**, which will be defined more exactly later. Two electrodes make up an electrochemical cell.

The branch of electrochemistry that utilizes the information gained from applying a fixed potential to an electrochemical cell and then measuring current is **amperometry**. Compounds are oxidized or reduced at the **working electrode**, producing electrons that can be measured as current and related to the amount of analyte. Amperometry is presently used in clinical laboratory science largely to determine the partial pressure of oxygen in the blood. **Coulometry** is a technique similar to amperometry; the main difference is that the current needed to completely convert a substance is measured and used to determine the concentration; alternatively, the current is not measured but is used in a titration with another means to detect the endpoint signal. Coulometry in

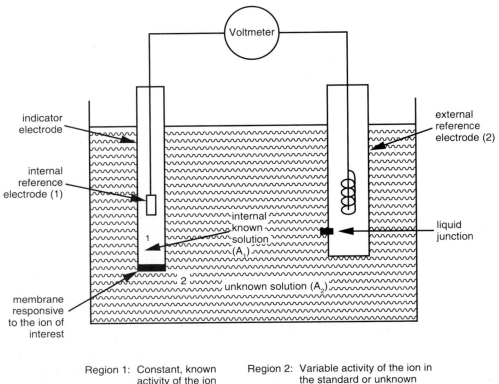

Region 1: Constant, known
activity of the ion
(A_1)

Region 2: Variable activity of the ion in
the standard or unknown
sample (A_2)

$$E_{meas} = E_{electrode\ 1} + E_{membrane} + E_{electrode\ 2} + E_{junction}$$

■ **FIGURE 4–1.**

Electrochemical cell.

laboratory medicine is chiefly applied to the determination of chloride.

POTENTIOMETRIC METHODS

Potentiometry is now common in clinical chemistry because of the popularity of ion-selective electrodes. As mentioned previously, the potential (E) of a single electrode cannot be measured, but the potential difference (ΔE) between two electrodes can be measured readily. In fact, electrochemistry in general always requires two electrodes or half-cells connected to a measuring device such as a volt-ohm meter (see Chapter 1). The circuit between the two half-cells and the meter is completed by a liquid junction (sometimes termed a "salt bridge"). More about the liquid junction later. A generalized depiction of an electrochemical cell is given in Figure 4–1.

The goal, of course, is to use electrochemistry to make useful measurements. Thus, one electrode must have a known potential; then the measured cell potential can give information about the other half-cell, which is chosen to vary depending on the activity of the ion of interest. The electrode (half-cell) with the known, constant potential is called the **reference electrode**; the electrode (half-cell) with the varying potential is called the **indicator electrode**.

The question must be asked: how would the first reference potential be determined? One electrode must have a known potential, then all other electrodes or half-cells would have a potential relative to the first. By convention, the standard, or "normal" hydrogen gas electrode (NHE) is assigned a potential of 0.00 V. The NHE half-cell is a wire connected to a platinum surface over which hydrogen gas is bubbled at 1 atmosphere of pressure. This electrode is immersed in a solution of hydrogen ions of activity 1.00, and the following half-cell reaction takes place:

$$H_2(g) \Leftrightarrow 2H^+ + e^- \quad E^\circ = 0.00 \text{ V}$$

The potential of all other half-cells may be determined when the half-cell in question forms an electrochemical cell (as depicted in Figure 4–1) with the NHE as the second half-cell. In this case, the unknown potential of the desired half-cell is exactly equal to the total cell potential measured by the voltmeter.

Always measuring the potential of a half-cell relative to the NHE is unnecessary. In fact, because of its cumbersome, unstable, potentially hazardous construction, the NHE is rarely used in practice. Other half-cells with known, reproducible, and constant potentials are available that serve as practical reference electrodes. The two most common half-cells are the saturated calomel electrode and the silver–silver chloride electrode. The **saturated calomel electrode (SCE)** contains a wire in contact with elemental mercury that is covered with a thin film of mercurous chloride (calomel). The

calomel is immersed in a solution of saturated potassium chloride (KCl). Figure 4–2A shows the SCE with an asbestos wick for a liquid junction pore. The half-cell reaction is:

$$Hg_2Cl_2 + 2e^- \Leftrightarrow 2Hg^\circ + 2 Cl^-$$

To keep the potential of this electrode constant, both temperature and chloride activity must be kept constant. The easiest way to accomplish the latter is to use saturated KCl.

SCEs, of course, require mercury; they also are hard to miniaturize and are sensitive to higher temperatures. Thus, the **silver–silver chloride electrode (Ag/AgCl)** is the more popular reference electrode, particularly for potentiometry. This electrode is constructed from a silver wire, or a platinum wire coated with silver, for which some of the silver is converted to silver chloride by electrolysis in hydrochloric acid. This wire is then immersed in a solution of known chloride ion concentration. The Ag/AgCl electrode is depicted in Figure 4–2B, with a porous Vycor glass junction. Its half-cell reaction is:

$$AgCl + e^- \Leftrightarrow Ag^\circ + Cl^-$$

Like the SCE, the potential of the Ag/AgCl electrode will be constant if temperature and chloride ion activity are held constant. Again, the easiest, most reliable way to maintain chloride activity is to saturate the solution with KCl and AgCl.

Several types of indicator electrodes exist in potentiometry; each style is useful for certain applications. All indicator electrodes possess a membrane that separates the inner electrolyte solution from the outer, unknown solution (refer to Figure 4–1). The characteristics of the membrane determine which analyte the electrode is capable of measuring; these characteristics also form

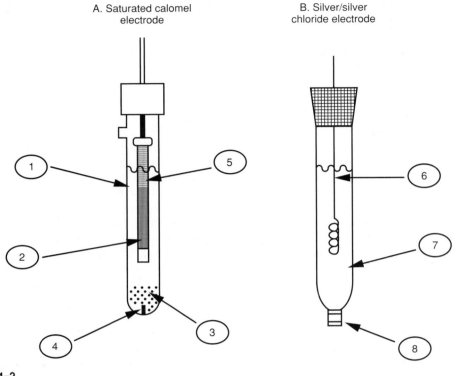

A. Saturated calomel electrode

B. Silver/silver chloride electrode

■ **FIGURE 4–2.**

Reference electrodes. 1, KCl solution; 2, mercury; 3, KCl crystals; 4, asbestos wick; 5, calomel; 6, Ag/AgCl wire; 7, KCl solution; 8, Vycor glass junction.

the basis for classifying indicator electrodes. The various indicator electrodes useful in clinical laboratory science are:

- glass membrane
- liquid polymer membrane
- precipitate-impregnated membrane
- solid-state membrane
- gas-sensing electrode
- enzyme electrode

Glass electrodes contain a specially designed thin piece of glass as the membrane. The layer of glass can be formulated so that it is sensitive to hydrogen ion; others are selective for sodium ion. **Liquid membrane electrodes** are constructed from po-

rous polymer membranes such as polyvinyl chloride into which a nonpolar liquid is soaked. A hydrophobic ion exchanger or neutral carrier ionophore that reacts selectively with the ion of interest is dissolved into the nonpolar liquid. *Precipitate-impregnated membranes* are somewhat similar, but the polymer is usually silicon rubber into which a solid precipitate containing the ion of interest is introduced. This type of electrode has been successful for anions such as chloride, in which the solid precipitate might be silver chloride. *Solid-state membrane electrodes* are another variation in which the active portion of the membrane is actually a solid crystal or salt pellet of the ion of interest. This crystal is secured at the base of the electrode and must be insoluble in the solvent to be encountered (usually aqueous samples). *Gas-sensing electrodes* are modifications of some of the aforementioned types, such as glass electrodes. By fashioning a membrane semipermeable to gases (such as Teflon) around the base of the glass electrode, the only portion of the sample encountering the glass membrane would be the gaseous portion. The most common example of a gas-sensing, potentiometric electrode is those selective for CO_2. Finally, *enzyme electrodes* utilize an immobilized enzyme as one of the layers of the membrane. In this way, the electrode can be made to respond to non-ionic analytes if the enzyme converts the analyte to a reactant that can be sensed by the basic electrode.

A thorough discussion of each type of indicator electrode is beyond the scope of this chapter. A few that are frequently encountered in clinical analysis will be described in more detail. Before that, however, we must remember our goal, which is to determine the concentration of the analyte of interest using these electrodes. At this point, we know that two half-cell electrodes—a reference and an indicator—can measure the potential difference between the electrodes. How does the potential relate to the analyte concentration?

Look again at Figure 4–1. The total cell potential measured by the meter is actually composed of four individual potentials: the potential from the inner reference electrode (1) of the indicator electrode, the potential across the membrane that is responsive to the analyte of interest, the potential of the external reference electrode (2), and the potential developed at the liquid junction. The potentials of the reference electrodes are constant by design (these two electrodes are most likely SCE or Ag/AgCl electrodes, as described earlier). The **junction potential** arises at the interface between inner elec-

trolyte fluid of the electrode (2) and the sample. The inner fluid is a solution containing Cl^- ions (saturated KCl for most reference electrodes). When cations and anions move at different rates through the "salt bridge" or the slowly porous frit ("liquid junction" on Figure 4–1), a potential is developed across this junction. KCl is a fortuitous choice as inner electrolyte for an additional reason other than keeping the chloride concentration constant for the reference electrode: K^+ and Cl^- have similar mobilities, thus minimizing the junction potential. Also, the high concentration of KCl will cause ion transport to be dominated by KCl. In any case, the junction potential will essentially be a constant. Therefore, the only potential changing the cell potential is that occurring across the membrane. $E_{membrane}$ is the key.

Figure 4–3 presents a magnified view of a small portion of the membrane. In part A, the membrane is at "equilibrium"; perhaps the electrode is encountering a flush solution, a reference fluid, or a storage solution. In this example, the activity of the ion of interest (X^+) is the same in the storage solution as in the solution inside the electrode body, and no concentration gradient exists across the membrane. Part B shows what happens when a sample or solution with a different concentration of the ion of interest is introduced. A concentration gradient now exists. Each ion has its own chemical energy. The increase in ions on the "test side" of the membrane causes more X^+ ions to be "extracted into" the surface of the membrane by the entity responsible for the membrane's selectivity for X^+, which leads to an increase in positive potential across that membrane. Hence a potential gradient also exists, which is measured by the voltmeter as a change in the cell potential. The ion concentration on the test side of the membrane is related to the cell potential by the

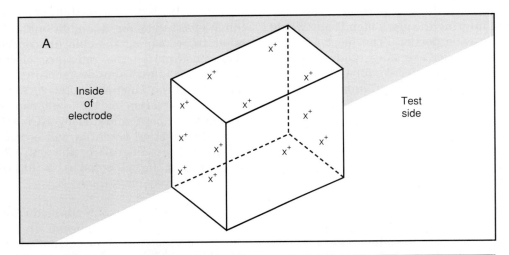

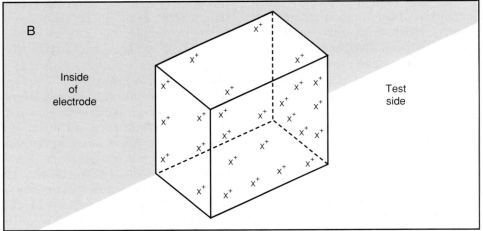

■ **FIGURE 4–3.**

Expanded view of the ion-selective membrane.

Nernst equation (expressed here for the case of an ion selective electrode):

$$\Delta E = \Delta E^\circ - \frac{RT}{nF} \ln a_x$$

where ΔE° = standard potential of the electrochemical cell

R = as constant

T = temperature, in degrees Kelvin

n = number of electrons involved in the electrode reaction

F = Faraday constant

$\ln$ = natural logarithm

a_x = activity of X^+, the ion of interest

At 25°C, and converting to common, base 10 logarithm, this equation simplifies to:

$$\Delta E = \Delta E^\circ - \frac{0.0591}{n} \log a_x$$

Armed with the Nernst equation and the fact that the other three potentials making up the cell potential of an ion-selective electrode system such as shown Figure 4–1 are constant, measurements of potential are directly related to the concentration of the analyte. In fact, the voltmeters can be calibrated so as to read out directly in concentration units, obviating the need for plotting of graphs and calculation of the unknown concentration. The meters should have a high internal resistance (high "input impedance," see Chapter 1) so as to not draw any current themselves and thus destabilize the system.

Clinical laboratory science makes significant use of potentiometry in blood gas and electrolyte determinations. Most pH electrodes use a glass membrane placed around an internal Ag/AgCl reference electrode. Glass membranes can be made selective for H^+ by manufacturing thin pieces of glass

from combinations of lithium oxide with silicates or oxides of heavy metals such as barium and lanthanum. The rest of the electrode body is glass as well, but this glass is not sensitive to H^+. The internal Ag/AgCl electrode is immersed in a buffered solution with constant Cl^- and H^+ activities. When the glass electrode encounters an unknown sample, H^+ from the sample combines with oxide sites in the membrane by an ion-exchange process with lithium. This exchange results in a difference of H^+ hydration on the outer surface of the membrane compared with the inner surface, where the H^+ activity is constant. This hydration—or concentration—difference causes a potential difference as well, which is related to the concentration of H^+ by the Nernst equation. For pH, the equation simplifies to

$$\Delta E = \Delta E^\circ + 0.0591 \text{ pH (at 25°C)}$$

Most blood gas instruments are thermostated to 37°C; at this temperature, the equation is

$$\Delta E = \Delta E^\circ + 0.0613 \text{ pH (at 37°C)}$$

The glass membrane can be and has been shaped in several forms. A glass bulb is common, but for determination of whole blood (when anaerobic conditions are advised), a flat surface or a glass capillary applicable to flow-through designs allowing very small sample volumes to be assayed is popular.

As mentioned, gas-sensing electrodes to measure the partial pressure of CO_2 gas can be fashioned from pH electrodes by placing a gas-permeable membrane around the glass electrode. The membrane is usually polypropylene or Teflon and will allow virtually any gas to permeate through it. These pCO_2 electrodes respond selectively to CO_2 gas and not to other gases because the outer membrane is separated from the glass electrode by a bicarbonate buffer solution. Only

CO_2 will have an impact on the buffer by forming carbonic acid and eventually hydrogen ion by the following reactions:

$$CO_2 + H_2O \Leftrightarrow H_2CO_3 \Leftrightarrow H^+ + HCO_3^-$$

Any change in pH of the buffer is directly related to how much CO_2 gas diffused across the gas-permeable membrane, which is proportional to pCO_2. These electrodes can be placed with the rubber membrane in contact with a narrow, flowing stream of sample, similar to the pH electrode configuration for whole blood instruments described in the last paragraph.

Another modification of glass pH electrodes is to change the composition of the glass membrane so the electrode responds to ions other than hydrogen. *Sodium electrodes* form the most common example of alternative glass membrane electrodes. They function similar to pH electrodes. Na^+ from the sample reacts with ion exchange sites selective for this ion on the outer membrane surface, and a potential difference develops that is proportional to the Na^+ activity. With these electrodes, sodium must be held constant on the inside of the glass membrane. Sodium electrodes of the liquid membrane type have also been developed and are gaining in popularity. As described, these electrodes typically include a neutral carrier ionophore in the membrane of nonsoluble liquid. The principle of how the measured potential develops and is related to the ion's concentration is similar to that of glass electrodes. The ion of interest from the sample encounters the outer surface of the membrane and reacts with the ionophore, changing the activity of this complex at the surface. The activity on the inner surface remains a constant by maintaining a fixed activity of the ion in the internal solution.

These liquid membrane electrodes are fairly ubiquitous in clinical chemistry, commonly used for potassium, calcium, and lithium electrodes as well as sodium. The ionophores or compounds responsive to the ion of interest are obviously different in each case, but the rest of the materials and features of these electrodes are similar to those already described. For *potassium electrodes*, the antibiotic valinomycin is most often used as the ionophore. Other molecules selective for the ions of interest are similar to valinomycin in that they have organic, ring-like, charged structures that produce cavities with binding characteristics favorable to this ion above other competing ions. The specific ionophore used in liquid membrane electrodes for each analyte will perhaps vary, depending on the manufacturer. *Chloride electrodes* have also recently been constructed using a liquid membrane approach, although a solid-state style using a crystal of silver chloride/silver sulfide has been more popular.

AMPEROMETRIC METHODS

As mentioned previously, **amperometry** is that branch of electrochemistry in which a fixed potential is applied to an electrochemical cell. This applied potential permits some compounds in the sample that come into contact with the electrodes to be oxidized or reduced. The potential serves as the generating or excitation signal; the response is the current measured. Molecules are oxidized or reduced at the working electrode, whose potential is controlled relative to a reference electrode such as an SCE or Ag/AgCl electrode, which were described earlier. Electrochemical techniques similar to amperometry include **voltammetry**, in which the potential is varied in some way and the current–potential relationship is monitored. The output of such a device is a voltammogram, a general example of which is shown in Figure 4–4. Another term often

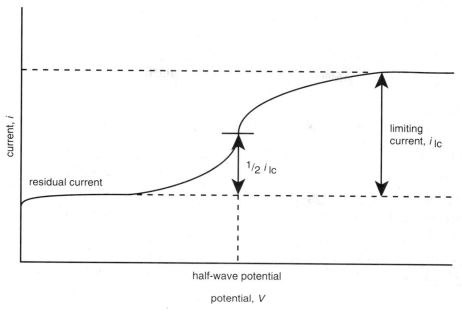

■ **FIGURE 4–4.**

A representative voltammogram.

used is polarography, which is a voltammetric technique using a working electrode of a continually renewable surface, such as the dropping mercury electrode.

Each amperometric technique is similar in that the applied potential and the measured current have a defined relationship based on the molecule(s) that react. When oxidation or reduction takes place, electrons are given off or consumed, respectively, producing a current. These methods can be quite sensitive, since the response originates as an electric current that can be amplified if necessary to produce a measurable effect for a small quantity of material reacted. Interference is an important consideration, since many electroactive species might be present in the sample that also oxidize or reduce at the applied potential. Specificity may be gained through a number of mechanisms, such as by surrounding the electrode with a semipermeable membrane

that keeps large molecules like proteins from poisoning the electrode. Only small molecules or analytes in the gaseous phase will get through the membrane and reach the working electrode.

The most common example of these amperometric techniques in clinical laboratory science is the pO_2 electrode, which is composed of a small platinum cathode and an Ag/AgCl anode placed in a supporting electrolyte—typically, a phosphate buffer—and enclosed by a gas-permeable membrane (e.g., polypropylene). A potential of about -0.6 V is applied to the cathode. Gases in the sample cross the membrane, diffuse to the cathode, and will be reduced if reactive at the applied potential. The only gas common in blood that will reduce at -0.6 V is oxygen. At this potential (well beyond oxygen's half-wave potential of -0.35 V), the amount of current flow is directly proportional to the amount of gaseous O_2 in the sample; i.e., the current meter can be calibrated so as to report the pO_2 value directly. Figure 4–5 is a schematic of the pO_2 electrode. The overall reaction at the cathode is given by:

$$O_2 + 2H_2O + 4e^- \rightarrow 4OH^-$$

Thus, for every molecule of O_2 reduced, four electrons of current will flow.

Amperometry is used in several other applications in laboratory medicine, most notably enzyme electrodes when oxygen, hydrogen peroxide, or some other electrochemically reactive entity is involved in the reaction. These electrodes consist of a membrane on which the enzyme of choice is immobilized. Glucose oxidase can be used to measure glucose, for instance. Glucose is oxidized to gluconic acid, and oxygen is consumed, as shown in the equation:

$$glucose + O_2 \rightarrow H_2O_2 + gluconic\ acid$$

The amount of oxygen reacted is directly related to the quantity of glucose present in the sample and can be monitored by an oxygen electrode fabricated much like that described in the previous paragraph. Alternatively, hydrogen peroxide that is produced can be detected at an amperometric electrode set to a potential at which H_2O_2 will oxidize, or a redox mediator can be coupled to the enzyme reaction on the inner side of the membrane. One of the redox couples can then be measured amperometrically.

A number of oxidase enzymes act in a similar way as the preceding equation, producing hydrogen peroxide. Thus, any substrate reacting with these enzymes can be detected by hydrogen peroxide amperometric probes. Clinically important examples include lactate, uric acid, ascorbic acid, and ethanol. Even cholesterol could be measured by such a method. Novel laboratory medicine applications of amperometry have also been suggested for urea, aspartate and alanine aminotransferase, and theophylline.

COULOMETRIC METHODS

Coulometry is an electrochemical technique related to amperometry, in that a single potential is applied between two electrodes and current flows because of an oxidation or reduction process. Two features are different, however. First, conditions are established so that *all* the substance of interest is electrochemically reacted. Second, instead of the current being measured, the *amount* of electricity (in coulombs = ampere second) produced by the process is quantified. The number of coulombs, Q, is proportional to the amount of substance produced or consumed at the working electrode, as given by Faraday's first law:

$$Q = z \cdot n \cdot F$$

where z is the number of electrons involved in the electrochemical reaction, n is the mole quantity of substance reacted, and F is the Faraday constant (96,490 coulombs/equivalent). Thus, if coulombs can be accurately and precisely measured, the concentration of desired analyte may be calculated. Two approaches to determining the amount of electricity are possible: controlled-potential coulometry, in which the current is monitored over the amount of time necessary to complete the electrolysis; or controlled-current coulometry, in which the current is kept constant and only the time needed to reach the end-point is measured. In either case, $Q = i \cdot t$, where i is the current and t is the time. Combining this relationship with the preceding equation gives

$$n = \frac{i \cdot t}{z \cdot F}$$

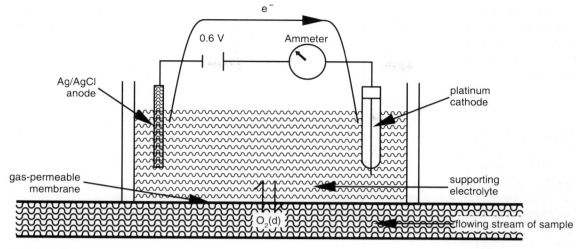

■ FIGURE 4–5.

The pO_2 electrode system.

In practice, controlled-current coulometry is more popular, particularly in clinical laboratory analysis, in which the most common application is the chloridometer, a coulometric approach for the determination of chloride concentration. When current is kept constant, the preceding equation illustrates that a direct proportion exists between the time measured and the amount of substance reacted. The chloridometer consists of two pairs of electrodes, one using coulometry to generate silver ions from a silver anode. The silver ions react with chloride ions (from the sample) and precipitate as AgCl. When all the chloride has precipitated, excess silver ions begin to appear. The second pair of electrodes sense the endpoint by detecting the presence of silver ions either potentiometrically or amperometrically. At that point, the generating electrodes are turned off and the time is measured. From the time, using an equation like the preceding, the concentration of chloride in the sample may be obtained.

PRACTICAL APPLICATIONS AND ISSUES IN CLINICAL LABORATORY ELECTROCHEMICAL ANALYSIS

Electrochemistry is the foundational technique for many of the critical care analytes in clinical chemistry today. Most if not all the devices available for the determination of blood gases and electrolytes depend on the electrochemical techniques just described. This chapter is not the place to list all these instruments, because modified and new versions of these systems are introduced regularly, and some of the manufacturers "disappear" through merger or acquisition. A listing of the firms currently active in supplying these instruments may be found in the yearly reference guides published for that purpose by some of the clinical laboratory societies or periodicals in the field (such as *Medical Laboratory Observer*).

Blood gas instruments have used electrochemical techniques for decades. Advances in the miniaturization of electrodes, flow-through design, maintenance-free construction, and computer control have produced improvements in performance, reliability, sample volume requirements, labor intensity, and speed of analysis. Many of these same improvements have also had an impact on the systems available for electrolyte analysis. In fact, because of their analytical quality, ease of use, and safety, ion-selective electrode methods have largely replaced flame photometry for sodium, potassium, and lithium. More diagnostic companies market ISE electrolyte instruments than make blood gas equipment. Some novel approaches to the design of these electrodes have been introduced, such as the disposable slide configuration of the Ektachem series of instruments (Eastman Kodak Company) (Fig. 4–6), but each depends on the same principles explained earlier.

Most of the techniques developed for electrolytes prior to ISEs used an *indirect* measurement, meaning that the sample is diluted prior to the actual analysis. Ion-selective electrodes are capable of determining the concentration of plasma sodium and other electrolytes without dilution of the sample. (It should be noted that then the activity of the ion is determined, *not* the concentration—which for most samples makes no practical difference to the clinical use of the results.) These direct potentiometric techniques provide several advantages but also generate some confusion. The advantages offered by direct methods over indirect approaches are:

- Clinically accurate results are obtained even when the plasma water percentage is altered
- Low volumes of reagent are consumed
- The sample is left intact for other use, such as further analysis downstream

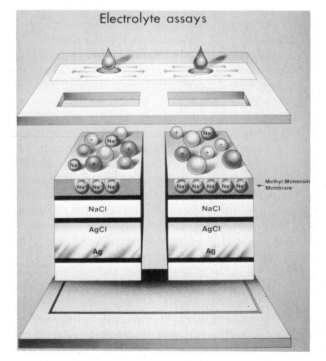

■ FIGURE 4–6.

Kodak Ektachem slide for ion-selective electrode.

- Determinations can use whole blood
- Combinations with multiple analytes are possible
- In vivo monitoring is feasible

The first of these advantages has been well recognized since the early 1980s and means that clinical conditions producing hyperproteinemia or hyperlipidemia will not give misleading sodium results. High lipid or protein causes falsely low results when sodium is determined using indirect techniques (whether ISE or not), owing to the displacement of plasma water, since almost all the sodium is in the aqueous phase. The second advantage may become increasingly important as efforts to reduce operating costs search out every possible resource for saving. The remaining advantages lead to applications that will be mentioned later.

The concern with or confusion from direct potentiometry revolves around the agreement of these results with those from more traditional, indirect methods (to be discussed in Part II of this chapter), particularly for plasma sodium in which concentrations are higher and any differences between the methods are noticeable. For the most part, this confusion is being resolved through a remarkable cooperative effort at standardization involving the major manufacturers, the National Institute for Science and Technology, and organizations such as the National Committee for Clinical Laboratory Standards.

When conducting determinations of data that will be used clinically, the medical care professionals involved must not limit their concern only to the analytical phase of the process. Other steps in the sequence of generating clinical laboratory results (the preanalytical and postanalytical aspects) must be considered as well. This point is particularly vital when reporting critical care analytes, such as electrolytes and blood gas parameters. Some of the issues of concern when determining these analytes include the syringe or container in which the sample is drawn, the kind and amount of anticoagulant used to maintain whole blood, how the sample is collected (e.g., with any stasis in the patient's blood supply, or any air in the sample container), the effect of hematocrit, whether to store the sample at all, and, if stored, whether the sample should be placed in a container of ice water. The importance of a few of these issues becomes clearer when some recent trends are contemplated, as in the next section.

RECENT AND FUTURE TRENDS

One of the key advantages of electrochemical techniques is the ability for simultaneous determination of virtually any number of analytes. This ability leads to production of instruments that amount to highly automated, multichannel, semirandom access machines suited for critical care chemistry. Instruments measuring electrolytes on samples of whole blood appeared in the early 1980s. By the mid-1980s, a few blood gas instruments began to add potassium determinations; other electrolytes followed quickly. Over a dozen different "combination analyzers" were available in 1993 from at least six international diagnostic companies. These devices are capable of determining the traditional blood gas analytes (pH, pCO_2, and pO_2) as well as one or more of the following: sodium, potassium, chloride, ionized calcium, lithium, urea, glucose, and lactate. Each battery of results can be obtained from a single injection of perhaps only 200 μL of whole blood in as little as 2 minutes or less. Virtually all the methods depend on electrochemistry.

Developments in the membranes used for ion-selective electrodes continue, both for the purpose of improving existing electrochemical methods and to produce electrodes capable of determining new analytes. In the latter category, an ion-selective electrode for ionized magnesium will be commercially available by the mid-1990s, added to existing systems measuring similar analytes such as ionized calcium. Novel ideas resulting in new membranes for analytes as common as H^+ have appeared at a steady pace. Most pH electrodes are made from glass membranes, as discussed above, but these can be somewhat troublesome unless used and maintained properly. Thus, technology using ion-sensitive field effect transistors (ISFET) for pH have been introduced and hold some promise, particularly for applications beyond clinical blood gas analysis.

Other ISFETs selective for analytes such as potassium and calcium are also becoming available. They have short response times and can be manufactured even smaller than typical ISEs. Hence, different ISFETs could be placed in sequence on a small chip, which might eventually serve as the sensor inside catheter tips for in situ analysis. A number of problems need to be resolved, however, not the least of which is the lack of a reliable ISFET reference electrode. Thus, these ISFET electrodes more likely may have an impact on existing or new instruments meant for in vitro use.

Improvements in anion-selective membranes have been rarer, although recent advances in electrodes for chloride, CO_2, and compounds as diverse as salicylate and heparin seem capable of making an impact. Finally, intriguing results are being reported with doped-polymer or ceramic electrodes, in terms of the breadth of analytes (limited only by the species with which the polymer is doped), wide applicability, and increased reliability and robustness, leading to potential cost savings.

A number of advances have occurred in the late 1980s and early 1990s in the development of devices for near-patient testing, including emergency laboratory service and physician office analysis. Many of these developments came about because of the use of electrochemistry. While these devices may offer advantages to patient care, particularly regarding convenience, they also present some problems. Most of these instruments, however, feature stability and easy maintenance, facilitating use outside the normal laboratory settings. For instance, instruments marketed by Mallinkrodt Sensor Systems include virtually everything needed for analysis—electrodes, reagents, and so on—in cartridges that are used and thrown away.

One of the problems nagging the whole field of clinical electrochemical analysis has been standardization of the measurements, as mentioned several times in this chapter. Fortunately, reference materials are now available from the National Institute of Science and Technology (NIST; formerly NBS) specifically to allow all electrolyte technology to have the same accuracy base. Standard reference material (SRM) 956 is fully calibrated for sodium and potassium, and efforts continue to develop a modified 956 that will include values for additional similar analytes. This work should reach fruition early in this decade as interlaboratory precision improves. Ultimately, patient care will continue to be enhanced through these and other efforts involving electrochemical sensors.

Part 2

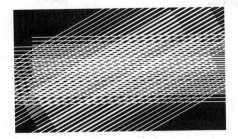

Emission and Absorption Spectroscopy

BARBARA J. CLEVELAND, MPH, MT(ASCP)

ELECTROMAGNETIC RADIATION

Certain orbiting electrons of atoms and molecules have limited numbers of energy levels; the lowest energy level is called the ground state. Electrons are excited to higher energy levels (electronic transitions) when supplied with sufficient energy. Lamps, lasers, flames, inductively coupled plasmas (ICP), and hollow cathode tubes are all examples of excitation sources. Energy is released in the form of heat, electromagnetic radiation, or both, when once-excited electrons relax and return to lower levels (ground state). The total energy of a molecule can be represented by:

$$E_T = E_{electronic\ transitions} + E_{vibrational} + E_{rotational}$$

When the energy released is in the form of electromagnetic radiation, a photon, $h\upsilon$, is created with an energy equal to the differ-

ence between the excited state and the lower energy level. Relaxation may also involve fluorescent or phosphorescent re-emission. Some compounds have the ability to absorb light energy and re-emit some of the energy in light of longer wavelengths; this is fluorescence. Both fluorescence and phosphorescence are discussed later.

Substances that are in the gaseous state behave as independent bodies and emit relatively few but specific radiating particles that are well separated from one another. The wavelengths formed are discontinuous, are essentially monochromatic, and are referred to as **line spectra**. Substances, such as solids and liquids, have atoms that are closely packed; their electrons are not capable of independent behavior, and the spectrum emitted is without sharply defined lines. This type of spectrum is called a continuous spectrum, and it contains all wavelengths over a wide range. It is important to

113

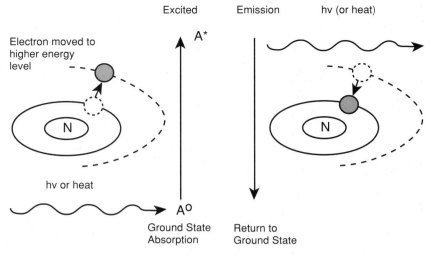

■ **FIGURE 4–7.**

Relationship between absorption and emission.

FLAME TECHNIQUES

In the process of absorption, the energy of photons, or heat, converts absorbing species to the excited form. This is depicted by the following equation:

$$A^0 + h\upsilon = A^* \text{ or } A^0 + \text{heat} = A^*$$

where A^0 is the ground state of the absorbing species, h is Planck's constant, υ is the frequency of oscillation, and A^* is the excited form of the absorbing species. The excited state is unstable and short-lived; the excitation energy is lost as photons of specific wavelengths or as heat. The following equation shows this; note that it is the reverse of the equation above:

$$A^* \rightarrow A^0 + h\upsilon \text{ (or heat)}$$

It should now be apparent that all elements are capable of absorbing heat and light energy, and when an element is subjected to a flame at least two things happen:

1. A^0, *ground state atoms absorb flame energy and become excited.*
2. A^*, *when these atoms revert to ground they emit radiant energy* (photon). *The wavelength of the emitted radiant energy is characteristic of the substance.*

The relationship between atomic absorption and flame emission is illustrated in Figure 4–7.

Flame Characteristics

Figures 4–8 and 4–9 illustrate the flame profiles for atomic absorption and flame

Also, a substance can absorb the same spectral line as can be emitted. We will soon see how both these phenomena are key to the principles of atomic absorption and flame emission photometry.

understand that substances excited by high energy, such as that seen in flame techniques, behave as gases and emit line spectra.

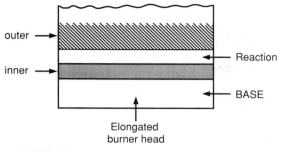

■ **FIGURE 4–8.**

Atomic absorption.

TABLE 4–1. ATOMIC ABSORPTION

PART OF THE FLAME	REACTION
Base	Evaporation
Inner cone	Disintegration
Reaction zone	Accumulation or oxidation
Outer mantle	No reaction or reduction

emission. First note that even though both applications use the flame, a different part of the flame is used for each application; also note that the flame parts are differently named; the outer cone or outer mantle of the flame for atomic absorption is different from that for flame emission. Tables 4–1 and 4–2 summarize the flame profiles for both types of flames.

Figure 4–10 illustrates the laminar flow or premix burner and probably gives a better view of what is happening in the flame for atomic absorption and flame emission, specifically pointing out nebulization and the areas of atomization and radiation.

Burners

The laminar flow or premix burner is the type most often used in atomic absorption and flame emission instruments. Its design facilitates the nebulization of the sample into small droplets that can be easily evaporated into the fuel/oxidant mixture; large droplets, which tend to cool the flame and reduce its effectiveness, are eliminated from the system and pass to the drain line. When the burner is used for atomic absorption, the burner head is elongated to introduce more atoms into the light path and thereby improve the sensitivity of the application.

Flame Temperature

The temperature of the flame is controlled by the fuel to oxidant ratio and the flow

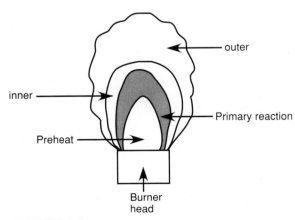

■ **FIGURE 4–9.**

Flame photometry.

TABLE 4–2. FLAME EMISSION PHOTOMETRY

PART OF THE FLAME	REACTION
Preheat zone	Temperature is increased by energy from primary reaction zone
Primary reaction zone	Primary combustion; merging gases heated to ignition temperature
Inner cone	Hot reducing atmosphere
Outer cone	Secondary combustion

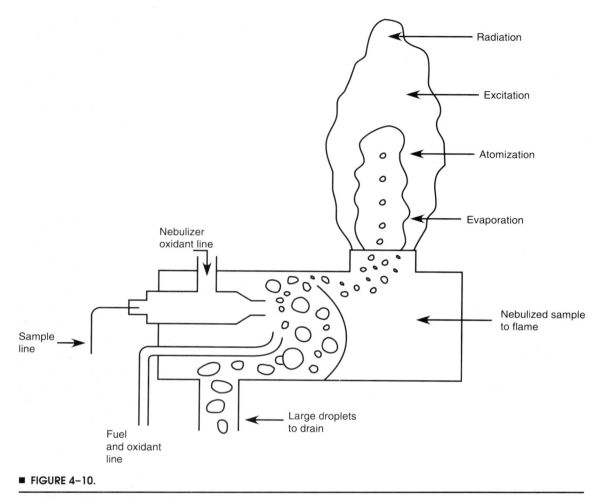

■ **FIGURE 4–10.**

Premix burner and nebulization process.

rate. This ratio determines whether the flame is an oxidizing or a reducing flame. An oxidizing flame has an excess of hot oxygen present and therefore promotes the oxidation of the atom. A reducing flame has an excess of fuel and reduced amounts of oxygen; this type of flame prolongs the life of ground state neutral atoms. Some examples of fuel/oxidant mixtures are presented in Table 4–3.

Because of the combustibility of oxygen,

air is used in the clinical laboratory as the oxidant for both flame emission and atomic absorption. Propane is generally the fuel of choice for flame emission photometry; acetylene is often used as the fuel for atomic absorption, depending on what is being analyzed. Some newer atomic absorption models use argon as the fuel.

We have now described electromagnetic radiation in terms of absorption and emission and have discussed the basic common-

TABLE 4–3. FUEL/OXIDANT MIXTURES

FUEL	OXIDANT	TEMPERATURE (°C)
Acetylene	Air	2275
Acetylene	Oxygen	3100
Propane	Air	1900
Propane	Oxygen	2700

alities between atomic absorption and flame emission. We now turn our attention to the specifics associated with atomic absorption, flame emission, and fluorescent techniques.

ATOMIC ABSORPTION

There are three major conditions for sample analysis under which the greatest sensitivity and selectivity may be achieved:

1. Maximal sensitivity is provided at the point of highest possible absorptivity.
2. A sharp absorption band contributes to maximal selectivity.
3. Radiant energy that is restricted to a particular wavelength band provides maximal sensitivity and selectivity.

These three conditions are met when **atomic absorption** spectroscopy is used. When the sample is introduced into the flame, it is converted to a gaseous, atomic state; each absorbing species is an atom, free of the vibrational and rotational properties associated with polyatomic ions and molecules. In this state, electronic transitions are at sharply defined wavelengths that produce line spectra. An un-ionized, unexcited atom will absorb light of a specific wavelength, a certain energy level. The absorption resonance lines are the same as the emission lines.

To be more specific, atomic absorption contains three major steps, summarized as follows:

1. A high energy source, e.g., a flame, converts the sample to an atomic vapor, which contains mostly ground state and some excited orbital electrons.
2. The wavelengths produced by the atomic vapor are characteristic of the element
3. The amount of light absorbed by the vaporized sample is proportional to the concentration of the sample.

Instrumentation

Now we must ask three questions. First, which wavelengths are best absorbed by the vaporized sample? Second, what are ways to provide these wavelengths? Third, how is maximal absorbance by the sample achieved?

The answer to the first question has already been given; the sample best absorbs wavelengths that are characteristic of it. If the vaporized sample contains magnesium, then wavelengths that are characteristic of magnesium will be absorbed. The more magnesium in the vaporized sample, the more magnesium light absorbed.

Hollow Cathode Lamp

Suppose a lamp is constructed so that the cathode filament is magnesium. Will the light from this lamp be maximally absorbed when passed through a vaporized sample containing magnesium? Yes. This is the answer to the second question and the basis for the construction of the **hollow cathode lamp**. A lamp containing calcium as the cathode element is used in determining calcium, a zinc cathode element for determining zinc, and so on. In short, the hollow cathode is the source of atomic line emission. The radiant energy is characteristic of the cathode element, and the gas in the tube is neon or argon. A diagram of the hollow cathode is shown in Figure 4–11.

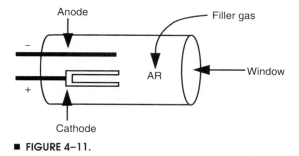

■ **FIGURE 4–11.**

Schematic diagram of hollow cathode.

This is a single-element hollow cathode lamp. Usually a different lamp is needed for each analyte in question. There are, however, multielement lamp sources. Such lamps usually contain no more than three elements, and the resonance lines of the elements are far apart so as not to overlap and interfere.

Also note that an element can produce more than one resonance line, thus more than one wavelength may be characteristic of the element, including lines emitted from the cathode. Sodium, for example, has absorption wavelengths of 330 nm, 589 nm, and 819 nm. These are also the emission wavelengths from the lamp as well as the excited sample. Calcium has absorbance wavelengths at 240 nm and 423 nm. The 423-nm wavelength is more sensitive and is therefore used to obtain maximal absorbance when calcium is analyzed by atomic absorption.

Modulation

Since the vaporized sample emits a resonance line at the same wavelength as it absorbs, a problem exists: distinguishing the absorption line produced by the hollow cathode from the emission line produced by the sample. This problem is overcome by the introduction of a modulation instrument, the rotary **chopper**. In principle, the direct current (dc) output from the hollow cathode is modified to alternating current (ac). The detector is then tuned to the same frequency and synchronized. The emission signal from the sample is dc, and the detector is unable to register it. In practice, modulation may be achieved by electrical as well as mechanical means. Using the electrical method, the power supply to the hollow cathode is ac or is rectified to pulsating dc. The synchronized detector will register only this signal.

A rotating disc, the chopper, can also be used to split the light from the hollow cathode mechanically into two beams, the reference beam and the sample beam, thereby creating a double-beam system. The disc is rotated at a controlled frequency; the light from the hollow cathode is alternately passed through the sample and reference paths. The reference path goes directly to the detector. The sample path goes first through the sample and then to the detector. The ratio between both paths is monitored; therefore, absorbed light is monitored. Figure 4–12 illustrates the mechanically modulated system for both the single-beam and double-beam configurations.

Burner Head

The burner type, previously discussed, is the laminar flow or premix burner. The head is elongated to allow more absorbing atoms in the light path. Burner problems are reduced or eliminated by controlling the gas flow for both oxidant and fuel, maintaining a steady flame, and keeping the burner head clean.

Wavelength Isolation and Detection

In general, a monochromator allows the passage of light of a particular wavelength. In the case of atomic absorption, this light may come from two sources: (1) the hollow

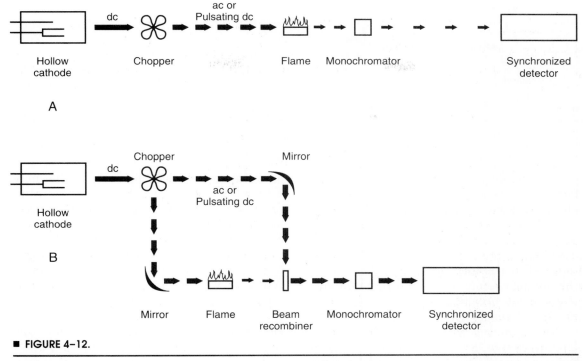

■ **FIGURE 4–12.**

A, Single-beam atomic absorption. *B*, Double-beam atomic absorption.

cathode, and (2) excited sample emissions. The monochromator and detector system are tuned so as to detect synchronized light (previously discussed in the section on modulation). The monochromator is generally a diffraction grating, although some instruments may use a prism, and the detector is generally a photomultiplier tube.

Peaking

We have seen from our discussion on flame characteristics that certain reactions happen in certain parts of the flame. This suggests that optical alignment is very important with flame techniques. It is especially important in atomic absorption if the instrument is designed to facilitate changing hollow cathode tubes and burner heads, which have movable parts. Peaking is the process of adjusting the cathode and the burner head in the optical system to obtain maximal output from the cathode and maximum absorption in the flame.

Interference

Four major types of interferences, chemical, ionization, matrix, and spectral, can occur with atomic absorption.

Chemical interference occurs when the flame cannot dissociate the sample into free atoms, which is necessary for absorption to occur. An example of this is in the measurement of calcium; in the presence of phosphate ions tight complexes of calcium phosphate are formed. This interference can be minimized or eliminated by adding lanthanum or strontium to the diluent to dis-

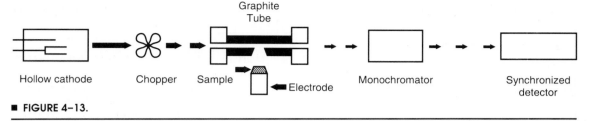

■ **FIGURE 4–13.**

Flameless atomic absorption.

place calcium from the complex, thereby forming a more stable complex with phosphate than with calcium.

Ionization interference occurs when atoms in the flame become ionized instead of remaining in the ground state; in this form they will not absorb the incident light from the hollow cathode tube. Addition of a substance that provides excess free electrons and is more easily ionized shifts the reaction to the formation of ground state atoms. Modification in the fuel combustion to lower the temperature of the flame will also minimize ionization interference.

Matrix interference occurs whenever the composition of the standard varies greatly from that of the test sample. This may be seen when the sample contains protein and the standard does not, or when there are difference in viscosity, solvent composition, and salt concentration between standards and samples. High concentrations of salt result in a decrease in the signal. To overcome matrix interference, many procedures use protein-containing calibrators as standards in an attempt to match the viscosity and composition of samples. Sometimes dilution is attempted to minimize the interference. Any procedure that minimizes the difference in composition between the standards and test samples will minimize matrix interference.

Spectral interference occurs when there is nonspecific, or background, absorption by materials other than the sample; this may be due to undisassociated molecular complexes and solids formed in the flame or residues formed on the burner head. A clean burner head will reduce this problem.

There also may be other sources of interference, such as continuous emission sources or emission interference. Background correction techniques tend to solve the problems associated with continuous emission sources. Modulation is used to correct emission interference.

Flameless Atomic Absorption

By replacing the burner head flame with a graphite furnace, as illustrated in Figure 4–13, another atomization process is introduced, that of flameless atomic absorption. The construction and use of the furnace insures uniform heating, increased sensitivity, and a lower detection limit. The graphite furnace is heated electronically to temperatures of up to 2700° C. At this temperature, trace elements and heavy metals can be detected.

During analysis, a small volume of the solution containing the analyte of interest is placed in the graphite tube where it is evaporated and ashed; it is then subjected to a temperature sufficient to cause atomization. Radiation from the source is passed through the system, and absorbance is observed.

FLAME PHOTOMETRY

Flame photometry, also called flame emission spectroscopy or atomic emission spectroscopy (AES), is the reverse of atomic absorption in that it is based upon the intensity of radiation emitted by excited atoms. To be more specific, metallic salts, such as sodium, potassium, and lithium, emit very specific wavelengths when burned in a flame. These wavelengths are characteristic of the element being burned. As previously mentioned, sodium has a major spectral line at 589 nm. Potassium's spectral line is at 767 nm, and lithium's is at 671. Increasing the thermal energy of the flame will cause more atoms to become excited and the intensity of the emission lines to increase. Likewise, the higher the concentration of the metallic salt in the sample, the greater the intensity of the characteristic wavelength in the flame. At a temperature controlled by the fuel/oxidant ratio and a constant flow rate, the concentration of a particular analyte can be determined, using flame photometry, by comparing its intensity with that of a standard.

Internal Standard

The preceding statement is the basic principle of flame photometry; however, it is not that simple. The excited sample in the flame is the light source for flame photometry. Unlike the light source in basic spectroscopy, the flame is not steady; it naturally flickers. By adding an **internal standard** (an additional element of known concentration) to the sample, the intensity of the spectral line of the unknown can be compared with that of the internal standard. When the flame fluctuates, the emission line from the internal standard and the sample also fluctuate, thereby canceling the fluctuation effect. It is important for the compound serving as the internal standard to

- be chemically pure and have a precisely known concentration,
- have a concentration of the same order of magnitude as the unknown element,
- have excitation potentials closely matched to those of the unknown element,
- have physical and chemical properties similar to those of the unknown element,
- have emission lines that are not close to that of the unknown, and
- not occur naturally in the unknown solution.

When lithium concentration was being determined by flame photometry, potassium was used as the internal standard. Lithium was previously used as the internal standard for sodium and potassium determinations until its increased use as a therapeutic agent removed it from the list of qualified candidates. Flame photometers are now being designed to use cesium as the internal standard. The basic design of the cesium internal standard flame photometer is illustrated in Figure 4–14. An example of how the internal standard ratio is used to determine the concentration of an analyte is:

Sodium concentration =

$$\frac{\text{sodium channel output}}{\text{cesium channel output}} (1.5 \text{ mmol/L}) (f)$$

where f is a response factor obtained by aspirating a solution with equal volumes of 1.5 millimolar sodium and 1.5 millimolar cesium.

Instrumentation

The basic spectrophotometer consists of a light source, lens, monochromator, sample

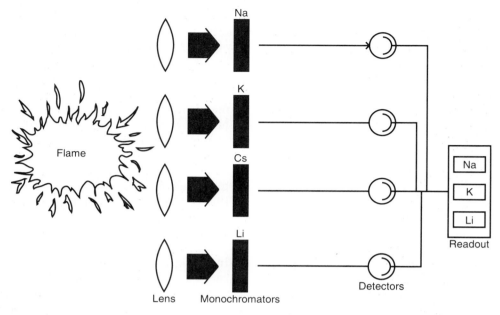

■ **FIGURE 4–14.**

Cesium internal standard flame photometer.

compartment, detector, readout device, and specifically arranged slits; this is also the case with the flame photometer. The major difference is that the light source and the sample compartment are together, in the burner assembly. The flame is the excitation source for the sample as well as the light source for the instrument. The atomizer-burner assembly has been discussed. In the ICP-AES (inductively coupled plasma–atomic emission spectroscopy), the ICP serves as the excitation source. The ICP is discussed later. It is mentioned here because of its relation to atomic emission spectroscopy.

Another major difference is in the multichannel arrangement, compared with the double-beam configuration of spectrophotometers. Newer instruments, used in the clinical laboratory, contain monochromators and detectors (phototubes or photomultiplier tubes) for sodium, potassium, lithium, and cesium. The choice of the detector depends on the intensity of the light reaching the detector. If the intensity is very weak, a photomultiplier tube generally will be used.

The major clinical application of flame photometry has been in the analysis of sodium, potassium, and lithium; however, this procedure is being replaced by the increasing use of ion-selective electrode technology.

INDUCTIVELY COUPLED PLASMA EMISSION SPECTROSCOPY

The concentration of the sample, using **inductively coupled plasma** (ICP) technology, is determined by measuring the intensity of the light produced by line spectra at discrete wavelengths. The sample is introduced as a fine mist (nebulized) into a hot argon gas. The temperature is extremely hot, approximately 8000° C; this evaporates the sample and destroys all chemical compounds. The remaining atoms are excited and ionized. The light emitted is at wavelengths that are characteristic for the element. Light intensity is used to determine the concentration.

Up to this point the instrument sounds much like that of most flame-type instruments. How is it different? The first difference is the plasma source and the temperature. The plasma source is argon gas, heated electrically by a radiofrequency oscillator; the temperatures reached are those approaching that of the sun, yet nothing is burning because argon is an inert gas. There is no danger of explosion or flashback.

Inductively coupled plasma is designed for multielement analysis and is most useful if there are more than five elements in a sample and several samples to analyze. All atoms in the sample emit light simultaneously and are measured at the same time.

Chemical interferences are small with ICP compared with other flame techniques. This is because of the temperature of the plasma and long residence time of the analyte in the plasma.

Many wavelengths are produced with emission spectroscopy, some quite close together. When flame techniques are used, especially to detect several elements and all characteristic wavelengths, spectral interference or poor wavelength resolution is a common problem. How does the ICP design solve these problems?

Spectral interference can be a problem with ICP. The spectral lines produced have a wide range of intensities, thereby being capable of producing stray light. The instrument design must be capable of little or no stray light. High-resolution spectrophotometers are those with very narrow bandpasses. In part, this can facilitate wavelength selection and elimination of spectral interference. However, a bandpass equal to or smaller than the physical line width of the ICP emission can contribute nothing more to the addition of resolution or the reduction of interference. Thus, to correct for spectral interference, instrument design includes high resolution, background correction, and selection of a line that is free of interference. The wavelength sensed by the detector is a function of the grating, a critical component in the optical system, which is selected by two major means: (1) the wavelengths can be changed by rotating the grating in a system with fixed entrance and exit slits, or (2) the detector and exit slit can be moved along a focal plane.

One ICP optical design uses a moving grating to select wavelengths at a fixed detector. In this case, misalignment of or damage to the grating will cause a large error in wavelength selection and, therefore, errors in analysis. Another system uses a fixed grating combined with a prism; this disperses light over two dimensions, allowing wide separation of wavelengths. The detector is moved to the wavelength of interest.

To illustrate the type of resonance lines produced by an element and the resolution that must be achieved by a good optical system, see Tables 4–4 and 4–5.

We have seen how important grating

TABLE 4–4. EXAMPLES OF CHARACTERISTIC SPECTRAL LINES

ELEMENT	SPECTRAL LINES (nm)
Aluminum	309.27
	308.22
	396.15
	226.92
Arsenic	193.70
	197.20
	228.81
	234.98
Zinc	213.86
	202.55
	206.20
	334.50

TABLE 4–5. ANALYSIS OF WAVELENGTHS

ELEMENT	WAVELENGTH
As	193.70
	234.98
Hg	194.16
	253.65
Se	196.03
Cr	205.55
	267.72

function is to wavelength selection. What about grating design? Let's briefly discuss two. A basic spectrophotometer may use the diffraction grating as a monochromator. With the diffraction grating, the incoming light will be at an angle, and some of the light will be reflected at an equal angle but on the opposite side of the grating normal. (Review diffraction grating.) The grating of an echelle grating is blazed at the same angle. Grating efficiency is high. However, there is an order overlap problem. This can be solved with the addition of a prism or second grating to disperse the light in a direction that improves resolution.

Nebulizer design is also critical to ICP performance. Designs common to ICP include the v-groove nebulizer, suitable for organics and oils, and the Hildebrand grid nebulizer (HGN), suitable for multielement analysis of high-salt digest or samples that are high in dissolved solids.

The ICP/Echelle Spectrometer, produced by Leeman Labs, Inc., is an example of the fixed optics, echelle grating prism, moving detector system (Fig. 4–15). A two-dimensional spectrum is created and detected by the moving detector. Other features include "state of the art" nebulizer design and purged optics, which allows it to detect a range of wavelengths from 178 nm to 800 nm, with a resolution range of 0.0075 nm to

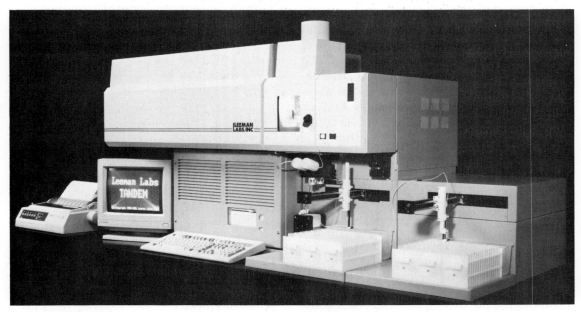

■ **FIGURE 4–15.**

ICP/Echelle spectrometers. (Courtesy of Leeman Labs, Inc., Lowell, MA)

0.024 nm. It may be automated to perform 42 samples per hour, detecting up to 18 elements. Other features include a wavelength library with approximately 30,000 wavelengths, special calculation abilities, and easy-to-use keyboard commands.

We discuss ICP because it uses the principles of absorption and emission spectroscopy in an advanced way. In addition to the ICP-AES, ICP technology as been applied to mass spectroscopy (ICP-MS). There are also attempts to couple its technology to high-performance liquid chromatography as well as gas chromatography. The instrument is not yet a part of the clinical laboratory; it is generally found in laboratories that analyze drinking water, waste water, ground water, hazardous waste, food contaminants, and trace elements (for whatever reason). Some specialized laboratories (toxicology) are becoming more involved in these types of analyses. It is very possible that the ICP will be a very important instrument in the future clinical laboratory.

CHEMILUMINESCENCE

Chemiluminescence is a chemical reaction that produces light. Therefore, chemiluminescence can be used as the label for an immunoassay, serving as a light enhancer to increase the output of photons. For example, peroxidase, as an enzyme immunoassay label, plus luminol (5-amino 2,3-dehydro-1,4-phthalazinedione) and enhancer (luciferin, 6-hydroxybenzothiazole) will yield water, oxidized luminol, and light. The photon emission is from 400 to 450 nm, and the reaction can be followed for up to 30 minutes or more. However, the system has disadvantages. Luminol requires a catalyst or strong reaction conditions, and the chemiluminescence can be a source of light interference.

Bioluminescence, an enzyme-catalyzed reaction that produces light, is believed to have some advantages over chemiluminescence because it requires specific enzymes. This system, however, suffers all the disadvantages associated with the use of enzymes.

Chemiluminescence can be a source of interference, especially with radioisotopes and liquid scintillation counting. When the chemiluminescent effect is high, it will add unwanted counts to the scintillation process. The effect is not constant and the count continues to drop over a period of time. The sample count is repeated to detect chemiluminescence, and readings are not taken until the count is stabilizes. Some of the more modern counters are able to correct for this interference.

FLUORESCENCE

Fluorescent spectroscopy makes use of radiant energy that is emitted by the analyte. Molecules absorb energy by forcing electrons from ground state molecular energy into higher-energy empty orbitals. These orbitals are filled by electron pairs with opposite spin directions. This is referred to as the singlet state (S). The first excitation level is represented by S_1 and the second excitation level by S_2. When the spins of excited electrons are unpaired, the excited state is called a triplet (T). This state may also have first level (T_1) and second level (T_2) excitation states. The ground state is represented by S_0. (See the energy level diagram in Figure 4–16). A molecule excited to a higher vibrational level may return to ground state by transferring excess energy to other molecules through collisions and by partitioning excess energy to other modes of vibration or rotation within the molecule. Possible transitions are S_2 to S_1 and S_1 to S_0, or S_1 to T_1 and T_1 to S_0. Some types of molecules can give off photons of radiant energy; the emit-

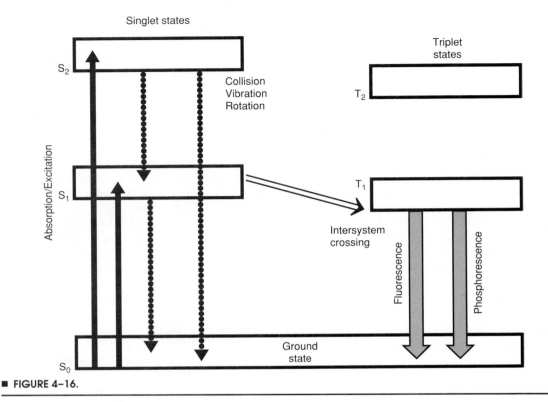

■ FIGURE 4–16.

Energy level diagram: Fluorescence.

ted photons are less energetic than the absorbed photons. Such molecules are called fluorophores. An S_1 to S_0 transition results in **fluorescence**; it is the immediate emission (10^{-8} sec) of light from a molecule after it has absorbed radiation. **Phosphorescence** is the delayed (10^{-2} to 100 sec) release of the absorbed energy; it is represented by a T_1 to S_0 transition.

The excitation light may be in the ultraviolet (UV) range and the emitted light may be in the visible range, or the excitation light may be in the short wavelength range of the visible spectrum and the emitted light may be in the longer wavelength range of the visible spectrum. The closer the excitation spectrum is to the absorption spectrum of a fluorescent compound, (the greater the portion of light that will be absorbed and proportionately emitted) the greater is the intensity of the fluorescence.

Instrumentation

How does instrument design for the fluorometer differ from that of the basic spectrophotometer? The basic fluorometer is illustrated in Figure 4–17.

Light Source

The first difference is in the light source. A high-intensity mercury or xenon arc lamp is used. Mercury lamps produce wavelengths at 254, 365, and 366 nm, as well as

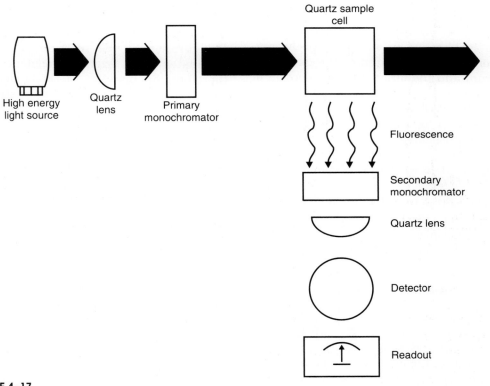

■ **FIGURE 4–17.**

Schematic of the basic fluorometer.

at other wavelengths. This lamp may be suitable for compounds with matching absorption bands but not for a wide range of other compounds or fluorescent labels. The xenon arc lamp emits a continuous spectrum from 200 to 800 nm and can be used to excite a wide range of compounds. Its main disadvantage is in its need for a specialized, stable-output power supply.

Monochromators

The instrument uses two monochromators, one for the selection of the excitation spectrum and the other for the selection of the emission spectrum. A fluorometer uses filters for wavelength selection. When gratings are used for wavelength selection, the instrument is called a spectrofluorometer.

Angle Configuration

Fluorescent light is measured at an angle, generally 90°, to the excited light. This is done to minimize the amount of excitation light that can reach the photodetector.

Sample Cells

Although round cuvets are sometimes used, rectangular sample cells are preferred to eliminate interference from the excitation source. These should be constructed of quartz or some special glass that does not absorb light in the excitation range. The absorption should be due to the sample, not the sample cell.

Detectors

Phototubes or photomultiplier tubes are used as the detectors, depending on the wavelength and intensity of the emitted light. If the emitted energy is high enough, a phototube may be used. If not, a photo-

multiplier is needed to increase the detection sensitivity.

Advantages

The advantages of fluorescence are in its sensitivity and specificity. The increased sensitivity is due to the fact that the emitted light comes directly from the sample. The specificity is increased because there is no interference from substances in the sample that absorb light and do not fluoresce. The configuration of the instrument virtually eliminates the original incident beam, therefore, fluorescence methods deal only with the sample and its characteristics.

Disadvantages

Three major disadvantages are associated with fluorescence methods: interference, sensitivity to environmental conditions, and self-absorption. These must be recognized and controlled for or corrected.

The most widely recognized interference is that of quenching. It is broadly defined as a reduction in the overall output of emitted light owing to the presence of a chemical or colored compound. This interference is encountered with liquid scintillation counting and results in a reduction in counting efficiency. A second type of interference is caused by the presence of other fluorescent compounds. This interference will add to the emitted light.

Sensitivity to the environment for the most part means sensitivity to pH and temperature. There is generally a decrease in fluorescence with increasing temperatures. There may be a pH range for fluorescence that includes a pH maxima.

At high concentrations, it is possible for the compound of interest to reabsorb the emitted light before it passes from the sample cell, thereby reducing the intensity of the emitted light. This is known as self-absorption.

Fluorescence Polarization

Fluorescence polarization measurements, fluorescence polarization immunoassay (FPIA), require molecular rotation, competitive binding, and an antigen tagged with a fluorescent dye (fluorescein) that has an electronic orientation such that the emitted light retains the initial orientation of the incident beam; it requires polarized light. Polarized light is light that travels in a single plane.

Molecules possess energy and tend to rotate in solution according to their size; the larger molecules rotate more slowly than the smaller molecules. An antigen-antibody complex is formed in the reaction; this is a large molecule compared with the free antigen molecules. When free fluorescent-antigen (a small molecule) is excited with polarized light (vertical light) in solution, it rotates rapidly and emits light in different planes; its original orientation is lost and there is a decrease in the intensity of vertically polarized light. The antigen-antibody complex is large; rotation is not as rapid, and much of the vertical orientation is maintained. The antigen/fluorescent-antibody complex absorbs the emitted light, fluorescence takes place, and there is an increase in the intensity of the polarized light at the detector. Remember, with competitive-binding assays, a high analyte concentration gives a low reading and a low analyte concentration gives a high reading. The same is true with FPIA. A high analyte concentration results in more free labeled antigen and thus a decrease in polarized antigen. The reverse is true for a low analyte concentration.

This approach is used for many procedures on the TDx and FLx instruments produced by Abbott Laboratories. The fluorescence that is produced by the excitation of the sample is emitted in all directions. The emission optical path is at an angle to the excitation source. The emitted radiation is passed through a filter that isolates the fluorescein emission from other radiation. The radiation from the emission filter is passed through a second filter, which completely absorbs the horizontal vibrations and very little of the vertical vibrations. The detector detects radiation that is vertically *polarized.*

SUMMARY

It has been suggested that the use in the clinical laboratory of flame photometry, atomic absorption, and fluorescence is diminishing. This is true to some degree but only because certain procedures are not yet a part of the clinical laboratory. Actually, the technology associated with these principles is dynamic and thus still advances.

Electrothermal atomic absorption spectrometry (ETAAS) continues to improve as the construction, type, and efficiency of the furnace improve. In addition to the graphite tube, other tube furnaces are available. These are constructed of molybdenum, tungsten, or glassy-carbon. Each has some major advantage associated with its use. For example, the tungsten-coil atomizer has less interference from chloride than does graphite when used to analyze certain metals. This might be a future consideration when metal toxicology becomes a major part of the clinical laboratory.

Fluorescence polarization techniques increased our ability to label compounds without using radiolabels. A routine chemistry, immunology, or toxicology therapeutic drug monitoring laboratory can now analyze many components that were once analyzed in specialized radioimmunoassay (RIA) laboratories.

What else might the future hold? Laser technology has been coupled with high-performance thin-layer chromatography for the detection of porphyrins, thereby using the fluorescent characteristic of porphyrins. Chemiluminescence and bioluminescence techniques have been coupled with high performance liquid chromatography. In addition to inductively coupled plasma (ICP) emission spectroscopy, we might find ourselves involved with furnace atomization plasma emission spectrometry (FAPES), laser-excited atomic fluorescence spectrometry (LEAFS), or even laser-enhanced ionization (LEI) spectrometry. As the clinical laboratory becomes more involved in biochemistry, cell biology, and DNA research and analysis, we are more likely to become involved with fluorescence detection of DNA fragments. In short, as basic principles become building blocks, laboratory techniques improve.

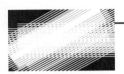

REVIEW QUESTIONS

Choose the BEST answer.

1. _____ is an electrochemical technique in which the basis of measurement is that the current required to convert a measured substance completely is proportional to that substance's concentration.

    a. voltammetry
    b. potentiometry
    c. coulometry
    d. amperometry

2. Measurement of a non-ionic analyte may be made possible if which of the following working electrodes is employed?

    a. gas-sensing
    b. enzyme
    c. liquid membrane
    d. ``a'' and ``b'' above

3. A pCO_2 electrode is a

    a. liquid membrane electrode.
    b. gas-sensing electrode.
    c. modified pH electrode.
    d. ``b'' and ``c'' above.

4. Valinomycin is used as the ionophore in which of the following ion-selective electrodes?

    a. Na^+
    b. K^+
    c. Cl^-
    d. CO_2

5. A technique used in the measurement of pO_2 is

    a. potentiometry.
    b. amperometry.
    c. polarography.
    d. voltammetry.

6. All the following statements are ad-

vantages of direct potentiometry, except:

a. There is good agreement with the indirect methods.
b. Low volumes of reagents are consumed.
c. Combinations with multiple analytes are possible.
d. The sample is left intact for other use, such as further analysis.

7. The flame technique in which a photon of light is emitted when an excited orbital electron returns to the ground state is

a. flame atomic absorption.
b. flame photometry.
c. flameless atomic absorption.
d. fluorescence.

8. Lithium is sometimes a part of the patient's serum sample because of its use in therapeutic drug monitoring. This is not always known by the technologist performing electrolyte analysis. What is the internal standard of choice to eliminate this problem?

a. potassium
b. sodium
c. lithium
d. cesium

9. The burner head of the atomic absorption flame is elongated to

a. allow more absorbing atoms in the light path.
b. increase emission potential.
c. pulsate the absorbing beam.
d. create nebulization.

10. Atomic absorption components designed to eliminate errors caused by measurement of flame light, espe-cially light of the specific wavelength emitted by the analyte, are

a. hollow cathode tube and photo-detector.
b. beam chopper and a tuned am-plifier.
c. flow rate controls for fuel and oxi-dant.
d. nebulizer and elongated burner head.

11. Quenching is the greatest problem in

a. nephelometry.
b. fluorometry.
c. atomic absorption.
d. UV spectroscopy.

12. Usually lanthanum is added to the diluent in the determination of calcium by atomic absorption to

a. remove phosphate interference.
b. reduce interference from back-ground emission.
c. serve as an internal standard.
d. improve atomization.

13. A chemical reaction that produces light is

a. atomic absorption.
b. flame emission.
c. phosphorescence.
d. chemiluminescence.

14. A _____ spectrum is produced by a single-element hollow cathode.

1. line
2. discontinuous
3. characteristic element
4. continuous

Which of these terms would make the above statement true?

a. 1, 2, and 3

b. 1 and 3
c. 2 and 4
d. 4 only
e. all of the above

15. An element serving as an internal standard for flame photometry must

1. be chemically pure and have a precisely known concentration and not occur naturally in the solution.
2. have physical and chemical properties similar to, and a concentration of the same order of magnitude as, the unknown element.
3. have excitation potentials closely matched to those of the unknown.
4. have emission lines that are not close to that of the unknown.

Which of these descriptions would make the above statement true?

a. 1, 2, and 3
b. 1 and 3
c. 2 and 4
d. 4 only
e. all of the above

16. Light that travels in a single plane is called _____ light.

1. scattered
2. fluorescent
3. transmitted
4. polarized

Which of these terms would make the above statement true?

a. 1, 2, and 3
b. 1 and 3
c. 2 and 4
d. 4 only
e. all of the above

BIBLIOGRAPHY

Part 1

Buckley BM, Russell LJ: The measurement of ionised calcium in blood plasma. *Ann Clin Biochem* 25:447–465, 1988.

Fonong T, Barber T: Determination of alanine aminotransferase and aspartate aminotransferase with immobilised enzymes and electrochemical detection. *Analyst* 113:1807–1810, 1988.

Koch DD: Electrolyte technology: Current and future. *J Med Tech* 2:40–43, 1985.

Ma S-C, Ynag VC, Meyerhoff ME: Heparin-responsive electrochemical sensor: A preliminary study. *Anal Chem* 64:694–697, 1992.

Mahoney JJ, Harvey JA, Wong RJ, Van Kessel AL: Changes in oxygen measurements when whole blood is stored in iced plastic or glass syringes. *Clin Chem* 37:1244–1248, 1991.

Mascini M, Palleschi G: Design and applications of enzyme electrode probes. *Selective Electrode Rev* 11:191–264, 1989.

Miller SM, Etnyre-Zacher P: Biosensors and diagnostic testing: Enzyme electrodes. *Clin Lab Sci* 2:169–173, 1989.

Moody GJ, Thomas JDR: Amperometric biosensors: A brief appraisal of principles and applications. *Selective Electrode Rev* 13:113–124, 1991.

Moody GJ, Thomas JDR, Slater JM: Modified poly(vinyl chloride) matrix membranes for ion-selective field effect transistor sensors. *Analyst* 113:1703–1707, 1988.

National Committee for Clinical Laboratory Standards: Standardization of sodium and potassium ion-selective electrode systems to the flame photometric reference method (tentative standard). NCCLS document C29-T. Vol 12, No 21. Dec. 1992.

Pace SJ, Hamerslag JD, Thompson DR: Thick-film multilayer ion sensors for biomedical applications (abstract). *Clin Chem* 38:940, 1992.

Toffaletti J, Ernst P, Hunt P, Abrams B: Dry electrolyte-balanced heparinized syringes evaluated for determining ionized calcium and other electrolytes in whole blood. *Clin Chem* 37:1730–1733, 1991.

Wang J, Dempsey E, Ozsoz M, Smyth MR: Amperometric enzyme electrode for theophylline. *Analyst* 116:997–999, 1991.

Worth HGJ: Measurement of sodium and potassium in clinical chemistry—a review. *Analyst* 113:373–384, 1988.

Part 2

Ackerman PG: *Electronic Instrumentation in the Clinical Laboratory.* Boston, Little, Brown, 1972.

Beauchemin D, Yves Le Blanc JC, Peters GR, Craig JM: Plasma emission spectroscopy. *Analyt Chem* 62(12):443R–464R, 1992.

Bender GT: *Principles of Clinical Instrumentation.* Philadelphia, WB Saunders, 1987.

Boumans PWJM: *Inductively Coupled Plasma Emission Spectroscopy*, Part 1 and 2. New York, John Wiley, 1987.

Hicks MR, Haven MC, Schenken JR, McWhorter CA: *Laboratory Instrumentation*, 3rd ed. Philadelphia, JB Lippincott, 1987.

Kaplan LA, Pesce AJ: *Clinical Chemistry: Theory, Analysis and Correlation*, 2nd edition. St. Louis, CV Mosby, 1989.

Lee LW, Schmidt LM: *Elementary Principles of Laboratory Instruments*, 5th edition. St. Louis, CV Mosby, 1983.

Skogg DA, West DM: *Analytical Chemistry*, 3rd edition. New York, Holt, Rinehart and Winston, 1979.

Willard HH, Merritt LL, Dean JA: *Instrumental Methods of Analysis*, 5th edition. New York, D. Van Nostrand, 1974.

CHROMATOGRAPHIC THEORY
GAS CHROMATOGRAPHY
HIGH PERFORMANCE LIQUID CHROMATOGRAPHY
THIN LAYER CHROMATOGRAPHY

Chapter 5

CHROMATOGRAPHY INSTRUMENTATION SYSTEMS

TIMOTHY G. McMANAMON, PhD, DABCC

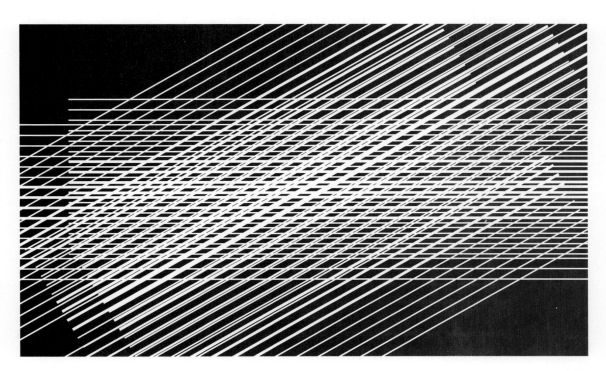

LEARNING OBJECTIVES

After studying this chapter, the student should be able to:

- Describe the fundamental processes of gas chromatography, high performance liquid chromatography, and thin layer chromatography.
- Describe the equipment used in each type of chromatography and list its function.
- Define the following terms:

  Theoretical plate
  Height equivalent of the theoretical plate
  Resolution
  Efficiency
  Retention volume
  Retention time
  Retardation factor

- Describe how quantitation is accomplished using chromatographic techniques.
- List the common clinical applications of chromatographic techniques.

KEY WORDS

Columns. The component in gas and liquid chromatography systems that houses the stationary phase, where the components are separated.

Chemical ionization. Reagent gas molecules are ionized by electrons. The ionized molecules interact with and fragment the sample molecules.

Efficiency. A mathematical concept that is determined by calculation of the height equivalent of a theoretical plate. The number generated is representative of the ability of the column to give good separation.

Electron ionization. Fragmentation of sample molecules by striking them with electrons.

Flame ionization detector (FID). A detector used in gas chromatographic systems, based on the principle that organic compounds are ionized in a flame; electrons are released and migrate to a detector, producing an electrical current that is amplified and measured.

Gas chromatography. A chromatographic system in which the mobile phase is a gas.

Gradient elution. A chromatographic technique in which the solvent composition of the mobile phase is varied throughout the analysis. The technique is used to change the polarity of the mobile phase while the analyte is eluting and helps improve the separation.

High performance liquid chromatography (HPLC). A modified liquid chromatography system that utilizes narrow, rigid columns with chemicals containing different functional groups that are bonded to a silica column to alter polarity.

Mobile phase. The solvent gas used in a chromatographic system that serves as the carrier of the compound through a column, i.e., through the stationary phase.

Normal phase. A chromatographic separation with a nonpolar mobile phase and a polar stationary phase.

Peak height ratio. The peak height of the analyte of interest divided by the peak height of the internal standard.

Peak resolution (R$_s$). The extent to which two peaks are separated in a chromatographic system; calculated by

$$R_s = \frac{2(t_B - t_A)}{W_A + W_B}$$

Quadripole mass filter. A mass analyzer that separates ions based on their movement through a field. The quadripole, four rods in a rectangular configuration, uses radio frequency in an electronic field.

Retardation factor (R$_f$). A measure of the relative distance a compound moves in a thin-layer chromatographic system. It is calculated by dividing the distance the analyte moved from the point of application by the distance the solvent moved from the point of application.

Retention time (t_R). The time it takes for a retained compound to elute from a chromatographic system.

Retention volume (v_R). The volume it takes for a retained compound to elute from a chromatographic system.

Reverse phase chromatography. A chromatographic separation accomplished with a polar mobile phase and a nonpolar stationary phase.

Stationary phase. The separating material that remains in a fixed position (liquid or solid).

Thermal conductivity detector (TCD). A detector used in gas chromatography systems that utilizes the principle of changes in heat conductivity (heat conduction) of a carrier gas caused by the sample eluting.

Thin layer chromatography (TLC). A chromatographic system in which flat beds or planar supports are used as the stationary phase.

Chromatography was first used in the 1850s by Runge, who developed methods for testing dyes and bleaches by spotting the mixtures on paper and producing color separations; however, he was unable to explain the process. The Russian scientist Tswett in 1903 first explained the separations that occurred; he is considered the father of chromatography. The word chromatography comes from two Greek words, *chroma* for color and *graphein* for write. Tswett used chromatography to separate colored plant pigments on a column of chalk. He described chromatography as "a method in which the components of a mixture are separated on an absorbent column in a flowing system."[1] Table 5–1 lists the milestones in the development of modern chromatography.

Today, chromatography can be defined as a system that separates the components of a mixture by interaction with stationary and mobile phases. As the **mobile phase,** which carries the solution to be separated, passes over the **stationary phase,** the components of the mixture interact with the stationary phase. The chemical and physical properties of the individual components determine their relative affinity for the stationary phase. Components of the solution

TABLE 5–1. MILESTONES IN THE DEVELOPMENT OF THE SCIENCE OF CHROMATOGRAPHY

1903	Chromatography explained by Tswett
1930s	Thin layer and ion exchange chromatography came into use
1940s	Development of partition chromatography and paper chromatography
1950s	Development of gas chromatography
1970s	Development of high performance liquid chromatography

with little or no affinity for the stationary phase move through the system quickly and are separated from the components that have greater affinity for the stationary phase. The components with greater affinity interact more with the stationary phase; therefore, they move through the system at a slower rate, separating them from the other components.

Modern chromatography can be divided into two broad classes: column and thin layer chromatography. In **column** chromatography, the stationary phase is contained within a column. The components are separated from each other as the mobile phase, either a liquid or a gas, carries the mixture through the column. The separated components are detected as they elute from the column. The stationary phase can be a liquid supported by a porous inert material or a liquid bound to the inner walls of a column, a porous adsorptive, or inert solid that has been packed into a column, an ion exchange resin, or a gel. The movement of the mobile phase through the column can be simply under the influence of gravity, in which a straight column is used and the mobile phase percolates from the top to the bottom of the column.

In **high performance liquid chromatography (HPLC),** the liquid mobile phase is pumped through the column under pressure, whereas in **gas chromatography** (GC) the gas pressure moves the gaseous mobile phase through the column. In **thin layer chromatography,** the stationary phase is a flat surface, and the mobile phase moves up the surface by diffusion, carrying the solution of interest, which is separated as the solvent front moves up the plate.

CHROMATOGRAPHIC THEORY

Figure 5–1 diagrams the chromatographic separation of a mixture made up of two com-

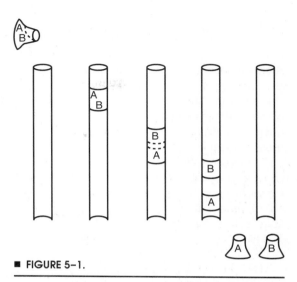

■ **FIGURE 5–1.**

Separation of components A and B on a packed column.

ponents, *A* and *B*. As the mobile phase moves *A* and *B* down the column, the components equilibrate between the mobile phase and the stationary phase. This equilibration is the same process that occurs in a separatory funnel when a substance partitions between the two liquids. In a separatory funnel, one equilibrium occurs; however, in a chromatographic system, many equilibrations take place as the components move down the column. This equilibrium, or partitioning, can be expressed mathematically as follows:

$$Dm = \frac{\text{amount of solute in the stationary phase}}{\text{amount of solute in the mobile phase}}$$

or

$$Dc = \frac{\text{concentration of solute in the stationary phase}}{\text{concentration of solute in the mobile phase}}$$

where Dm is the mass distribution ratio and Dc is the concentration distribution ratio. If *A* and *B* have different Dm or Dc values, the two components will be separated by the time they reach the end of the column.

The components are detected eluting from the end of the column by a chemical or physical process, and the bands are recorded on a chromatograph, as shown in Figure 5–2. Since the components are in a band within the column, the amount of the component eluting at a given time is a gaussian distribution, resulting in an elution curve commonly termed a *chromatographic peak*.

The volume of mobile phase that passes through the column from the introduction of the solute until the band emerges from the column is called the **retention volume** (v_R). In dealing with a chromatogram, as in Figure 5–2, it is more convenient to refer to the **retention time** (t_R) than to the retention volume, because the chart speed is known and the time is easy to calculate. The retention volume can be calculated by multiplying the retention time by the flow rate of the mobile phase.

As noted earlier, a solute undergoes a large number of equilibrations as it moves through the column. Each of these equilibrations is called a *theoretical plate*. This terminology is borrowed from fractional distillation, in which the number of plates is a measure of the system's ability to separate components with different boiling points. The separating ability of a chromatographic

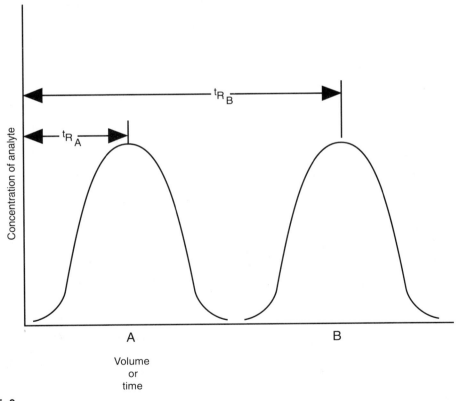

■ **FIGURE 5–2.**

Chromatographic elution curve for the complete separation of components A and B. The retention time is indicated by t.

system is also described in terms of theoretical plates. In a chromatographic system, the number of theoretical plates, n, is calcuted using the following formula:

$$n = 16\left(\frac{v_R}{W}\right)^2 = 16\left(\frac{t_R}{W}\right)^2$$

where v_R and t_R are the retention volume and retention time, respectively, and W is the width of the peak at the baseline. The units of W must match the units of the numerator when calculating theoretical plates. As the length of a chromatographic column increases, more theoretical plates are possible; therefore, n increases with column length.

The **efficiency** of a chromatographic system can be determined from the *height equivalent of a theoretical plate,* abbreviated HETP or h. This is calculated by dividing the length of the column (L) by the number of theoretical plates (n).

$$h = \frac{L}{n}$$

The lower the value of h, the better the column efficiency and the better the separation. Typically, values of h are in the range of 1 mm.

Two bands may not be completely separated before emerging from the column, and the two peaks overlap on the chromatogram, as illustrated in Figure 5–3. The extent to which these two peaks are separated is the

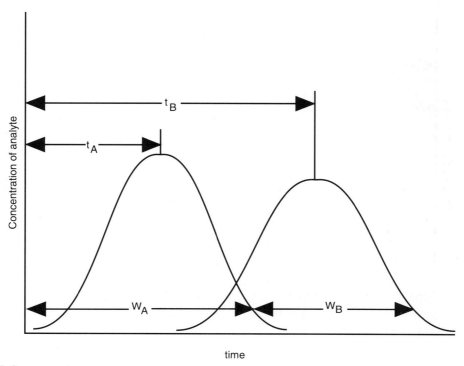

■ **FIGURE 5–3.**

Chromatographic elution curve for the incomplete separation of components A and B. The peak width is indicated by W_A and W_B.

peak resolution, R_s, which is calculated from the following formula:

$$R_s = \frac{2(t_B - t_A)}{W_A + W_B}$$

where t_B and t_A are the retention times of the two overlapping peaks, and W_A and W_B are the widths of the two peaks at the baseline. An R_s of 1.0 indicates an area of overlap of approximately 2 percent, whereas an R_s of 1.5 or more indicates an overlap of less than 0.1 percent.

Column chromatographic methods can be used for both qualitative and quantitative analysis. Qualitative analysis is accomplished by comparing the retention time of the unknown to the retention time of known standards that have been analyzed on the same system. When conducting a qualitative analysis, it is important to remember that compounds can co-migrate, thus two compounds can have the same retention time. To prevent an erroneous identification, an interference study should be conducted to identify compounds that co-migrate with the compound of interest.

Quantitative analysis is conducted with the use of an internal standard, which is a compound with chemical and physical properties similar to the analyte compound. A constant volume of the internal standard is added to the patient sample, as well as to the standards and controls, before any sample preparation is performed. Any variations or inconsistencies that occur to a given standard or sample during the preparation and chromatographic separation are corrected for by the internal standard. The area under a chromatographic peak is related to the amount of the compound present, and, therefore, is an indication of the concentration in the original patient sample. In the laboratory, the peak height is used for determining the concentration rather than the area, because it can be measured easily with a ruler, although most modern chromatographic systems include a computerized integrator that can determine either peak area or peak height as well as retention time.

To determine the concentration of the compound of interest in the patient sample, a set of standards of known concentration is analyzed to generate a standard curve (Fig. 5–4). For each of the standards, a **peak height ratio** is calculated by dividing the peak height of the analyte of interest by the peak height of the internal standard. The peak height ratios are then graphed against the standard concentrations. By calculating the peak height ratios for the controls and patient samples, the unknown concentrations can be determined from the standard curve.

Another approach is to determine a factor for each of the standards by dividing the peak height ratio by the standard concen-

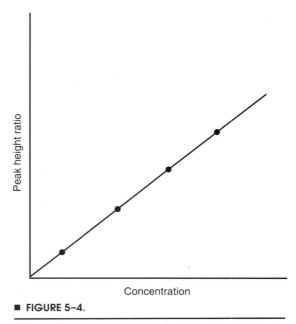

■ **FIGURE 5–4.**

Calibration curve relating concentration to peak height ratio.

tration. The peak height ratios of the controls and the patient samples are divided by the average factor to determine the unknown concentration. Many computerized integrators determine the concentration of the unknowns from the standard data. In any chromatographic system, it is best if a minimum of three standards are included in each day's analysis.

GAS CHROMATOGRAPHY

A gas chromatograph, as diagrammed in Figure 5–5, is made up of three main components: the injector, the oven that holds the column, and a detector. The injector (Fig. 5–6) provides a means to introduce the sample onto the column and is basically a tube that fits onto the head of the column. At the top of the injector is a self-sealing silicone rubber septum that can be pierced with a needle to inject the sample onto the column. Once the needle is pulled out, the septum seals the hole, preventing gas from escaping from the column through the injector.

The injection can be accomplished in one of two ways: either manually with a syringe or automatically with an autosampler. The manual method requires a glass syringe with a very fine needle. Injection volumes are in the order of 1 microliter; therefore, great care must be taken when drawing up the solution to be injected. Air bubbles within the sample would alter the volume being injected and could cause interference with the chromatography. Because of the inherent variability associated with using a syringe, it is imperative that an internal standard be used in any procedure involving manual injections.

When an autosampler is used, the samples are placed in small vials and sealed with a septum. The vials are placed on the autosampler and the needle of the autosampler goes into the vial and removes the programmed volume of liquid. The needle moves to the injection port of the gas chromatograph and precisely injects the sample

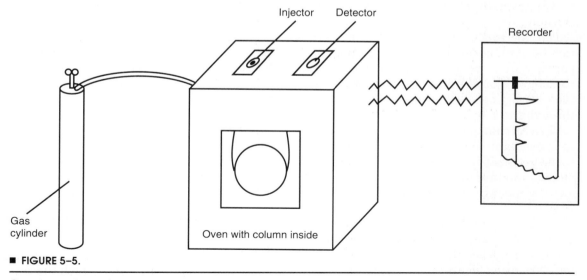

■ **FIGURE 5–5.**

Gas chromatograph.

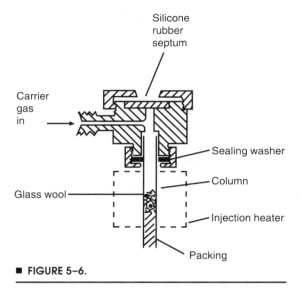

■ **FIGURE 5–6.**

Diagram of an injector for gas chromatography. (From Willett JE: *Gas Chromatography*. Chichester, England, John Wiley and Sons, 1987, p 20.)

onto the column. The advantages of an autosampler over a manual syringe are a significant decrease in the variability of volumes injected onto the column and the ability to load the autosampler and walk away, thus reducing the labor component of the analysis.

The injector is maintained at a temperature above that of the oven in order to vaporize the analyte solution immediately; therefore, a gaseous sample is introduced to the carrier gas, which carries the sample through the column.

The chromatographic column is contained in a constant temperature oven. The temperature must be high enough to keep the analyte mixture in the gaseous state but below the point at which the column packing would break down. The higher the temperature, the faster the components will move through the column. Lowering the temperature will lengthen the retention time, allowing for more complete separation of the bands and better resolution. Fluctuations in

the oven temperature can cause variations in the retention time of the components, making the identification and quantitation difficult if not impossible.

Some analyses use *temperature programming* to improve the separation. In temperature programming, the mixture is injected onto the column at an oven temperature slightly below the boiling point of the component of interest, allowing the higher boiling, potentially interfering components to elute first. After a defined time interval, the oven temperature is raised at a constant linear rate to a temperature above the boiling point of the components of interest, which allows better resolution of the peaks of interest.

The column traditionally was made of a glass tube 4 mm in diameter and approximately 1.5 meters long, which was coiled to fit into the oven. Many columns are still made of glass, but stainless steel is also popular. One end of the column is attached to the injector and the other to the detector. The mobile phase, known in gas chromatography as the *carrier gas,* flows through the column at a pressure of approximately 40 psi. The two most common carrier gases are helium and nitrogen, although argon, hydrogen, and carbon dioxide have been used. The column is filled with the stationary phase, often called the *column packing*. This packing is a finely divided solid that is either an adsorbent itself or is coated with a thin film of a nonvolatile liquid. Packed columns are still used today.

Another type of column in wide use today is the *open tubular column,* more commonly known as a *capillary column* because of the small diameter, typically ranging from 0.1 to 0.5 mm internal diameter. These columns are made of quartz or fused silica. The stationary phase is attached to the walls of the column, leaving an open lumen through the middle of the column through which the carrier gas passes. Capillary columns range in length from 15 meters to as long as 100 meters. The liquid stationary phase can be coated onto the smooth inner walls of the column or can be coated onto a thin layer of small support particles attached to the inner wall of the column. The long length of the column and the straight path of the carrier gas through the column results in much better resolution than is attainable with a packed column (Fig. 5–7).

The stationary phase for either type of column can be a liquid or a solid. The liquid stationary phase must be nonvolatile, thermally stable, and chemically unreactive. Separation with a liquid stationary phase is based on the volatility and solubility of the components being separated. Solid stationary phases are made of alumina, carbon black, silica gel, zeolite, or porous polymers. With the solid phases, separation is based on the differential adsorptivity of the components with the stationary phase.

Once the components of the injected mixture have passed through the column, the detector measures their presence. Detectors measure physical rather than chemical properties of the components because it is easier to turn a physical property into an electrical signal. Several types of detectors are available, from the simple **thermal conductivity detector (TCD)** to the sophisticated mass spectrophotometric (MS) detectors.

The TCD detector utilizes a *Wheatstone bridge* (Fig. 5–8), employing the property that the heat loss from a wire in a constant stream of gas is related to the thermal conductivity of the gas. Two arms of the Wheatstone bridge are made of wire, which is heated. One of the heated arms is in a stream of pure carrier gas while the other is in the effluent stream from the column. When a component elutes from the column, the thermal conductivity of the gas decreases; therefore, the rate of heat loss from the wire increases. This increase in heat

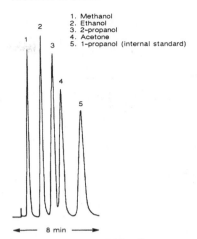

Alcohols in Blood

1. Methanol
2. Ethanol
3. 2-propanol
4. Acetone
5. 1-propanol (internal standard)

← 8 min →

Column:	Porapak Q and R 1:1, (80/100 mesh) 6 ft x 1/8 in. ss
Carrier:	μ (He) = 30 ml/min
Oven:	150°C
Injection:	0.16% v/v of each component in water
Detector:	FID

Serum Drug Screen

1. Ethclorvynol
2. Methyprylon
3. Butalbital
4. Amobarbital
5. Pentobarbital
6. Secobarbital
7. Glutethimide
8. Phenobarbital
9. Methaqualone
10. Amitriptyline
11. Imipramine
12. Cyheptamide (ISTD)
13. Phenytoin
14. Diazepam

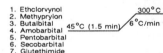

45°C (1.5 min) → 6°C/min → 300°C

← 22 min →

Column:	Ultra 2 (Cross-Linked 5% Phenyl Methyl Silicone) 50 m x 0.32 mm x 0.52 μm film (HP Part No. 19091B-115)
Carrier:	μ (H₂) = 80 cm/sec
Oven:	Temperature program listed above
Injection:	1 μl, splitless
Detector:	FID

■ **FIGURE 5–7.**

Comparison of a GC chromatographic using a packed column (top) and a capillary column (bottom). (Courtesy of Hewlett Packard Company, Avondale, PA, 1990.)

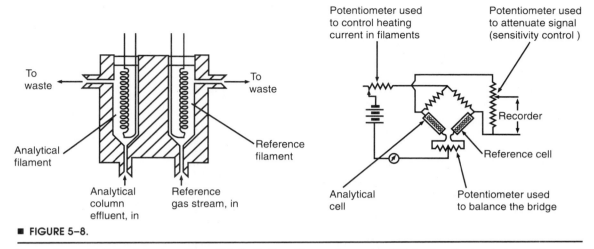

■ **FIGURE 5-8.**

Thermal conductivity detector. (From Willett JE: *Gas Chromatography.* Chichester, England, John Wiley and Sons, 1987, p 28.)

loss causes an imbalance in the Wheatstone bridge. The recorder measures the amount of resistance needed to bring the bridge back into balance, which is recorded on the strip chart as a chromatogram.

The **flame ionization detector (FID)** (Fig. 5–9) is the universal detector for organic compounds. Hydrogen is mixed with the carrier gas, which is usually helium, and the mixed gases are burned in air supplied from an external source. Analyte molecules eluting from the column are burned in the flame and produce electrons. The electrons migrate to electrodes in the detector, producing an electrical current that is amplified and measured. The current produced is proportional to the carbon content of the organic molecules entering the flame from the column. Like the TCD detector, the FID is inexpensive to purchase and operate. The FID must be kept clean, which is a relatively simple procedure.

The detectors discussed thus far tell only when a component elutes from the column and how much is present. The mass spectral detector (MS), in addition to when and how much, also provides information on the chemical structure of the eluting compound. When the effluent enters the MS, it is ionized, breaking it down into its molecular components, called fragments. These fragments are then separated according to their molecular weight and detected. The molecular weight of the fragment is graphed against the relative abundance present to produce a mass spectrum of the compound, which can be interpreted and the compound identified.

The ionization is accomplished in one of two ways: either **electron or chemical ionization.** In electron ionization, the effluent enters a chamber maintained at very low pressure, typically 10^{-8} torr. Electrons that collide with the analyte molecules are passed through the chamber. These electrons have sufficient energy to break all the bonds in the molecule. When a molecule is bombarded with these electrons, it will fragment in a reproducible pattern. Chemical ionization utilizes a high pressure environment, typically 1 torr, to which a reagent gas is introduced. The electrons ionize the

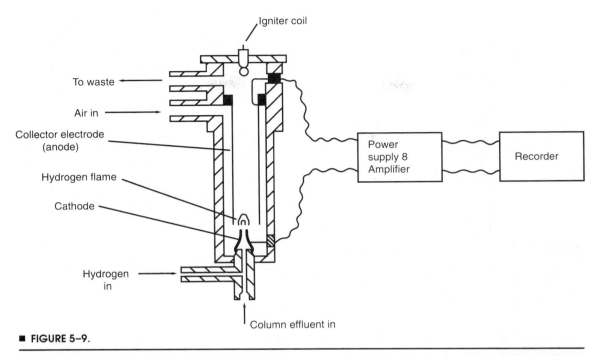

Igniter coil

To waste

Air in

Collector electrode
(anode)

Hydrogen flame

Cathode

Hydrogen
in

Column effluent in

Power
supply 8
Amplifier

Recorder

■ **FIGURE 5–9.**

Flame ionization detector. (From Willett JE: *Gas Chromatography*. Chichester, England, John Wiley and Sons, 1987, p 35.)

reagent gas molecules, which interact with the effluent molecules and cause fragmentation. With chemical ionization, more molecules remain intact, which provides more information concerning the molecular weight of the compound.

The fragments are drawn into the separation portion of the mass spectrophotometer. The most commonly used separating device is the **quadripole mass filter** (Fig. 5–10), which is made up of four rods (poles) surrounding the path of the fragmented ions. Both radio frequency and direct current are passed between the rods. Fragments with energy levels identical to the frequency and current travel through the filter, emerging from the far end of the quadripoles. If the frequency and current do not match the energy level of the fragments, the fragment will not maintain a straight flight

path but will crash into the poles and be neutralized. By varying the frequency and current, the fragments can be separated based on their mass-to-charge ratio, which for practical purposes is the molecular weight of the fragments. A detector at the end of the quadripole collects the fragments and converts them into an electrical signal that is amplified and processed by the computer.

The mass spectrophotometer can be operated in one of two modes. In the *scan mode* (Fig. 5–11), the frequency and current are varied over the entire range of energies (i.e., molecular weights) to determine the total mass spectrum of the eluting compound. Using a computerized library, the identity of an unknown compound can be determined by comparison with spectra of known compounds.

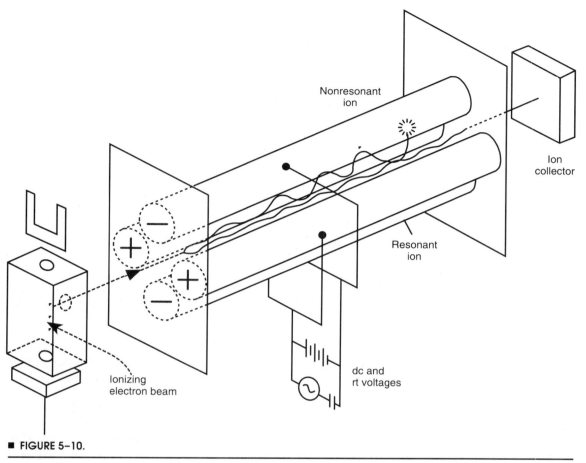

Nonresonant
ion

Ion
collector

Resonant
ion

dc and
rt voltages

Ionizing
electron beam

■ **FIGURE 5–10.**

Ionization chamber and quadripole mass filter from a mass spectrophotometer. (From Willard HH, Merrit LL, Dean JA: *Instrumental Methods of Analysis*, 5th ed. New York, D. Van Nostrand Company, 1974, p 476.)

The *single ion monitoring (SIM) mode* is used when testing for a known analyte, such as a drug in a urine sample. In the SIM mode, the frequencies and currents are set to monitor only one to three of the major fragments known to exist in the compound of interest; therefore, the signal occurs only when the compound of interest has passed through the mass spectrophotometer. The SIM mode can be used for quantitative analysis. The internal standard is a deuterated or tritiated form of the compound of interest that will chromatographically co-elute with the analyte. Because of the deuterium or tritium, the molecular weight of the internal standard fragments is 1 or 2 mass units higher than the analyte fragments. The mass spectrophotometer can monitor the specific energies for the analyte and for the internal standard, yielding abundant information for both. The ratio of analyte peak to internal standard peak is used to calculate the concentration in the original sample.

Gas chromatography is used in the clinical laboratory mainly in the area of toxicology. Gas chromatography with FID is exten-

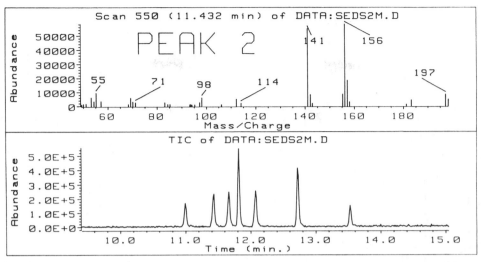

■ **FIGURE 5–11.**

Gas chromatographic—mass spectrophotometric scan. (Courtesy of Hewlett Packard Company, Avondale, PA, 1990.)

sively used as the instrument for measuring alcohol in body fluids. The alcohol analysis can be conducted in one of two ways. The sample can be directly injected onto the column; however, the large number of other compounds in biologic fluids can interfere with the chromatography and lead to shortened column life because of contamination. The other way to perform this analysis is by using *head space GC,* which is accomplished by placing the sample in an autosampler vial and sealing the vial. The vial is placed in an autosampler equipped with an incubator. The sample is warmed to volatilize the alcohol. An equilibrium is formed between the gaseous alcohol in the air space above the sample—i.e., the head space and the sample. After sufficient time for the equilibration to occur, the needle of the autosampler removes a portion of the head space gas and injects it onto the column. The head space technique eliminates the nonvolatile components of the sample before injection; therefore, a cleaner chromatogram

is obtained, and the column life is extended because the contamination is nearly eliminated.

Gas chromatography with MS detection is the definitive method of drug testing because of the high specificity. Any positive drug screen that needs to undergo judicial scrutiny must be confirmed by GC-MS. A disadvantage of GC is that the analyte species must be volatile to be analyzed. Most drugs, however, are not volatile; therefore, they must be made volatile by being extracted from the sample and chemically altered to make the compound volatile. The alteration called derivatization is accomplished by chemically adding or changing a functional group on the drug molecule to create a volatile compound.

HIGH PERFORMANCE LIQUID CHROMATOGRAPHY

High performance liquid chromatography (HPLC) was developed to maximize the performance of liquid chromatography, which until the advent of HPLC had been done in columns that relied on gravity for moving the mobile phase. The knowledge gained in the development of GC was combined with the knowledge of liquid chromatography to produce the high performance liquid chromatograph, which is diagrammed in Figure 5–12. The HPLC is made up of an injector, a pump to move the mobile phase through the column at high pressure, a column, and a detector.

In classic column chromatography, the stationary phase was made of a polar substance, such as silica, and the mobile phase was made of a nonpolar solution. The combination of polar stationary phase and nonpolar mobile phase is referred to as the **normal phase.** In HPLC columns, chemicals with different functional groups are bonded to the silica to alter the polarity. Long carbon chain molecules are often used in this process, with an 18-carbon chain being the most common. These bonded columns are referred to by their carbon number; therefore, the 18-carbon chain is called a C-18 column. The attachment of the carbon chains yields a stationary phase that is nonpolar; therefore, the mobile phase must be polar. This combination is called **reverse phase chromatography.**

In gas chromatography, the analyte molecules interact only with the stationary phase and are simply carried along by the mobile gas phase. In HPLC, however, the analyte molecules interact with both phases. A partition occurs between the two phases, based on the polarity of the phases and the analyte molecules. Recalling that like dissolves like, nonpolar molecules partition into the stationary phase; therefore, their movement through the column will be slowed while polar molecules will remain in the mobile phase and elute from the column first. The mobile phase can be an aqueous-organic mixture, a buffer solution, or a mixture of organic solvents.

Gradient elution is used in HPLC for the same purposes as temperature programming is used in GC. In gradient elution, the solvents in the mobile phase are not premixed but are mixed by a solvent handling system that varies the proportions of each solvent in the mobile phase throughout the analysis. By changing the proportions of the solvents, the polarity of the mobile phase is changed; therefore, altering the partitions occurring within the column often can improve the separation.

The mobile phase moves through the column under pressure produced by the pump. The pressure that develops is dependent on

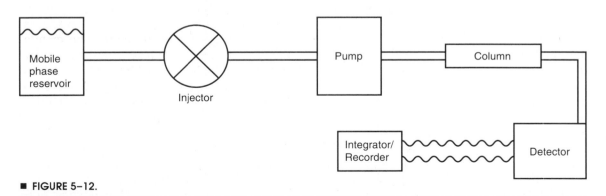

■ **FIGURE 5–12.**

Diagram of a high performance liquid chromatograph.

the length of the column, the particle size of the stationary phase, the viscosity of the mobile phase, and the flow rate of the mobile phase.[2] Typically, an HPLC operates at a pressure of 350 to 1500 psi and a flow rate of 1 to 5 mL per minute.

The sample is introduced into the column through an injector. The typical injector is a mechanical device with load and inject positions. While set in the load position, a sample loop in the injector is filled using a syringe. When the injector is moved to the load position, the mobile phase flows through the sample loop and carries the sample onto the column.

HPLC columns, made of stainless steel, have a typical internal diameter of 4.5 mm and are up to 25 cm long. These columns are packed with modified silica particles that have diameters of 3, 5, or 10 μm.

The most common detector used in HPLC is a spectrophotometer. The effluent from the column passes through a flow cell in the spectrophotometer. A wavelength is selected at which the compounds of interest absorb. A common wavelength is 254 nm, because all aromatic compounds and many other organic compounds absorb at this wavelength. Some detectors have a fixed wavelength, but more commonly variable wavelength detectors that cover the visible and ultraviolet spectrum are used. When a compound elutes from the column into the flow cell, an absorbance change is recorded as a chromatographic peak. The spectrophotometer functions as a selective detector because compounds that elute from the column but do not absorb at the chosen wavelength are not detected. Mass spectrophotometric detectors are available for use with HPLC but have not found wide application in the clinical laboratory.

HPLC is still used in the clinical laboratory in the area of therapeutic drug monitoring (TDM) and endocrine testing, although most of these tests are now performed by immunoassay techniques. An advantage of HPLC over immunoassays is its ability to monitor more than one drug or metabolite in one analysis. The disadvantages include the length of time required to perform the analysis; the requirement that the compound be soluble, which in clinical testing is not usually a concern but can be overcome by derivatization, expensive equipment, and the need for highly trained and skilled technologists.

THIN LAYER CHROMATOGRAPHY

The role of thin layer chromatography (TLC) in the clinical laboratory must not be overlooked. Thin layer chromatography still has wide applications in drug testing and fetal lung maturity testing.

The stationary phase is coated in a thin layer onto a glass or plastic plate. The extracted sample, along with standards of the analytes of interest, is applied to the bottom of the plate. The plate is placed in a jar that has a small amount of mobile phase in the bottom. Only a small portion of the bottom of the plate near the point of application is immersed in the liquid. The mobile phase diffuses up the plate, carrying the applied sample with it. As the solvent front moves up the plate, the compounds contained in the sample are separated. The plate is removed from the jar when the solvent front approaches the top of the plate. The mobile phase is evaporated off the plate, and the plate is treated chemically or physically to visualize the separated compounds, which can be identified by comparison with standard spots analyzed on the same plate. To determine that a spot is consistent with the standard, the spot must match the standard in position, size, and color. A great deal of expertise is required to interpret TLC plates.

In GC and HPLC, compounds are compared based on retention volume or time. In TLC, neither volume nor time are factors; therefore, the distance the compound travels up the plate is used to compare compounds. This distance is called the **retardation factor,** or R_f, which is calculated by dividing the distance a compound moved from its origin by the total distance the solvent front moved.

SUMMARY

Chromatographic techniques remain an important part of the clinical laboratory because of their ability to separate compounds for specific identification and sensitive quantitation. Chromatographic techniques have several disadvantages, including lengthy sample preparation and analysis times, and they require highly skilled technologists, but these drawbacks are countered by the amount of information a chromatographic technique provides and by its flexibility to adapt to the analysis of different compounds. The modern clinical laboratory has entered an era in which purchased kits are used for most analyses; however, with chromatography, clinical laboratory scientists at the bench can still develop a procedure from start to finish and implement it within their laboratory.

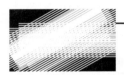

REVIEW QUESTIONS

Choose the best answer.

1. Reverse phase chromatography refers to chromatography in which

   a. cations are exchanged.
   b. the mobile phase is polar and the stationary phase is nonpolar.
   c. the stationary phase is polar and the mobile phase is nonpolar.
   d. the least polar solute elutes first.

2. A chromatographic technique in which various solvents are introduced into the mobile phase as the compound elutes through the system

   a. causes changes in the polarity of the mobile phase.
   b. promotes improved separation of compounds.
   c. is known as gradient elution.
   d. all the above are correct.

3. All the following are characteristic of gas chromatography except:

   a. Lowering the temperature of the oven will lengthen the retention time.
   b. Resolution improves as the column length increases.
   c. Separation depends on both solubility and volatility of the compound.

d. The flame ionization detector is the detector of choice for all compounds separated by GC.

4. A quadripole is found in which of the following detectors?

   a. Electron capture.
   b. Mass spectrophotometry.
   c. Thermal conductivity.
   d. Flame ionization.

5. The major advantage of HPLC over immunoassay techniques is

   a. length of analysis.
   b. ability to measure multiple drugs in one analysis.
   c. need for highly trained and skilled technologists.
   d. all of the above.

6. The retardation factor (R_f) is calculated by

   a. the ratio of the distance the compound moves divided by the distance the standard moves.
   b. the ratio of the distance the compound moves divided by the total distance the solvent moves.

c. the ratio of the distance the solvent moves divided by the distance traveled by the compound.
d. the ratio of the distance the standard moves divided by the distance the solvent moves.

REFERENCES

1. Braithwaite A, Smith FJ: *Chromatographic Methods,* 4th edition. London, Chapman and Hall Ltd, 1985.
2. Lindsay S: *High Performance Liquid Chromatography.* Chichester, England, John Wiley and Sons, 1987.

BIBLIOGRAPHY

Fritz JS, Schenk GH: *Quantitative Analytical Chemistry,* 4th edition. Boston, Allyn and Bacon, 1979, pp 347–395.
Jonsson JA: Common concepts of chromatography. *In Chromatographic Theory and Basic Principles.* New York, Marcel Dekker, 1987.
Karasek FW, Clement RE: *Basic Gas Chromatography—Mass Spectrometry: Principles and Techniques.* New York, Elsevier Publishing Company, 1988.
Willard HH, Merrit LL, Dean JA: *Instrumental Methods of Analysis,* 5th edition. New York, D. Van Nostrand Company, 1974, pp 455–495, 522–560.
Willett JE: *Gas Chromatography.* Chichester, England, John Wiley and Sons, 1987.

Chapter 6

ELECTROPHORETIC INSTRUMENTATION SYSTEMS

JAMES E. LOVE, JR., PhD, MBA
KORY M. WARD, PhD, MT(ASCP)

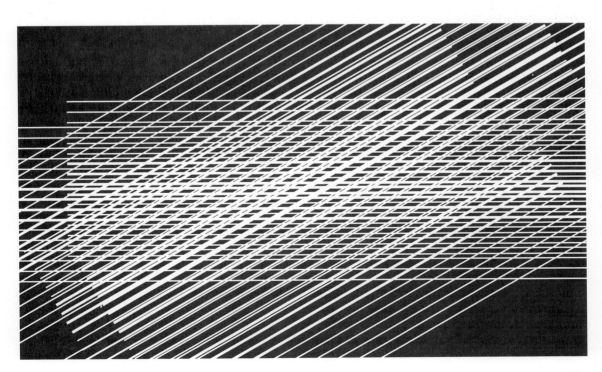

LEARNING OBJECTIVES

After studying this chapter, the student should be able to:

- Describe the function of each component of an electrophoresis system.
- List some important features to be considered in selecting a densitometer.
- State at least three possible causes of distorted band patterns and their corrective actions.
- Identify at least one stain application for each electrophoresis.
- Describe the principles involved in at least two enhanced or newly developed electrophoretic techniques.
- Summarize the advantages of automation of electrophoresis.

KEY WORDS

Ampholytes. Low molecular weight (300 to 1000 daltons) amphoteric polyaminocarboxylic acids used in isoelectric focusing electrophoresis to create stable pH zones.

Appraise. A densitometer manufactured by Beckman Instruments, Inc., Brea, California.

Automatic indexing. A feature on a densitometer that automatically advances the electrophoresis strip, which contains multiple sample channels, from one channel to the next.

Capillary zone electrophoresis. Also referred to as capillary electrophoresis (CE) or high performance capillary electrophoresis (HPCE), this analytic technique combines high performance liquid chromatography and conventional electrophoresis in a single system.

Cathode. The negatively charged pole that attracts more cationic proteins.

Delimiting. A feature in automated electrophoretic systems that allows for deletion, or suppression fractions, and adjustment of the scanned baselines or slopes.

Densitometer. A modified spectrophotometer that determines the intensity of each band of an electrophoretogram.

Electroosmotic flow. A bulk flow of fluid resulting from excess of positively charged ions in the direction toward the cathode that enhances the separation of the charged ions.

Endosmosis (electroendosmosis). The slowing, retardation, or reversal of protein migration when the support medium becomes negatively charged because of the adsorption of hydroxyl ions from the buffer.

High resolution protein electrophoresis. An electrophoresis technique that employs a specialized agarose gel (low content of sulfate and carboxyl groups) under high voltage to achieve greater specificity in protein separation.

Isoelectric focusing electrophoresis (IFE). A high resolution electrophoresis technique in which proteins migrate through a pH gradient, with the aid of ampholytes, to their respective isoelectric points (pls).

Paragon. An electrophoresis system manufactured by Beckman Instruments, Inc., Brea, California.

REP. An electrophoresis and densitometry system manufactured by Helena Laboratories, Beaumont, Texas.

Two-Dimensional (2D) electrophoresis. An electrophoretic process that applies a two-stage approach to separation of proteins. Separation is accomplished first based on charge and then upon molecular mass.

Wick flow. The upward movement of buffer through both immersed ends of a membrane to replace lost moisture. This phenomenon can reduce separation and lead to compression of the final band patterns.

INTRODUCTION

Electrophoresis is one of the most powerful tools available for the separation and quantitation of macromolecules. In the clinical laboratory, it is essentially used to separate proteins, isoenzymes, lipoproteins, and hemoglobins in various body fluids.

Early uses of this technique began with the study of colloidal proteins placed in a U-shaped tube into which buffer was added. When electrical current was applied, the proteins moved at different rates into the vertical arms of the tube, forming refractable boundaries, hence the term *moving boundary technique*. The later use of filter paper and starch gel as support mediums and the resulting distinct and stable separations found in zone electrophoresis increased the application of this technique.

With the advent of improved support mediums, buffers, and automation, electrophoresis has evolved from a strictly research commodity to an extremely versatile and useful approach to clinical problems. Today, it represents one of the most innovative and growing methods of analysis. Its promise and potential are still unfolding.

This chapter explains the basic principles of electrophoresis, followed by a discussion of each of its major components. Common problems in electrophoretic methods and possible solutions are discussed, ending with descriptions of the latest improved or new techniques and some of the more advanced state-of-the-art systems.

BASIC PRINCIPLES OF ELECTROPHORESIS

. . . In Theory

Charged particles in a support medium will migrate toward the electrode with the opposite charge when an electric field is applied. Particles carrying a positive charge will migrate toward the cathode (negative electrode), and particles carrying a negative charge will migrate toward the anode (positive electrode). Since many organic molecules are amphoteric (can be either positively or negatively charged), their charge in solution and the magnitude of the charge can be altered by varying the pH. Amphoteric molecules such as proteins will have a net positive charge if the pH of the solution is below the protein's isoelectric point, at which the net molecular charge is zero. Above the isoelectric point, the protein will have a net negative charge.

The mobility, or rate of migration, is influenced by a number of factors: (1) *Migration of the charge.* The greater the net charge, the more swiftly the molecule will move. (2) *Size of the molecule.* Larger molecules tend to move more slowly. (3) *Properties of the support medium.* Support medium with small pores will act as a molecular sieve and separate particles not only by charge but also by size. Increased viscosity of medium retards mobility as well as the degree of adsorption. (4) *Strength of the electric field.* The greater the voltage, the more rapid the migration. (5) *Endosmosis.* A special property of the support medium that results in a flow of solute and solvent particles against the flow of the separating molecules. This phenomenon will be discussed later in greater detail. (6) *Ionic strength of the buffer.* Lower ionic strength buffers favor more rapid migration. (7) *Temperature.* Increasing the temperature will increase the rate of migration.

Many of the factors that affect migration are highly interrelated and can be expressed mathematically. The driving force, F (in newtons), exerted upon a molecule of net charge, q (in coulombs), when placed in an electric field is given by:

$$F = \frac{E}{d} q \qquad (1)$$

where E is the applied electromotive force in volts per meter, and d is the distance in meters across the support medium through which the molecule will migrate. This force, however, is opposed by a friction, or resistance, that is characteristic of the solution in which migration occurs. The opposing force, F′, expressed by Stokes' law,

$$F' = 6\pi r \eta \upsilon \qquad (2)$$

where F′ is the counterforce, r is the radius in meters of the migrating molecule, η is the solution viscosity in newtons-seconds per square meter, and υ is the velocity of the migrating molecule in meters per second. At constant velocity, F′ counteracts F, such that

$$\frac{E}{d} q = 6\pi r \eta \upsilon \qquad (3)$$

By rearranging equation 3,

$$\upsilon = \frac{Eq}{d6\pi r \eta} \qquad (4)$$

it can be seen that the velocity is directly proportional to the voltage and net charge but inversely proportional to the size of the molecule and solution viscosity.

Another mathematical expression of migration defines electrophoretic mobility, m, as the distance, d, travelled by a molecule in time, t, under applied electromotive force, E, such that

$$m = \frac{d}{tE} \quad \text{or} \quad m = \frac{\upsilon}{E} \qquad (5)$$

As this expression might suggest, a molecule will travel the same distance in half the time by doubling the voltage. Owing to the influence of other factors, this is only partly true. Volts multiplied by time, however, can provide a rough estimate of how changing these factors will affect the migration.

Both the pitfalls and promise of electrophoresis rest in an understanding and manipulation of the factors that affect migration. For example, increasing the ionic strength of the buffer may improve resolution, but the accompanying increase in temperature may denature heat-labile proteins. An increase in voltage may decrease operating time but cause increased current and heat that may distort migration patterns. The user must strike a balance among the various factors to achieve the separation desired.

. . . In Practice

As shown in Figure 6–1, a typical electrophoresis system consists of a covered chamber, support medium, buffer, power supply, and densitometer (not shown). The procedure usually begins with the preparation of reagents and filling both sides of the chamber with buffer. Support media, such as cellulose acetate, may require presoaking in the buffer solution. The medium is placed over the bridge and into the chamber so that opposite ends of the medium are in contact with the buffer. Sample is spotted onto the medium, and the power supply is turned on and adjusted to constant voltage or constant current. After a determined length of time, the medium is removed, placed in a fixative, and stained. Excess stain is removed and the medium dried. It is now ready to be scanned in a densitometer.

SYSTEM COMPONENTS

Sample

Serum and plasma are the most common biologic specimens applied to electrophore-

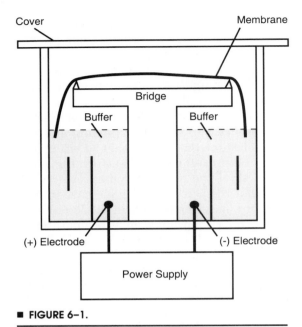

■ FIGURE 6-1.

Diagram of an electrophoresis chamber. (From Clinical Laboratory Product Comparison System: *Electrophoresis Equipment.* Plymouth Meeting, PA, Emergency Care Research Institute, April 1991, p 3. ©1991, ECRI. Duplication in whole or in part by any means or for any purpose is prohibited.)

sis in clinical applications, followed by urine and cerebrospinal fluid (CSF). Other body fluids that can provide diagnostically useful information are from the pleura, pericardium, peritoneum, and synovial membrane. Even tears may be used.

Whether a sample requires pretreatment may depend on the concentration of the molecules to be separated, possible interferents, the support medium, and the information to be collected. Fluids such as urine and CSF, which are ultrafiltrates of plasma, usually contain small quantities of proteins. These fluids may require concentration of the protein before electrophoresis. Urines may also require centrifuging or dialyzing or both to remove undesirable mineral salts, biliary salts, and pigments. If the urine will be placed on polyacrylamide gel with the addi-

tion of sodium dodecyl sulfate, a concentration step is not needed. Body fluids such as synovia may contain various substances that confer viscous properties to the sample. Viscosity can affect the separation, and several dialyses may be necessary. When the molecules of interest are insoluble or tend to aggregate, pretreatment with urea, glycerol, or a nonionic detergent may be needed.[1]

The sample is usually placed directly on the medium where it is absorbed. Commercially available media may have slots or holes for the discrete placement of the sample. The amount of sample applied may range from 0.3 to 25 µL, depending on the concentration of the analyte and the type of support medium. A tracking dye is sometimes added to the sample to indicate when the electrophoresis should be terminated. These dyes have high mobilities and migrate at a rate faster than any of the molecules to be separated. Bromphenol blue is commonly used in alkaline buffer systems, whereas methylene green or methylene blue is appropriate for acid systems.

Buffers

Buffers serve two important functions: (1) they fix and maintain a constant pH that determines the net charge on the molecules and thus the direction of migration; and (2) they conduct current.

There are a few important considerations in choosing the appropriate buffer. First, the buffer must not react with the sample. Interactions of this kind can vary the rate at which molecules of a single pure species will migrate. The result can be the artifactual appearance of two migrating species in place of one. Second, the pH chosen should charge but not denature the molecules of interest. Most clinically useful proteins are separated in an alkaline environment (pH, 8 to 9), which provides a negative charge to the molecules. Third, the ionic strength of the buffer must be considered. Buffers of low ionic strength result in faster rates of migration. As the ionic strength increases, the concentration of buffer ions surrounding the migrating molecule increases, thus slowing its movement. This hindrance produces sharper band separations. But the advantage can be offset by an increase in heat, because of the increased availability of current carrying buffer ions. This heat can denature heat-labile proteins. High ionic strength buffers can be used effectively under conditions of controlled reduced temperature.

Of the many buffers available for electrophoresis, the barbital buffers and the *tris*-boric acid–EDTA buffers are the most commonly used.

Support Media

Although electrophoresis has and can be performed in a wholly liquid support medium, the inability to stabilize and manipulate the material after separation can be a real disadvantage. Most techniques today use some form of membrane or gel.

Two major influences on the migration of molecules are associated with support media. These factors may have a bearing on which support medium to use. The two factors are **endosmosis** (also called **electroendosmosis**) and **wick flow.**

Endosmosis occurs when the support medium becomes negatively charged because of the adsorption of hydroxyl ions from the buffer. The negatively charged surface attracts positive ions from the buffer. When current is applied, the positive ions move toward the cathode, against the flow of the negatively charged molecules (e.g., proteins) moving toward the anode. Depending on the strength of the charge on the molecule and the magnitude of the endosmosis, the proteins can be slowed, remain immobile, or be pushed toward the cathode (Figure 6–2). On media such as cellulose acetate or agarose gel, certain species of globulins are swept behind the point of application. The effect of endosmosis can be reduced in agarose by the addition of sucrose or sorbitol, which increases the osmolality and makes the gel almost free of endosmosis.

The heat generated during electrophoresis enhances evaporation of liquid from the support medium. Wick flow is the upward movement of buffer through both immersed

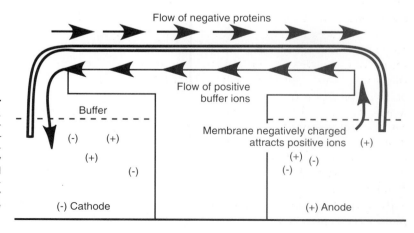

■ **FIGURE 6–2.**

The process of endosmosis. (From Clinical Laboratory Product Comparison System: *Electrophoresis Equipment.* Plymouth Meeting, PA, Emergency Care Research Institute, April 1991, p 2. ©1991, ECRI. Duplication in whole or in part by any means or for any purpose is prohibited.)

ends of the membrane to replace lost moisture. This flow adds distance to molecules moving toward the center of the membrane and retards molecules moving away from the center. The net result can be a reduced separation and lead to compression of the final band patterns.

Agarose Gel. Among the various types of gels with clinical applications, agarose gel is probably the most widely used. Unlike agar gel, which is composed of agarose and agaropectin, agarose gel does not contain acid sulfate and carboxylic acid groups. In neutral and alkaline buffers, these groups contribute to considerable endosmosis. Agarose gel is generally free of ionizable groups and experiences little endosmosis. However, some commercially available lots of agarose gel still contain some residual charged groups in varying quantities. This is not to-

tally undesirable because it allows the investigator to select the degree of endosmosis to suit the electrophoretic separation.

Compared with other support media, agarose gel offers a number of other advantages. For example, a well-known characteristic of paper is that it absorbs proteins, and all proteins are not absorbed equally. This results in a distortion of the final bands. Agarose gel has a lower affinity for proteins than paper has, and absorption is not a problem. Agarose also gives sharper resolution than cellulose acetate. Although both agarose and cellulose acetate yield 5 to 6 bands in routine serum protein electrophoresis, the increased resolution of agarose gel has provided much more information, especially in the gamma globulin region. Agarose will also accept a larger sample size. Figure 6–3 exemplifies the differences ob-

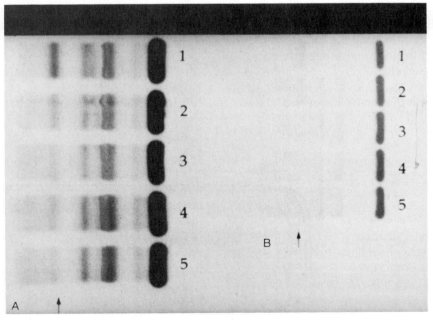

■ **FIGURE 6–3.**

Paragon agarose gel vs. cellulose acetate. A = Paragon agarose gel; B = cellulose acetate. (Courtesy of Beckman Instruments, Inc., Brea, CA.)

served in pattern resolution and sensitivity between agarose gel and cellulose acetate for serum protein electrophoresis. This attribute, combined with its increased resolution, results in greater sensitivity for detecting unusual proteins, such as oligoclonal bands.

One final advantage of agarose is its native clarity. Cellulose acetate is opaque and must be cleared (made transparent) for densitometry. Agarose is optically clear.

Cellulose Acetate. Cellulose acetate membranes are the result of the reaction between cellulose and acetic anhydride. The product is a dry, brittle film of interlocking cellulose acetate fibers. Commercially prepared membranes contain approximately 80 percent air space, which, when filled with buffer, makes the membrane quite pliable. Presoaking with buffer is a common prerequisite with this medium.

Cellulose acetate is a more homogeneous, chemically uniform medium than is paper. It also tends to be stronger and have a more uniform pore size. Protein absorption is minimal, and sharp, well-defined bands can be obtained. Although it is opaque, it can be cleared for densitometry with a solvent mixture. The solvent partially dissolves the cellulose acetate fibers, leaving the stained protein fractions on the transparent background.

An advantage of cellulose acetate is that it can be stored for long periods of time and retrieved for scanning at a future date. Also, proteins separate more quickly on cellulose acetate.

Polyacrylamide Gel. The routine use of polyacrylamide gel electrophoresis (PAGE) in the clinical laboratory is generally limited to the separation of alkaline phosphatase isoenzymes. This gel has many applications in research and exhibits extraordinary resolving power.

Polyacrylamide gel is formed by the reaction of "activated" acrylamide molecules that produce long polymer chains. Alone in solution, these chains do not coalesce. Gel formation requires that the chains cross-link to one another by inclusion of N,N'-methylene-*bis*-acrylamide (Bis for short). Varying the pore size is a function of changing the concentration of acrylamide, which determines the extent of cross-linkage.

As with other gels, the migration of molecules can be hindered by the size of the pores. But it is the relative ease with which the pore size can be altered that gives polyacrylamide its resolving properties. If the pore size is large, almost all serum proteins will migrate unhindered, and separation will be according to charge. As pore size becomes progressively smaller, molecular sieving becomes a factor as the larger molecules are slowed down and separation is not only by charge but by size. Over 20 serum proteins can be routinely seen on PAGE, and over 1100 different proteins have been detected in certain bacterial species.[2]

Methods employing PAGE are almost as varied as the number of available pore sizes. Electrophoresis can be conducted using horizontal slabs, vertical slabs, or vertical cylinders (rods). Figure 6–4 is an example of alkaline phosphatase isoenzyme separation on polyacrylamide gel. In the two-dimensional technique, proteins are separated in one direction, usually in cylinders, and then the cylindrical gel is attached to a slab so that separation occurs in a second direction. The complexity of the patterns can be such as to require computer assistance to scan and map.

Starch Gel. Starch gel is composed of granules containing amylose and amylopectin. When a concentrated suspension of these granules is heated in an aqueous solution, a viscous solution is formed that sets to gel upon cooling. It shares with polyacrylamide the capacity to separate molecules by size and charge. But unlike PAGE, the wide range of pore sizes and consistency is diffi-

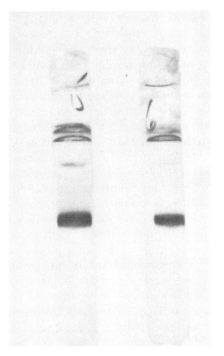

■ FIGURE 6–4.

Polyacrylamide gel separation. (From Ward KM, Cockayne S: Enzymology. *In* Anderson SC, Cockayne S (eds): *Clinical Chemistry: Concepts and Applications.* Philadelphia, WB Saunders, 1993, p 263.)

cult to achieve, which in turn makes it difficult to obtain reproducible results. Another disadvantage is its opaqueness, making densitometry difficult. Starch gel can be made relatively transparent by overnight soaking, but quantitation may still be somewhat inaccurate.

Although this gel provides a degree of resolution exceeded only by PAGE, its disadvantages have limited its routine clinical use.

Paper. Paper electrophoresis is only of historical interest in the modern clinical laboratory. Although high in tensile strength and low in cost, it will absorb some proteins. This results in broad bands and poor reso-

lution. The time required for separation can be lengthy.

Current uses of paper are generally restricted to the separation of low molecular weight molecules, such as amino acids.

Power Supply

Power supplies provide energy to the electrodes that results in the movement and separation of the molecules. They operate at either constant voltage or constant current. Depending on the type of power supply, adjustments can be made from 0 to 500 volts or 0 to 100 milliamperes.

Since diffusion (blurred bands) increases with the square root of time, it is often advantageous to complete electrophoresis as quickly as possible. When adequate separations are possible in 30 minutes or less, constant voltage is recommended at high settings. However, as the voltage is kept constant, current will increase because of the thermal agitation of dissolved ions. This is accompanied by an unwanted increase in temperature. When longer separation times are required, constant current is preferred to minimize the increase in temperature.

Stains

A variety of stains and techniques are available for visualizing the various fractions and bands once they have migrated. The choice of stains is often a matter of what works best for a given substance under a particular set of conditions.

One of the most commonly used stains for cellulose acetate protein separations is ponceau S. As a bright red dye, it absorbs light strongly at 525 nm. Ponceau S has a greater affinity for albumin than gamma globulin, but it shares this characteristic with other protein dyes. Coomassie brilliant blue R250 is another widely used protein dye that has replaced amido black (naphthol blue black) for some investigations because of its greater sensitivity and because it can be used with ampholyte gels such as polyacrylamide. Some dyes, though fine for protein, are not suitable for use with ampholyte-containing gels because of their reactivity toward these particles.

Proteins that are high in lipid or carbohydrate content may not stain well with certain dyes. Lipoproteins are best visualized with fat stains such as oil red O. This stain also absorbs at 525 nm. Schiff's reagent is another stain that is used to visualize both lipoproteins and glycoproteins. It absorbs in the range of 545 to 555 nm.

Enzymes are often visualized by coupling the reaction catalyzed by the enzyme to a chemical reaction, which generates a product that can be detected by its fluorescence or by its color. Lactate dehydrogenase, for example, can be demonstrated by incubating the medium with a mixture containing lactate and NAD^+. The NADH that is generated can be detected by its fluorescence when excited by ultraviolet light at 365 nm. Alternatively, the NADH can reduce a tetrazolium salt to form a colored formazan.

A summary of commonly employed stains appears in Table 6–1.

DENSITOMETRY

After the proteins or other compounds have been separated and stained, there are

TABLE 6–1. COMMONLY EMPLOYED STAINS

SUBSTANCE	STAIN	COMMENTS
Proteins	Ponceau S	Less sensitive than amido black, but more specific for proteins
	Bromphenol blue, light green SF	Low sensitivity but can be used with ampholyte gels
	Coomassie brilliant blue	Can detect less than 0.2 μg of protein; can be used with ampholyte gels
	Silver stain	At least 10 to 50 times more sensitive than others; different proteins give different colors
	Stains-All (cationic carbocyanine dye)	General sensitivity, including phosphoproteins
	Amido black 10B	Very sensitive stain
Lipoproteins	Sudan black B	
	Oil red O	
	Coomassie brilliant blue R250	Used with SDS gels
Glycoproteins	PAS (periodic acid–Schiff)	Best for neutral glycoproteins; 2 to 3 μg of carbohydrate detectable
	Stains-All	Best for sialic acid–rich glycoproteins
Nucleic acids	Stains-All	Best for RNA, DNA, and mucopolysaccharides
	Silver stain	
	Ethidium bromide	Fluorescent bands with DNA; less than 10 ng detectable
Enzymes		
Dehydrogenases	NADH	
	Nitro blue tetrazolium chloride	
Esterases, cholinesterases	Beta-naphthyl esters and tetrazotized O-dianisidine	
Phosphatases	Naphthylphosphate and fast blue B	

From Brewer JM: *Clinical Chemistry:* Theory, Analysis, and Correlation. St. Louis, CV Mosby, 1984.

essentially two ways to quantify the amount of dye in each individual band. In the *elution method*, the support medium is cut into sections that contain the separated bands. The dye in each band is then eluted by means of a solvent, and the amount of color in the eluted solution is measured on a photometer. The relative proportion of each band is determined by the intensity of its color. This method assumes that all proteins will bind the dye to the same extent, which may not be true. Also, this method may not be appropriate for certain support media. The second method of quantitation is *densitometry*, which is the focus of this section.

In densitometry, the intensity of the color of each band is measured directly from the strip or gel as the medium is moved past an optical system similar to that of a photometer. If the support medium is not transparent, it must be cleared. As previously mentioned, cellulose acetate is opaque and is most often cleared with an acid-alcohol mixture.

The similarities between a photometer and a **densitometer** extend to their basic components, which include a light source, a monochromator, a device to move the medium or provide analysis over a given area, an optical system, and a photodetector.

To produce incident light containing all the wavelengths that may be needed, at least two light sources are often used. For measurements in the visible portion of the spectrum (approximately 380 to 750 nm), the light source is usually a tungsten filament bulb. Tungsten bulbs, however, do not supply sufficient radiant energy for measurements below 320 nm. Fluorescence measurements require an ultraviolet light source, such as a deuterium or hydrogen lamp. Deuterium lamps tend to be more stable with a longer life than hydrogen lamps.

To isolate the desired wavelength, the radiant energy from the light source must be sent through a monochromator. Monochromators are of various types, including filters, prisms, and diffraction gratings. The specific wavelength leaving the monochromator is then passed through a slit to restrict the amount of light reaching the support medium.

Depending on the model of densitometer, two optical modes are possible: absorbance or fluorescence. In the absorbance mode, the unabsorbed light is reflected from the medium as the bands pass through a secondary slit to a photodetector. In the fluorescence mode, the bands are radiated with ultraviolet light, which stimulates the emission of visible fluorescent light. The fluoresced wavelength is in turn passed through a secondary slit and onto a photodetector.

Photodetectors transform light into electrical energy. Four principal types are used in densitometers. Photodiodes and phototubes convert photons of light into an electrical current that is proportional to the amount of impinging light. Photomultiplier tubes and phototransistors, in addition, can amplify the electrical current. They have extremely rapid response times and are very sensitive.

The signal leaving the photodetector is a function of the optical density of the sample, which is related to its analyte concentration. In most densitometers, the support medium is moved through the light at a fixed rate so that each fraction, according to its location and density, can be recorded on an x-y plotter as in Figure 6–5. The graph (electrophoretogram) represents multiple density readings taken at various points to determine the dispersion of sample fractions.

The sample fractions can be further quantified by determining the area under each peak. This can be done in several ways. If the curves are plotted on cross-sectional paper, the number of squares under each peak can be counted. Another method is to cut out each peak with scissors and weigh them. The weight of each peak is taken as propor-

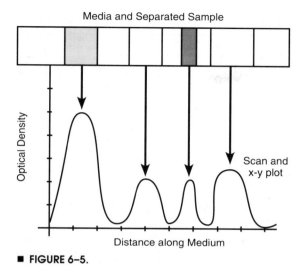

■ **FIGURE 6–5.**

The x-y plot of a separated sample. (From Clinical Laboratory Product Comparison System: *Densitometers, Laboratory, Scanning.* Plymouth Meeting, PA, Emergency Care Research Institute, April 1991; p 3. ©1991, ECRI. Duplication in whole or in part by any means or for any purpose is prohibited.)

tional to the area. Still another method is using a geometric device called a planimeter that calculates the area under the curve.

Advanced but more simple densitometers have some form of automatic built-in integrators for determining the area under the curve. A linear traverse or zigzag integration of the total protein scan in Figure 6–6*A* is illustrated in Figure 6–6*B*. In these densitometers, an electromechanical assembly operates a pen tracing across a series of horizontal lines. The smaller the area under the curve, the fewer horizontal lines are crossed. If the number of horizontal lines crossed under each curve is divided by the total number of lines crossed, the fractional contribution of each peak to the total is obtained. Multiplying these values by the total protein as determined by another analytical method will give the concentration of protein in each peak, as shown in Table 6–2. The more sophisticated densitometers use

microprocessors to carry out all necessary integration and computation functions.

Epstein suggests a number of features that should be considered in choosing a densitometer:[3]

(1) Ability to scan electrophoresis support lengths of 25 to 150 mm.

(2) Capability of automatic gain control to prevent the most intense peak or zone of an electrophoretogram from going off scale.

(3) Automatic background zeroing capability for background correction, which allows the instrument to choose the lowest background point in the electrophoretogram as baseline so that minor peaks will not be lost or "cut-off."

(4) Variable wavelength control, either as a continuously variable monochromator or

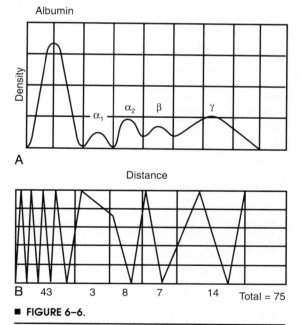

■ **FIGURE 6–6.**

A, The x-y plot of a total protein scan. *B,* The zigzag integration of the total protein scan. (From Clinical Laboratory Product Comparison System: *Densitometers, Laboratory, Scanning.* Plymouth Meeting, PA, Emergency Care Research Institute, April 1991, pp 3 and 4. ©1991, ECRI. Duplication in whole or in part by any means or for any purpose is prohibited.)

TABLE 6–2. CALCULATION OF SAMPLE FRACTION PERCENTAGE AND CONCENTRATION

ANALYTE FRACTION	% CALCULATION	%	CONCENTRATION
	Total protein = 7.1 g/dL		
Albumin	43/75	57	(.57 × 7.1) = 4.1 g/dL
α_1	3/75	4	(.04 × 7.1) = 0.3 g/dL
α_2	8/75	11	(.11 × 7.1) = 0.8 g/dL
β	7/75	9	(.09 × 7.1) = 0.6 g/dL
γ	14/75	19	(.19 × 7.1) = 1.3 g/dL

as variably selectable interference filters, to allow operation in the 400- to 700-nm range.

(5) Variable slits from 0.1 × 2.0 to 0.2 × 10.0 mm.

(6) An integrating device.

Desirable but not essential:

(7) Computerized integration and print-out.

*(8) **Automatic indexing,** a feature that automatically advances the electrophoresis strip, which contains multiple sample channels, from one channel to the next.*

(9) Built-in diagnostics (microcomputerized) for instrument troubleshooting.

(10) A choice of one of several (commonly three) scanning speeds.

SOURCES OF ERRORS AND OTHER PROBLEMS

Improvements in technique, automation, and the quality of support media have made electrophoresis a more robust and reliable procedure. Many of the remaining problems, such as disproportionate staining of proteins and zone truncation in fixed slit densitometry,[4] do not present simple solutions and are beyond the scope of this text.

What is offered in Table 6–3 are common problems and possible solutions associated with electrophoresis. With proper technique and attention to the following guidelines, many of these problems can be avoided.

Sample Application. Avoid overapplication of the sample. Overfilling the sample well may cause distorted bands. Some procedures call for a very specific amount of serum that can be delivered with a micropipet. Other procedures may use a template. Still others procedures use a twin-wire applicator. The wire should be clean and straight. Be careful not to overload the wire with excessive serum. These wires also come in different sizes. Make sure to use the correct size.

Buffers. Buffers that are contaminated or too old may result in unusually short migration patterns. They should be refrigerated when not in use to avoid growth of microorganisms. They can be used directly from the refrigerator. Buffers used in large volume apparatuses (700 to 1000 mL) can be reused if two conditions are met: (1) the polarity of the electrophoretic cell is switched after each run; and (2) the buffer is refrigerated between runs. This practice may be followed for up to four electrophoretic runs.[3] Discard buffers used in smaller volumes after each use.

Support Media. Handle support media with care. Avoid fingerprints or other contamination before the medium is cleared

TABLE 6-3. POSSIBLE PROBLEMS AND CORRECTIVE ACTIONS IN ELECTROPHORESIS

SYMPTOM	POSSIBLE PROBLEM	POSSIBLE CORRECTION
MIGRATION		
No migration	Power supply not connected or electrodes connected backward	Check circuit
	Support medium not in buffer	Make sure medium is in contact with buffer
	Wrong pH	Check pI of protein and pH of buffer
Short-length migration	Voltage too low	Increase voltage
	Run time too short	Increase run time
	Buffer old or contaminated	Change buffer
Long-length migration	Voltage too high	Decrease voltage
	Run time too long	Decrease run time
	Buffer old or contaminated	Change buffer
Slow migration	High molecular weight	Use support with a larger pore size
	Low charge	Change pH to increase charge
	Ionic strength too high	Dilute buffer
	Voltage too low	Increase voltage
Migration in wrong direction	Polarity reversed	Reverse polarity
BAND PATTERNS		
Band tailing	Too much sample	Decrease sample
	Voltage too high	Decrease voltage
	Wrong buffer	Check buffer
	Subunit dissociation or adsorption to support	Use different support; try different pH
	Salt in sample	Check sample for salt; dialyze against buffer
Weak bands	Not enough sample	Increase sample volume
	Staining time too short	Increase staining time
	Too much clearing	Decrease clearing time
Diffuse bands	Support too wet when sample applied	Remove excess liquid
	Run time too long	Decrease run time
	Wrong buffer	Change buffer
	Poor technique in applying sample	Check sample application technique
Bowing on edges	Overheating or drying out of support	Humidify chamber; check buffer ionic strength
Thin, sharp bands	Molecular weight of sample very high for support pore size	Use support with larger pore size
UNUSUAL BANDS		
Increased β-globulin	Hemolyzed sample	Repeat on unhemolyzed sample
Band between α_2 and β_2 globulin	Hemoglobin-haptoglobin complex	None
Grossly wide albumin band	Drug-bound albumin	None

Compiled from references 1, 3, 4, 25 and 26.

and dried. If presoaking is required, insert the medium into the buffer slowly so that no air bubbles will be trapped. Lightly blot the gel on filter paper to remove excess liquid. Applying sample to an excessively wet gel may result in diffuse bands.

Stains. Most stains can be reused several times. As a guideline, 100 mL of a staining solution can be used for a combined total of 387 cm² (60 inch²) of cellulose acetate or agarose gels. Replace the stain if leaching of the protein-stained bands occurs in the 5 percent acetic acid wash or clearing solutions.[3]

NEW DEVELOPMENTS AND ENHANCED TECHNIQUES

Isoelectric Focusing

Isoelectric focusing (IEF) is a technique capable of very high resolution. It is performed much like other electrophoretic methods, except the separating molecules migrate through a pH gradient. The gradient is created with the aid of a group of compounds called **ampholytes.** These are mixtures of low molecular weight (300 to 1000 daltons) amphoteric polyaminocarboxylic acids. The anode of the electrolytic cell is placed in a solution of acid and the **cathode** in a solution of base. The space between the cells is filled with the solution of ampholytes. The ampholytes in the area close to the anode will carry a net positive charge, and those close to the cathode will have a net negative charge. When the current is applied, the ampholytes will be repelled by the electrodes and rapidly migrate according to their effective mobilities to an area where the pH is equal to the **isoelectric point (pI)** of that particular ampholyte. The ampholytes are now electrically neutral, and migration ceases in the order of their isoelectric points. Because of their high buffering capacity, the ampholytes create stable pH zones so that when the more slowly migrating proteins reach their respective pI zones, migration ceases. The protein zones tend to be very sharp because the pI of a protein is confined to a narrow pH range and the pH gradient is at equilibrium. Any diffusion of the ampholyte or protein toward the anode or cathode will result in the formation of a net charge on the molecule, causing it to migrate back to the place where its net charge is 0.

There are notable advantages to isoelectric focusing, the most salient being its resolving power. Using narrow-range ampholyte mixtures, macromolecular species differing in pI by only 0.02 pH units can be distinguished. Under more specific conditions, it is possible to separate macromolecules that differ in pH units by as little as 0.001 pH units.[5] The technique can also be used to help characterize a macromolecule by determining its isoelectric point. This is most easily done by measuring the pH in the gradient at the position of the band of interest. Since a molecule will migrate from any point in the gradient to its pI, the point of sample application is not so important. In fact, it is a common practice to mix the molecules to be separated with the ampholyte solution. Other variables such as time and voltage may also assume less importance, within limits, since the band patterns are stabilized at the isoelectric point and there is little or no band diffusion.

The basis for separation in isoelectric focusing is by net charge. Any molecular sieving effect by the support medium will interfere with the final band pattern. Therefore, only highly porous gels should be used. Polyacrylamide gel is the medium of choice for most analytic work and is widely used. Although agarose gels have a larger pore size, they have not been well used in the past owing to high endosmosis. This problem has essentially been resolved with the

■ **FIGURE 6–7.**

Isoelectric focusing: alkaline phosphatase isoforms.

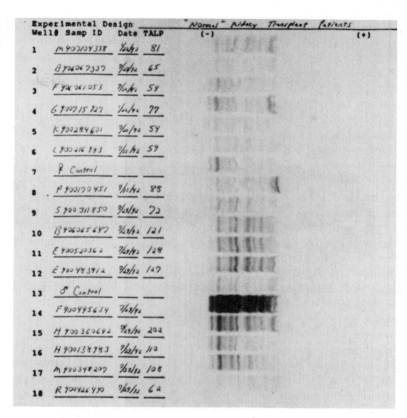

availability of specially prepared endosmosis-free materials. Isoelectric focusing methods have been adapted for use on both agarose and cellulose acetate.

Clinical Application

The clinical utility of IEF is still being realized as attempts are made to standardize separations so that highly reproducible results are obtained. IEF has been used to study acid phosphatase isoenzymes in both red blood cells[6] and serum.[7] A useful feature of IEF is that very small amounts of tissue can be implanted directly into the gel without further modification or pretreatment. Using this or similar techniques, proteins have been studied from biopsied material.[8] Isoforms of creatine kinase have also been examined by IEF.[9–12] The latest application of this technique has been to separate alkaline phosphatase into isoforms[13] (Figure 6–7). Although high resolution protein electrophoresis is widely used to detect oligoclonal bands in cerebrospinal fluid, a recently commercialized IEF system has been used for this same purpose.[14]

High Resolution Protein Electrophoresis

The technique for what has since become known as **high resolution electrophoresis (HRE)** was first published with the title "Agarose Gel Electrophoresis" in 1972 by B.G. Johansson,[27] and again in 1979 by J.O. Jeppsson[28] as a proposed selected method. The technique involves the use of agarose gel under high voltage (greater than 250 volts). To exclude the overgeneration of heat, the system is water cooled.

The agarose, with its relatively low content of sulfate and carboxyl groups, exhibits low endosmosis. Since it can easily accommodate proteins with sizes up to 10^6 daltons, the gel allows almost free migration of all plasma proteins except chylomicrons, very low density lipoproteins, immune complexes, and fibrinogen polymers.

Instead of the traditional 5 protein bands observed on cellulose acetate, 15 or so bands can be separated routinely. The exact number and nature of the bands depend on the purity of the agarose and the buffer composition. The number of bands detected can also be a function of the stain employed. Stains like amido black 10B and buffalo black are commonly used, but they show a greater affinity for one type of protein over another and can detect proteins only in the sample whose concentration exceeds 30 to 50 mg/dL. Coomassie brilliant blue is slightly more sensitive, but it requires that samples with a low protein content be concentrated prior to separation. Silver staining can detect proteins in concentrations as low as 100 μg/dL and permits visualization of protein bands without preliminary concentration of the sample.

Clinical Application

High resolution electrophoresis received less than enthusiastic acceptance when it was initially introduced, as clinicians pondered the usefulness of the additional bands and the more complicated protein patterns. Since then, it has evolved into a highly regarded diagnostic tool in selected situations.

In the area of CSF electrophoresis in demyelinating disease, HRE has been considered the most effective single diagnostic test for the diagnosis of multiple sclerosis. Despite the fact that the detection of oligoclonal bands is not entirely specific for multiple sclerosis, the value of this information is well documented.[15–17] At least 90 percent of patients with multiple sclerosis will demonstrate oligoclonal banding at some time during the course of their disease.[18]

Another area in which HRE has been uniquely useful is in the initial detection of some lymphoproliferative disorders, especially light chain disease. This monoclonal gammopathy can be particularly difficult to diagnose, but HRE can provide an early indication of the pathologic process, even in the absence of clinical symptoms.[20]

The separation and characterization of urinary proteins of both glomerular and tubular excretion is well suited to the properties of HRE. The information provided has been found useful in understanding renal function and disease.[18, 20, 21]

Two-Dimensional (2D) Electrophoresis

Two-dimensional electrophoresis represents the ultimate in electrophoretic resolving power. O'Farrell successfully resolved over 1100 proteins from lysed *Escherichia coli* cells and suggested that a mixture containing up to 5000 proteins could be adequately separated.[2]

The technique is a two-stage approach, based on the separation of proteins by two distinctly different physical or chemical properties. In its most powerful application, the protein mixture is first subjected to isoelectric focusing on a 1- to 6-mm diameter gel in a capillary tube. As with isoelectric focusing, the proteins are separated according to charge in a pH gradient. Since the resolving power of IEF is greater than 0.01 pH unit, very precise separations are possible. The gel is then carefully removed from the tube and placed across the top of a slab gel. It is usually held in place with either polyacrylamide or agarose gel for the second-dimension separation, which will take place at right angles to the first.

The next separation is usually by polyacrylamide gel, using sodium dodecyl sulfate (SDS) to separate the proteins by molecular mass. SDS is an ionic detergent that binds to proteins at the rate of 1.4 g of SDS per gram of protein. When bound, this highly charged detergent changes the helical structure of the protein and overwhelms the intrinsic charge. With each protein carrying a net charge per unit mass that is approximately constant, electrophoretic mobility becomes a function of molecular weight. On polyacrylamide gel, the effect is strictly molecular sieving such that the larger the molecule, the slower the mobility. The molecular weight of the unknown proteins can be determined by comparing their mobilities with those of protein standards of known molecular weight. After separation, the proteins can be visualized by staining or by detecting a fluorescent or radioactive label.

While the presence of SDS will interfere with dyes such as amido black, the removal of SDS is not a prerequisite for adequate staining, depending on the desired outcome. Coomassie blue R250, xylene cyanine brilliant G, and acid-fast green FCF have been used successfully.[1] The more sensitive silver staining does require the removal of SDS.

Fluorescent and radioactive labeling are techniques that involve the pretreatment of proteins, usually prior to separation, with either a fluorescent marker or a radioactive isotope, such as ^{3}H, ^{14}C, ^{32}P, ^{35}S, or ^{131}I (hydrogen, carbon, phosphorus, sulfur, iodine). Both techniques are highly sensitive and capable of detecting as little as 10 ng of protein or less. The fluorescent-labeled proteins can be visualized under ultraviolet light and photographed. Proteins carrying radioactive isotopes are visualized by autoradiography, in which the gel is exposed to sensitive x-ray film.

Ordinary densitometric scanning of two-dimensional gels is not too effective because of the complexity of the information to be gained. Two-dimensional mapping is best achieved by some form of automatic scanning and data handling equipment. Scanning is usually handled by a video camera connected to a computer of varying sophistication. The use of "expert systems" has been invaluable in measuring and interpreting these complex patterns.

Clinical Application

The tremendous potential of this technique has been investigated for over a decade, especially its power to study changes at the molecular level. For a number of complex reasons, it has not been accepted into general diagnostic use. Harrison and associates have proposed several routine indications for which two-dimensional electrophoresis would be useful: (1) resolution of diagnostic immunoprotein characterization ambiguities with oligoclonal or multiple monoclonal band patterns; (2) alpha-1-antitrypsin phenotyping; (3) apolipoprotein E phenotyping; (4) detection of certain genetic deficiency states; and (5) routine phenotyping of polymorphic serum proteins in other genetic diseases.[22]

Capillary Electrophoresis

Capillary electrophoresis (CE), also called **capillary zone electrophoresis** (CZE) and high performance capillary electrophoresis (HPCE), represents one of the newest breakthroughs in separation techniques. It has been favorably compared with the strengths of both high performance liquid chromatography and conventional electrophoresis as a single system that yields rapid, automated, and efficient analysis of complex mixtures.[23]

A typical CE system as shown in Figure 6–8 consists of a fused silica capillary, two electrolyte buffer reservoirs, a high voltage power supply, and a detector linked to some form of data acquisition equipment. The sample is introduced into the capillary by either the pumping action of the moving fluid within the capillary (electrokinetic injection) or by creating a pressure difference between the inlet and outlet of the capillary (hydrostatic or displacement injection). For best resolution, sample volumes are typically small, in the nanoliter to picoliter range. When voltage is applied, molecules in the sample are separated under the influence of **electroosmotic flow.** This bulk flow of fluid results from the excess of positively charged ions at the inner surface of the capillary. Positively charged ions emerge early because both the electroosmotic flow and the motion of the ion are in the same direction toward the cathode. The electroosmotic flow will also move negatively charged ions toward the cathode, but they tend to emerge at a much slower rate. Several different types of modes of separation by CE appear in Table 6–4. As the ions move toward the capillary outlet, detection takes place on-line, as with HPLC. A number of different types of detectors can be used, including optical (absorbance or fluorescence), conductivity, electrochemical, mass spectroscopy, or radioactivity detectors.

Advantages of CE over conventional electrophoresis and HPLC are its microvolume analysis, resolving power, and speed. Figure 6–9 shows a comparison of agarose gel electrophoresis to CZE. Using nanoliter quantities of sample, complex mixtures can be separated with a theoretical plate number (an empiric measure of column efficiency) approaching 1 million.[19] Many separations are completed in less than 10 minutes, compared with the hours sometimes required by conventional electrophoresis. Key to CE's resolving ability and speed is the high applied voltages it uses. This is possible because the capillaries used have such a high surface-to-volume ratio that heat is efficiently dissipated by transfer through the capillary walls.

With all its strengths, CE is not without major challenges to overcome. One is its limited sensitivity. While its ability to detect mass is excellent, the sample volumes are so small that molar detection limits are only comparable to gel electrophoresis or HPLC.

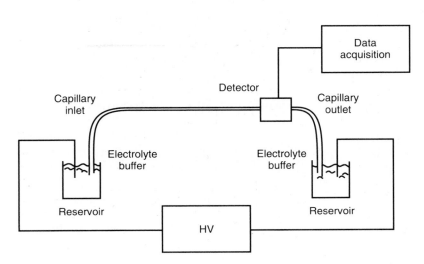

■ **FIGURE 6–8.**

Diagram of a capillary electrophoresis system. (From Burolla VP, Pentoney SL, Zare R: High performance capillary electrophoresis. *Am Biotech Lab* 7(10):20–26, 1989.)

TABLE 6–4. MODES OF CAPILLARY ELECTROPHORESIS

NAME	BASIS OF SEPARATION	REFERENCE
Free-zone capillary electrophoresis	Electrophoretic mobility	J.W. Jorgenson and K.D. Lukacs, Science **22**, 226 (1983)
Micellar electrokinetic capillary chromatography	Partitioning into detergent micelles, charge	S. Terabe, K. Otsuka, K. Ichikawa, and T. Ando, Anal Chem **56**, 113 (1984)
Isoelectric focusing	Isoelectric point	S. Hjerten and M. Zhu, J Chrom **346** 265 (1985)
Chiral separation	Enantiomeric structure	E. Gassman, J.E. Kuo, and R.N. Zare, Science **242**, 813 (1985)
Gel electrophoresis: Polyacrylamide gel electrophoresis	Size, charge	A.S. Cohen et al., Proc Natl Acad Sci **85**, 9660 (1988)
Sodium dodecyl sulfate polyacrylamide gel capillary electrophoresis (SDS-PAGE)	Size	A.S. Cohen and B.L. Karger, J Chrom **397**, 409 (1987)

From Banks P: Capillary electrophoresis: The small bore comes to the fore. *J NIH Research* 2(1):88, 1990.

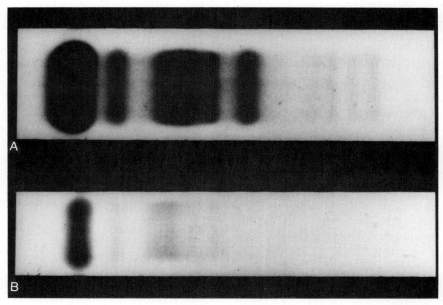

■ **FIGURE 6–9.**

Comparison of capillary zone electrophoresis *(A)* with agarose gel electrophoresis *(B)* of serum proteins. (Courtesy of Beckman Instruments, Inc., Brea, CA.)

There are also concerns about sample throughput, since samples can be run only one at a time.

Clinical Application

Hundreds of publications detail the application of CE to biomedical analysis. One of the most successful reports to establish the potential utility of CE for clinical diagnostic applications demonstrated equivalent, if not better, separation of serum proteins and hemoglobin variants by CE in a fraction of the time of conventional electrophoresis.[24] This same study also analyzed urine and CSF with equally successful results, without having to concentrate the sample. Expectations are high that this method will become a widely accepted tool within the biomedical community.

STATE-OF-THE-ART ELECTROPHORESIS SYSTEMS

Today, highly automated electrophoresis systems are utilized for separation of proteins and enzymes when rapid turnaround time is desired. These systems include the power supply, incubator, dryer, densitometer, and a computerized data management system. In other words, manufacturers can provide a complete internal system for electrophoresis development and densitometry. All operations—voltage adjustment, timing of the run, mechanical transfers of the gels, temperature control, and scanning—are controlled via a computer.

Consolidation of custom-configured work stations for processing more than one gel at a time can be seen with the Beckman **Paragon** electrophoresis system and the Beckman **Appraise** densitometer (Beckman Instruments, Inc., Brea, California), as well as the Helena **REP** electrophoresis system (Helena Laboratories, Beaumont, Texas). Figure 6–10 illustrates how work stations may be organized.

For automated electrophoresis systems, the process begins with loading the patient samples and control materials either directly into wells on the gels, or by filling small disposable specimen cups as illustrated in Figure 6–11. Once the sample wells are filled and the buffer is added, the REP system utilizes a "built-in" buffer reservoir, thereby eliminating the need to make, mix, or measure buffers. Gels have molded-in ridges that also serve as buffer reservoirs. Substrates for enzyme procedures may be prepared and placed into an appropriate vial holder on the instrument, if required.

To commence the electrophoresis process, the desired tests are selected from simple display options, utilizing a CRT (cathode ray tube) and the manufacturer's customized computer software program, as seen with Figure 6–12. A test determination, such as lipoprotein electrophoresis, is highlighted by the technologist. At this point the technologist has the opportunity to accept or edit the existing preprogrammed parameters. Additionally, a "user-defined" mode is typically available for the storage of the modified parameters. Now the run can be initiated, and the patient demographic information can be entered simultaneously.

While the gels are undergoing the electrophoresis process, the functions of substrate dispensing, gel transfers, temperature control, and scanning are all automated. Proteins, isoenzymes, hemoglobins, and lipids can be separated and scanned within 15 to 45 minutes, depending upon the electrophoresis system employed and the application chosen. While the scanning function is taking place, the technologist can edit the scans in a random fashion. Single keys, as shown in Figure 6–13, allow for addition, deletion, or suppression of fractions; adjustment of

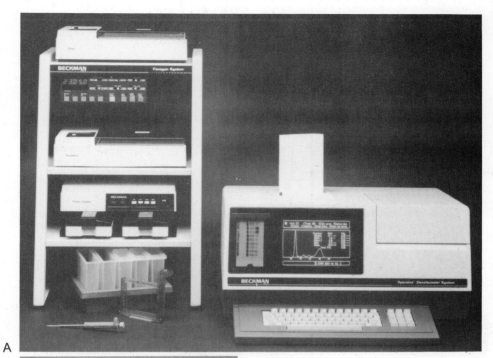

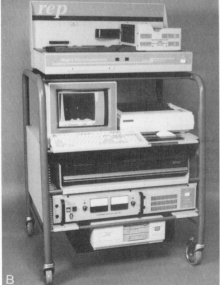

■ **FIGURE 6–10.**

Power Stacker stations for automated electrophoresis. A, Beckman Paragon Electrophoresis System and Appraise densitometer. (Courtesy of Beckman Instruments, Inc.,
Brea, CA); B, Helena REP ® Automated Electrophoresis System (Helena Laboratories).
(Courtesy of Helena Laboratories, Beaumont, TX.)

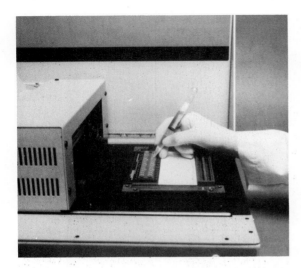

■ **FIGURE 6–11.**

Loading patient samples into specimen cups for automated delivery to the gels with the REP system. (Courtesy of Helena Laboratories, Beaumont, TX.)

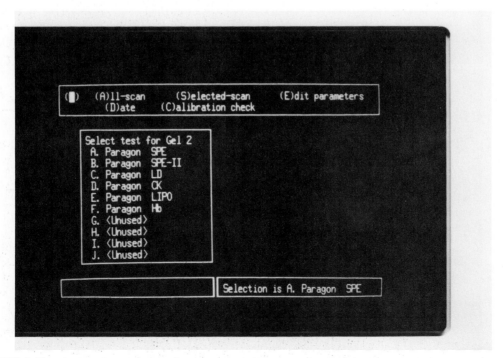

■ **FIGURE 6–12.**

CRT test menu display for microprocessor-controlled electrophoresis. (Courtesy of Beckman Instruments, Inc., Brea, CA.)

■ FIGURE 6–13.

Computer key pad options for editing densitometry scans. (Courtesy of Beckman Instruments, Inc., Brea, CA.)

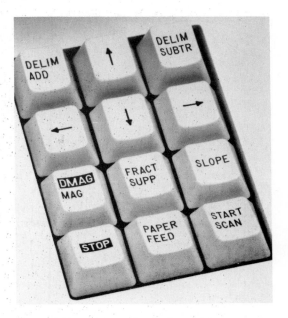

the baseline or slope; and magnification or restoration of patterns. Since the patterns can be viewed first on the display monitor, modifications such as **delimiting** can be made prior to printing (Figure 6–14).

These highly automated electrophoresis systems contain elaborate database management systems for reporting and interpreting patient results. Figure 6–15 is an example of a typical patient report. The re-

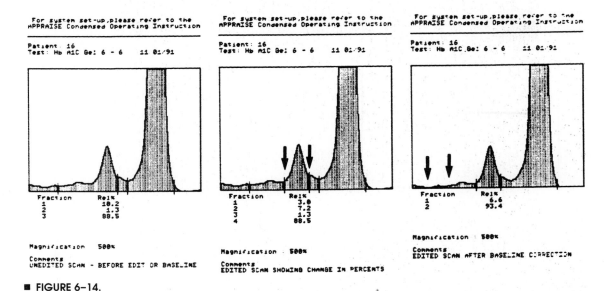

■ FIGURE 6–14.

Scans demonstrating the editing of delimits and baselines. (Courtesy of Beckman Instruments, Inc., Brea, CA.)

```
================================================================
                 C O M M U N I T Y   H O S P I T A L
                 2 O O   S .   C E N T R A L   D R I V E
                      A N Y T O W N ,   U S A
                  DR. S. HAMILTON, PATHOLOGIST
                  T. JONES, CHIEF TECHNOLOGIST

================================================================
================================================================
   NAME         :MARTIN, JAMES        SPECIMEN DATE:01-29-88
   AGE          :65                   SPECIMEN TYPE:SERUM
   SEX          :M                    IGG          :2050
   DOCTOR       :BURKE                IGA          :50
   HOSPITAL #   :4321                 IGM          :45
   DIAGNOSIS    :MONOCLONAL GAMMOPATHY
================================================================
================================================================
```

Test: SPE   Gel 1 - 6   1-29-1988

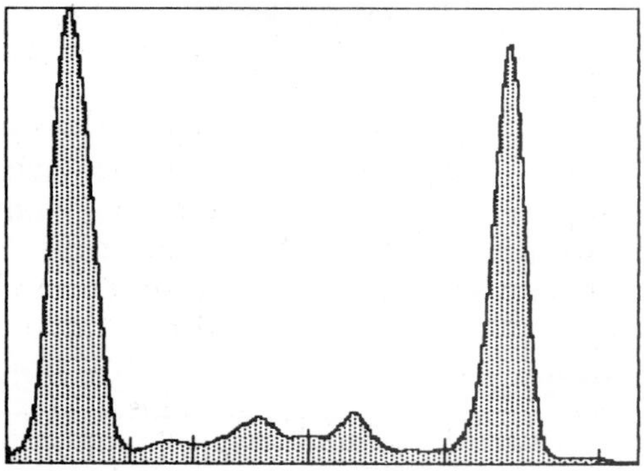

Fraction	Rel%		G/L	
Albumin	47.6	--	4.28	
Alpha 1	2.4		0.22	
Alpha 2	7.1	-	0.64	
Beta	6.5		0.58	
Gamma	36.5	+++	3.28	+++

Total G/L : 9.00   A/G: 0.91

Reference Ranges:

Fraction	Rel%		G/L	
Albumin	56.4	- 71.6	3.97	- 5.34
Alpha 1	1.8	- 4.5	0.11	- 0.32
Alpha 2	7.3	- 15.0	0.53	- 1.12
Beta	6.1	- 11.5	0.42	- 0.87
Gamma	7.8	- 18.2	0.53	- 1.37

```
================================================================
```

INTERPRETATION: MONOCLONAL SPIKE PRESENT IN THE GAMMA REGION. SUGGEST SERUM AND URINE IMMUNOFIXATION TO CHARACTERIZE MONOCLONAL PROTEIN.

Reviewed by: _____ Date: _____

```
================================================================
```

■ **FIGURE 6–15.**

Serum protein electrophoresis report. (Courtesy of Beckman Instruments, Inc., Brea, CA.)

port usually includes the title of the test; patient demographics; a graphic display of the scan; scan data including but not limited to user-defined fraction names, reference ranges, and calculated ratios for serum protein electrophoresis; an interpretative analysis that includes suggestions for possible diagnoses, follow-up tests, and other diagnostic considerations like prognosis or treatment.

Automated electrophoresis systems provide rapid turnaround time, excellent reproducibility, lower reagent costs per test, and the capability to produce customized report forms. Further, this type of system makes it easier to monitor quality control and retrieve data for research.

SUMMARY

Simply stated, electrophoresis is the movement of charged molecules in an electromagnetic field. Mobility or rate of migration is influenced by the molecules's net charge and size. Other analytical variables affecting the rate of migration are the properties of the support medium, strength of the electromagnetic field, endosmosis, ionic strength of the buffer, and temperature. Various mathematical equations have been developed that express the interrelationships of all these factors. Practical aspects of electrophoresis, however, are of more concern to the laboratory worker than is theory.

The system components for performing electrophoresis and an electrophoretic scan include the sample, a buffer, a support medium, a power supply, and a densitometer. Stains may be necessary when visualization of the bands is desired. Many procedural steps are required to perform electrophoresis. These include reagent preparation (buffers, stains, and so on), sample application, placement of the buffer and the gel (support medium) into the electrophoretic chamber, application of the substrate or stain and clearing solution, gel transfer to the incubator or drying oven, and final transfer to the densitometer. Therefore, numerous features must be considered when selecting an electrophoresis procedure and apparatus. Specific features also should be considered when selecting a densitometer for purchase. These include the ability to scan a variety of support lengths, automatic gain control adjustment, automatic zeroing capability, variable wavelength control, variable slits, and the incorporation of an integrator. Other desirable but not essential features include computerized integration and printout, automatic indexing, built-in computerized troubleshooting, and choice of scanning speeds.

Since the technique of electrophoresis was first employed, improvements in technique, automation, and the quality of the support media have made it a more robust procedure. Many remaining technical problems still remain, especially with manual operations. These common sources of error are associated with sample application, buffer preparation and storage, handling of the support medium, and the preparation, application, clearing, and storage of stains.

New developments in the field include isoelectic focusing, high resolution protein electrophoresis, two-dimensional electrophoresis, and capillary zone electrophoresis. Capillary zone electrophoresis is actually a combination of two technologies: electrophoresis and high performance liquid chromatography.

Over the years, aspects of the electrophoresis procedure have become automated. Most notable has been the quantitation of the zones via densitometry scanning. The new state-of-the-art electrophoretic systems on the market today have essentially automated all the labor-intensive steps of electrophoresis. In addition, computer-controlled data management systems have become an integral component of these systems. Now there is on-line time, voltage, and temperature control, which leads to extremely reproducible results.

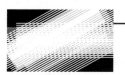

REVIEW QUESTIONS

Choose the BEST answer.

1. All the following are characteristic of two-dimensional electrophoresis, EXCEPT:

   a. Involves separation of proteins by two different properties, chemical and physical.
   b. High resolution.
   c. Fewer bands are produced.
   d. Involves separation of proteins at their isoelectric point.

2. Electroosmotic flow results in all of the following, EXCEPT:

   a. A bulk flow of fluid toward the cathode that enhances the separation of the ions.
   b. Movement of positively charged ions toward the cathode.
   c. Movement of negatively charged ions toward the cathode.
   d. Movement of positively charged ions toward the anode.

3. A diffuse band pattern may be corrected by

   a. increasing the sample volume.
   b. decreasing the voltage.

   c. decreasing the run time.
   d. choosing a different stain.

4. All the following are advantages of automated electrophoresis systems, EXCEPT:

   a. Rapid turnaround time.
   b. Excellent reproducibility.
   c. Greater specificity.
   d. Lower reagent costs per test.

5. The major advantage for choosing Coomassie brilliant blue as a stain for proteins is

   a. its analytic sensitivity.
   b. its fluorescent capabilities.
   c. that it can also stain RNA and DNA.
   d. its selectivity for low molecular weight proteins.

6. A number of essential features should be considered when selecting a densitometer. From the following, select which feature is **desirable,** not essential:

   a. An integrating device.
   b. Automatic indexing.

c. Variable wavelength control.
d. Ability to scan electrophoresis support lengths of 25 to 150 mm.

REFERENCES

1. Andrews AT: *Electrophoresis: Theory, Techniques, and Biochemical and Clinical Applications.* New York, John Wiley & Sons, 1977.
2. O'Farrell PH: High-resolution two-dimensional electrophoresis of proteins. *J Biol Chem* 250:4007–4021, 1975.
3. Epstein E: Electrophoresis. *In* Tietz N (ed): *Textbook of Clinical Chemistry.* Philadelphia, WB Saunders, 1986.
4. Artiss JD, Epstein E, Kiechle FL, et al: Potential problems in serum protein electrophoresis. *Clin Lab Med* 6:427–440, 1986.
5. Cooper TG: *The Tools of Biochemistry.* New York, John Wiley & Sons, 1977.
6. Anderson CJ, Shamberger RJ: High voltage electrophoresis and isoelectric focusing of red cell acid phosphatase isoenzymes for use in paternity classification. *Clin Chem* 311:1006, 1985.
7. Mack DO, Reed VL, Smith LD: Isoelectric focusing of serum prostatic acid phosphatase. *Clin Chem* 33:927, 1987.
8. Thompson BJ, Burghes AHM, Dunn MJ, et al: The application of direct tissue isoelectric focusing to the human skeletal muscle. *Electrophoresis* 2:251–258, 1981.
9. Chapelle JP: Serum creatine kinase MM sub-band determination by electric focusing: A potential method for the monitoring of myocardial infarction. *Clin Chim Acta* 137:273–281, 1984.
10. Heinbokel N, Srivastava LM, Goedde HW: Agarose gel isoelectric focusing of creatine kinase (EC2.7.3.2) isoenzymes from different human tissue extracts. *Clin Chim Acta* 122:103–107, 1982.
11. Panteghini M: Serum isoforms of creatine kinase isoenzymes. *Clin Biochem* 21:211–218, 1988.
12. Williams J, Marshall T: Heterogeneity of serum creatine kinase isoenzymes MM in myocardial infarction: Standardization of patterns using cord blood serum. *Clin Chem* 34:398–401, 1988.
13. Randolph JA, Lott JA, Tsei RJ, Thomas TM: Serum alkaline phosphatase (ALP) isoforms as an early detection of the complications in liver transplantation (TX). *Clin Chem* 38(6):978, 1992.
14. Wybo I, Van Blerk M, Malfait R, et al: Oligoclonal bands of cerebrospinal fluid detected by Phast-System isoelectric focusing. *Clin Chem* 36:123–125, 1990.
15. Bloomer LC, Bray PF: Relative value of three laboratory methods in the diagnosis of multiple sclerosis. *Clin Chem* 27:2011–2013, 1981.
16. Gerson B, Cohen SR, Gerson JM, et al: Myelin basic protein, oligoclonal bands, and IgG in cerebrospinal fluid as indicators of multiple sclerosis. *Clin Chem* 27:1974–1977, 1981.
17. Keshgegian AA, Coblentz J, Lisak RP: Oligoclonal immunoglobulins in cerebrospinal fluid in multiple sclerosis. *Clin Chem* 26:1340–1345, 1980.
18. Killingsworth LM: High resolution protein electrophoresis. A clinical overview with renal and neurological case studies. Beaumont, Texas, Helena Laboratories, 1983.
19. Lauer HH, McManigill D: Capillary zone electrophoresis of proteins in untreated fused silica tubing. *Anal Chem* 58:166–170, 1986.
20. Killingsworth LM, Cooney SK, Tyllia MM: Protein analysis: The closer you look, the more you see. Part I: Plasma protein patterns. *Diag Med* Jan/Feb, 47–59, 1980.
21. Killingsworth LM: Clinical applications of protein determinations in biological fluids other than blood. *Clin Chem* 28:1093–1102, 1982.
22. Harrison HH, Miller KL, Powell D, et al: Clinical applications of high resolution two-dimensional electrophoresis (2DE) of proteins: Comparative analysis by 2DE of proteins in high resolution agarose electrophoresis (HRE) bands and current medical indications for 2DE analysis of serum proteins. *Clin Chem* 35:1083, 1989.
23. Burolla VP, Pentoney SL, Zare R: High performance capillary electrophoresis. *Am Biotech Lab* 7(10):20–26, 1989.
24. Chen FA, Liu C, Hsieh Y, et al: Capillary electrophoresis—a new clinical tool. *Clin Chem* 37:14–19, 1991.
25. Brewer JM: Electrophoresis. *In* Kaplan LA, Pesce AJ (eds): *Clinical Chemistry; Theory, Analysis and Correlation.* St. Louis, CV Mosby, 1984.
26. Ferris CD: *Guide to Medical Laboratory Instruments.* Boston, Little, Brown, 1980.
27. Johansson BG: Agarose gel electrophoresis. *Scand J Clin Lab Invest* 29, suppl. 124: 7–19, 1972.
28. Jeppsson JD, Laurell CB, Franzén B: *Clin Chem* 25:629–638, 1979.

Chapter 7

AUTOMATED INSTRUMENTATION (GENERIC)

LINDA KASPER, MS, MT (ASCP) SC

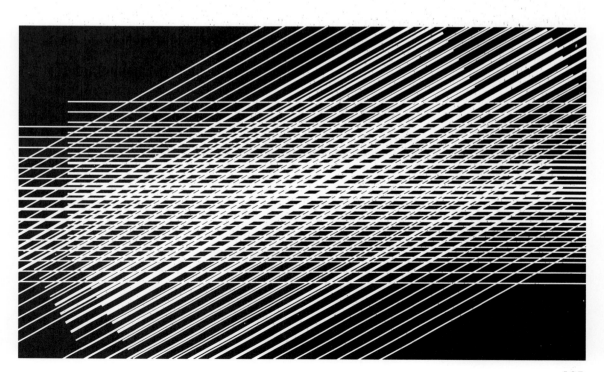

LEARNING OBJECTIVES

After studying this chapter, the student will be able to:

- Identify factors that led to the development of laboratory instruments.
- Explain why automation was more rapidly developed to perform chemistry assays.
- Discuss reasons why instrumentation has altered the ways in which physicians utilize laboratory services.
- Describe how instrumentation has led to new roles and responsibilities for laboratorians.
- List several functions accomplished by microprocessor units in laboratory instruments.
- Discuss advantages of using bar code technology in laboratory testing.
- Discuss problems associated with currently available robotic systems.
- Distinguish between laboratory turnaround time, testing turnaround time, and therapeutic turnaround time.
- List the advantages and disadvantages of closed reagent systems.
- Identify features of laboratory instruments that should be considered by purchaser.
- List criteria for selecting calibration materials.
- Compare advantages and disadvantages of wet and dry reagent systems.
- Discuss advantages of using closed tube sampling systems.

KEY WORDS

Batch analyzer. Instrument designed to perform the same test or a group of tests on multiple patient samples during each analytical run.

Bidirectional interface. Allows two-way communication via computer linkage between the laboratory information system (LIS) and any on-line instrument.

Calibration. Prescribed steps performed to establish testing parameters and instrument conditions that provide precise and accurate results.

Centrifugal analyzer. A batch analyzer utilizing centrifugation to mix reagent(s) and sample in a self-contained rotary cuvet assembly.

Closed reagent system. User can purchase reagents only from instrument manufacturer.

Closed tube sampling. Designed to allow sampling of patient specimen without opening tubes, resulting in cost savings and reduced biohazardous risks for operator.

Diagnostic programs. Software programs designed to assess instrument function and to report malfunctions to operator.

Downtime. Time during which instrument is not capable of producing patient results that can be reported.

Expert system. A type of information system programmed to solve problems, such as interpretation of test results and/or diagnosis by established criteria.

Laboratory information system (LIS). Computerized system that transmits many types of laboratory information, including work lists and patient test results. More complex systems allow bidirectional communication between laboratory and patient care units.

On-site testing. Laboratory testing performed in same location and at same time as patient is seen by physician.

Open system. Reagents and consumable supplies can be purchased from any available vendor.

Robotic system. A mechanized device designed to perform repetitive tasks with a high degree of precision and accuracy.

Satellite testing. Testing performed in locations other than main laboratory site, such as critical care unit.

Test menu. Identifies names of tests offered by an instrument.

Test profile. A group of tests designed to provide information about specific organ function or disease process.

Turnaround time. Typically refers to time required to produce test result once sample arrives in laboratory.

Workload. Quantity of work accomplished by an instrument, a laboratorian, or an entire laboratory staff in a defined time.

INTRODUCTION

This chapter of introduction to automation will examine the impact of instrumentation on clinical laboratory practice by considering the following questions: Why was automation necessary? What groups of individuals have been most influenced by advances in laboratory automation? How has computer technology influenced laboratory automation? How has automation changed the testing process? In general, how has technology been applied to testing in various laboratory disciplines? Finally, what are the most important features of an instrument in today's laboratory?

WHY WAS AUTOMATION NECESSARY?

Prior to the late 1950s, laboratory analyses were performed with time-consuming and often labor-intensive techniques. Hence, the amount of time required to produce a test result was dependent upon the number of requests for that analyte, the time inherent in the method, and the speed at which the laboratorian could perform the tasks associated with the assay. As advancements were made in clinical laboratory services, both the number of developed assays and the number of requests for those assays increased. Using only manual methods, it became humanly impossible for existing laboratory personnel to handle the increased workload efficiently, and in particular, to provide results within time limits that were compatible with patient care needs. There were two choices: hire additional personnel or find ways to automate some of the tasks involved in the testing process, with the expectation that automation would improve the efficiency, or the number of test results produced per salary dollar, of existing personnel.[1]

The first significant automated instruments were introduced into the chemistry and hematology sections of the clinical laboratory. Early manual assays for biochemical analytes were primarily based on the knowledge of chemical reactions and the principle of light absorption. The challenge facing instrument designers involved combining these concepts with automated mechanisms that could take over some of the repetitive tasks performed by laboratory personnel (basically sample and reagent measurement, mixing, incubation, and readout). There were at least two reasons why automation was readily introduced into chemistry. First, existing assays could be adapted to automation. Technically, these assays involved pipetting and mixing specified volumes of sample and reagents, coupled with some type of readout capability. Biochemical test results are usually reported as numerical data, and changes in light intensity could be easily converted for the readout device. In addition, biochemical analytes make up a majority of the total number of test requests for most laboratories, therefore more pressure was exerted on that section of the laboratory to improve turnaround time.

The first automated instrument for biochemical analytes, the AutoAnalyzer, was introduced in 1957 by Dr. Leonard Skeggs in cooperation with Technicon.[2] The instrument employed a pump and a variable-sized tubing system to bring sample, reagents, and air bubbles together in a continuously flowing stream. At the end of the reaction time a colorimeter/recorder interface provided a readout that could be converted to a reportable result. The number of specimens analyzed per hour was determined by sampler cams. The cams were interchangeable to provide different ratios of sampling time:air time (wash time in later generations of the instrument). Cam specifications were optimized for each assay. Once the sample tray was loaded and the instrument operation initiated, the laboratorian could concentrate on translating data from the recorder into reportable results.

Early models of the AutoAnalyzer focused on automating the most routinely requested analytes (glucose, blood urea nitrogen, and electrolytes). Each test requested required its own sample aliquot, and the instrument performed the same test on multiple samples. The flexibility of a given instrument was limited to changing cams on the sampler module to provide a different sample:air ratio, to changing pump tubing for different sample:reagent volumes, and to changing filters in the colorimeter for wavelength selection. The early systems were not conducive to fast turnaround of STAT requests unless the instrument was dedicated to one test. The number of tests that could be assayed around the clock without recalibration for each new batch of samples was also limited. In spite of these limitations, the number of test results completed in 1 hour increased as much as 20-fold when compared with manual assays for the same analyte. For any given assay, sample handling and data management became the primary determinants of productivity, or the work produced per hour of staff time.[1, 3]

One year earlier, in 1956, Coulter Electronics had introduced an automated cell counter for the hematology laboratory. The first model required individual dilutions and independent assays for total white cell and red cell counts. The instrument saved hours of staff time because it could perform these two counts much faster than a laboratorian could perform two separate dilutions of the blood, load two sides on each of two hemocytometers, and count the cells under a microscope.[4]

From these early beginnings, automated systems have been introduced into every area of the laboratory. The impact of laboratory technology has been heightened and expanded by the developments in computer technology, and in today's laboratory, the microprocessor is an integral component of most instruments. Bearing little or no resemblance to their predecessors, each new generation of instruments offers larger test menus and more sophisticated technology aimed at providing more results in less time.

WHAT GROUPS HAVE BEEN MOST INFLUENCED BY LABORATORY AUTOMATION?

Within the health care environment, three groups have been significantly influenced by advances in laboratory automation: physicians, laboratorians, and patients.

Physicians

As technology advanced, physicians increasingly demanded improved laboratory services. Their dependence on test results also increased and was related to several external factors, including medical care reimbursement, malpractice lawsuits, and the nature of the patient case load.

Prior to the widespread availability of health insurance, physicians were limited in their access to laboratory testing, in part by the patient's ability to pay for the services. As automation was being introduced into clinical laboratories, the third party reimbursement system expanded to cover medical care expenses that originally had been borne by the patient or otherwise not provided. Once health insurance was made readily available to the general public through employer benefit programs or private insurance carriers, out-of-pocket medical expenses became less of an issue to many patients. Physicians were at liberty to manage patient care using a comprehensive

health care system that included automated laboratory services. This practice went largely unchanged until the early 1980s, when sharply rising health care expenses forced changes in reimbursement programs. Federal reimbursement of medical care for the elderly was altered to include diagnosis-related groups and other cost-containment features. Some predicted that requests for laboratory tests would decrease. However, the predicted negative impact of this legislation did not occur. Instead, the number of test requests has continued to increase.

Another factor that has promoted the physician's utilization of laboratory services has been the increased incidence of malpractice suits. Many physicians practice "defensive medicine," often ordering what might be considered unnecessary tests simply as added protection in the event of a lawsuit. Today, as health care costs continue to rise at a rate of 20 to 30 percent annually, stronger emphasis is being placed on cost containment. One of the outcomes is shorter hospital stays for inpatients. As a result, the patients in the hospital are more critically ill from diseases that are accompanied by a complexity of problems. Consequently, they require a broad, rapid response support system that includes highly automated laboratory services.[3, 5]

Improved technology combined with efforts to contain increasing health care costs have been two prime driving forces in moving toward ambulatory care. In large ambulatory care centers, physicians need and expect prompt same-day service from today's laboratory. Physicians in private practice have a similar need.

Some of the factors that promote ambulatory care also foster laboratory testing in physicians' offices. Simple push-button desk-top analyzers provide testing capability with minimally trained personnel for the one- or two-physician office. Larger group practices may have more sophisticated instruments run by a dedicated laboratory staff. In ambulatory care centers and in physicians' offices, these instruments are capable of providing fast, accurate results, making it possible for the physician to have rapid access to a variety of test results by the time the patient is seen. This is convenient for both patient and physician because diagnostic and therapeutic decisions can be made while the patient is in the office. Initiation of, or changes in, therapy can be discussed with the patient in person rather than by phone several hours later or in a follow-up visit several days later.[6] By testing in the office, physicians have become competitors for testing volume and revenue. An estimated 90 percent of physicians' offices perform some laboratory testing, making this the most rapidly expanding segment of the laboratory industry.[6–9] For the physician in private practice, automation has provided the convenience of **on-site testing,** improved the quality and efficiency of practice, and provided another source of income.

Laboratorians

Technology has revolutionized laboratory practice and led to different expectations of performance for those laboratorians who are responsible for day-to-day tasks. As users of laboratory services have pressed for increased efficiency, productivity, precision, and accuracy, laboratorians have had to rely on a combination of instrumentation and computer technology to meet those demands. Technology, however, changes rapidly, and a new generation of instruments appears approximately every 5 years.[10] This forces laboratory personnel to be adaptable and to engage in life-long learning.

Existing roles of the laboratorian have changed, and new roles have been assumed. A laboratorian performs a manual method as a direct, hands-on participant in producing the resulting data. The advancement of technology has promoted the laboratorian to a data analyzer/manager. Once laboratorians checked out reagent problems; they now operate instruments, analyze and interpret data, and perform preventive maintenance and basic instrument repair. Laboratorians have had to develop more sophisticated problem-solving skills because of the increasing complexities of problems associated with automation.

Technology has increased the testing capacity of the laboratory far beyond what a few technologists could accomplish using manual methods. Simultaneously, the number of tasks that need to be done has increased as well. Test menus offered by large instruments are beginning to cross traditional lines of discipline-specific testing. An instrument may be capable of performing assays that were typically provided by different sections of the laboratory, i.e., routine chemistry, special chemistry (drug and hormone testing), and coagulation. Newly developed assays focus on measuring analytes that have not been measured previously. As increased options become available, instrument operators must then broaden their skills and knowledge base in order to incorporate these new tests into their area of responsibility.

In addition to managing workflow operations and information processing, laboratorians serve as educators and consultants. The laboratorian's role as an educator will expand to include training nonlaboratory personnel to utilize instruments in decentralized locations and teaching patients to use home-testing devices. Laboratorians will be responsible for implementing and monitoring quality control and quality assurance programs for these same testing environments and will serve as consultants to the users. They may also serve as consultants to physicians with office laboratories, as well as instrument manufacturers.[11] These factors contribute to the ever-changing role of the multiskilled laboratorian.

The production side of automation has had another impact on the laboratorian. The industrial setting provides opportunities for employment in research/development, quality control, user education, customer service, and sales. These expanded employment opportunities have resulted in an exodus of many trained personnel from hospital laboratories and have, in part, contributed to the current shortage of laboratory workers. Rather than reducing the need for personnel, each successive model of an instrument is more complex and sophisticated than the previous one. This increases the need for better trained laboratorians who can adapt to performing in a variety of environments.[12]

Patients

Today's health care consumers are more interested and educated in personal health care matters than their ancestors. To the extent that automation has increased the availability and convenience of laboratory testing as a component of comprehensive health care, it has had an impact on the consumer's view of health care.

Some factors that have contributed to the consumer's heightened awareness of the importance of personal health care, and in particular preventive health care, include health fairs, mass screenings, and employee wellness programs. Automation has been made available to the general public through on-site cholesterol and glucose testing as major components of health fairs and screening programs. In the late 1980s, the American Heart Association, in cooperation with local health care personnel and industrial representatives, conducted large cholesterol screening programs as part of its public ed-

ucation program. Through these programs, individuals were voluntarily tested for total cholesterol and educated about "good" and "bad" cholesterol. Some institutional and corporate wellness programs offer periodic test profiles that include screening for risk factors for heart disease, occult blood, and kidney and liver function.

As consumers became more educated, they demanded improved access and quality service from the health care system. Ideally, patients visit their physicians and have access to testing and therapeutic services at the same location. Laboratory technology has made it possible to improve testing capabilities; and this, together with the economics of cost containment, gives consumers access to testing in ambulatory care centers, in STAT laboratories in emergency centers, and in their own private physician's laboratory. The rapid turnaround time has decreased the time between testing and initiation of therapy.

Automation has allowed home testing for some individuals with chronic disorders. For example, many diabetics are able to monitor their blood glucose at home, transmit the data to the physician's office via a modem, and receive same-day feedback on adjustments in diet and therapy based on the individual's projected physical activities. This adds an extra dimension of freedom to the patient's lifestyle and promotes a level of self-care that reduces the complications of a chronic disease process. Retail sales from the home testing market are projected to exceed 1 billion dollars in 1995.[13]

Laboratory automation has contributed simultaneously to the complexity and the quality of health care. Latest developments show a trend toward monitoring analytes at, or near, the patient's bedside. Bedside testing is advantageous in any critical care area, where rapid decisions and therapeutic responses are required.[14] In one institution, a robotic system performs testing, and a laboratorian in another location monitors and verifies the operation via a computer interface. Such systems result in significant savings of time and personnel. It is not necessary to transport the specimen to the laboratory receiving area, and the amount of hands-on time required of the laboratorians is reduced.[15, 16] To accomplish testing in this manner it requires a complex network of instrumentation and computerization. These types of systems are being proposed as one solution to replace the additional trained personnel that would be required to staff **satellite testing** areas, such as critical care units.

In the decade of the nineties, budget restrictions and personnel shortages will continue to challenge laboratories to find new ways to do more with less. Automation will be a critical dimension of the level of success that laboratorians are able to achieve in facing this challenge.

While many of the complex problems brought about by automation still need solutions, quality has improved. The improved precision, increased efficiency, and improved turnaround time have contributed to more accurate results and faster decision making by physicians regarding diagnosis and treatment.

Although it has provided laboratorians with the tools and technology to do more work in shorter periods of time (improved efficiency and productivity), automation has also contributed to the rise in health care costs. Instruments designed to be major work stations cost thousands of dollars. Another cost factor involves the personnel, reagents, and consumable supplies required to operate the instrument over its lifetime of usefulness. When assessing the influence that automation has on health care costs, of primary interest to the laboratory is the cost of producing individual patient results.[17]

HOW HAS COMPUTER TECHNOLOGY INFLUENCED LABORATORY AUTOMATION?

The advancement of laboratory automation has been greatly facilitated by the introduction of computers in the 1960s and the subsequent explosion in computer technology. Computers are critical to the efficient operation of any laboratory. Requests for laboratory testing can be generated via computer terminals located at nursing stations that are either linked to the laboratory information system (LIS) or to the hospital information system that networks with the LIS.

Sample identification systems have been greatly improved by computer technology. As tests are requested via the LIS, a set of collection labels is printed with numeric or bar code accession numbers. If a manual requisition system is still in use, one of the labels is applied to the requisition. The remaining labels can be used as specimen labels for the original patient sample, aliquot labels, slide labels, and so on.

Once the accession number is generated and a sample is collected, all testing operations for that sample remain linked to that accession number until the results have been reported and verified to the LIS.

A major advantage of computerized sample identification systems is the reduction in human error. In manual systems, laboratory personnel were responsible for generating accession numbers and transcribing requests from the requisition to log sheets and then to worksheets. All specimens and aliquot containers had to be labeled. Completed results were transcribed from worksheet to requisition. Each time the information had to be transcribed to a new location, another opportunity occurred for human error to be introduced into the system.[18]

If bidirectional interface is available between the LIS and laboratory instruments, worklists from the LIS can be downloaded to the instrument computer. Otherwise, test requesting must be done using a keyboard or touch screen. The latter option doubles the work effort since each test must be requested twice. Unfortunately, many laboratories still function under such a system.

The development of the microchip made it possible to build in microprocessors as integral components of instruments. Microprocessors are responsible for numerous tasks in the testing process, and when more than one is present in an instrument, multiple tasks can be handled simultaneously. Inside the laboratory, computers simultaneously control such operations as start-up, calibration, testing mode, and reagent dispensing. Computers monitor equipment functions, such as optical system stability and temperature control. Computers communicate malfunctions to the operator. Computers facilitate delta checks (comparison of present result with most recent result).[19]

The entire process of data management is computer controlled, whether it involves data conversion and calculation prior to the reporting of a result or simply the transmission of a completed result to the LIS. The LIS disseminates the patient data summary to a terminal, to a hard copy chart report, or to a computerized medical record system. As physicians are able to have access to results from terminals prior to receipt of chart copies, the number of telephone calls to the laboratory is reduced. This is another step in increasing the efficiency of the staff.[20]

Another component of information systems that is emerging in clinical laboratories is the **expert system.** Expert systems are programmed to solve problems. These systems are capable of providing interpretive and diagnostic feedback to physicians and can also be integrated into the testing operation of the laboratory.[21, 22]

Repair of instruments or updating operational programs may be as simple as changing a computer board or a microchip.[11] Modem technology allows communication between manufacturer and user for such purposes as downloading new software to the instrument and for running **diagnostics programs** for technical assistance.

Personal computers (PCs) are also an important tool in the laboratory. A recent survey indicated that 83 percent of the 1462 respondents used personal computers in their laboratory. The primary task performed on the PC by most respondents was word processing. PCs can provide the data base for inventory control, quality control, quality assurance, workload recording, and productivity studies, as well as other parameters. Many laboratorians are not achieving the full benefit of their PCs.[23]

Computer systems can be networked to provide an avenue of communication between the laboratory and other areas of the hospital for a multitude of purposes, including patient locater lists, admission/discharge summaries, purchasing, billing, and so on.

HOW HAS THE COMBINATION OF AUTOMATION AND COMPUTERS CHANGED THE TESTING PROCESS?

A primary goal for any laboratory should be to automate as many repetitive tasks as possible, thus relieving personnel to perform other functions. The overall impact should demonstrate increased efficiency and throughput, improved precision, reduced errors, and lower labor costs per test. Each new generation of instruments is designed to assume an increasing role in performing the varied tasks of the testing process. As the performance of these tasks moved from manual to automated mode, many changes occurred. Some of these tasks include patient identification, sampling, measuring reagents, mixing, incubation, readout, calculating, and recording of results.

Patient Identification

In a manual system of testing, the assay and the record-keeping components include numerous opportunities for human error to occur. For many years, in-patient identification has been achieved by a wrist band attached to the patient on admission and worn for the duration of the hospital stay. Prior to collecting a blood sample for laboratory testing, information on the wristband is compared with the patient data on the requisition. Careful attention to detail is required to prevent an error in identification.

Bar coding technology has the potential to solve this problem, but this identification system is still in its infancy in clinical laboratories. A bar code is defined as "an array of parallel, rectangular bars and spaces that together represent data characters in a particular symbology."[17] The three bar code systems that are primarily used by instrument manufacturers are Code 39, Codabar, and Code 2 of 5.[24] Several problems prevent full utilization of bar code technology in the laboratory. The laboratory industry lacks standardization of coding systems, i.e., no code is uniformly recognized by all instruments. Variations in the quality of stock labels may cause printing or reading problems. Some reading problems can be attributed to the poor quality of readers on some instruments. Finally, there is a lack of integration of bar coding into the total health care plan of a given institution.[25]

Ideally, an integrated bar code system would include automatic patient identification through bar coding of wrist bands. Bar codes would be incorporated into the collection label, and portable readers would confirm a positive match of the coding on the wrist band and the collection label. A bidirectional interface between the laboratory information system and laboratory instruments would allow downloading of test requests. Instruments would read the bar code label and match patient data with test request(s).

Sampling and Measuring Reagents

Many laboratories still use a manual system of sample processing. These systems require many steps and are very labor intensive. Even though minimally skilled individuals are often assigned these tasks, this remains a significant contributor to slower turnaround time as well as to the number of human errors made in the laboratory. In chemistry laboratories, samples must be centrifuged, and aliquot containers must be prepared. After centrifugation, sample is transferred to aliquot containers. This represents a critical step in which transfer errors can be made. In addition, personnel are exposed to the risk of infection with multiple handling and aliquoting of samples.[26]

Some laboratories are developing automated sample processing systems. Robotics, conveyor belt systems, and bar codes are main features of these systems.[27-31] Robotic technology has been more widely used in industry than in clinical laboratories. While a **robotic system** can perform repetitive tasks precisely and accurately to reduce human errors and biohazardous risks, many problems still remain. A robot frees a laboratorian to do other tasks, but it does not usually work any faster. In general, robots are not easily programmed by the user. Present models are expensive, and each model requires unique space considerations. Because of the different needs and different physical facilities of individual laboratories, market standardization is difficult.[15, 16]

In the ideal automated sample processing system, primary sample tubes would be loaded on an instrument (preferably by robotics). The instrument scans the bar code, matching it to the previously downloaded test request(s), and analysis begins.[25]

Once the sample reached the testing area, manual procedures required a clean pipet and at least one clean testing container for each individual sample being tested. This required adequate glassware support services or a large supply of disposables.

Three types of pump systems are commonly used in automated sampling devices: syringe, peristaltic, and pneumatic. The sampling system should be designed to eliminate carryover between patient samples. This may be accomplished by incorporating an internal/external wash of the probe between patients, by using disposable tips, or by using an inert material that coats the probe but does not mix with the patient's sample nor interfere with the assay. A properly functioning automatic sampler will accurately measure the required volume each time; therefore, random access analyzers must be equipped with a sampling device that is capable of changing the volume of delivery very quickly.[17]

During sampling, the technologist can perform other tasks, resulting in significant savings in personnel costs. The cost of an automated assay will also be influenced by the amount of consumable supplies required in the sampling/testing process. It should be noted that some centrifugal analyzers require that sample and reagent measurement occur external to the analyzer. The measurement, or pipetting, may be done by an automated device, but the technologist must transfer the rotor containing the sample and the reagent(s) to the analyzer unit. This reduces the efficiency of both the instrument and the technologist.

As an additional aid to the laboratorian, some automated sampling devices are designed to monitor the measurement of sample volume. These monitoring devices detect the difference between air and liquid by measuring differences in conductivity, by using visible or infrared wavelengths to measure optical differences, or by using light-sensitive diodes.[17]

Mixing

The task of mixing in manual assays was accomplished by gentle swirling, by inversion, or by a variety of mechanical mixers or shakers. Automated mixing in wet reagent systems may use peristaltic pumps with mixing coils, magnets, centrifugal force, or mechanical devices. The exact time when mixing begins and ends, the length of time for mixing, as well as how vigorously mixing occurs, is built into the computer program. This greatly increases method precision. Dry reagent systems do not require mixing. Instead, a small volume of sample is applied to the reagent strip or slide, and the liquid rapidly spreads through the matrix of the test area.

Incubation

The purpose of the incubation step in an assay is usually to provide a waiting period designed to allow for measurement of reaction rates or to allow a reaction to come to completion. The waiting period may be accomplished at room temperature or in some prescribed temperature-controlled environment, such as 37°C. An instrument's ability to maintain a constant temperature in the testing chamber and to perform at optimal levels may be hampered by the heat generated from the instrument during operation. If an instrument requires a narrow tolerance of variation in room temperature and yet generates a large amount of heat during routine operation, the laboratory may be required to install additional hot air exhausts or air handling (cooling) units.

Readout

Successive models of instruments brought improvements in readout capabilities. The calibrated numerical scales, such as the % T/absorbance scales of early spectrophotometers, were followed by servo motors that provided direct numerical readouts for results. The next generation of instruments was equipped with light-emitting diodes (LEDs) that provided optional modes of readout, e.g., absorbance or concentration. The introduction of computers brought cathode ray tube (CRT) screens that displayed results in a variety of formats and that were linked to printers that provided a hard copy of each patient's results.

Technology has advanced far beyond the cuvet and simple filter capability. A number of automated systems use test packages designed as self-contained units capable of accommodating an assay from the time the sample is added and mixed with reagents until the readout is complete. Two examples are the Dupont aca and the Kodak EK-TACHEM. The aca forms the cuvet in the reagent pack, whereas the EKTACHEM reads directly from the slide. Both automatically deposit used test packages into the instrument's waste container. Centrifugal analyzers use disposable rotors in which readings are taken directly from the cuvet wells.

As long as a reaction mixture can be delivered to a readout station, any number of measurement technologies can be adapted to testing. Some of the specific principles that have been adapted to provide readout capability include light absorption, light re-

flectance, ion-selective electrodes, coulometry, potentiometry, and light scattering. A multitude of immunoassay and laser applications have also been developed. Bichromatic measurements reduce the influence of interfering substances. These applications have improved method sensitivity and specificity, making it possible to measure analytes that are present in very low concentrations—a feat not possible with older manual methods.

Calculating and Recording

Manual data manipulation by the technologist has been significantly reduced. In medium-to-large laboratories, data management is largely achieved via microcomputers and laboratory information systems. Calibration curves, calculations, and other mathematical manipulations of data are programmed functions and are used by the system to convert a patient's raw data into reportable results.

A permanent copy of each patient's results may be printed for laboratory records or maintained on discs. When a laboratory information system is in operation, large instruments are usually on-line. Some interfaces are unidirectional and only allow transmission of patient results to the LIS. Bidirectional interfaces allow communication between the instrument and LIS in both directions. In either case, patient results are transmitted to the LIS, and all patient data are formatted for the permanent medical record. Prior to becoming a part of the permanent record, completed results may be retrieved at any time by physicians at a computer terminal networked to the LIS.

Reagent and Sample Volume

Significant reductions in the reagent volume and the sample volume required for an assay have resulted from advances in automation. Precise volumes of sample can be delivered by micropipets or probes with little or no carryover between sample deliveries.[17] Final reaction volumes in manual methods ranged from 5 to 50 mL, compared with 300 to 600 μL in automated wet chemistry assays. The current trend is toward dry chemistry methodology, in which sample volumes as small as 1 or 2 μL are possible.[22] These reductions in sample volumes reduce the amount of specimen to be collected and are of particular importance in a pediatric patient population.

Turnaround Time

One of the driving forces behind the development of laboratory automation was the demand for faster response, or **turnaround time,** for test results. Zaloga divides turnaround time into three categories: laboratory time, testing time, and therapeutic time.[14] According to his definition, laboratory time refers to the time required to produce a result once the specimen reaches the laboratory. Testing time includes collecting, transporting, and assaying the sample. Therapeutic time begins when the physician requests the test and ends when the physician makes a therapeutic decision or takes an action based on the test result. Therapeutic time is obviously a critical component of quality patient care, and the value of any laboratory test is first determined by its individual therapeutic turnaround time.[14, 20] The laboratory time of a manual method was limited by the sample handling system, by the number and complexity of steps in the procedure, by the reaction time involved, and the speed at which the laboratorian could perform the tasks associated with the assay. The laboratory time in a highly automated laboratory will be determined primarily by the time spent in proc-

essing the sample and the speed at which the instrument can provide individual results.

The extended overall turnaround time for those low volume tests that were only performed once or twice weekly severely limited their therapeutic usefulness. As manufacturers continue to develop expanded **test menus** with improved specificity and sensitivity, physicians will be able to obtain results for a number of rarely ordered tests just as readily as for a blood glucose.

HOW HAS TECHNOLOGY BEEN APPLIED TO TESTING IN VARIOUS DISCIPLINES?

The types of instruments that have been successfully introduced into specific areas of the laboratory have been determined by a number of factors. Manufacturers determine whether a system will be open or closed. An **open system** allows the user to obtain reagents and consumable supplies from any available vendor. This allows the user to negotiate for the best price. With the purchase of a **closed reagent system,** the owner is committed to purchasing only the instrument manufacturer's reagents and supplies. Advantages of a closed system include the convenience of dealing with only one vendor, improved stability of reagents, and longer calibration times on the instrument. However, a closed system is usually more costly to operate, since there is no competition to hold prices down. The current trend is toward closed systems.[11, 31, 32]

Chemistry analyzers can be divided into two basic categories: random access and batch. Random access analyzers process test requests in order of receipt, without regard to their position in a sample tray. These analyzers use a single analytic path for all testing.[33] Tests are performed on a sequential basis as they are requested.[19] These analyzers are most convenient for integrating STAT requests into a routine workload.

Batch analyzers process all tests of one type for a given number of samples or process the same group of multiple tests on a predetermined number of samples. Once initiated, testing proceeds to completion in a set sequence. Some batch analyzers, such as the AutoAnalyzer, utilize multiple paths to assay the maximum number of analytes available. However, each time a group of samples is analyzed, each sample is carried through every analytic path without regard to test request. This results in wasted sample and wasted reagents. When these types of instruments are used to assay a defined battery of tests **(test profile),** the turnaround time is determined by the slowest testing time in the group of tests. **Centrifugal analyzers** are batch analyzers that use a single analytic path determined by the analytic method. Only one test can be done at a time. The order of testing is predetermined by the sequence of samples in the carousel. Batch analyzers are not conducive to large volumes of STAT requests. Specific chemistry instrumentation is discussed in Chapter 8.

Since 1958, automated cell analyzers have advanced rapidly. Today's models perform a complete blood count, including a blood cell profile, or differential. Every laboratory that provides hematology services utilizes some type of counter for total blood cell counts, but not everyone uses the automated differential result. Some still resort to manual microscopic identification and enumeration of white cells and evaluation of red cell morphology. This is a labor-intensive task. Lack of precision on replicate analyses by the same individual or between individuals has been documented. Manual differentials involve counting 100 cells, while automated instruments count thousands of cells and therefore provide much more precise results. Tentative standards established by the National Committee on Clinical Laboratory Standards require instruments to perform normal leukocyte differentials as well as or better than a laboratorian can. The question must then be raised: Why do some laboratorians continue to perform manual blood cell profiles when an instrument can do it with more speed, more precision, and with equal accuracy? Additionally, some question the usefulness of a differential in any situation other than a suspected abnormality.[34]

Each new generation of cell counters provides additional parameters of data for red cells, white cells, and platelets. Scientists are attempting to improve the usefulness of these data by correlating these new parameters with disease states.[34] The principles and features of the four most popular systems will be discussed in Chapter 9.

Microbiology laboratories have been slower to adopt automated systems. Systems are available to identify common gram-positive and gram-negative bacteria, using a combination of growth curves and computer analysis of biochemical profiles. The results are available within a few hours, compared with the 24-plus hours needed when using a manual system. Some instruments are capable of providing the identification and minimum inhibitory concentration (MIC) of antibiotics for each organism tested. Semiautomated blood culture systems were initially based on radiometric principles. Newer versions used infrared spectrophotometry to detect growth, and a recent prototype is based on the colorimetric measurement of the CO_2 produced by growing microorganisms.[35-37]

One of the newest technologies that is rapidly expanding in microbiology testing is the DNA probe. Probes are designed to detect specific nucleic acid sequences that are unique to a given microorganism.[37] This technology has been applied to other areas of testing, including genetic disorders.

During the past two decades a tremendous amount of research and development has centered on the concept of immunoassays. The first to be introduced was radioimmunoassay.[38] Radioassays were initially employed in hormone testing and were automated in the early 1970s. Today many of these radiolabeled assays have been replaced by enzyme- or fluorescent-labeled assays, as well as chemiluminescent assays, making immunoassays one of the most widely used analytical techniques in today's laboratory. For example, random access instruments utilizing chemiluminescent immunoassay technology offer test menus that include hormones, tumor markers, and drug monitoring. Advantages of nonisotopic immunoassays include improved sensitivity, stability, and safety, as well as potential for incorporation into automated systems. The development of monoclonal antibodies has had a major impact on testing capabilities. This technology made it possible to produce large supplies of antibodies that possessed a unique and narrow antigenic specificity.[4, 11]

Automated nephelometric assays are available to quantify immunoglobulins. Microtiter technology has combined with fluorescent immunoassay and enzyme-linked immunosorbent assay (ELISA) to provide automated serologic testing for the first time.

Flow cytometry has the ability to analyze thousands of cells per sample and is utilized to analyze cell surface markers and to quantify the DNA content of cells, providing data that can be used in evaluating malignant disease processes.[39, 40]

Detailed manual methods and extensive record keeping have been characteristic of blood bank laboratories since their beginning. Both were designed to reduce the risk of transfusion errors. In modern blood banks, automation is available for blood typing, for direct and indirect antiglobulin testing, and for antibody screening. The cross-match can also be performed; however, in high volume, rapid response laboratories, the efficiency will be reduced by the number of different donor cells used in testing the requested number of transfusable units. Incorporation of automated bar code technology and computers for data management should reduce record-keeping errors as well as improve efficiency.[41]

Automated pheresis units allow capture of white cells or platelets when component therapy is critical. Autologous blood lost during surgery can be salvaged and processed for return to the patient as packed red cells or filtered whole blood.[41]

WHAT ARE THE MOST IMPORTANT FEATURES OF AN INSTRUMENT IN TODAY'S LABORATORY?

When purchasing any instrument for the laboratory, a number of important features should be considered. Throughput, or the number of samples analyzed per unit time, is an important selling feature. Laboratorians are always seeking increased throughput to allow more results to be produced in a shorter time. The buyer should determine whether the advertised throughput is based on the number of samples per hour or the number of tests per hour. If it means samples per hour, does the number include calibrators, controls, and patients, or just patients? If it means tests per hour, the test mix may be critical to maximal output. For example, if the throughput is advertised at 1000 tests per hour, will the instrument perform any combination of 1000 tests, or will it only analyze 1000 tests of a few selected quick and easy assays? The time delay from sampling to available result is critical in high-volume testing areas, and STAT testing capability is a must in today's laboratory.

The size and flexibility of the test menu

will determine an instrument's adaptability to a routine, STAT, or routine and STAT testing environment. The user needs the broadest menu possible, but the size of the test menu should be supported by maximum usability of its particular tests. It may not be cost effective to tie up positions on the menu for infrequently ordered tests. Ideally, the more flexibility the user has in determining or changing the test menu, the better. If the menu is solely established by the manufacturer, the flexibility is reduced and costs may be increased, particularly if some test selections are rarely used.

The cost of obtaining the instrument is a critical decision. Should it be purchased outright, leased with intent to purchase, or only leased? An ongoing expense is the supplies and reagents consumed by the test volume for that instrument. Also contributing to overall costs is the time required for preparing and calibrating the instrument to begin analyses. The amount of hands-on time required by the operator may be a major cost factor. Hands-on time may include start-up and shut-down, loading new sample trays, resupplying consumables, normal operation, and preventive maintenance or repair activities, each of which contributes to personnel costs applied to the instrument. An instrument that has large periods of **downtime** (nonproductive) contributes to increased costs. Personnel time is required for repair, and during this period of time, income is not being generated.

Calibration of an instrument involves a number of considerations. In addition to the ease with which the instrument is calibrated, the manufacturer's recommended frequency of calibration is significant. Calibration may be required on a daily basis, or the instrument may remain accurate and stable for periods of up to 6 months, depending on the instrument. On most instruments the microprocessor monitors the status of calibration and either automatically recali-

brates or alerts the operator that recalibration is necessary. Ideally, an instrument remains in stand-by calibration mode. This means that the instrument is continuously available for immediate start-up when patient samples arrive. Time and supplies used to recalibrate for every new patient or batch of patients are lost revenue and decreased productivity and efficiency. Calibration materials should be easily obtainable, be available in adequate supply, and remain in stable condition for acceptable periods of time.[42]

Reagent supplies come from a variety of sources. Although some of the earlier instruments allowed for in-house reagent preparation, most new systems include patented reagents as part of the package. Reagent systems may be based on wet or dry technology. Wet reagents are usually less expensive than dry reagents; however, more personnel time is required for preparation. Calibration is usually required more frequently. Some instruments that use wet reagents are equipped with probes that sense levels of liquid and make it possible to monitor reagent supplies and detect insufficient samples. Some probes sense the amount remaining in the reagent containers; others function by monitoring the amount used from a starting volume that was input by the laboratorian.[17] These probes may be connected to alarm systems that alert the operator when reagent supplies are nearing depletion or when the sample probe senses that it has aspirated something other than liquid.[43] Some instruments use bar codes for reagent identification, monitoring expiration dates, and inventory control. One recently introduced chemistry analyzer is equipped with a microchip that manages the reagent system.* The microchip contains calibration data and bar code data for the current reagent lot number, including expi-

---

*Nucleus by Nova Biomedical, Waltham, MA.

ration dates. Reagent usage is also monitored.

The current trend is toward dry reagent systems, which have many advantages over wet systems. Costs are higher than wet reagent costs; however, in-house preparation time is at a minimum because reconstitution is not required. This results in time savings for personnel and reduced opportunities for human error to occur in the preparation process. Dry reagents offer simpler testing operations because most involve single-step assays. Systems that rely totally on dry reagents usually incorporate the reagents with some type of support matrix, such as a strip or a slide. The prescribed amount of reagent required for an individual assay is a component of this self-contained unit. A small volume of sample is added to the reagent area; the instrument then processes the test and discards the used slide or strip into a waste container on board the instrument. Biohazardous waste disposal is easier and safer, because the instrument waste container can be emptied into the appropriate container for autoclaving and disposal. Some self-contained wet reagent systems have a similar disposal system; however, the wet system requires more space. Dry reagents tend to be more stable, thereby providing longer shelf lives. Large supplies of single lot numbers are possible, and calibration is usually required less frequently. Dry reagents require less storage space than liquids.[11, 19, 32]

Some disadvantages with dry reagent systems: The user is usually limited to a single vendor for consumables, a factor that contributes to the higher costs.[19] The test menu of an instrument using dry reagent technology may not be as broad as that of a wet reagent system. New test development by the user is possible with wet reagents but rarely achievable with dry systems.[17]

The capability of sampling directly from a closed primary specimen tube with bar code labeling is important for several reasons. The amount of personnel time required for sample processing is reduced. This reduces the opportunity for human error as well as labor costs per patient sample. It ensures a closed system for the sampling process. This improves safety because it reduces personnel exposure to biohazardous risks. Savings in consumable supplies are realized from two perspectives. Aliquot containers are not required. The amount of consumable supplies required for disposing of biohazardous materials according to Universal Precautions guidelines is also reduced.[19]

Automatic redilution and reassay of an out-of-range sample is important, particularly to a closed primary tube sampling system. The advantages of increased safety and reduced personnel time are lost if a laboratory worker is required to open the tube to obtain a sample for a dilution.

Closed-tube sampling systems should accommodate multisized specimen containers. The system must be capable of penetrating the tube cover, controlling carryover between samples, and sensing fluid levels.[26]

A new instrument should improve the workflow. The goal is to handle the **workload** with the least number of work stations. Ideally, a new instrument would reduce the present number of work stations and free personnel who can be assigned to other tasks. This has the net effect of reducing some of the negative impact of a personnel shortage in a given work area.[10, 44]

Laboratory automation and computer technology have combined to increase efficiency and productivity, to improve standardization of testing, and to reduce opportunities for human errors in testing and data management. Laboratorians have been provided with tools to improve accuracy and to reduce turnaround time, both of which are critical to quality patient care.

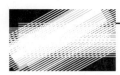

REVIEW QUESTIONS

Choose the best answer.

1. Laboratory instruments were developed more readily for clinical chemistry assays because

   a. other areas were slow to recognize the benefits of automation.
   b. many existing manual procedures could easily be adapted to an automated system.
   c. these instruments did not require precise measurements.
   d. manufacturers had no interests in other areas.

2. Which of the following can be achieved with bar code technology?

   a. Increased accuracy in patient identification.
   b. Reduced hands-on time in sample processing.
   c. Decreased human error in transmitting test results.
   d. All of the above.

3. Which of the following is not usually controlled by the microprocessor unit of an instrument?

   a. Sequence in which patient samples are loaded.
   b. Start-up and calibration procedures.
   c. Testing mode.
   d. Data management.

4. Which of the following has prevented widespread use of robotic systems in laboratory instruments?

   a. Robotics are expensive.
   b. Robotics do not perform at an acceptable level of accuracy.
   c. Robotics are not easily programmed by user.
   d. a and c.
   e. b and c.

5. The time elapsed between specimen arrival in the laboratory and the reporting of a result best defines

   a. laboratory turnaround time.
   b. overall turnaround time.
   c. testing turnaround time.
   d. therapeutic turnaround time.

6. One advantage of using a closed reagent system is

   a. reduced costs.
   b. access to multiple vendors.
   c. longer calibration times on instruments.
   d. easier use by operator.

7. Which of the following features should be considered when evaluating an instrument for purchase?

   a. Cost of consumables.
   b. Downtime.
   c. Throughput.
   d. Size/flexibility of test menu.
   e. All of the above.

8. All of the following are advantages of closed tube sampling EXCEPT:

a. Reduced sample processing time.
b. Reduced costs.
c. Reduced biohazardous risk.
d. Reduced sample volume required.

REFERENCES

1. Aller RD: Maintaining the quality of laboratory services in a cost-containment environment. *Clin Lab Med* 5(4):623–634, 1985.
2. Skeggs LT: An automated method for colorimetric analysis. *Am J Clin Pathol* 28:311–322, 1951.
3. Krieg AF: Laboratory information systems from a perspective of continuing evolution. *Clin Lab Med* 11(1):73–82, 1991.
4. Hardwick DF, Morrison JI: *Directing the Clinical Laboratory*. Field & Wood Medical Publishers, Inc., 1990, pp 56–66.
5. Rock RC: Why testing is being moved to the site of patient care. *Med Lab Obser* (Special Issue), September, 1991, pp 2–5.
6. Statland BE: Tests performed in physicians' office laboratories. *Lab Med* 17:335–336, 1986.
7. Kroger JS: An internist's view of the physician's office laboratory: New opportunities, new challenges, and new responsibilities. *Lab Med* 17:327–329, 1986.
8. Miller SM, Etnyre-Zacher P: Biosensors and diagnostic testing: Enzyme electrodes. *Clin Lab Sci* 2:169–173, 1989.
9. Statland BE, Moskowitz MA: Why office testing? *Clin Lab Med* 6(2):205–209, 1986.
10. DeCresce RP, Lifshitz MS: Integrating automation into the clinical laboratory. *Clin Lab Med* 8(4):759–774, 1988.
11. Burtis CA: Advanced technology and its impact on the clinical laboratory. *Clin Chem* 33:352–357, 1987.
12. Felder RA, Boyd JC, Margrey K, et al: Robotics in the medical laboratory. *Clin Chem* 36:1534–1543, 1990.
13. Starrs C: Technology rises to the occasion: The growth of home testing. *Clin Lab Sci* 2:330–333, 1989.
14. Zaloga GP: Evaluation of bedside testing options for the critical care unit. *Chest* 97:185S–190S, 1990.
15. Felder RA, Boyd JC, Savory J, et al: Robotics in the clinical laboratory. *Clin Lab Med* 8(4):699–711, 1988.
16. Hard R: Robots: Can they help solve the technologist shortage? *Hospitals* 65(12):56, 58, 1991.
17. Lifshitz MS, DeCresce RP: New technologies in chemistry instrumentation: The basis for clinical chemistry automation. *Clin Lab Med* 8(4):623–631, 1988.
18. Rhoton D: Developing a microcomputer-based laboratory management system. *Clin Lab Sci* 1:218–220, 1988.
19. DeCresce RP, Lifshitz MS: Chemistry instrumentation: Part II: Reagent systems, liquid handling capabilities and microprocessor-based control systems. *Lab Med* 17:395–399, 1986.
20. Winsten D: Why spend the money? Justification for laboratory information systems. *Clin Lab Med* 11(1):105–121, 1991.
21. Connelly DP, Bennett ST: Expert systems and the clinical laboratory information system. *Clin Lab Med* 11(1):135–151, 1991.
22. Duben-von Laufen J, Bishop ML: Automation in clinical chemistry: Discrete analyzers. *J Med Technol* 2:221–226, 1985.
23. Jahn M: Personal computers in the clinical laboratory. Part I: Available in most labs, fully utilized by few. *Med Lab Obser* August, 1991, pp 24–31.
24. Garza D, Murdock S, Garcia L, Trujillo JM: Bar codes in the clinical laboratory. *Clin Lab Sci* 4:23–25, 1991.
25. Weilert M, Tilzer LL: Putting bar codes to work for improved patient care. *Clin Lab Med* 11(1):227–239, 1991.
26. Columbus RL, Palmer HJ: The integrated blood-collection system as a vehicle into complete clinical laboratory automation. *Clin Chem* 37:1548–1556, 1991.
27. Bond LW: Consideration of laboratory parameters in design and implementation of automated systems with barcoding. *Clin Chem* 36:1583–1584, 1990.
28. Goldolphin W, Bodtker K, Uyeno D, Goh L: Automated blood-sample handling in the clinical laboratory. *Clin Chem* 36:1551–1555, 1990.
29. Maffetone MA, Watt SW, Whisler KE: Automated specimen handling: Bar codes and robotics. *Lab Med* 21:436–443, 1990.
30. Nabb D: A systematic approach to materials handling in clinical laboratories. *Clin Chem* 36:1576–1578, 1990.
31. Whisler K, Maffetone M, Watt S: Automated systems for positive specimen identification and sample handling. *Clin Chem* 36:1587–1588, 1990.
32. Decrese RP, Lifshitz MS: Selecting laboratory instrumentation, Part II. *Med Lab Obser* March, 1989, pp 73–75.
33. Lifshitz MS, DeCresce RP: Automation of routine chemistry analysis. *Clin Lab Med* 8(4):633–642, 1988.
34. Schoentag RA: Hematology analyzers. *Clin Lab Med* 8(4):653–673, 1988.
35. LeBeau LJ: Roots of automation in microbiology: An introduction. *Am J Med Technol* 49(5):299–301, 1983.
36. Thorpe TC, Wilson ML, Turner JE, et al: BacT/Alert: An automated colorimetric microbial detection system. *J Clin Microbiol* 28(7):1608–1612, 1990.
37. Tierno PM, Hanna BA: Automated and rapid meth-

ods in clinical microbiology: Past, present, and future. *Clin Lab Med* 8(4):643–651, 1988.

38. Berson SA, Yalow RS: Quantitative aspects of the reaction between insulin and insulin-binding antibody. *J Clin Invest* 39:1996–2006, 1959.

39. Camenson G, Patterson MJ: Application of flow cytometry to malignant disease. *Clin Lab Sci* 2:223–226, 1989.

40. Michael BS, Davis BG: Automation in immunology. *J Med Technol* 2:213–216, 1985.

41. Polan CS: Automation in blood banking and hemotherapy. *Clin Lab Med* 8(4):675–687, 1988.

42. Lifshitz MS, DeCresce RP: Clinical laboratory instrument selection. *Lab Med* 21:367–370, 1990.

43. Lott JA: Strengthening the weak link in lab services. Presented at Central Indiana Clinical Biochemistry Forum/Ohio Valley Section of American Association of Clinical Chemistry, Indianapolis, September 21, 1991.

44. DeCresce RP, Lifshitz MS: Selecting laboratory instrumentation, Part I. *Med Lab Obser* February, 1989, pp 76–83.

HISTORICAL REVIEW
Manual Systems
Dedicated Instruments
Sequential Batch Systems
Fixed Profile Systems
Centrifugal Analyzers
Batch Systems
STAT Systems
Random Access Analyzers
THROUGHPUT AND OPERATING CYCLES
ANALYZER SUBSYSTEMS
Liquid Handling
Sampling
Reagent Systems
Optical Systems
Computers
STAT Testing

C h a p t e r   8

CLINICAL CHEMISTRY AUTOMATION

ROBERT P. DE CRESCE, MD, MBA
MARK S. LIFSHITZ, MD

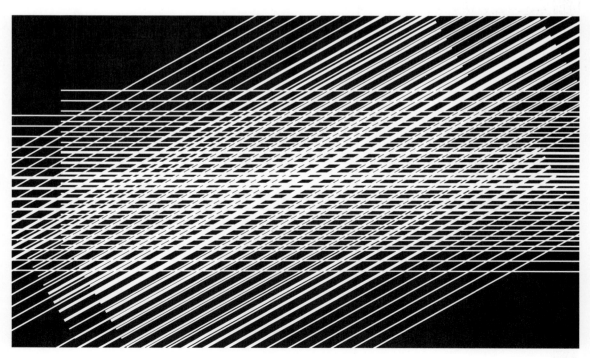

LEARNING OBJECTIVES

After studying this chapter, the student will be able to:

- Describe the difference between random access analyzer and batch analyzer.
- Define the advantages of centrifugal analysis.
- Describe the changes that the Technicon AutoAnalyzer brought to the clinical chemistry laboratory.
- Identify all of an analyzer's subsystems and explain their function.
- List the advantages and disadvantages of both dry and wet reagents.
- Define the term *carry-over.*
- Describe the difference between open and closed reagent systems.
- Define biosensors and describe one advantage they have brought to testing.
- List the functions of microprocessors in an instrument.

KEY WORDS

Batch systems. Analyzers that perform large numbers of single tests.

Centrifugal analyzers. Analyzers that use centrifugal force to join sample and reagents together.

Dedicated instrument. An instrument that is dedicated to perform one or two tests.

Fixed profile systems. A sequential system that performs a specific number of tests at one time.

Manual systems. Laboratory tests that are performed manually.

Random access analyzers. Analyzers that process different tests simultaneously and discretely.

Sequential batch system. Automated system that automatically adds samples and reagents to an analytical stream for a particular test.

STAT systems. Systems that are dedicated to performing only STAT tests.

Today's clinical chemistry analyzers are the products of many technologic developments over the past 30 years. Many technologic changes were revolutionary, whereas others were enhancements of pre-existing technology that significantly improved daily laboratory operations. This chapter chronicles the development of the state-of-the-art chemistry analyzer and discusses the operational benefits and limitations of the technology used in these highly sophisticated systems. This information should be used to analyze and compare different instruments in order to make intelligent purchase decisions. Though virtually all analyzers in today's market meet technical specifications, their performances may differ significantly from one laboratory setting to another. Ultimately, the performance level determines how satisfied a laboratory is with its purchase. Understanding how a system works can help determine which analyzer is best suited to a specific setting.

HISTORICAL REVIEW

The modern chemistry analyzer has evolved over the years. Here is a short review of the various systems that culminated in today's instrument. For the most part, the goal of these systems was to automate the tasks involved in performing a test or to provide an enhanced method of analysis.

Manual Systems

The earliest clinical laboratory tests were performed manually. One example is the Ortho-Toluidine glucose method, in which sample and reagent are mixed together in an individual cuvet. After a suitable incubation time at the appropriate temperature, the reaction is read in a spectrophotometer. This may involve transferring the contents to a specialized cuvet if performed in a reaction cell, or the reaction cell itself may act also as the cuvet. This type of procedure has obvious limitations: inaccurate sample and reagent metering, poor control of reaction timing, imprecision introduced at the spectrophotometer level, and operator variation. Further, throughput is limited even if many tests are run together. For all these reasons, alternatives to manual procedures were sought.

Despite its shortcomings, manual testing had several potential advantages: the ability to customize test conditions and use a separate cuvet for each test to eliminate the possibility of sample carryover, to vary reagent and sample addition times and volumes, and to process tests in any order (i.e., randomly or in batch). These benefits were not available on early automated devices and began to reappear with the introduction of today's sophisticated systems.

Dedicated Instruments

The earliest automated instruments were often dedicated to running one or two analytes in a highly automated manner. These devices were often flame photometers that performed sodium and potassium analyses. Mechanical diluters eliminated what were previously manual sample preparation steps. They also had automatic, albeit crude, data reduction systems that eliminated manual result calculations and potential errors. These systems offered obvious benefits: improved precision, fewer calculation errors, and enhanced throughput. The primary operational drawback of these systems was that they were inflexible, i.e., they were dedicated to running specific tests. Dedicated analyzers capable of performing only one or two tests are still found in the laboratory today. They include instruments that perform analyses such as lead and ionized calcium. These systems represent automation perfected to perform a specific test and tailored to achieve optimal results. However, the tradeoff is a loss of flexibility, which is not always required.

Sequential Batch Systems

One of the most important developments in the clinical laboratory was the introduction of the Technicon AutoAnalyzer. This system offered unique advantages that far outweighed its disadvantages.

The AutoAnalyzer allowed the laboratory to perform a single test in a fully automated fashion. The system automatically added sample and reagent, using mechanical pipets and pumps. Instead of single cuvets, the system used a dedicated analytic channel in which each assay was performed sequentially. Sample mixed with reagent flowed through this channel; different samples were separated by air segments; and the reaction eventually flowed through a cuvet where the reaction was measured. This eliminated manual sample addition. The system could sequentially analyze multiple samples loaded on a carousel, though the operator could not walk away since instrument functions had to be monitored continuously. Nonetheless, throughput was increased, and productivity was improved. The earliest AutoAnalyzers had virtually no data reduction capabilities, though this was added to future systems.

This analyzer offered many benefits. Tests could be performed relatively easily, and a high throughput was possible. Samples could be continuously added to the instrument as long as it was in operation, which meant that batches did not all have to be started at the same time. Furthermore, automation greatly improved precision. Labor expended to run assays fell, and high-volume testing became a reality in the laboratory. However, these advantages came at a price. Compromises had to be made in the reaction conditions to adapt methods to the format of the analytic system. Furthermore, it took considerable time to set up the systems and to change from one analyte to another. **Carryover** also was a problem, because there was a single analytic channel and a flow-through cuvet. Nonetheless, these **sequential batch systems** were the revolutionary laboratory development of the 1950s and blossomed in the 1960s.

Fixed Profile Systems

Fixed profile systems evolved from sequential batch systems. Technicon pioneered this market with the introduction of the SMA 6/60 instrument, followed by the SMA 12/30 and SMA 12/60. These instruments used the same technology as the AutoAnalyzer except that there were multiple channels. In essence, an SMA 12/60 consisted of 12 separate sequential batch channels, each dedicated to a single analyte. This was a major step forward in the development of instrumentation. Suddenly laboratories could produce large test panels, easily and conveniently. Advantages included high throughput and greater productivity (when all tests of the panel were desired), extremely low variable reagent cost per panel, and a dramatic decrease in the labor required to run a test. The disadvantages were related to the technology itself: carryover and method limitations. As the name implies, the profiles were fixed and all tests were performed on every specimen even if it was not ordered. In other words, tests could not be selected. Furthermore, it took a long time to start up the analyzer and shut it down. And since reagents constantly flowed through the system when it was turned on, it was not economical to run the system for a few samples. Thus productivity and throughput were high when running large batches of specimens. However, the system was not suited to run sporadic samples during off-hours. Thus efficiency was gained at the cost of flexibility and availability. Nevertheless it was a suitable compromise, given other alternatives. The market for fixed profile systems was not limited to Technicon, although they completely dominated the field. In the history of automated systems, these instruments are landmarks. They also contributed to the development of commercial laboratories and hospital laboratories, since they could produce a large volume of work at very low variable cost.

Fixed profile systems remained popular for nearly two decades. Because of this, a number of variations developed. Most famous was the Technicon SMAC system. This computerized instrument performed a fixed battery of tests at very high speed. Because of its computer capabilities, it could modify profiles by choosing from the 20-test menu. This was accomplished by performing the test and suppressing the result of the assay(s) that were not wanted. The Auto-Chemist, followed by the PRISMA from Sweden, also allowed the operator to select tests, but the system was cumbersome and infrequently used. The BMD 8700, which was a rework of the HYCELL-M, offered extremely high speed with some test selectivity. The American Monitor Parallel was the most recent of the group, and it offered both test selectivity and relatively small sample requirements, compared with the other members of the group. All these systems eventually fell out of favor because of outmoded technology, poor mechanical reliability, or obsolete computer systems. They also could not deliver the flexibility and ease of use required by the laboratory of the 1980s and 1990s.

As a class, fixed profile analyzers performed best when processing many samples in batch. Systems took a long time to set up and shut down, and standby capabilities were limited. Even though all of the systems could perform tests extremely fast, hospital laboratories could not offer profiles around the clock because these systems were too costly to run sporadic samples during off-hours. Thus the high throughput was usually confined to a burst early in the morning and perhaps late in the afternoon. These instruments had inherent shortcomings in the hospital market (which receive samples throughout the day and night), which were not as important a factor in the commercial laboratory (since samples arrived in one large batch).

Centrifugal Analyzers

Centrifugal analyzers represented a major technologic improvement. These systems provided chemists with the ability to perform multiple reagent additions under specifically timed conditions. True kinetic enzyme measurements became possible. The instruments allowed tremendous flexibility in test performance and reagent selection.

Centrifugal analyzers also had the capability to perform tests very rapidly, often in less than 3 minutes. Sample volume requirements dropped from milliliter to microliter amounts; this was also a function of the more precise pipeting systems.

With these scientific advantages came two major drawbacks. The first was the batch nature of the system. All samples of a single test had to be run at the same time. Thus, to run a 12-test panel required 12 separate runs. If a rotor held 30 specimens and 40 profiles had to be run, at least two runs of each analyte were needed. Even though the actual analysis time was short, total time to produce a profile was much longer. The other issue was labor utilization and cost. Unfortunately, each rotor on a system had to be loaded separately, which required significant technologist intervention. Elaborate work lists were also required to keep track of where each specimen was loaded and when a result was expected. Control and **calibrator** costs were high because of the multiple runs. In summary, the technical advantages of centrifugal systems had to be contrasted with the inefficiencies inherent in the batch processing mode. These issues remain today; most centrifugal instruments are used as specialty instruments rather than primary laboratory analyzers.

Batch Systems

Batch processing systems were popular in the early to mid 1970s. Examples of systems like this are the American Monitor KDA and the Abbott ABA 100. These systems let the operator run a large number of samples of a single test in a relatively short period of time. In this regard they shared some of the characteristics of the centrifugal analyzers, although they lacked some of their method flexibility. Batch systems generally had high throughput and relatively low reagent costs. Some systems, such as the KDA, could produce many hundreds of results per hour of a single test. Unfortunately, tests had to be produced in batches, which, as with the centrifugal analyzers, greatly compromised true productivity. This was because the high throughput came in bursts; considerable time was required to change over from test to test, and profiling was laborious. Laboratories that lacked a computer system were inundated with paperwork, since a patient's results from different batches had to be collated; this was very labor intensive.

STAT Systems

No discussion of the evolution of chemistry analyzers would be complete without mentioning the introduction of STAT analyzers—instruments designed to produce small profiles rapidly and in high volume. This market was defined in the late 1970s and early 1980s by the Beckman ASTRA. This system could perform from one to eight tests on a selective basis from a fixed menu. The use of special electrode technology and rapid colorimetric methods allowed the instrument to perform eight tests in under 2 minutes on a single sample. ASTRA was a collection of separate modules supported by a single mechanical probe system and computer. The instrument was able to operate 24 hours per day with minimal reagent waste. Calibration was automatic for the electrode-based tests, and the modular design allowed rapid replacement of defective or damaged parts.

The arrival of the ASTRA did two things. First, it replaced the SMA 6/60 as the premier instrument in hospital laboratories for performing electrolyte panels. This was mainly because of the ease of operation of the ASTRA and its excellent standby capabilities. The second major effect was the introduction into the laboratory of an instrument that could be used around the clock for high-volume tests and also for individual assays. This 24-hour testing capability, first provided by ASTRA, has become an increasingly important feature and one that is routinely expected today. The main drawback of ASTRA was its limited menu of eight analytes.

Random Access Analyzers

In recent years, the random access analyzer has grown in popularity. These analyzers can handle on a random basis both sample and reagent without regard to their placement in the carousel. This type of operation implies several unique characteristics that differentiate it from other instruments. The random access analyzer does not have channels dedicated to performing a single test. Instead, it has a single analytic pathway for all testing. The configuration must be flexible enough to take into account each test's unique parameters, such as wavelength, number and time of readings, sample and reagent volume, and so on. The system must also be able to process different tests simultaneously as they pass through the channel, since tests are initiated sequentially based on the request and are not batched. Last, random access analyzers perform testing discretely, usually in a separate cuvet. Throughput is determined by the number of tests run per hour, not by the number of samples per hour.

Do all random access systems adhere exactly to the above description? No. In fact, the definition of a random access system is even subject to interpretation. However, most instruments that are called random access incorporate the most important characteristics of a random access system though they do not, strictly speaking, process tests in this manner. Should this matter to the purchaser or operator? Not really, so long as the analyzer meets customer needs.

The most common variation of a random access system is the so-called optimized batch system. This is typically an instrument that automatically optimizes throughput by running minibatches of the same test. Though these systems can also run in true random access mode, this usually diminishes throughput. When running in optimized mode, tests with the longest incubation time are started first and those with the shortest time are started last. Instruments often use this operating method because it reduces mechanical movements (e.g., eliminates washing reagent probes between each specimen since the minibatch comprises one test) and therefore reduces processing time. As the batch size grows, throughput increases, and as the size of the batch falls, throughput is reduced. Similarly, some instruments impose a time penalty when a STAT sample interrupts a routine run. This is because the optimal processing mode is interrupted and must be reinitiated.

THROUGHPUT AND OPERATING CYCLES

Throughput is one of the most widely used, and unfortunately misused, terms in automation. We define it as the maximum number of tests that an instrument can perform when operating in the steady state. This is invariably a theoretical number since it requires an ideal test mix, constant availability of specimens, and a running start so the system can reach a steady state situation before timing starts. Instrument purchase decisions are often based on theoretical throughput; this can lead to disappointment. A better indicator of instrument performance is productivity. This is the ability of an instrument to perform a defined workload in a given period of time. Invariably, productivity is less than throughput, but it is a better indicator of overall performance. Productivity depends on test mix, a very important factor and one that varies from one laboratory to another. Instrument dwell time is also important. Dwell time is the amount of time between the initiation of the test and the completion of the analysis. This definition is imprecise since it often depends on what constitutes the beginning of a test. For our purposes, dwell time excludes related instrument tasks (e.g., preparing or pouring-off sample, loading, test selection, and so on) and preanalytic time, but it includes time spent in actual testing (e.g., adding the first reactant, be it sample or reagent). For example, if reagent is added before sample, dwell time begins with the addition of reagent. Preanalytic time is the interval between starting the run and the beginning of the dwell time. During this period the instrument may reinitialize its components before a run, wash cuvets, reoptimize processing, position the sample, read the sample bar code, and so on. Preanalytic time varies from one analyzer to another.

To fully appreciate the throughput capabilities of an analyzer, it helps to understand operating cycles. Most instruments have an analytic and a sample cycle; these may be the same or different. The analytic cycle is the rate at which a test can be initiated. Since it is an inherent instrument characteristic, it cannot be modified. For instance, a device with a 12-second analytic cycle theoretically can run 300 tests per hour; similarly, a 5-second cycle will provide a throughput of 720 seconds per hour. Random access analyzers are test based, so throughput is determined by how many tests can be initiated in an hour. Compare this with sample-based profilers. Their throughput is based on the sample cycle. So, an analyzer with a sample cycle of 12 seconds runs 300 samples per hour, regard-

less of the number of tests ordered on each sample.

Several factors can reduce the theoretical throughput of an instrument. When a reagent or sample blank is needed for a test, it uses a cycle that would otherwise be used for a reportable result. Similarly, a two-reagent addition test might require separate analytic cycles for each reagent; this effectively halves the throughput for those tests. Last, if reagent must be added or changed or if cuvets must be replaced, the instrument operation may be interrupted, further reducing throughput.

The sample cycle is the rate at which a new specimen can be introduced into the analyzer. It is often longer than the analytic cycle, thereby reducing throughput when a single test is ordered on sequential samples. For instance, if the sample cycle is 20 seconds and the test cycle is 5 seconds, throughput will vary from 180 to 720 tests per hour, depending upon whether one or four or more tests are ordered per sample.

The ISE (ion-selective electrode) cycle is often used by manufacturers to overstate an instrument's throughput. ISE modules that are integral to the operating cycle produce several electrolyte results instead of a single photometric chemistry result. ISE modules that are additive to the operating cycle use a separate pipet for sample aspiration; electrolyte results augment the basic chemistry output—that is, a chemistry analytic cycle is not used. Most chemistry systems achieve their highest throughput when running a typical seven- or eight-test panel composed of electrolytes (run by ISE) and photometric tests.

From the preceding discussion, it should be clear that test mix is an important factor in determining the net throughput of a device. Though an approximation of net throughput often can be calculated, the most accurate method of determining net throughput is by actually timing an instrument from the start of operation to the completion of results for a given mix of tests.

From the perspective of the operator, the unattended cycle is also important. It represents the period during which an instrument can be run without operator intervention. Several factors can limit the unattended cycle, such as a sample carousel or a reaction disc that can hold only a small supply of specimens or cuvets, respectively. Systems that use individually packaged reagents also will require more operator interaction, as will instruments that have limited on-board reagent capacity that requires switching reagent trays in order to complete a profile.

ANALYZER SUBSYSTEMS

Liquid Handling

All fully automated laboratory analyzers require a mechanism to reduce carryover between samples and different reagents, ensure the delivery of adequate volume, aspirate and dispense sample and/or reagent, and monitor reagent inventory. Liquids are usually handled by a pump that can meter microliter quantities precisely. A pump controller determines the timing and the volume of liquid that is moved.

Historically, the volume of liquid delivered could not be easily adjusted. Mechanical devices had to be manually inserted or removed in order to vary the length of the pump arm to deliver different volumes. This was time consuming and imprecise. The development of the step motor allowed sample and reagent volumes to be adjusted electronically rather than mechanically. Step motors are DC-powered, microprocessor-regulated devices that precisely control the pump. A screwlike mechanism converts the shaft revolutions into pump action. The major advantages of step motor–controlled

pumps are very precise liquid metering and the ability to change delivery volumes rapidly. The former characteristic allows delivery of microliter quantities of sample and reagent with great precision (coefficients of variation less than 1 percent); the latter characteristic allows tests with different reaction parameters to run on the same analytic pathway, such as in a random access analyzer.

The most common form of liquid handling device is the syringe pump. As noted, it is usually combined with a step motor. Peristaltic pumps are useful in delivering larger liquid volumes; they use rotating spokes to force pump tubing against an immovable platen. Pneumatic pumps use air pressure to force liquids through valves at a constant rate; this is especially useful when large volumes must be delivered in a relatively short time.

Another interesting approach to handling liquids is the solid state fluidics system developed by Instrumentation Laboratory.[1] Reagents and samples flow through and mix in solid acrylic blocks that are precision machined with interconnecting channels. The design eliminates many of the typical problems associated with tube-based systems and reduces maintenance requirements, sample and reagent volume, and the size of the instrument.

Since automated instruments must access sample and reagent in fairly rapid succession, they need to incorporate a method for reducing or eliminating liquid carryover. To reduce surface wetting during aspiration, most probes are coated with Teflon. Many instruments also limit the depth of immersion of the probe. These methods are often used in conjunction with a probe cleaning system that washes the probe internally and externally. Some instruments can eliminate all carryover completely. For instance, the EKTACHEM analyzers eliminate sample carryover by using a disposable plastic tip, whereas sample-based profilers that use dedicated reagent channels and dispensers eliminate reagent carryover by their very nature.

Another approach to eliminating carryover is the development of a patented liquid fluorocarbon, referred to as "random access fluid."[2] This immiscible material coats the interior and exterior surfaces of the probe, thereby preventing carryover. Because the material is inert, it does not affect the ensuing analysis.

Liquid level–sensing devices are needed to ensure that adequate sample or reagent is aspirated. Fluid handling mistakes can result in erroneous results. A variety of techniques are used, including changes in capacitance and resistance. The latter detects the difference in conductivity between air (low) and liquid (high). Other instruments sense liquid by first introducing a wave and then detecting oscillations. Optical detectors can also be used; they sense the difference in visible or infrared light transmission between air and liquid. Some devices use light-sensitive diodes in the probes to detect that a sufficient volume was aspirated.

Sampling

All instruments must be able to identify samples properly. In the most simplistic sense, this identification might consist of a cup position on a carousel that is manually correlated with the patient ID by the operator. More sophisticated techniques have reduced sample handling errors and streamlined processing by providing varying degrees of enhanced sample identification. For instance, an identification method might use a binary-coded sample carrier, or require the operator to place specimens in a designated position, or identify samples by a unique binary code on the tray. Though

these enhanced identification methods reduce errors, they do not provide sample identification.

Positive sample identification is best achieved by using a **bar code;** this can be used to identify a patient throughout a hospital stay. In the ideal situation, a bar code label should be placed on the sample at the time of collection; this is becoming more commonplace in hospitals. Bar coded labels are often printed with the phlebotomy draw list. However, many times bar codes are affixed to the sample at the laboratory receiving area or at the chemistry workstation.

A bar code is an array of parallel, rectangular bars and spaces that together represent data characters in a particular symbology. Several different bar code formats exist, including Interleaved 2 of 5, Code 39 (Code 3 of 9), and Codabar. Bar codes must be printed on paper with a high reflective index in order to be read by a laser scanner. Most bar codes are read several times to prevent misreads, a condition wherein the data output from the reader does not correspond to the data encoded in the bar code. This may be due to unwanted dark areas in the spaces, as from printing errors or dirt. Many bar codes use check digits to minimize the likelihood of a misread. These are characters included within the symbol whose value is used to perform a mathematical check on the preceding data.

Bar codes are of tremendous value in high-speed instruments. This is especially true when there are many tests to choose from and different ones may be ordered with each sample. Bar codes are typically used (1) to identify the sample in a positive way, thereby eliminating the need to have worksheets and match cup numbers to results, and (2) with a host computer to allow rapid transfer of data between the instrument and the laboratory. Laboratories that have two-way interfaces obtain the greatest benefit. These interfaces typically allow the instrument to read the bar code and identify the specimen. The analyzer then queries the host computer for the orders on that patient, which are automatically downloaded from the host to the analyzer. At the completion of testing, the instrument "uploads" the data to the host computer. Bar coded samples also aid in processing STAT specimens, since they can be freely switched with other samples without having to consider tray location. In other words, the STAT can be placed in the next position to be scanned and aspirated; the sample occupying that position can be moved elsewhere without regard to tray location.

To realize the full potential of positive sample identification through bar code labeling, an instrument should also be able to sample directly from the primary (blood collection) tube. Otherwise, sample must be poured into cups, and the likelihood of error increases. Primary tube sampling speeds processing, saves time and money, and, in combination with bar codes, virtually guarantees the proper identification of the sample. A variant of this is closed-tube sampling. This is popular on hematology instruments and is also available on Baxter's Paramax 720 ZX. This feature greatly diminishes the chance of technologists coming in contact with serum or whole blood and simplifies storage, since leakage problems are minimized.

Reagent Systems

The development of new reagent systems has simplified the operation and enhanced the capability of clinical chemistry analyzers. In the past, reagents were best classified based on physical characteristics, i.e., liquid or dry. Liquid reagents were run on "open" chemistry analyzers, meaning the system was nonproprietary so reagents could be purchased from third party vendors. Dry reagents were run on "closed" analyzers, meaning the system was proprietary so reagents were available from only one vendor. In recent years, these arbitrary distinctions between reagent systems no longer hold true, in that many liquid systems are closed or semiclosed. Perhaps the most accurate way to classify today's reagent systems is as open or closed. Closed systems may be subdivided into liquid and dry reagents.

Traditional open liquid reagent systems offer several advantages, such as flexibility in designing or adapting new methods, provided the laboratory's instrument parameters can be modified. A wide variety of tests are available from multiple manufacturers, including urine and cerebrospinal fluid (CSF) chemistries, drugs, hormones, and other immunoassays. This wide availability prevents "reagent lock-in" and prices usually are competitive, so these systems are especially attractive in high-volume settings such as commercial laboratories.

In general, liquid reagents cost less than those prepared by proprietary methods. However, this does not mean that the overall operating cost associated with liquid reagents is less; other factors must be considered, such as calibration, outdating, and labor. Liquid reagent systems may require daily calibration for some analytes. However, many liquid reagent systems now offer calibration stability of a month or longer. In the past, most liquid reagents had to be reconstituted, leading to a potential source of error. Now, most current systems either eliminate this source by providing ready to use (i.e., liquid) reagent or by simplifying the reconstitution process through providing premeasured liquids to combine in the reagent container. Liquid reagent systems can be rendered closed or partially closed based on the packaging. Proprietary packaging precludes one from running another vendor's reagents. Other systems may allow third party reagents but often without all the benefits of their own reagent system, such as bar coding, automatic expiration tracking, and so on.

By their very nature, dry reagent systems are closed. They offer long shelf-life and on-board stability, owing in part to a manufacturing process that can produce large reagent lots. Calibration is often extended to several months. Dry reagents are also automatically reconstituted or activated on board the instrument, eliminating all operator sources of error and promoting convenience and ease of use.

Dry reagent systems also have limitations. These systems are proprietary, that is, they are developed by a manufacturer for exclusive use on a single instrument or family of instruments. The user is locked-in to the manufacturer's reagents, usually resulting in a higher reagent cost per test than for liquid systems. This is probably due to the lack of competition and the payback required for the research and development of the system. Another potential drawback is test menu, since there may be a limit to the number and type of assays that are available (or can be adapted) for a particular system. Immunoassays, for instance, are more readily available on liquid systems than on dry ones. Last, there is no user flexibility in developing new tests when dry reagents are used.

The demarcation between dry and liquid reagents is not as clear as it used to be. Most dry reagent systems are liquid chemistry–based, that is, they are reconstituted on board the instrument. In most instances, it is the reagent packaging that confers its uniqueness. A variety of dry reagent systems are available, but the only fully automated dry chemistry random access analyzer is the Kodak EKTACHEM family of analyzers. These systems are based on multilayered film technology; all the chemicals required for the reaction are layered onto a slide.[3] The only liquid used in the system is patient sample (and reference fluid for electrolytes). Reflectance spectrophotometry is used to read the reaction since there is no liquid medium to read.

Other dry systems use liquid chemistries. For example, the Baxter Paramax,[4] the venerable DuPont aca, and the DuPont Dimension ES are really liquid systems that reconstitute dry reagents on board the analyzer. The Paramax uses tablets, whereas the Dimension has special multiwelled FLEX cartridges. Chem 1 + reagent cassettes are activated before they are loaded on board.[5] These and other such systems are prepackaged dry (and in some cases liquid) reagents to perform the tests in a liquid medium that uses transmittance spectrophotometry. All the aforementioned systems are closed, or proprietary, meaning the reagents can be purchased only from the original vendor. Generally they are protected by patents on either the reagents or the packaging, which prevent competitors from copying the system.

Bar codes have played an increasingly important role in reagent management for open and closed systems. Typically, bar coded reagent containers identify reagent name and amount, lot numbers, and calibration factors. This facilitates reagent handling and prevents the operator from placing a reagent container in the wrong location. It also allows the user to place several reagent containers of the same type on an instrument, so that when one container is depleted, the second is started automatically. Some analyzers can also monitor online expiration dates and lot calibration; if either is exceeded, the reagent is not used.

Which reagent system is better—open or closed? There is no clear-cut answer. Liquid reagents are potentially less expensive and more flexible than dry systems, but the economies are not guaranteed, especially at low to medium volumes. Dry systems are usually more expensive for reagents alone, but the savings in labor and preparation time often outweigh the extra cost. Similarly, calibration tends to be more stable with closed systems because of the nature of the reagent manufacturing process, and this also has financial implications. The choice requires a detailed analysis of the particular laboratory's situation, since there are no simple solutions.

Optical Systems

At the core of every instrument is a method of sensing the chemical reaction; a transmittance or reflectance spectrophotometer is generally used for this purpose. In transmittance spectrophotometry, light passes through liquid and then strikes a detector; results are calculated based upon Beer's law. In contrast, reflectance spectrophotometry requires a solid phase reagent; light is reflected from the solid phase and strikes a detector. Results are calculated by a complex set of empirically derived formulas.

The basic elements of a spectrophotometer are a light source, monochromator (to supply light of a single wavelength), and detector. The most common light source used for routine chemistry applications is the tungsten-halogen lamp. It emits a continuous spectrum of light from 360 to 950 nm; the light is of high radiant energy per watt consumed. Some instruments use a xenon flash lamp, which produces short bursts of high-intensity light; this prolongs the lifetime of the lamp. Lasers are powerful sources of monochromatic light; they are used in specialized applications that require enhanced sensitivity and specificity.

All light sources, other than lasers, must be able to select out a single wavelength for measurements. A high-grade interference filter with a bandpass of less than 10 nm is generally used for this purpose. For those

analyzers using transmittance spectrophotometry, glass or plastic cuvets are used, which may be disposable or reusable. Instruments that reuse cuvets require a mechanically complex wash station and a high-grade water supply; although this may add to the overall purchase price of an instrument, it usually reduces ongoing operating costs.

After passing through the cuvet, light is measured by a detector such as a photodiode or photomultiplier tube (PMT). A photodiode is a semiconductor form of a barrier cell; it is very stable and durable and does not require an external power source. However, it does require intense light, which makes it unsuitable for situations in which the light beam is split. On the other hand, PMTs can amplify a light signal; this lets them detect low-intensity light beams. They also require an external power supply and are more expensive than photodiodes.

Recent advances in solid state electronics and manufacturing techniques have provided current instruments with optical systems that are compact, more reliable, simpler, and more adaptable than those in older models. However, some of the most significant improvements have not related to the individual components of the optical system but rather to their configuration.

Traditional optical systems were usually arranged in a double-beam in-space or double-beam in-time configuration. In the former system, a single light source is split into two separate detection systems that allow for simultaneous parallel measurements between reference and sample. In the latter design, a light beam is split in two and then directed out-of-phase to a single detector. Until recent years, it was common for a clinical instrument to incorporate several optical systems, each with its own light source. Not only did this add to the overall size of the instrument, it also required frequent calibration.

With the availability of fiberoptics, light

from a single source can be efficiently split into multiple beams and transmitted over longer distances than in traditional optical systems. A multiple-beam configuration usually requires PMTs, since the light intensity of each split beam is relatively low. The advantage of this configuration is that a single light source can be used to illuminate multiple cuvets. This is a particularly useful feature when the reaction track and detector stations are arranged in a linear path; it permits multiple reactions to be simultaneously monitored. Another advantage of light guides is that they allow the optical system to be located at a distance from the detector stations, and in a location that is easily accessible for maintenance.

Another significant advance has been in multiwavelength monitoring. Whereas traditional systems have used a fixed wavelength or selected one from several discrete filters, newer arrangements can monitor multiple wavelengths continuously. For instance, rapidly spinning filter wheels do not stop at a specific wavelength during the reading. Instead, all available wavelengths pass sequentially through each cuvet; the detector takes readings on all wavelengths and the instrument's computer discards those that are not necessary for the analyte being measured.

Linear diode array optics provide simultaneous measurement of multiple wavelengths.[6] In this configuration, polychromatic (full spectrum) light is passed through the cuvet; the transmitted light is then dispersed by a grating into multiple wavelengths. Diodes are arranged in a linear array to detect the transmitted light; by virtue of its position within the array, each diode detects a single wavelength. A major advantage of this system is that it has no moving parts, since the diode array is fixed in position; this makes it more reliable than conventional systems. Diode arrays also provide a rapid means of collecting data at many more wavelengths than would be possible with a filter wheel.

Multiwavelength monitoring capabilities provide new ways of analyzing measurement data. Bi- and trichromatic corrections can be performed to eliminate interference from hemolysis or lipemia. Also, multiple reactions can be run in the same cuvet, provided each is monitored at a different wavelength.

Recently, much attention has been focused on a new type of sensing technology, biosensors. These devices are microelectronic devices that use a biologic molecule, such as an antibody or enzyme, as a sensing element. Biosensors are advantageous because they are a reagent-free method of analysis and can provide simultaneous measurements of several analytes, all from a single whole blood specimen. A compact hand-held device was recently introduced to the market by i-Stat Corporation.

Computers

Perhaps the most significant technology leap has been in the area of computers. Without these advances, the full potential of newly developed reagent, optical, and liquid handling systems could not be realized. The basis of computers is the microchip—miniaturized transistors on a silicon chip. The microprocessor is the central processing unit of a computer and is contained on a single chip.

Microprocessors perform multiple functions in an instrument. Many of these are transparent to the operator. Microchips are responsible for data management operations, including reduction of raw data such as optical readings, matching cup position with results, collating patient results with demographic data, reporting, and data retrieval. A second function is process control, that is, coordinating the activities of various subsystems. For instance, microprocessors must control the precise timing of robotic arms so that pipeting and dispensing correspond to reaction turntable movements; this insures proper liquid handling and optical readings that match a given cuvet. Microprocessors also enable instruments to assume different operating modes and to optimize the time of processing through the use of sophisticated algorithms.

Many instruments use several microprocessors, each dedicated to performing specific functions. This configuration confers the ability to perform multiple functions simultaneously (multitasking). For instance, instruments can perform real time quality control. If a control value is out of range, the instrument can notify the operator automatically and often suggest a course of action. Multitasking also allows test ordering, results editing, and data retrieval to occur while the instrument is in full operation reading test reactions.

Increasingly powerful computers have also introduced more user-friendly display environments, such as window environments, as well as a host of other helpful features, including management reports (e.g., statistics), automated maintenance and quality control records, correlation studies, and custom-defined reports. In many instances, the data management capabilities of the analyzer overlap those of the host computer. Ultimately, the degree to which an analyzer's computer capabilities are helpful depends on whether or not a laboratory has a host computer and how it is used.

STAT Testing

The ability to run routine and STAT samples on the same instrument has been the goal of many laboratory directors and managers. While certainly possible with many modern instruments, compromises are necessary. STAT testing implies a short dwell time for the first result and sufficient throughput to eliminate the queuing effect. However, since STAT tests are generally less frequent than routine tests, the availability of the instrument at a given time rather than its actual output per unit time is most important. Routine processing has different demands. Total throughput and productivity for a given test mix are most important. The actual amount of time required to process an individual analyte is less important than the volume produced per unit time. High-volume systems tend to have high throughput and often a long (10 to 15 minute) dwell time before the first result is available—not an optimal arrangement for STAT tests. Systems that are designed for STAT use, such as the Beckman CX-3, or for high-volume work, such as the Hitachi 747-200, are designed to optimize their respective functions. Many systems for the clinical laboratory are necessarily a compromise between these designs; they perform both functions more or less well but rarely excel at either.

SUMMARY

The choice of an instrument requires careful analysis of the needs and future plans of the laboratory, as well as its workflow. For the most part, instruments work to the extent that they meet analytic specifications. However, their performances may differ significantly from one laboratory setting to another. Understanding how a system works can help determine which analyzer is best suited to a specific setting.

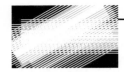

REVIEW QUESTIONS

Choose all the responses that are true.

1. The early autoanalyzers (sequential batch systems) played an important role in the chemistry laboratory during the

   a. 1940s and 1950s.
   b. 1950s and 1960s.
   c. 1960s and 1970s.
   d. None of the above.

2. Centrifugal analyzers offered

   a. true end-point analysis.
   b. two-point analysis.
   c. multiple wavelength analysis.
   d. true kinetic enzyme measurements.

3. Examples of a batch system are

   a. American Monitor KDA.
   b. Kodak Ektachem.
   c. Abbott ABA 100.
   d. a and b are correct.
   e. a and c are correct.

4. The correct definition for throughput is

   a. The maximum number of tests an analyzer can perform in a 24-hour period.
   b. The maximum number of samples an analyzer can perform in a 24-hour period.
   c. The maximum number of tests an analyzer can perform when operating in a steady state.
   d. The maximum number of tests an analyzer can perform in a given hour.

5. Primary tube sampling is defined as

   a. sample directly from collection tube.
   b. sample directly from bar coded cup.
   c. sample from analyzer's primary tube.
   d. none of the above.

6. A dry reagent system can be found on which of the following?

   a. Miles DAX systems
   b. Beckman systems
   c. Olympus systems
   d. Kodak EKTACHEM systems
   e. Baxter Paramax system
   f. Dupont Dimension ES system

7. Light from a single source that can be split into multiple beams and transmitted over longer distances than traditional optical systems defines

   a. photodiode.
   b. fiberoptics.
   c. photomultiplier tube.
   d. linear diode array optics.

REFERENCES

1. De Cresce RP, Lifshitz MS: New instrumentation preview. Cellect hematology analyzer. *Lab Med* 17:624–626, 1986.

2. Smith J, Svenjak D, Turrell J, et al: An innovative technology for "random-access" sampling. *Clin Chem* 28(9):1867–1872, 1982.

3. Shirey TL: Development of a layered-coating technology for clinical chemistry. *Clin Biochem* 2:147, 1983.

4. Driscoll RC, Edwards RB, Liston MD, et al: Discrete automated chemistry system with tableted reagents. *Clin Chem* 29:1609–1615, 1983.

5. Cassady M, Diebler H, Herron R, et al: Capsule chemistry technology for high-speed clinical chemistry analyses. *Clin Chem* 31:1453–1456, 1985.

6. De Cresce RP, Lifshitz MS: Chemistry instrumentation: New technology for the 1980s and beyond. *Lab Med* 17:267, 1986.

BIBLIOGRAPHY

Lifshitz MS, De Cresce RP: *Understanding, Selecting, and Acquiring Clinical Laboratory Analyzers.* New York, Alan R. Liss, Inc., 1986.

Narayanan S: *Principles and Applications of Laboratory Instrumentation.* Chicago, ASCP Press, 1989.

The Instrument Report (newsletter). Applied Technology Associates, 839 West Belden Avenue, Chicago, IL 60614.

TECHNOLOGIES
Electronic Impedance
Light Scattering
Light Scatter and Absorbance
INSTRUMENTS
Coulter STKS
Technicon H-1
Sysmex NE-8000
Cell-Dyn 3000
Serono System 9000+
Cobas Argos 5 Diff
ISSUES

Chapter 9

AUTOMATED HEMATOLOGY ANALYZERS

DONALD J. GARTNER, MS, MT (ASCP) SH
JOHN R. SNYDER, PhD, MT (ASCP) SH

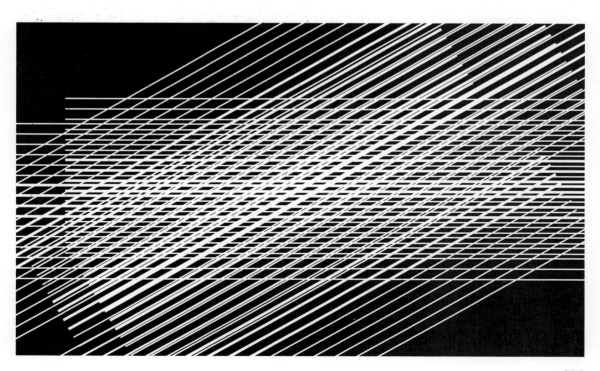

LEARNING OBJECTIVES

After studying this chapter, the student should be able to:

- Define terminology associated with automated hematology analyzers and principal components of these systems.
- Describe and contrast electrical impedance and light scattering as basic technologies used in automated hematology analyzers.
- Describe different principles for analyses used by various hematology instrumentation.
- Identify characteristic features for hematologic analyses used by the Coulter STKS, Technicon H-1, Sysmex NE-8000, Cell-Dyn 3000, Serono System 9000+, and Cobas Argos 5 Diff automated systems.
- Describe special issues related to flagging abnormal or questionable results and interpretive statements.

KEY WORDS

Argos 5 Diff. An automated hematology analyzer using cytotechnology, resistivity, and optical density measurements to produce a 26-parameter report.

Auto-Reporter 3. An optional module for the Coulter STKS analyzer for generating laboratory and chart reports.

Cell-Dyn 3000. An automated hematology analyzer that uses a flow cytometer to determine a white cell count and differential as well as aperture resistance to count red cells and platelets.

"Coincidence" error. An error in analyzers using the electronic impedance principle in which two or more cells simultaneously enter the aperture separating the internal and external electrodes, resulting in one pulse.

Conductivity analysis. A method used in cell counting based on the electrical conductivity difference between particles in a suspension and the diluent as measured between two electrodes.

Coulter STKS. An automated hematology analyzer that uses aperture impedance to enumerate cells and platelets and to measure cell volume. A five population white cell differential is produced using a combination of aperture impedance, conductivity, and laser light scatter.

Double Hydrodynamic Focusing System. A patented measurement process of the Cobas Argos 5 Diff analyzer that uses two successive measurements on each cell—electronic resistance and optical absorbance.

Electrical impedance. A principle for cell counting based on cells acting as insulators momentarily increasing the resistance in an electrical path between two electrodes.

Flow cytometer. An instrument that uses light scatter methodology for making multiple measurements of individual cells in a flowing fluid.

Hemogram. A group of hematologic direct analyses usually including hemoglobin, erythrocyte count, and leukocyte count.

Hydrodynamic focusing. A process in which a stream of isotonic sheath fluid is used to arrange cells in single file and channel them through a counting chamber with an orifice only slightly larger than a leukocyte.

Lobularity index. A ratio of polymorphonuclear nuclei (PMNs) to mononuclear nuclei (MNs) indicates the degree of nuclear segmentation.

Matrix-Plot. A high-resolution charge produced by the Cobas Argos 5 Diff analyzer, in which collected signals from successive measurements of electronic resistance and optical absorbance are computerized and categorized.

Multiangle Polarized Scatter Separation (MAPSS). A high-resolution flow cytometer used in the Cell-Dyn 3000 to differentially classify white cells.

Parallel analysis. A comparison of results for select analytes between different analyzers and/or methodologies.

Scatter measurements. A methodology for analyzing cell characteristics using a focused beam of light that is interrupted (scattered) when cells are encountered in a flowing fluid.

Scatterplots. A display of data points or cells classified by two or more measurable characteristics. This is used to identify the presence of abnormalities in subpopulations, primarily from conductivity.

Sweep flow technology. A modification in the Coulter STKS anaylzer that improves platelet count accuracy by preventing red cell recirculation.

Sysmex NE-8000. An automated hematology analyzer using aperture impedance to focus cells hydrodynamically for counting and sizing. A five population white cell differential is produced using aperture impedance, radiofrequency measurement, and differential cell lyses.

System 9000+. An automated hematology analyzer using impedance counting and sizing to produce an 18-parameter hematology report.

Technicon H-1. An automated hematology analyzer using laser light to count and size cells. White cells are differentiated into four populations using light scatter, peroxidase staining, and differential lyses.

VCS. An acronym for volume (V), conductivity (C), and laser light scatter(s) describing the technology used in multiple measurements for leukocyte differentials in the Coulter STKS.

The automation of hematologic tests in the clinical laboratory has advanced remarkably in the last three decades. Prior to the mid-1950s, hematology tests were performed manually using basic laboratory equipment: the hematocrit was measured as a packed cell volume using a centrifuge; hemoglobin was measured using a spectrophotometer; white blood cells, red blood cells, and platelets were enumerated using a hemocytometer chamber and microscope; and a white cell differential count was performed on a stained blood smear using a microscope.

Although labor intensive, the measurements of hemoglobin and hematocrit and cell counts by these earlier manual methods were accurate and reliable by clinical diagnostic standards. The manual leukocyte differential, however, suffered from numerous analytic variables. The quality and method of smear prepared as well as the quality of stain and slides used compromised the accuracy and precision of manual differentials. The procedure suffered from variations in standardization of technique ranging from level of magnification to the quality of microscope used. In addition, technologist training and experience as well as a fatigue factor detracted from accuracy and precision.

Advances in hematology automation first focused on counting erythrocytes, leukocytes, and platelets. Early instruments using a darkfield optical scan, light scatter, or electrical impedance measurements were unable to count these different cell types simultaneously and hence are sometimes referred to as "single-parameter" instruments. In the mid-1960s, Coulter Electronics introduced an instrument capable of simultaneous white and red cell counts as well as determinations of mean red cell volume (MCV) and hemoglobin. From these data, calculations for hematocrit, mean cell hemoglobin (MCH), and mean cell hemoglobin concentration (MCHC) were possible.

Automation of leukocyte differentials occurred at a slower pace. Image recognition and flow-through instruments using cytochemical or volume criteria eventually developed. While image processing instrumentation is generally being phased out, flow-through instruments using cytochemical and volume criteria for differentiating leukocytes have evolved to multiple part leukocyte classification systems. These instruments are capable of accurately classifying routine leukocytes with greater speed and precision than afforded by manual techniques. The current sophistication in leukocyte differential technology is enhanced by new sample handling systems and patient data integration systems.

The purpose of this chapter is to describe the basic technologies used in automated hematology instrumentation, to provide an overview of some of the major instruments on the market, and to identify special issues related to flagging abnormal or questionable results and interpretive statements. Specific instruments described include the Coulter STKS, Technicon H-1, Sysmex NE-8000, Cell-Dyn 3000, Serono System 9000+, and Roche Cobas Argos 5 Diff.

TECHNOLOGIES

The technologies developed to automate hematology procedures use one of two physical properties as the principle of operation: **electrical impedance** or light scattering. The principle of electrical impedance is based on the electrical conductivity difference between particles in a suspension (cells in a fluid) and the fluid (diluent). By contrast, the light-scattering methodology uses a focused beam of light that is interrupted (scattered) when cells are encountered in a flowing fluid.

Electronic Impedance

The principle of electronic impedance was first introduced in the 1950s by Joseph and Wallace Coulter and has consequently become known as the Coulter principle. This principle was described earlier in Chapter 3, Particle Counters, but is reviewed briefly here to describe its use with automated hematology systems. The electronic impedance principle is the basis for many of the automated hematology systems on the market today.

Figure 9–1 is a simple drawing of the measuring apparatus used in electronic impedance systems. A blood sample is diluted in an electrolyte solution such as saline. The electrolyte solution is a good conductor of electrical current, while cells in the solution are relatively poor conductors. To establish an electronic current flow, two electrodes are used: one, the external electrode is located in the blood cell suspension; the other, an internal electrode, is located in a hollow glass tube containing a small opening (aperture or orifice) enabling passage of the blood cell suspension in limited volume between the two electrodes. Cells suspended in the electrolyte are made to pass through the aperture by creating a vacuum inside the aperture tube. When a current flow is established between the internal and external electrodes, the cells, acting as insulators, momentarily increase the resistance of

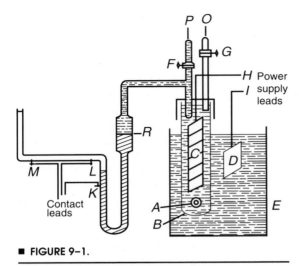

■ **FIGURE 9–1.**

The Coulter principle: electronic impedance; a manometer measuring section and control section with electrodes. (After Mattern CFT, Brackett FS, Olson BJ: Determination of number and size of particles by electrical gating: Blood cells. *J Appl Physiol* 10:56, 1957.)

the electrical path, generating pulses that can be counted.

It is possible for two or more cells to enter the aperture simultaneously, resulting in one pulse. This results in a **"coincidence" error,** for which a correction had to be made on early instrumentation. Newer instrumentation employs sophisticated circuitry and other techniques to decrease coincidence error. In addition, cells may recirculate back into the sensing zone, causing erroneous pulses. To correct for this error, more recent instrumentation uses circuitry to "edit" out unusually shaped electronic pulses. The reduction in errors resulting from coincidence has been achieved by decreasing the size of the aperture, decreasing the concentration of cells, and using a sheath fluid.

Each pulse spike is proportional to the size of the particle that produces it. Consequently, the size of particles to be counted can be established by setting the size to be analyzed, using a threshold to set size limits electronically above which the pulse is analyzed and below which it is ignored.

Electronic impedance as a technology has also been developed for leukocyte differential analysis. By using lysing agents to strip away or shrink a cell's plasma membrane and cytoplasm, "bare" nuclei from cells can be counted as they pass through the aperture. The type of leukocyte can be determined on the basis of the size of the remaining bare nuclei. In this manner, subpopulations of cells can be determined as a use for screening differentials. Counts and differentiation of five cell populations are possible, using specific reagents to alter the cell nucleus and cytoplasm.

Light Scattering

The second major technology used for cell analysis is a light-scattering methodology. Cells pass through a flow cell on which a beam of light is focused. Light is scattered in all directions as the cells interrupt the beam. Photodetectors sense and collect the scattered rays at specific angles as individual cells pass through the sensing zone. Cell counts and size information are determined by the analysis and conversion of the scatter data into digital form.

The instruments that use light-scatter methodology for making multiple measurements of individual cells in a flowing fluid are termed **flow cytometers** (Fig. 9–2).

The flow cell used in this type of instrumentation is made of quartz rather than glass since quartz is transparent and does not bend light passing through it. Quartz allows ultraviolet light to pass through the flow cell where cell counting and cell characteristics are measured. The light source is a laser (*light amplification by stimulated emission of radiation*), which emits a single wavelength. Since laser light is coherent

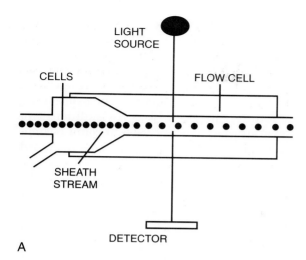

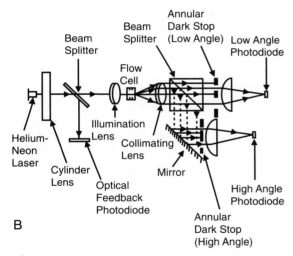

■ **FIGURE 9–2.**

Flow cytometer: light scatter; cytometer measuring differential light scattering. (Courtesy of Miles Inc., Tarrytown, NY.)

flow cell is filled with a sheath fluid that surrounds the stream of sample cells passing through the flow cell. The sheath fluid prevents the flow cell from being coated by substances, such as reagents or cell stroma, that would bend the rays of light entering the flow cell. The sheath fluid also facilitates laminar flow (cell particles flowing in parallel lines through the flow cell without mixing with the surrounding sheath fluid) and hydrodynamic focusing (rapid flow of the cell sample resulting in a narrow stream permitting separation and alignment of cells into a single file for passage through the sensing zone).

Photodetectors (photodiodes and photomultiplier tubes) are used in the sensing zone of the flow cell to detect light scatter by a particle. Defraction of light yields a forward low-angle light scatter used for measuring cell volume. Structure inside the cell is measured by forward high-angle light-**scatter measurements.** RBC (volume versus hemoglobin concentration) and WBC (volume versus nuclear lobularity) are measured using a combination of low- and high-angle forward scatter known as differential scatter. Nuclei and cytoplasmic granules determine the intensity of right-angle light scatter.

Light Scatter and Absorbance

A modification of the light scatter technology is to employ specific staining of some cells. When this technology is used, there are three distinct steps: the cytochemistry for the preparation of the blood cells; the cytometer in which the actual measurement of specific cell properties takes place; and the use of algorithms to convert measurements into usable results for cell classification, cell count, and cell size. This technology uses a darkfield optical method to count and classify leukocytes for differentials.

(traveling in phase where wave peaks and valleys are together), it enables the detection of interference with little light spread. Cells scatter light in all directions, including defraction (bending around corners), refraction (bending because of a change in speed), and reflection (light rays turned back by the surface or boundary of an obstruction). The

Light is scattered through the opening around the darkfield disc as cells pass through the sensing zone. The light scatter is measured with a photodetector, which results in signals or pulses representing the number of cells passing through. With the absorbance channel, as a stained cell passes through the sensor some light is absorbed, leaving less light hitting the photodetector. This light absorption is measured as proportional to the amount of staining. By employing different stains for different cell types, a differential of leukocytes can be calculated.

INSTRUMENTS

It is clear that the recent development of hematology analyzers has led to enhanced accuracy, improved precision, and faster, more automated analysis. Various reports in the literature have attempted to compare various automated hematology analyzers for operational and quantitative differences. Usually, the comparison includes identification of an existing instrument for **parallel analysis** as well as a comparison with manual methods. In this section, a description of three of the major types of automated hematology analyzers is given, followed by a briefer description of three more recent analyzers.

Table 9–1 compares the Coulter STKS, the Technicon H-1, and the Sysmex NE-8000. The Coulter STKS analyzer uses aperture impedance to enumerate white cells, red cells, and platelets, as well as measuring cell volume. In addition, this analyzer produces a five-population white cell differential count using a combination of aperture impedance, conductivity, and laser light scatter. The Technicon H-1 uses laser light at two different angles to count and size cells. Using tungsten light scatter, proxidase staining, and differential lyses, white cells are differentiated into four major pop-

ulations. The Sysmex NE-8000 uses aperture impedance technology with a sheath fluid to focus cells hydrodynamically for counting and sizing. A five-population differential is produced by combining aperture impedance, radiofrequency measurement, and differential cell lyses. In addition, two separate channels are used to count eosinophils and basophils, which are subtracted from the total granulocyte count.

Coulter STKS

Coulter Electronics has long been a leader in hematology instrumentation. As described earlier, the Coulter principle remains the basis for most hematology cell counters. The **Coulter STKS** continues the tradition of using electronic impedance technology with added dimensions for analysis to produce a differential. Introduced in 1987 and first shipped in 1989, the Coulter STKS uses three simultaneous measurements: volumetric impedance for size, high-frequency electromagnetic energy for nuclear and granular constituents, and laser light scattering for surface structure, shape, and granularity.

For the basic **hemogram** component, three values are measured directly: red blood cells (RBCs), white blood cells (WBCs), and hemoglobin. From a whole blood sample, two aliquots are prepared with isotonic diluent. One aliquot is delivered to an RBC aperture bath for calculation of RBCs and platelets. The other aliquot is placed in a WBC bath where a lytic agent is added to break down the RBC stroma and release hemoglobin. Each bath contains three sensing apertures for counts. Both count and size information are generated in triplicate through electronic impedance in the form of pulses. These counts are statistically analyzed for agreement—then averaged. Agreement between two of the counts is required

TABLE 9–1. COMPARISON OF SELECTED AUTOMATED HEMATOLOGY ANALYZERS

	COULTER STKS	TECHNICON H-1	SYSMEX NE-8000
Overview	Three independent simultaneous measurements: 1. Volumetric impedance (size) 2. High-frequency electromagnetic energy (nuclear and granular constituents) 3. Laser light scattering (surface structure, shape, and granularity)	Two channels: 1. Perox channel (NE, LYM, BA, MO, EO, LUC) Light scattering Myeloperoxidase activity 2. Basophil/lobularity channel Cell-specific lysing reagent Laser light Scattering (size, counting)	Three detector blocks: 1. GR, LYM, MO detector block Direct current (DC) (size) Radiofrequency (RF) (nuclear size and density) 2. EO detector block Cell-specific lysing reagent and temperature regulation (counting by a DC) 3. BA detector block Cell-specific lysing reagent and temperature regulation (counting by a DC) • Formula: NE = GR − (EO ± BA)
Detection Method	Impedance, light scatter, sheath, conductivity, cytochemical	Laser and tungsten lamp, cytochemical sheath	Resistance, sheath
Number of Parameters			
RBC	7	8	7
WBC	7–11	15	4
PLT	2	2	4
Sample Size (μL)	100 or 175	100 or 150	200
WBCs Sample	8.2×10^3	10×10^3	Varies with WBC count
Sampling System	Open or auto cork piercing	Open or auto cork piercing	Open, manual, or auto
Throughput/Hr	109	60 (100+)	119
Graphics	Cytogram, histogram, nomogram	Cytogram/histogram	Histogram
Startup Time (min)	0–5	40–160 sec	0–5
Barcode	Yes	No	Yes
Data Storage Patient	1000	Yes	300
QC	Yes	Yes	60×9 files

GR = granulocytes; NE = neutrophils; LYM = lymphocytes; MO = monocytes; EO = eosinophils; BA = basophils; LUC = large unstained cells. (From Payne BA: Instruments for automation of the differential. In Lotspeich-Steininger CA, Stiene-Martin EA, Koepke JA (eds): Clinical Hematology: Principles, Procedures, Correlations. Philadelphia, JB Lippincott, 1992.)

for valid averaging. A display is provided for all three counts for each parameter.

After the leukocyte information is obtained, hemoglobin concentration is measured by the amount of light transmittance, using a hemoglobinometer. The STKS system uses Coulter's patented log-fitting platelet algorithm. The algorithm eliminates RBC interference while capturing macrothrombocytes. Size distribution histograms of WBC, RBC, and platelet popula-tions are illustrated by pulse heights. Other values are calculated, including the MCV (mean corpuscular volume) and RCDW (red cell distribution width) derived from the RBC histogram, the mean platelet volume (MPV) and platelet distribution width (PDW) derived from the platelet histogram, and hematocrit, MCH (mean corpuscular hemoglobin), and MCHC (mean corpuscular hemoglobin concentration) calculated from measured and derived values.

The Coulter STKS uses a new approach to WBC differential analysis—Coulter **VCS** technology. VCS is an acronym for volume (V), conductivity (C), and laser light scatter (S). All three measurements are performed simultaneously in the VC analysis chamber. Thousands of particles are individually analyzed with each instrument cycle, providing high statistical accuracy.

VCS technology provides a complete differential count (DIFF) on whole blood without pretreatment; the DIFF remains stable in samples stored for up to 24 hours. The VCS uses a stream of isotonic sheath fluid to arrange cells in single file and channel them through a counting chamber with an orifice only slightly larger than a WBC; this process is called **hydrodynamic focusing.** One major difference between VCS and previous Coulter cell counters is that it measures WBC in a near-native state. This is done by first gently lysing red blood cells (RBC) with Erythrolyse and then adding an antilysing agent, Stabilyse, to neutralize the lytic action. WBC surface and cytoplasmic characteristics remain intact, and the cell remains about the same size as it is in vivo. This approach differs from the differential shrinkage techniques used by some competitors and earlier Coulter models.

After the RBC are lysed, the WBC are directed to the triple transducer where three measurements are simultaneously but independently taken in the flow cell. The cylindrical measurement chamber gradually narrows toward the center. Hydrodynamic focusing maintains a stable environment for the cells as they pass through the sensing area. About 8000 WBC are analyzed in a typical specimen.

By using volume, conductivity, and scatter measurements, VCS classifies WBC. Volume measurements are based on the Coulter principle for sizing cells, which measures the change in electrical resistance as a particle suspended in diluent passes through a small opening or aperture. Cells are poor electrical conductors, i.e., they impede the flow of current; on the other hand, the diluent is a good electrical conductor. When two submerged electrodes are positioned on opposite ends of an aperture, current flows through the diluent between the electrodes. As diluent is drawn through the aperture, current remains constant except when a nonconductive particle (cell) passes through the aperture. The cell causes a rapid rise in resistance as the buffer (conductor) is displaced by the cell (nonconductor). This change in resistance appears as an electrical pulse, which is sized and counted. The size of the peak corresponds to the cell volume (large cells displace more buffer than small cells), and the number of peaks corresponds to the number of cells passing through the aperture. The instrument records the size of each cell as it passes through the chamber. Different cell types, e.g., small lymphocytes and mature basophils, may be the same size. So this property alone cannot be used to classify cells. However, simultaneous measurements of volume and conductivity provide additional information that differentiates these cells.

Conductivity uses a high-frequency electromagnetic probe to measure a cell's internal structure. Though cell walls do not conduct low frequency current (used for volume sizing), they do conduct high frequency current so changes are related to a cell's intracellular granules, nuclear composition, and intracellular matrix. So, conductivity differs according to the type of WBC and its size. Since cell volume and conductivity are measured simultaneously, the VCS system can differentiate similarly sized cells based on their nuclear differences. Coulter uses **conductivity analysis** of cytoplasmic and nuclear content to determine a new parameter: cell opacity.

The last measurement, laser light scatter, is a function of cell surface characteristics and internal structure. The STKS uses a 0.8 HeNE air-cooled laser that is cooler, more precise, and more reliable than early systems that used a tungsten-halogen lamp to measure light scatter. Light is directed into the sensing chamber where forward light scatter is measured at a 10° to 70° angle. Coarsely granular cells scatter more light than finely granular ones. This helps the instrument differentiate granulated cell populations.

Each cell's size, nuclear structure and surface, and internal characteristics are plotted within a three-dimensional matrix. Then, the WBC is classified according to these properties; it is not classified based on cell distribution data. **Scatterplots** help spot abnormalities, derived primarily from conductivity. Lymphocytes, granulocytes, and monocytes are the prominent populations.

The DIFF stability plays an important role in determining whether a fully automated complete blood count (CBC) is suitable for a laboratory. Some instruments have been popular in hospitals and commercial laboratories with large outpatient populations because the counts remain stable for over 24 hours, a requirement for samples often arriving by courier many hours after collection. Most methods based on differential sizing (e.g., Coulter STKR) have had stabilities under 24 hours and often closer to 8 hours. Coulter claims that the STKS DIFF is stable up to 24 hours and supports this with independent studies submitted to the FDA for product clearance. A recent STKS evaluation confirmed this by reporting that DIFFs were stable in K_2EDTA anticoagulated blood samples for between 18 and 24 hours when stored at 20°C and for longer periods when stored at 4°C and aspirated immediately.

The STKS is a bench-top system that produces a full hemogram and a complete five-part DIFF. It combines features of the VCS system for DIFFs and the STKR for cell counting (based on the Coulter principle) and sample management capabilities. The analyzer can process up to 109 samples per hour when running a complete blood count (hemogram and DIFF) or 138 samples per hour when running only a hemogram. Typical throughput is closer to 120 samples when running only the hemogram. Samples are loaded into a large capacity automatic closed tube sampler; alternatively, an open tube can be manually introduced. The STKS consists of the following modules: power supply, dilutor, analyzer, and data management system (DMS). Reagents are stored externally and are fed into the instrument on demand. There are two major options: the **Auto-Reporter 3** and a color graphics printer.

Besides VCS, the STKS includes several other hardware enhancements. Coulter has improved its RBC and platelet (PLT) measurement systems. Axial flow draws most cells through the apertures along the optimal path. Pulse Edit Technology identifies cells traveling along a nonoptimal path and eliminates their abnormal pulses, thus ensuring size measurement integrity.

Platelet count accuracy is achieved through the use of **sweep flow technology,** which prevents red cell recirculation within the counting area. An individualized log-fitting algorithm further ensures accurate platelet counts even in the presence of microthrombocytes and schistocytes. The algorithm also eliminates microcytic RBC interference and captures macrothrombocytes.

RBC, WBC, and PLT are measured by impedance; hemoglobin is measured photometrically at 525 nm by the cynmethemoglobin method. The STKS uses a reagent blank for each determination; both signals are compared prior to computing the final result. The major sources of error in this channel are severe lipemia (interference with the actual photometric reading), extremely high WBC counts, and rare RBC abnormalities that make them highly resistant to lysis.

A scatterplot pattern enables the technologists to identify the presence of abnormalities in subpopulations with this instrument. In addition, a comprehensive white cell flagging system calls attention to specific abnormalities. Figure 9–3 illustrates a scatterplot pattern for the identification of abnormalities in subpopulations.

Both a laboratory report and chart report are generated from the Coulter STKS, as illustrated in Figure 9–4. The laboratory report calls attention to white cell, red cell, and platelet abnormalities and also quantifies anisocytosis, microcytosis, macrocytosis, hypochromia, and poikilocytosis. Table 9–2 illustrates the definitive flags that can be set on the laboratory report for confirmation of abnormalities.

Technicon H-1

The Technicon Corporation has continued its development of hematology analyzers from its earlier versions of the Technicon Hemalog D and the Technicon H-6000. Like these predecessors, the **Technicon H-1** uses the principle of flow cytometry. Table 9–3 shows the features of the Technicon H-1. The system performs complete blood counts for both red cells and white cells as well as platelets. Mature white blood cells are differentiated, and both red cell and white cell morphology are quantified.

The Technicon H-1 analyzer follows three distinct steps:

- Cyto-chemical reactions prepare the blood cells for analysis.
- A cytometer measures specific cell properties using differential light scattering.
- Computer algorithms convert these measurements into the usual hematologic re-

sults of cell classification, count, size, and hemoglobinization.

As illustrated by block diagram in Figure 9–5, the H-1 system consists of four channels: hemoglobin, peroxidase, red cell/platelet, and basophil/lobularity or "nuclear" channel. Sampling can be from either a closed or open specimen tube. The sample is then split four ways to enter each of the four channel reaction chambers. After the reaction chambers, cells are measured one-by-one as they pass through flow cells in optics benches. Red cell/platelets and basophils are analyzed using helium-neon laser optics in the same flow cell. Tungsten light optics are used in the peroxidase channel. Results from the hemoglobin reaction chamber and colorimeter and these two optics are sent to a computer for result processing, data analysis, and internal consistency checks. After calculations are completed, the final results are printed out on a ticket, and numeric plus histogram and cytogram results are displayed on a cathode ray tube (CRT). Additionally, a graphic screen printer can print anything that appears on the CRT.

The schematics for each of the four channels are shown in Figure 9–6. In the hemoglobin channel, the method used is a modification of the manual cyanmethemoglobin procedure. After a surfactant in the diluent reagent lyses the red blood cells, releasing hemoglobin, the protein moiety is denatured and heme is solubilized and combined with cyanide. Hemoglobin is then measured in this mixture, using a colorimeter at 546 nm.

In the peroxidase channel, red blood cells are lysed and white cells are fixed with formaldehyde. A chromagen and hydrogen peroxidase substrate are added, yielding dark precipitate forms when peroxidase is present in the primary granules of leukocytes. Since neutrophils, eosinophils, and monocytes contain varying amounts of peroxidase, the intensity of staining will vary with

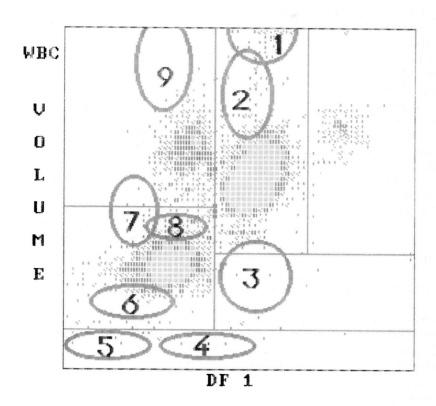

1. Suspect Blasts
2. Suspect Immature Granulocytes
3. Aged and Damaged Neutrophils
4. Giant Platelets
5. Nucleated Red Blood Cells
6. Variant Lymphocytes
7. Suspect Blasts
8. Variant Lymphocytes
9. Suspect Blasts

■ **FIGURE 9–3.**

Coulter STKS scatterplot pattern. (Courtesy of Coulter Corporation, Hialeah, FL.)

Chartable Report.

Laboratory Report.

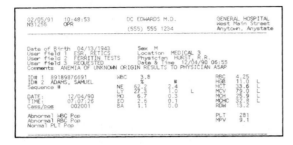

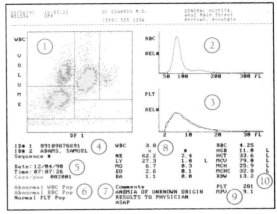

1. WBC scatterplot.
2. RBC histogram.
3. Platelet histogram.
4. Sample I.D. and demographics.
5. Date and time of sample analysis.
6. Sample status.
7. Comment field.
8. Differential results in # & %.
9. RBC and plt results.
10. High and low action flags.

Suspect and Definitive flag information is operator selectable.

■ **FIGURE 9–4.**

Coulter STKS laboratory report and chart report. (Courtesy of Coulter Corporation, Hialeah, FL.)

TABLE 9–2. COULTER CLASSIFICATION CHART

	WBCs	RBCs	PLATELETS
Instrument-defined suspect classifications: (lab report only)	Immature grans/bands Variant lymphs Blasts Review slide	Nucleated RBCs Dimorphic RBC population Micro RBCs/RBC fragments RBC agglutination	Platelet clumps Giant platelets
User-defined abnormalities: definitive flags (lab report only)	Leukopenia Leukocytosis Neutropenia Neutrophilia Lymphopenia Lymphocytosis Monocytosis Eosinophilia Basophilia	Anisocytosis (quantitative +, + +, + + +) Microcytosis (quantitative +, + +, + + +) Macrocytosis (quantitative +, + +, + + +) Hypochromia (quantitative +, + +, + + +) Poikilocytosis (quantitative +, + +, + + +) Anemia Erythrocytosis Pancytopenia	Thrombocytopenia Thrombocytosis Large platelets Small platelets
User-defined high and low action limits (chartable report only)	All WBC parameters	All RBC parameters	All platelet parameters

(Courtesy of Coulter Corporation, Hialeah, FL.)

TABLE 9–3. TECHNICON H-1 SYSTEM FEATURES

One workstation	CBC, platelets, full 5-part differential, RBC morphology ``flags,'' WBC ``flags,'' plus lymphocyte subsets
Complete 5-part differential	Differentiation and quantitation by cytochemical technology of neutrophils, lymphocytes, monocytes, eosinophils, and basophils
RBC morphology	Patented techniques utilizing laser-based optics and cytochemistry permit evaluation of RBCs on a cell by cell basis. Provides RDW, HDW, anisocytosis, macrocytosis, microcytosis, anisochromasia, hypochromasia, and hyperchromasia
Micro sample	100-μL sample from any size collection tube in the open tube mode
	Optional closed-tube sampling available for increased operator safety
	Minimal reagent use
Computer-controlled	Self-prompting; menu driven; on-board QC and system diagnostics; automatic cross-checks for results validation; RS232C standard interface; single-key stroke mode selection
Multiple report formats	Choose from standard ticket or optional graphic screen printer for hard copy results, including histograms and cytograms
Lymphocyte subset analysis	Utilizes immunoperoxidase methodology coupled with standard H-1 system delivery and detection modes; requires no additional instrumentation

RDW = red cell distribution width; HDW = hemoglobin distribution width. (Courtesy of Miles Inc., Tarrytown, NY.)

cell type. Lymphocytes and large unstained cells do not contain peroxidase, hence they are unstained. The stained cells are measured when the effluent is passed through a sheathed stream flow cell in a tungsten-light cytometer optics channel. Cells are analyzed one at a time by passing an extremely narrow stream past a pair of detectors. One detector is darkfield and is sensitive to light scatter; the other detector is brightfield and is sensitive to the degree of staining. Each cell is plotted on a cytogram as a point defined by the levels of light scatter and absorption. Enhanced computer technology enables a pattern recognition system to isolate cell clusters, count the cells in each cluster, and classify them on the basis of information stored in the computer memory.

The basophil/lobularity (nuclear) channel measures the conformation of the nucleus in white cells. In this channel's reaction chamber, the membranes and cytoplasm of neutrophils, eosinophils, lymphocytes, and monocytes are removed by a surfactant at low pH, leaving bare nuclei. Since the membranes of basophils remain intact, a specific basophil count can be performed. A laser-based cytometer is used to distinguish leukocytes by differences in nuclear shape with light scattering at two angles, low (0° to 5°) and high (5° to 15°). Low-angle scatter measures size; high-angle scatter measures lobularity of nuclei. A ratio of polymorphonuclear nuclei (PMN) to mononuclear nuclei (MN) provides an index of the degree of nuclear segmentation. Hence, a low **lobularity index** (PMN:MN) suggests a "left shift."

In the RBC/platelet channel, a buffered reagent isovolumetrically spheres and fixes red cells and platelets. Using the same laser-based optical assembly as was just described for the basophil/lobularity channel, light scatter is measured at low and high angles to determine volume (size) and optical density (hemoglobin concentration) of each cell. Separate histograms are created for each RBC volume and hemoglobin concentration, then merged into a red cell cytogram. From the direct measurements of hemoglobin, RBC count, and mean corpuscular volume (MCV), additional parameters can be obtained from the histograms, including red cell distribution width (RDW), cellular hemoglobin concentration mean (CHCM), hemoglobin distribution width (HDW), he-

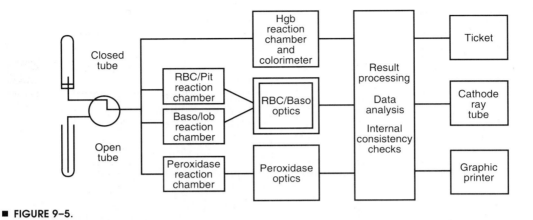

■ **FIGURE 9–5.**

Technicon H-1 system: block diagram. (Courtesy of Miles Inc., Tarrytown, NY.)

matocrit (HCT), mean corpuscular hemoglobin (MCH), and mean corpuscular hemoglobin concentration (MCHC). The high-angle detector is used to measure platelets, resulting in a platelet histogram and "mean" platelet volume (MPV), the mode of the measured platelet volumes.

A recent expansion of the H-1 analysis is lymphocyte typing. By using an immunoperoxidase system, the peroxidase cytometer channel can be used to isolate and count pan T, helper T, and suppressor T and B cells.

Figure 9–7 shows both a screen-printed laboratory report with data on all channels, including histograms and cytograms, and a traditional ticket report with flags for both RBC and WBC abnormalities. This system of flags for abnormal morphology alerts the operator that additional review may be required, such a the microscope examination of a stained smear. Some flags indicate the presence (+) of an abnormality; other flags quantify the abnormality (+ to + + +). Six morphology flags grade for severity of volume (size) in terms of anisocytosis, microcytosis, and macrocytosis; and hemoglobinization (color) in terms of anisochromia, hypochromasia, and hyperchromasia. Other flags prompting action related to white cell

counts and morphology are shown in Table 9–4.

Sysmex NE-8000

The **Sysmex NE-8000** hematology analyzer is manufactured by TOA Medical Electronics Company of Kobe, Japan, and is marketed by Baxter Healthcare Corporation through its Scientific Products Division in the United States. Using automated rack sampling and bar code sample identification features, the NE-8000 is a closed tube, walkaway hematology analyzer capable of producing 23 hematologic parameters, including a full hemogram and five-part differential. Earlier Sysmex cell counters used the electronic resistance principle, measuring DC current across an electrode. To classify white cells, special buffers were applied to shrink leukocytes selectively so they could be classified by nuclear size. This resulted in a three-population differential: neutrophils, lymphocytes, and mixed. These early systems were unable to classify basophils, eosinophils, or immature neutrophils.

The NE-8000 exhibits expanded capabilities over earlier systems by using radio fre-

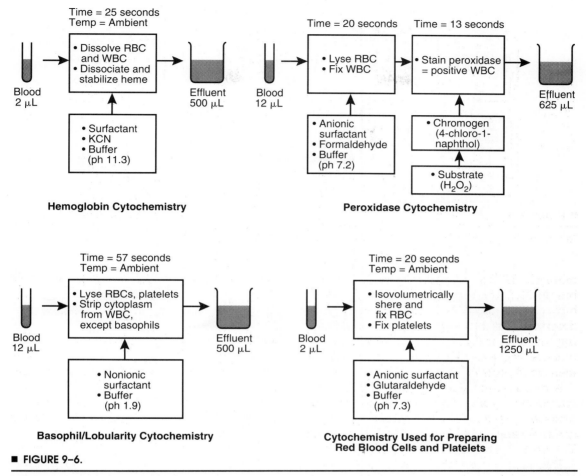

Hemoglobin Cytochemistry

Time = 25 seconds
Temp = Ambient

Blood
2 µL

• Dissolve RBC
and WBC
• Dissociate and
stabilize heme

Effluent
500 µL

• Surfactant
• KCN
• Buffer
(ph 11.3)

Peroxidase Cytochemistry

Time = 20 seconds

Time = 13 seconds

Blood
12 µL

• Lyse RBC
• Fix WBC

• Stain peroxidase
= positive WBC

Effluent
625 µL

• Anionic
surfactant
• Formaldehyde
• Buffer
(ph 7.2)

• Chromogen
(4-chloro-1-
naphthol)

• Substrate
(H_2O_2)

Basophil/Lobularity Cytochemistry

Time = 57 seconds
Temp = Ambient

Blood
12 µL

• Lyse RBCs, platelets
• Strip cytoplasm
from WBC,
except basophils

Effluent
500 µL

• Nonionic
surfactant
• Buffer
(ph 1.9)

**Cytochemistry Used for Preparing
Red Blood Cells and Platelets**

Time = 20 seconds
Temp = Ambient

Blood
2 µL

• Isovolumetrically
shere and
fix RBC
• Fix platelets

Effluent
1250 µL

• Anionic surfactant
• Glutaraldehyde
• Buffer
(ph 7.3)

■ **FIGURE 9–6.**

Technicon H-1 system: channel schematics. (Courtesy of Miles Inc., Tarrytown, NY.)

quency (RF) and direct current (DC) to perform a five-part differential. Special buffers help identify eosinophils and basophils. Red cells and platelets are counted using the DC (electronic resistance) method with hydrodynamic focusing to reduce coincidence error. As in other instruments described earlier, hemoglobin is measured by the cyanmethemoglobin method. Capable of analyzing 120 samples per hour, the NE-8000 presents results as interpretive reports, histograms, and a WBC scattergram.

One factor distinguishing the NE-8000 from the Coulter STKS and Technicon H-1 systems described earlier is the combined use of DC and RF for cell counting, sizing, and classification. Figure 9–8 illustrates four in a single transducer chamber; cells passing through the aperture are subjected to both direct current and a radio frequency. When a cell passes through the aperture, a DC voltage spike is produced proportional to the cell's internal volume, since the cell membrane is poorly conductive. By contrast, the RF signal passes through the cell

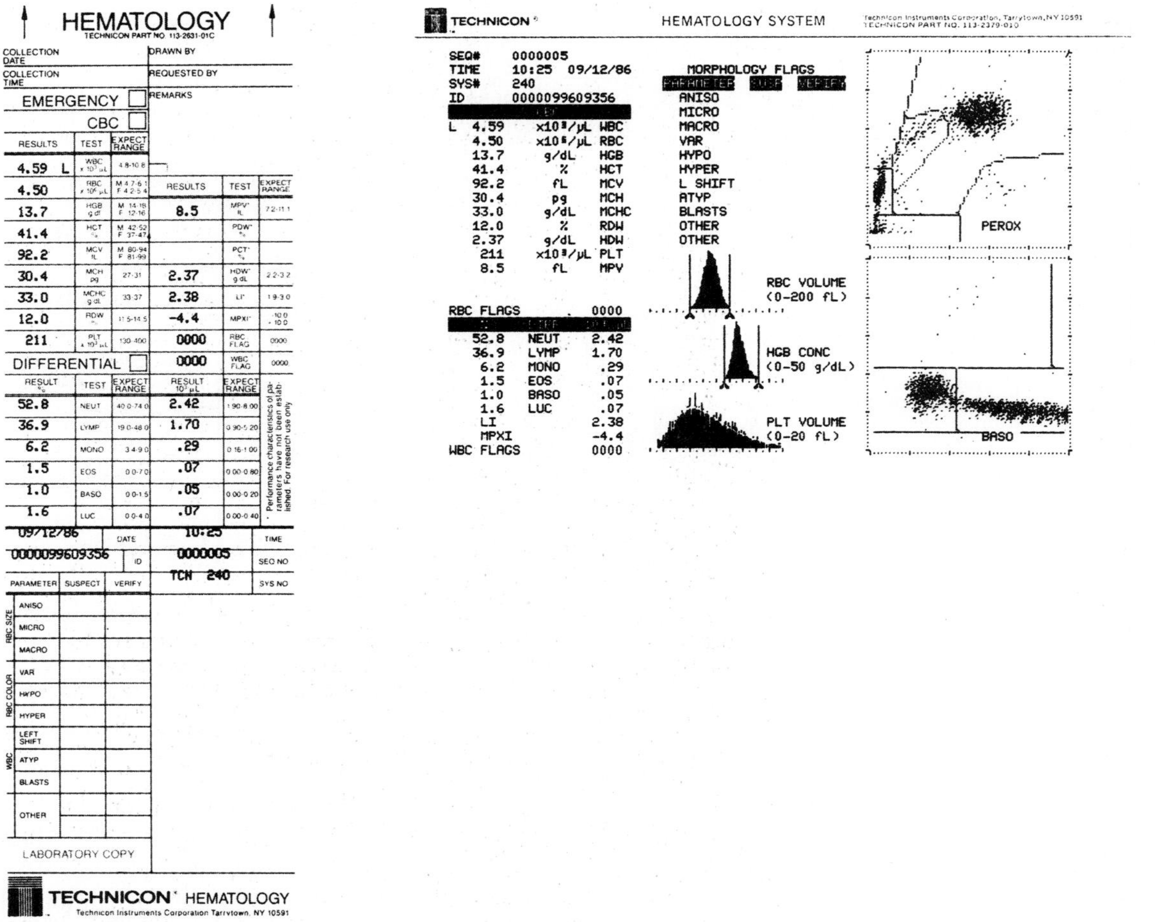

■ **FIGURE 9–7.**

Technicon H-1 laboratory report and chart report. (Courtesy of Miles Inc., Tarrytown, NY.)

TABLE 9–4. TECHNICON H-1 WHITE BLOOD CELL (WBC) DIFFERENTIAL
REVIEW CRITERIA

FLAGGING*	LAB ACTION
Abnormal cytograms (with or without other flags)	Review smear† if any abnormal clustering, excess noise, or valley failures occur on perox or baso channel.
LUC %	Accept <4% with no WBC flags; with flags, follow criteria listed below. If LUCs > 4%, review smear; if atypical lymphocytes, append LUCs with ''atypical lymphs'' comment; if large lymphocytes or agranular monocytes, add back to lymph or mono % and absolute counts, respectively; if abnormal cells, do manual differential count; >4% LUCs should be reported only when commented as atypical lymphs.
LS	If + in combination with normal absolute neutrophil count and normal cytogram, verify H-1 results. Review + + or + in combination with absolute neutrophil <1.5 × 10⁹/L or >10.5 × 10⁹/L or abnormal cytogram, or other WBC flags. If smear review confirms that left shift is due to bands only or <2% metamyelocytes, add ''slight left shift'' comment to the differential report. Greater than 2% metamyelocytes, or any less mature cells such as myelocytes or promyelocytes, must be enumerated and reported separately.
Atyps	If LUCs ≤4% and normal cytogram, verify H-1 results. If LUCs >4%, review smear. If atypical lymphocytes seen, append LUCs with ''atypical lymphs'' comment. If blasts or abnormal cells are present, perform manual differential count.
Blasts	Review smear. If blasts or abnormal cells are present, perform manual differential count. Otherwise, verify H-1 results.
Other	
N	Scan for NRBCs or large or clumped platelets. Correct WBCB (WBC basophil lobularity channel) if NRBCs >5/100 WBCs and report manual differential count. Report WBCB instead of the WBCP (WBC peroxidase channel) if giant platelets are present and do not report the H-1 absolutes if the WBC substitution did not occur.
IG	Review smear. Perform manual differential count, if necessary.
NF-B/NF-P	Review smear. Perform manual differential count, if necessary.
NF-H	Dilute, return, correct results.
NF-L	If WBC count <1.0 × 10⁹/L, comment as ''insufficient cells for differential.'' If WBC count >1.0 × 10⁹/L, review smear. Perform manual differential count, if necessary.
WBC	If WBC count >80 × 10⁹/L, dilute for H-1 differential count.
Asterisked differential	Review smear. Perform manual differential count, if necessary.

*LUCs indicates large unstained cells; LS, left shift; Atyps, atypical lymphocytes; NRBCs, nucleated red blood cells; N, NRBCs or large platelets; IG, immature granulocytes; NF, no fit; B, basophil lobularity channel; P, peroxidase channel; H, high; and L, low.

†Manual smear review will be defined as follows: WBC review-scan approximately 50 WBCs on 50 × oil. A 100-cell manual differential count should be done only when necessary. If a manual differential count is necessary, absolute counts should not be calculated and reported.

From Miles MK, Exton MG, Hurlbut TA, Cousar JB: White blood cell differentials as performed by the Technicon H-1. Lab Med 22:99, 1991.

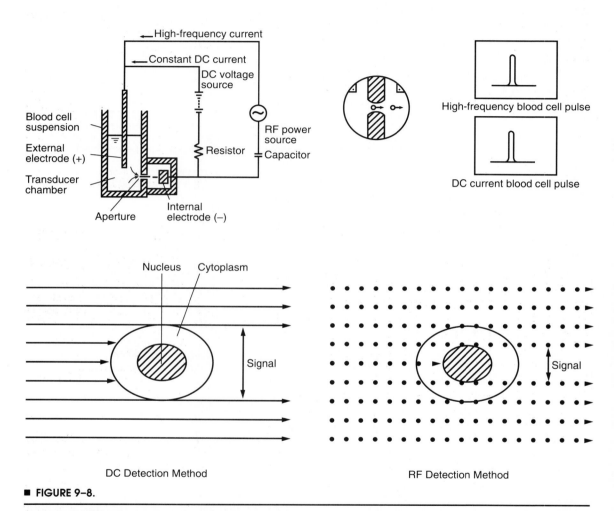

■ **FIGURE 9–8.**

Sysmex NE-8000 DC and RF detection methods. (Courtesy of Baxter Healthcare Corporation, McGaw Park, IL.)

membrane but is resisted by the cell nucleus and cytoplasmic granules. Consequently, the DC voltage spikes measure both the number of cells and the size of the cells; the RF signals measure the sizes and density of the nuclear material. By plotting RF and DC spikes, the NE-8000 is able to separate granulocytes, lymphocytes, and monocytes far more precisely than would be possible by the DC method alone.

Basophils and eosinophils are counted separately, using special agents to alter other cell populations. Heat and chemical reactions lyse red cells and shrink all cells except basophils, which are subsequently counted by the DC detector. Similarly, another buffer is used to shrink all cells except eosinophils before counting. By subtracting the basophil and eosinophil counts from the total granulocyte count, a neutrophil count is computed.

A separate DC detector with hydrodynamic focusing is used to count red cells and platelets. The laminar flow technique in hydrodynamic focusing lines up the cells for more precise counting, avoiding spurious counts from the same cell being counted more than once. Automatic discriminators set upper and lower threshold limits of the particle distribution.

The NE-8000 produces five histograms and a WBC scattergram to provide the operator with useful clinical information for the identification of abnormal samples. Figure 9–9 shows the positioning of normal cell populations on a scattergram. The lower half of this figure shows the location of possible abnormal cells. The five histograms include WBC, RBC, PLT, EO, and BASO. An example of a patient with atypical or variant lymphocytes is shown in Figure 9–10.

Like other automated hematology analyzers, the NE-8000 has a variety of flags to prompt the operator to consider whether additional action is necessary. Table 9–5 lists

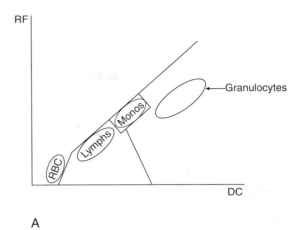

A

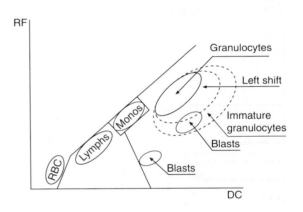

B

■ **FIGURE 9–9.**

Sysmex NE-8000 WBC scattergram. (Courtesy of Baxter Healthcare Corporation, McGaw Park, IL.)

flags that are displayed on the NE-8000 screen and appropriate subsequent actions.

Cell-Dyn 3000

The Unipath **Cell-Dyn 3000** is an automated, bench-top blood cell counter that measures and calculates 22 blood cell parameters. Over a decade ago, earlier, less

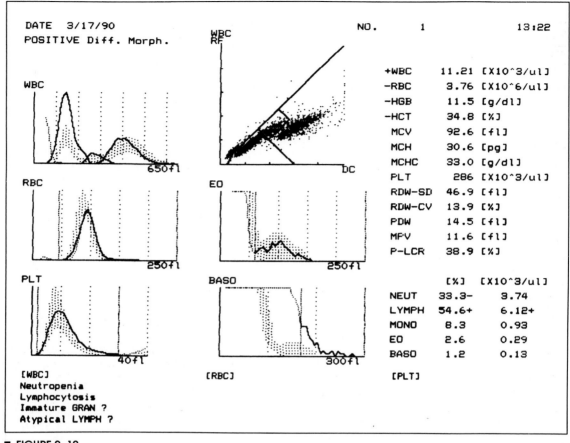

FIGURE 9-10.

Sysmex NE-8000 WBC scattergrams and histograms for a patient with atypical or variant lymphocytes. (Courtesy of Baxter Healthcare Corporation, McGaw Park, IL.)

sophisticated versions of this instrument were marketed by Sequoia Scientific to physicians' offices. The Cell-Dyn 3000 incorporates a flow cytometer to determine the white cell count and five-part differential. Red cells and platelets are counted and their volume measured by an adaptation of the widely used aperture resistance transducer. Hemoglobin concentration is measured by an accelerated version of the cyanmethemoglobin method.

A unique feature of the Cell-Dyn 3000 is the high resolution flow cytometer used to classify white cells differentially. The laser beam of this flow cytometer is shaped into a uniformly wide "top hat" profile and centrally focused on a quartz flow cell (Fig. 9–11). This design is the foundation for **multiangle polarized scatter separation (MAPSS)** providing even illumination across a narrow sample stream to maintain stability. While traditional flow cytometers use forward light scattering (0°) and orthogonal light scattering (90°) to differentiate granulocytes, lymphocytes, and monocytes, the MAPSS technology adds two additional

TABLE 9–5. SYSMEX NE-8000 DIFFERENTIAL SUSPECT FLAGS

MESSAGE	PARAMETER(S)	ACTIONS
WBC SUSPECT FLAGS		
Blasts?	WBC scattergram/BASO histogram	Make film, report manual differential if indicated.
Immature GRANs?	WBC scattergram/BASO histogram	Make film, report manual differential if >5% immature cells, >15% bands. Ignore WBC flags for known HGB and HCT on MICU, SICU, traumas, PAR, OR, open hearts.
Left shift?	WBC scattergram	Make film, report manual differential if >5% immature cells, >15% bands.
Atypical LYMPHs?	WBC scattergram	Make film, report manual differential if <5 yr. and WBC <3.0, or >12.0; 5 yr.-adult >20% of LYMPH population.
NRBC?	WBC scattergram	Adults: Make film, report manual corrected WBC count. If <3 days old, ignore flag or make film only if ordered.
Monocytosis?	Ratios: User-established limits	>20%—verify with film.
Eosinophilia?		>10%—verify with film.
Basophilia?		>5%—verify with film.
RBC SUSPECT FLAGS		
RBC agglutination or elevated MCV?	MCHC, MCH, RBC, RU (%)	Warm, reanalyze.
Turbidity/HGB interference?	MCHC, HGB/HCT mismatch	Examine plasma for lipemia, hemolysis, icterus. Correct HGB, calculate indices.
HGB Defect?	MCV, RDW-CV	Make film if <70 MCV, >5 million RBCs. Save blood and report. Copy.
Fragments?	MCV, RDW-SD, PU flag, PU (%)	Make film, report if indicated.
Dimorphic Population?	MP flag	Make film. Save blood and report. Copy.

(Courtesy of Baxter Healthcare Corporation, McGaw Park, IL.)

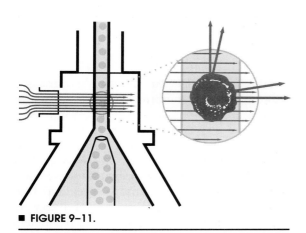

■ **FIGURE 9–11.**

Cell-Dyn 3000 multiangle polarized scatter separation. (By permission of Abbott Diagnostics, Abbott Park, IL.)

dimensions. Narrow-angle light scattering (10°) to resolve basophils and depolarized light scattering (90°) to resolve eosinophils eliminate the need for cytochemical staining or monoclonal tagging. A report from the Cell-Dyn 3000 is shown in Figure 9–12.

Serono System 9000+

The **System 9000+** automated hematology analyzer is marketed and serviced by Serono-Baker Diagnostics. This is an 18-parameter analyzer providing results for WBC, RBC, HGB, HCT, MCV, MCH,

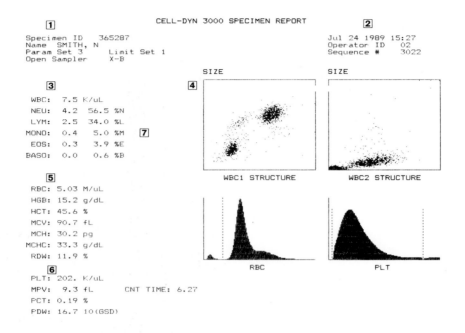

■ **FIGURE 9–12.**

Cell-Dyn 3000 sample report. (By permission of Abbott Diagnostics, Abbott Park, IL.)

MCHC, PLT, RDW, MPV, PCT, PDW, lymphocytes (# and %), monocytes (# and %), granulocytes (# and %), eosinophils less than 10 percent, basophils less than 3 percent, and three histograms (WBC, RBC, and PLT).

The System 9000+ simultaneously analyzes RBC/PLT and WBC for a throughput of up to 60 samples per hour. The instrument uses impedance counting and sizing, a patented automatic reverse air purge/fluidic flush system, automatic sample probe and sample valve rinse, and a multiple counting/proprietary flow monitor.

COBAS HELIOS 5 DIFF

Roche Diagnostics Systems offers a 26-parameter hematology analyzer called the COBAS HELIOS 5 DIFF. This analyzer is capable of analyzing 120 samples per hour, producing a full CBC plus total WBC differential, and flagging of analytic and mor-

■ **FIGURE 9-13.**

COBAS HELIOS 5 DIFF double hydrodynamic focusing system. (By permission of Roche Diagnostic Systems, Branchburg, NJ.)

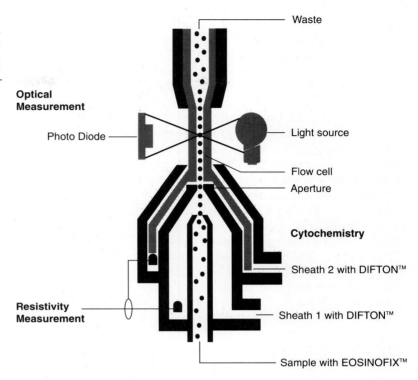

phologic variations. The three-part interpretive differential includes lymphocytes, monocytes, granulocytes, and estimates for eosinophils and basophils.

The COBAS HELIOS 5 DIFF incorporates cytochemistry, resistivity, and optical density measurements in a patented **double hydrodynamic focusing system.** During analysis, an aliquot of whole blood is mixed with a specific patented reagent. The resulting cytochemical reaction lyses red cells, stabilizes white cells in their native form, and uses an eosinophil-specific stain. In the double hydrodynamic focusing system, two successive measurements are made on each cell: electronic resistance and optical absorbance (Fig. 9–13). Collected signals are computerized and categorized into a high-resolution chart called **Matrix-Plot.** This chart plots relationships between size and morphologic detail, separating neutrophils, lymphocytes, monocytes, and eosinophils. Atypical lymphocytes and large immature cell populations are also quantified. Basophils are counted in a specific channel using cytochemistry and electronic impedance.

ISSUES

The six automated hematology systems just described include those most widely used in the field at the time of this writing. The salient characteristics were discussed for each to provide a foundation for various technologies and system outputs.

Some general issues that are not instrument-specific may alert the user to potential problems. In some instances, lyse-resistant red cells can alter both hemoglobin values and cell counts. For instruments that rely on the presence of nuclei to indicate leukocytes, the presence of nucleated red cells will falsely elevate these counts. In some conditions, platelets have a propensity for clumping, obviously altering a platelet count but equally important altering cell counts and potentially changing hemoglobin determinations. Hemoglobin determination also can be altered by the presence of lipids in the plasma, since a colorimeter is used to measure cyanmethemoglobin.

As new instruments become available, it is important to be aware of published comparative reports and to compare these new technologies with those they are expected to supersede. The National Committee for Clinical Laboratory Standards offers guidelines for comparison of leukocyte differential counting. As noted earlier, a number of published studies have compared the automated hematology analyzers discussed in this chapter. Comparing the Technicon H-1, Sysmex NE-8000, Coulter STKS, and Cell-Dyn 3000, Buttarello and colleagues found imprecision very low among all analyzers for neutrophils and leukocytes. However, for other white cell populations, precision decreased as the presence percentage decreased. Monocyte differentiation appears to be a particular problem, whether comparing instrumentation with manual counts or comparing monocyte percentages with different automated instruments. Swaim suggests that automated hematology analyzers be compared for:

1. Accuracy, the degree of agreement between analyzer values for each cell type and values determined by a reference method;
2. Imprecision, the within run replication of values; and
3. Clinical sensitivity, values falling within

TABLE 9–6. REFERENT LEVELS OF THE REFERENCE METHOD DIFFERENTIAL

	RANGE (CELLS × 10⁹/L)
A. CELL TYPE	
Segmented plus band neutrophils	1.40–6.50
(band neutrophils)	0.00–0.70
Mature lymphocytes	1.00–3.60
Monocytes	0.00–0.70
Eosinophils	0.00–0.40
Basophils	0.00–0.10
Differentials above or below these limits are classified as distributionally abnormal	
B. ABNORMAL MORPHOLOGY	
Variant lymphocyte (for the H-1, any value for LUCs 4%)*	0.02
Metamyelocyte	Any
Myelocyte	Any
Promyelocyte	Any
Blast	Any
Nucleated red blood cell (NRBC)	Any
Other: Plasma cells, smudge cells, other abnormal cells (e.g., hairy cells, Sézary cells, and other specific abnormal cells)	
	Any

*Manufacturer's recommended level. (From Swaim WR: Laboratory and clinical evaluation of white cell differential counts. Am J Clin Pathol 95:381, 1991.)

referent limits for absolute numbers of each cell type (Table 9–6).

SUMMARY

This chapter has described the principal technologies and major instrumentation currently used for automated hematology analysis. The technology of electrical impedance remains widely used in many instruments. However, light scattering using a flow cytometer, is also popular. Many of the newer instruments employ both technologies, with modifications of each to maximize the benefits and overcome shortfalls of the other.

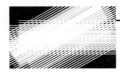

REVIEW QUESTIONS

Choose the one correct answer.

1. When measuring hemoglobin photometrically by the cyanmethemoglobin method in automated hematology instrumentation, all of the following are major sources of error *except*

   a. rare RBC abnormalities making cells highly resistant to lysis
   b. severe lipemia
   c. extremely high WBC counts
   d. immature granulocytes

2. In conjunction with the light-scattering principle, specific cytochemical staining of cells can be used to differentiate leukocytes using a darkfield optical method. This differentiation is based on

   a. electrical impedance
   b. absorbance
   c. volume
   d. conductivity

3. The Coulter STKS analyzer uses a high-frequency electromagnetic probe to measure a cell's internal structure through conductivity analysis of cytoplasmic and nuclear content. This parameter is called

   a. cellular granulation
   b. lobularity index
   c. cell opacity
   d. cellular resistance

4. Sweep flow technology on the Coulter STKS analyzer prevents red cell re-circulation by improving the accuracy of

   a. white cell counts
   b. platelet counts
   c. white cell differentials
   d. hemoglobin determination

5. The Technicon H-1 analyzer consists of four channels, including all of the following *except*

   a. electrical impedance
   b. hemoglobin
   c. ``nuclear'' channel
   d. peroxidase
   e. red cell/platelet

6. The Technicon H-1 analyzer can be used to isolate and count pan T, helper T, suppressor T, and B cells by using

   a. a histogram of leukocytes
   b. an immunoperoxidase system
   c. an electrical impedance
   d. a lobularity index

7. With the Technicon H-1 analyzer, a low lobularity index (PMN:MN) suggests

   a. a ``left shift''
   b. an increase in eosinophils
   c. more than 40% lymphocytes
   d. hypersegmented neutrophils

8. A distinguishing factor of the Sysmex NE-8000 analyzer to the Coulter STKS

and Technicon H-1 analyzers for cell counting, sizing, and classification is the combined use of

a. electrical impedance and laser light scatter
b. direct current and radio frequency
c. laser light scatter and cytochemical staining
d. radio frequency and laser light scatter

9. The Multiangle polarized scatter separation (MAPSS) used in the Cell-Dyn 3000 to differentiate white cells uses which form of light scattering to classify eosinophils, eliminating the need for cytochemical staining or monoclonal tagging?

a. forward light scattering (0°)
b. orthogonal light scattering (90°)
c. depolarizing light scattering (90°)
d. narrow light scattering (10°)

10. Scatterplots display cell distribution data to

a. help spot abnormalities in white cell populations
b. compare red cell indices
c. match hemoglobin and hematocrit values
d. identify equipment malfunctions

11. When compared through parallel analysis, the leukocyte population least precisely measured by automated hematology analyzers is

a. segmented neutrophils
b. lymphocytes
c. monocytes
d. basophils
e. eosinophils

12. Which of the following abnormalities

may falsely elevate leukocyte counts in instruments relying on the presence of nuclei to indicate leukocytes?

a. atypical lymphocytes
b. "left shift" granulocytes
c. lipemic plasma
d. nucleated red cells

REFERENCES

Banez EL, Bacaling JH: An evaluation of the Technicon H-1 automated hematology analyzer in detecting peripheral blood changes in acute inflammation. *Arch Pathol Lab Med* 112:885–888, 1988.

Barnard DF, Barnard SA, Carter AB, Patterson AY, Machin SJ: An evaluation of the Coulter VCS differential counter. *Clin Lab Haematol* 11:255–266, 1989.

Barnard DF, Barnard SA, Carter AB, et al: Detection of important abnormalities of the differential count using the Coulter STKR blood counter. *J Clin Pathol* 42:772–776, 1989.

Breakell ES, Marchand A, Marcus R, Simpson E: Comparison of performance for leukocyte differential counting of the Technicon H6000 system with a manual reference method using the NCCLS standard. *Blood Cells* 11:257–279, 1985.

Buttarello M, Gadotti M, Lorenz C, Toffalori E, Ceschimi N, Valentini A, Rizzoti P: Evaluation of four automated hematology analyzers. *Am J Clin Pathol* 97:345–352, 1992.

Clarke PT, Henthorn JS, England JM: Differential white cell counting on the Coulter counter Model S Plus IV (three population) and the Technicon H6000; A comparison by simple and multiple regression. *Clin Lab Haematol* 7:335, 1985.

Coulter Electronics, Inc: *Product Reference Manual for S + IV,* PN 4235328. Hialeah, Florida, 1983.

Coulter Electronics, Inc: *Coulter Counter Analyzer Model S-Plus STKR Manual,* PN 4235547. Hialeah, Florida, June, 1986.

Coulter Electronics, Inc: *Reference Manual for STKS,* PN 42359030. Hialeah, Florida, 1989.

Cox CJ, Habermann TM, Payne BA, et al: Evaluation of the Coulter counter model S-Plus IV. *Am J Clin Pathol* 84:297–306, 1985.

DeCresce R: The E-5000. *Lab Med* 17:6, 1986.

Hyder DM: *Clinical Study on Sysmex NE-8000 Five-Part WBC Differential: A Hematology Monograph.* McGaw Park, Illinois, Baxter Diagnostics, 1989.

Jones AR: *Evaluation of the Coulter VCS automated differential counter—a hematology flow cytometer.* Hialeah, Florida, Coulter Electronics, 1988.

Krause JR: Automated differentials in the hematology laboratory. *Am J Clin Pathol* 93(Suppl 1):S11–S16, 1990.

Krause JR, Costello RT, Krause J, Penchasky L: Use of the Technicon H-1 in the characterization of leukemias. *Arch Pathol Lab Med* 112:889–894, 1988.

Miers MK, Exton MG, Hurlbut TA, Cousar JB: White blood cell differentials as performed by the Technicon H-1: Evaluation and implementation in a tertiary care hospital. *Lab Med* 22:99–106, 1991.

National Committee for Clinical Laboratory Standards: *Tentative standard for leukocyte differential counting.* NCCLS H20-T, Vol 4(11). Villanova, Pennsylvania, 4:257–312, 1984.

Nelson L, Charache S, Wingfield S, Keyser E: Laboratory evaluation of differential white blood cell count information from the Coulter S-Plus IV and Technicon H-1 in patient populations requiring rapid "turnaround" time. *Am J Clin Pathol* 91:563–569, 1989.

Newman-Smith A, Gillion R, Thurrell W, Baughan ASJ: An evaluation of the Sysmex M2000 haematology analyser. *NHS*. London, Procument Directorate, May 1988.

Payne BA, Pierre RV: TOA E-5000 multiparameter automated hematology analyzer. *Am J Clin Pathol* 88:51, 1987.

Pierre RV: The routine differential leukocyte count vs. automated differential counts. *Blood Cells* 11:11–23, 1985.

Pierre RV, Payne BA, Lee WK, et al: Comparison of four leukocyte differential methods with the National Committee for Clinical Laboratory Standards (NCCLS) reference method. *Am J Clin Pathol* 87:201, 1987.

Poulsen KR, Bell CA: Automated hematology: Comparing and contrasting three systems. *Clin Lab Sci* 4:16–17, 1991.

Proceedings of the Technicon H.1 Hematology Symposium. Tarrytown, New York, Technicon Instruments Corporation, October 11, 1985.

Reardon DM, Hutchinson D, Bradey L, Trowbridge EA: Automated haematology: A comparative study of cell counting and sizing using aperture impedance and flow cytometric systems. *Med Lab Sci* 44:320–325, 1987.

Reardon DM, Hutchinson D, Preston FE, Trowbridge EA: The routine measurement of platelet volume: A comparison of aperture-impedance and flow cytometric systems. *Clin Lab Haematol* 7:251–257, 1985.

Ross DW, Bently S: Evaluation of an automated hematology system (Technicon H-1). *Arch Pathol Lab Med* 110:803–808, 1986.

Rumke CL: The statistically expected variability in differential leukocyte counting. *In* Koepke JA (ed): *Differential Leukocyte Counting.* Skokie, Illinois, College of American Pathologists, 1978, pp 39–45.

Shapiro MF, Hatch RL, Greenfield S: Cost containment and labor-intensive tests: The case of the leukocyte differential count. *JAMA* 252:231–234, 1984.

Simson E, Ross DW, Kocher WD: *Atlas of Automated Cytochemical Hematology.* Tarrytown, New York, Technicon Instruments Corporation, 1989.

Swaim WR: Laboratory and clinical evaluation of white blood cell differential counts. *Am J Clin Pathol* 95:381–388, 1991.

Sysmex/TOA Medical Electronics: *Manual for Sysmex NE-8000.* 1988.

Van Wersh JWJ, Bank C: A new development in haematological cell counting: The Sysmex NE-8000, automation for cell count and physical five-part leukocyte differentiation. *J Clin Chem Clin Biochem* 28:233–240, 1990.

Verwilghen RL: Standardization and cell counting in haematology: ICSH document. *Biochem Clin* 14:1179–1181, 1990.

Warner BA, Reardon DM: A field evaluation of the Coulter STKS. *Am J Clin Pathol* 95:207–217, 1991.

Warner BA, Reardon DM, Marshall DP: Automated hematology analyzers: A four-way comparison. *Med Lab Sci* 47:285–296, 1990.

Warren JS, Davis RA: Evaluation of the Technicon H-1 hematology system. *Lab Med* 18:316, 1987.

Watson JS, Richard AD: Evaluation of Technicon H-1 hematology system. *Lab Med* 18:316–322, 1987.

Wenz B, Ramirez MA, Burns ER: The H-1 hematology analyzer: Its performance characteristics and value in the diagnosis of infectious disease. *Arch Pathol Lab Med* 111:521–524, 1987.

Chapter 10

AUTOMATION IN CLINICAL MICROBIOLOGY

GEORGE T. TORTORA, PhD

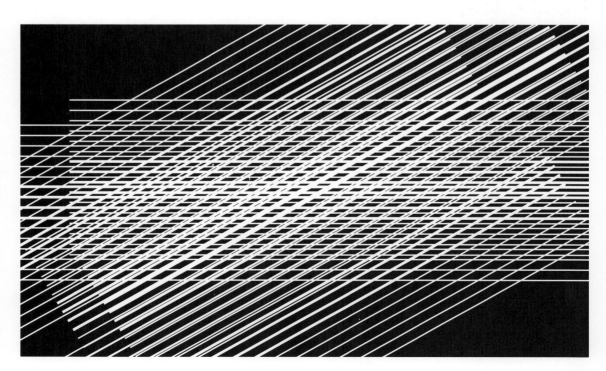

After studying this chapter, the student should be able to:

- Describe, in general terms, the conventional method of microbial identification and list three problems with this technique.
- Differentiate between multistep and unistep identification procedures and enumerate their advantages and disadvantages.
- List and define five techniques that can detect microbial growth.
- Explain the principle of operation of three automated blood culture systems and identify their advantages and/or disadvantages.
- Describe how the Vitek system determines the positivity or negativity of biochemical reactions.
- Differentiate between the concepts of likelihood and percent probability in identifying microbes with the Vitek system.
- Explain how the minimal inhibitory concentration of an antibiotic is calculated by the Vitek system.
- Describe how fluorescent-tagged compounds are used in the MicroScan Rapid Panels to determine biochemical reactions and antimicrobic susceptibilities.
- List several advantages of the ALADIN systems' use of video pixels in interpreting microbial growth.
- Describe the process of ``quenching'' used by the Sensititre Microbiology Systems for detecting substrate utilization.
- List five noncultural techniques used for the detection and/or identification of microorganisms.

KEY WORDS

Acridine orange. A fluorochrome that binds to nucleic acid. Its primary use is in highlighting bacteria in blood cultures.

Colorimeter. A device for estimating the percentage of a colored substance in a solution.

0.5 McFarland turbidity standard. A turbidity standard equivalent to 1.5×10^8 cells/ml.

Minimal inhibitory concentration (MIC). The minimum concentration of antimicrobial agent needed to yield a 99 percent reduction in colony-forming units (microbial colonies) of a microbial suspension.

Nephelometer. An instrument that measures light scattered at 90°C from the primary beam.

Optical density (absorbance). Microbes in solution refract and deflect light from passing through a solution. By using a device such as a colorimeter or spectrophotometer, turbidity can be expressed in units of absorbance.

Spectrophotometer. An instrument that measures the intensity of light. It can be used to measure turbidity in units of absorbance.

Susceptibility testing. Determining an antibiotic's capability of killing or suppressing the growth of microorganisms.

Turbidity. Cell (microbial) suspensions appear turbid because each cell scatters light. The amount of turbidity is proportional to the quantity of microbes present.

INTRODUCTION

History

The techniques of Koch heralded the beginnings of what has been called "the golden age of bacteriology." Along with his discovery of *Bacillus anthracis* in 1877 as the causative agent of anthrax came the establishment of the scientific basis for associating a microorganism with a disease, known thereafter as Koch's postulates. Koch solidi-

fied broth media with gelatin in 1881 and utilized the pour plate technique to isolate pure cultures of microorganisms from a mixed culture. This technique proved to be a vast improvement over the dilution method designed by Lister. The development of that indispensable stain by Gram in 1884 allowed separation of the microbial population into two categories based on tinctorial characteristics. The introduction of agar by Hess in 1891 served as a landmark in bacteriology, enabling the incubation of cultures above the melting point of gelatin and solving the problem of isolation of bacteria that liquefied gelatin, thus completing the development of the basic techniques used to this very day by all clinical microbiology laboratories.

The field of microbial physiology developed from a need by the early bacteriologists to succeed in the cultivation and identification of microorganisms involved in disease. Investigations of the actions of bacteria on a variety of substrates, producing a whole range of metabolites, led to what is commonly referred to as "classic," or "conventional," biochemical tests. Combining these techniques with serologic tests and animal pathogenicity tests, the bacteriologists of that time achieved heroic results, elucidating the bacterium–infectious disease connection for some 20 diseases, including anthrax, gonorrhea (1879), typhoid fever (1880), suppuration (*Staphylococcus,* 1879; *Streptococcus,* 1880), tuberculosis (1882), cholera and diphtheria (1883), tetanus (1884), pneumococcal pneumonia (1884), meningitis (1887), *Salmonella* food poisoning (1888), gas gangrene (1892), plague (1894), botulism (1896), dysentery (1898), syphilis (1903), and whooping cough (1906).

Thus, these basic techniques, i.e., the use of microscopic morphology and tinctorial characteristics, macroscopic morphology on agar medium, and "biochemical testing," supplemented on occasion with serologic tests, remain today as the mainstay for identifying bacteria commonly encountered in the clinical laboratory.

The discovery of penicillin by Fleming in 1928, and the development of production methods by Florey, Chain, and others in the 1940s, heralded the beginning of the antibiotic age. By the late 1950s it was apparent that the bacteria would not cooperate by remaining uniformly susceptible to penicillin or the newer antimicrobial agents available. The clinical microbiology laboratory took on the added responsibility of providing antimicrobial susceptibility studies on isolates from patients suffering from a variety of infectious diseases.

Changing Face of Clinical Microbiology

What has changed since those early days? As a result of those early heroic efforts, it became a common practice to draw up a list of "pathogens," microorganisms that caused infectious disease, and a list of "nonpathogens," organisms that did not cause disease. As the science and practice of medicine evolved, elaborate surgical and invasive diagnostic techniques were developed. The study of microbiology advanced as well, and a better understanding of the host-parasite relationship developed.

It became apparent that whether or not an infectious disease developed did not depend solely on properties of the microorganism, but rather on the complex relationship of the host and its ability to counter microbial colonization, invasion, or the production of toxic products. Consequently, consideration of the interaction between the host, the microbe, and the environmental existence of the organism assumed an important place in the equation that determined the establishment of infectious disease in a given host. By following this logic, it has become evident that placement of the host, i.e., the patient in a hospital setting, with its own unique environmental flora, often multiresistant to antibiotics, while simultaneously executing a variety of invasive techniques, or dispensing any of a number of immunosuppressive drugs, resulted in the establishment of infectious disease with relatively avirulent microorganisms.

The tragedy of the AIDS epidemic has brought this lesson home as nothing else could. The current literature is filled with reports of isolation of organisms from AIDS victims that were not previously described as causing or being involved with infectious disease. The infectious processes range from sepsis with organisms used in the production of fermented foodstuffs (*Leuconostoc mesenteroides*)[1-4] to diarrhea due to blue-green algae contracted while swimming in tropical waters.[5] Infections with microbes possessing pathogenic potential widespread in nature, yet rarely encountered among the healthy population, suddenly have become common occurrences, forcing upon the laboratory the necessity of becoming adept at the recognition, isolation, and identification of such organisms. The microorganisms currently encountered in the compromised patient include a wide variety of both procaryotes and eucaryotes, including, as examples, *Cryptococcus neoformans, Mycobacterium avium* complex, and *Pneumocystis carinii.*

The current use of DNA homology techniques to discover the relatedness of groups of organisms originally classified by the techniques discussed earlier, i.e., morphology, physiology, and serology, has uncovered new relationships among microorganisms with consequent reclassification, leading to the establishment of new taxonomy and nomenclature. As a result of this new technology, hardly a month goes by that the clinical microbiologist is not forced into learning a new name, or rethinking the relationships between old and familiar groups of organisms, adding yet another dimension to the problems facing the clinical microbiology laboratory.

Needs

Conventional, or classic, approaches to the identification of microbes utilized a variety of organic sources of carbon and simple methods to determine metabolic end-products. These methods included the use of pH indicators to detect acid end-products or use of an organic compound as the sole source of carbon, or the use of a reagent to detect intermediary or end-compounds. The familiar "IMViC" acronym typifies this type of testing, in which I stands for indole production from tryptophan; M is methyl red, a pH indicator; V connotes the Voges-Proskauer reaction, a test for acetoin (also known as acetyl-methyl-carbinol); i is for euphony; and C stands for the utilization of citrate as the sole carbon source. This group of tests served originally to differentiate between two members of the coliform group of bacteria—those that fermented the carbohydrate lactose.

This concept expanded through the years so that the laboratories utilized an ever-increasing number of biochemical tests. Laboratories used different methodologies for preparation of many of these substrates and developed highly individualistic interpretation schemes to reach a final identification. This made interlaboratory comparisons difficult at best.

The time to final identification varied. Often delays were created by making the identification a multistep process, inoculating only a small number of substrates initially, followed by an incubation period of at least 18 to 24 hours, which was then followed by another decision-making process, and so on. Quality control efforts were substantially below the standards of today, and often the least qualified technical individual was relegated to making media upon which all the subsequent decisions of more qualified senior technologists were made! Because of the increasing complexity of the tasks given to the clinical microbiology laboratory, the working methods, and the increasing workload, it became clear that changes in the approach were needed.

During the late 1960s, a transition occurred from the classic multistep procedures to more modern single-step procedures, spurred, no doubt, by newer, more stringent requirements for quality control by regulatory agencies. Standardization and quality control were stressed with the introduction of systems addressing, at first, identification of members of the family Enterobacteriaceae. These first-generation systems consisted of a series of miniaturized tubes with individual substrates, multicompartment tubes or plates, and discs or strips of paper impregnated with dehydrated substrates. These systems were a distinct improvement over classic procedures, eliminating errors of quality control inherent in in-house prepared media, shortening incubation periods, providing more data rapidly, organizing the identification schemes based on increased numbers of tests, and providing standardized methodology.

However, each system demonstrated some difficulties with identification, because the substrates were not always identical to ones used by Edwards and Ewing in their *Manual of the Enterobacteriaceae,* even though the identification schemes were based on their techniques. This led to the development of the second-generation unistep procedures, or kits. Commercial efforts to resolve these problems included the incorporation of highly sophisticated computer-generated identification bases specific for each system. The result was the establishment of systems that yielded more reliable and consistent identifications. Other advantages were the inclusion of additional groups of microorganisms, reaction endpoints made readable after 4 hours' incubation, and finally the ability to mechanize or automate inoculation procedures and interpretation of test results.

The development of automation in clinical microbiology lagged far behind the progress made in automating the chemistry and hematology laboratories, because of the inherent difference between these disciplines. In many ways microbiology remains tied to those procedures introduced and developed by Koch and Hess. We must still isolate the microorganisms from mixed culture for the majority of the automated procedures, and we still use media solidified by the addition of agar!

PRINCIPLES OF DESIGNING AUTOMATED INSTRUMENTS

All automated instruments designed to detect the presence of microorganisms, to measure their quantity, and to determine their identification or antimicrobial susceptibility must use some detection technique to observe and record changes in population density, metabolite production, or a combination thereof.

Detection of Microbial Growth

Turbidity

Changes in **turbidity** of a broth medium inoculated with microorganisms indicate growth. When the laboratorian visually compares an uninoculated broth medium with one that has been inoculated and incubated, it becomes readily apparent that microbial growth has taken place. Turbidity results when the particles (microorganisms) in suspension refract and deflect light passing through the suspension, reflecting the light back into the observer's eyes. Some instruments designed to measure turbidity determine the **optical density** (OD) by comparing the amount of light that passes through the suspension (the percent transmittance) to the amount of light passing through the same liquid minus the suspended particles (microorganisms), in the same manner as the laboratorian compares inoculated and uninoculated broth medium. A photoelectric sensor or photometer then converts the light that it receives to a quantifiable electrical impulse. Turbidity measurement also can be accomplished by using the principle of nephelometry, or light scatter. The photometer in a **nephelometer** is placed at angles to the suspension. The suspension is illuminated by either an incandescent bulb or a laser beam, and the resulting light scatter, produced by the microorganisms in suspension, is measured. The number and size of the organisms or particles in suspension determine the amount of light scatter.

Colorimetry

As stated earlier, the measurement of the end-products of microbial metabolism by conventional techniques frequently relies on color changes of pH indicators. These measurements can be automated by utilizing the principles of colorimetry. Measurements by a **colorimeter** determine the kind and amount of light transmitted or absorbed by a solution. Absorbance, also termed *optical density (OD)* in the older literature, is a measurement of the amount of light that is blocked or absorbed by a solution. The term *transmittance* refers to the measurement of the amount of light that passes through a solution and is expressed as a percentage (% T).

Measurement of CO_2

The end-product of microbial metabolism of a carbon source is carbon dioxide (CO_2). Several automated techniques have been developed to detect microbial metabolism and therefore growth. One of the earliest used the technique of measuring the production of radioactive carbon dioxide gas from ^{14}C-labeled substrates, including glucose, amino acids, and alcohols. Owing to regulations governing the handling of radioactive substances and the cost involved in their disposal, a later development took advantage of infrared **spectrophotometer** to measure CO_2. The latest concept involves the detection of CO_2 colorimetrically in an indicator sequestered from the growth medium by a CO_2-permeable membrane.

Bioluminescence

The light reaction that takes place in fireflies is due to the conversion of the substrate luciferin to oxyluciferin and light, catalyzed by luciferase and driven by the dephosphorylation of ATP (adenosine triphosphate). A luminometer is used to measure the amount of light generated by this reaction. The amount of light the reaction produces when luciferin is present in excess is proportional to the ATP present in the solution. There is no need for a light source, as in a photometric system. By selective release of ATP from bacterial cells in suspension, quantification can be achieved.

Fluorometry

Microbial metabolism can be detected and quantified by conjugating fluorophores to substrates. When the organism metabolizes the substrate, the fluorogenic markers are released and create measurable fluorescence. This method is said to produce a more sensitive reaction than is possible by the standard method of measurement of a pH shift.

Blood Culture

One of the more critical specimens received in clinical microbiology laboratories is blood for culture. The treatment of septicemia or bacteremia requires rapid recognition and initiation of rigorous appropriate treatment. Any patient admitted with a fever of undetermined origin is a candidate for multiple blood cultures. The presence of blood in the broth medium obscures developing turbidity and requires that microscopic examination be made and that subcultures to solid media be prepared under appropriate incubation conditions. Often the large amount of cells and cellular debris obscures faintly staining gram-negative organisms such as *Haemophilus influenzae,* so that a special stain such as **acridine orange** is needed to visualize the organism, and a fluorescent microscope is required.

In a large teaching hospital or tertiary care medical center, the volume often exceeds 15,000 to 20,000 blood cultures annually. Approved protocols for examination of blood cultures require Gram stain and subculture at 24 and 48 hours, and final subculture at 7 days. If this is multiplied by aerobic and anaerobic broths, the total number of operations on 15,000 blood cultures is 90,000 microscopic examinations and 90,000 subcultures annually! This has led to the development of the first automated blood culture instrument.

AUTOMATED MICROBIOLOGY SYSTEMS

BacTec 460 (Radiometric)

Principle of Operation

The principle of operation, as described earlier, is the release of $^{14}CO_2$ from ^{14}C-labeled substrates. The $^{14}CO_2$ is detected in the headspace (gas atmosphere in a closed bottle over the liquid medium) by the instrument specifically designed to do so.

System Description

The BacTec 460 instrument (Becton-Dickinson) was designed to utilize the radiometric technique (Fig. 10–1). The culture medium consists of specially modified tryptic soy broth in a closed bottle sealed by means of a rubber septum. Various formulations of medium are provided by the manufacturer for aerobic and anaerobic culture, as well as for recovery of wall-deficient microbial forms and microorganisms from blood containing antibiotics. The atmosphere provided for aerobic culture consists of 5 percent CO_2 and air, whereas that provided in anaerobic bottles is 5 percent CO_2 and nitrogen. The bottles are inoculated, incubated on a shaker, and periodically sampled.

Operating Procedures

The bottles are removed from the incubator, the rubber septum is decontaminated with 70 percent alcohol, and the bottles are placed in specially designed holders on the sampling tray. Once the sampling process is started, the sequence of testing is controlled by the electronics of the instrument. The sampling tray is designed to move the holders containing the culture bottles to a sampling head. An electrical element heats two sampling needles for a specified time to remove any contamination. The needles then move downward and puncture the rubber septum that seals the bottle. The appropriate (aerobic or anaerobic) gas mixture flushes the headspace gas to an ionizing chamber where the amount of radioactive carbon dioxide is determined. If the reading is above a preset threshold, which takes into account metabolism by cellular elements of the blood, the microbiologist removes the bottle for microscopic evaluation and subculture for subsequent identification and **susceptibility testing.** A warning light on the front of the control panel corresponding to the position of the bottle indicates when the reading is above a preset threshold. In addition, a printout is generated listing the readings for all the bottles when a run is completed. There is also an alpha numeric display for each bottle as the sampling is

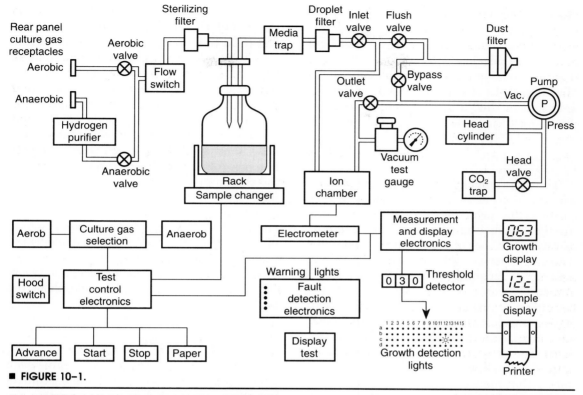

■ **FIGURE 10–1.**

Flow of the headspace gas, after displacement by aerobic or anaerobic mixtures, to the electrometer and subsequently to the electronics that convert the $^{14}CO_2$, released by microbial metabolism to a growth index. (Courtesy of Becton-Dickinson Diagnostic Instrument Systems, Sparks, MD.)

completed. Sampling time for each bottle is 1 minute, and the sampling tray holds up to 60 bottles at any one time.

Advantages/Disadvantages

Advantages. Since the amount of labor required to sample each bottle manually to determine whether or not microorganisms are present is considerable, a large savings in labor costs is realized by limiting the microscopic and cultural examination to only the bottles demonstrating microbial metabolism through production of $^{14}CO_2$. In addition, limiting the handling of the bottles manually reduces the chances of contamination. Time to detection for positive cultures is shortened, and detection of fastidious, or wall-deficient, microorganisms is enhanced.

Disadvantages. The major disadvantage to the radiometric technique lies in the guidelines for disposal of radioactive isotopes. Carbon-14 is a very weak beta-emitter, and the medium contains only 2 microcuries of activity; however, the autoclaved used bottles must be disposed of by a licensed handler separately from the other waste generated by the clinical microbiology laboratory. This increases waste disposal costs and requires more labor for separate handling of the waste.

BacTec 660 (Nonradiometric)

A nonradiometric technique for blood cultures was developed by Becton Dickinson Instrument Systems to obviate some of the disadvantages of the radiometric system. In addition to this, a design was created that further reduced culture bottle manipulation.

Principle of Operation

The nonradiometric design that evolved from the earlier radiometric design retained some of the principles of operation, mainly needle sterilization by heat and sampling through the use of two needles that puncture a rubber septum, with subsequent headspace flushing with either aerobic or anaerobic gas mixtures. The aerobic mixture was changed to 2.5 percent CO_2, with the balance consisting of air, and the anaerobic mixture was made up of 5 percent CO_2, with the balance nitrogen. The headspace gas is routed to an infrared spectrophotometer that measures the amount of CO_2. As in the radiometric system, the reading above a preset threshold indicates microbial metabolism. For the most part, this system has replaced the earlier radiometric methodology for blood cultures. Many laboratories have adapted the older instrument for use in their mycobacteriology section as a means of decreasing the time required to detect growth of *Mycobacterium* species.

System Description

The BacTec 660 system consists of a sampling unit controlled through a dedicated computer. Trays containing up to 60 aerobic or anaerobic culture bottles are removed from the incubator and placed in the sampling module. A command to test is generated through the computer keyboard, and the sampling tray is moved into position. An ultraviolet light provides sterilization of the

test area, while a heating unit surrounds the sampling needles for sterilization. The test head then automatically positions itself over each bottle to be tested, lowers to puncture the rubber septum, and samples the headspace gas. The headspace gas is routed to an infrared spectrophotometer that measures the level of CO_2 and sends a signal to a central processing unit, which creates a relative growth index. An incubator unit with two integral shakers, which serves as a base for the sampling head, provides a convenient space-saving method for incubation. The computer memory programmed for either a 5- or 7-day protocol prompts loading of the appropriate tray. Patient demographics are entered into the computer; these provide a convenient method of specimen tracking and data storage for the length of the protocol.

Operating Procedures

The microbiology technologist begins each day with a computer-directed quality control procedure. Prompted by the computer, the trays are loaded in sequence. At the end of sampling each tray, a computer printout of the positive culture bottles is rendered, enabling the technologist to perform the necessary procedures while the next tray is sampled. If any special readings are required, a "special procedures" tray may be processed off protocol at any time during the day. At the end of the day a printout of the cultures that have completed the 5- or 7-day protocol is produced. These cultures are then discarded, making room for new cultures.

Advantages

The nonradiometric BacTec has the obvious advantage of ease of disposal of completed culture bottles. Once sterilized, they can be discarded with the regular microbiology waste. The instrument allows for a shorter sampling period (30 seconds vs. 60 seconds for each bottle) and less manual manipulation of the bottles, since each tray contains 60 bottles and is incubated just below the test unit. The sampling head moves into place over the bottles to be sampled, unlike the radiometric version, thus providing a simpler procedure. In addition, the needle sterilizer is more efficient, surrounding the needles with heat for a longer period. The ultraviolet bulb provides for sterilization of the test area, including the tops of the bottles. Each set of needles is located within the holder so that the rubber septum is punctured in a different site each day, further reducing chances of contamination.

BacT/Alert (Organon Teknika)

The BacT/Alert (Organon Teknika) is a blood culture instrument that provides continuous monitoring of blood cultures while they are incubating with continuous agitation.

Principle of Operation

The principle of operation for the BacT/Alert involves the measurement of microbially produced CO_2 by means of a colorimetric sensor placed in the bottom of each culture bottle and separated from the growth medium by a CO_2 permeable membrane. The sensor changes from green to yellow in the presence of microbial metabolism. A light-emitting diode provides a light source to the bottom of each bottle. Changes are then monitored by means of a reflectometer capable of detecting slight color changes in the colorimetric sensor. Detection of CO_2 production is based on a computer-driven algorithm that monitors initial CO_2 production during the microbial growth phase and the total level of CO_2 produced. By relying

on changes in CO_2 production, the instrument can differentiate between microbial growth and CO_2 produced by blood components.

System Description

The BacT/Alert microbial detection system consists of modules capable of handling up to 240 bottles and a data management system. Each data management system is capable of handling up to four modules with a capacity of 960 samples.

Operating Procedures

The specially designed culture bottles are placed in the receptacles containing the LEDs and reflectometers. The patient demographics are entered into the computer. The data management system receives information from the detection system and signals when a culture becomes positive. The system incorporates bar-coding to enhance specimen tracking.

Advantages

This system totally eliminates the need for mechanical methods to position culture bottles for sampling and eliminates the need for gas and sampling needles, providing a significant reduction in labor. Further, monitoring of cultures is continuous. Cultures that became positive during the night can be immediately attended to when the laboratory staff arrives, reducing the turnaround time.

IDENTIFICATION AND SUSCEPTIBILITY SYSTEMS

Fully Automated Bacteriology Identification Systems

System Description

The Fully Automated Bacteriology Identification Systems (Vitek Systems), available

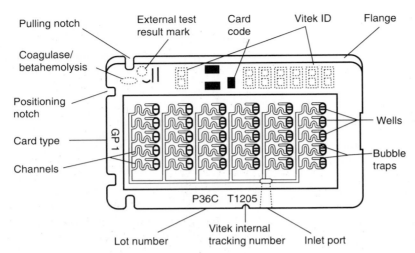

Pulling notch · External test result mark · Card code · Vitek ID · Flange · Coagulase/betahemolysis · Positioning notch · Card type · Channels · GP 1 · P36C T1205 · Wells · Bubble traps · Lot number · Vitek internal tracking number · Inlet port

■ FIGURE 10–2.

The Vitek test card has 30 wells containing either substrates for microbial identification or antimicrobials for susceptibility tests. Channels for distribution of the microbial suspension and smaller wells that trap air bubbles are molded into the card. Codes indicating the card type are printed on the card, and an embossed area is provided for entering the sample number. (Courtesy of Vitek Systems, Hazelwood, MO.)

from bioMerieux, utilize plastic cards (test kits) measuring approximately 57 mm. (2.25 inches) by 90 mm. (3.5 inches) by 3.2 mm. (0.13 inches), each containing 30 wells (Fig. 10–2). These cards contain either substrates for microbial identification or antibiotics for susceptibility testing. A number of different cards are available for identification, including GNI (gram-negative identification), GPI (gram-positive identification), EPS (enteric pathogen screen), UID-1 and UID-3, (enumeration and identification of organisms in urine), YBC (yeast identification), NHI (*Neisseria, Haemophilus* identification), and ANI (anaerobe identification). The latter two consist of wells containing chromogenic substrates designed to react with preformed enzymes when inoculated with a heavy suspension of the test organism. The design of the NHI and ANI cards, therefore, does not depend on growth within the wells and must be read visually with the reactions entered manually into the computer.

A number of susceptibility cards are available with a variety of antibiotics for either gram-positive or gram-negative organisms. In addition, a large user may design its own susceptibility panel for gram-negative bacteria if an order for a minimum of 1000 cards is placed.

The instrument for reading the cards and recording and interpreting the results consists of several modules, including one or more Reader/Incubator modules, a card Filling Module/Sealing unit, a computer, a printer, and a terminal. Reader/Incubator modules, available in 30-, 60-, 120-, or 240-card capacity, process the cards. Depending on the capacity, each Reader/Incubator holds from 1 to 8 trays, each capable of containing 30 cards. A sampling unit removes each card once an hour, whereupon a light source directs light through the wells to a reader. The data are transmitted to the computer, which records and interprets the readings. The system is a dynamic one, measuring changes in transmitted light as the organisms grow. As microbial growth changes the turbidity or the color of the indicator, depending on the test, the percent change in transmitted light is recorded.

The determination of positive and negative wells for gram-negative and gram-positive identification differs in certain details.

In general, raw value readings are recorded for each well once an hour and stored in the computer. Once the initial readings have been recorded, the percent change in light transmission is calculated for each well once an hour. The percent change is compared to a unique threshold for each well. If the change is equal to or greater than the threshold, a positive reaction is recorded. If the calculated change is less than the threshold, the well is considered negative until the next reading, when the change is recalculated and compared with the threshold again.

Gram-Negative Identification. The GNI card contains a growth control well, a decarboxylase negative control well, a polymyxin B well, and 27 substrates. The decarboxylase reactions are determined after the percent change of the negative control well has been subtracted from the change of each decarboxylase well. If the organism proves to be a glucose nonfermenting gram-negative rod, the lactose well is compared with two thresholds, one with a lower value for determining the lactose reaction and one with a higher value for determining the 10 percent lactose reaction. An oxidase test is performed on the isolate and entered manually on the card; a positive result is recorded by the instrument as part of the data base, while the absence of a mark is considered negative.

Final organism identification is reported at 4, 5, 6, 7, 8, 9, 10, 13, 15, or 18 hours after the GNI card is placed in the Reader/Incubator. The final hour for identification of glucose-fermenting gram-negative rods is usually at hour 13 but may be extended if the glucose well becomes positive at a later hour. The final hour for attempted identification of glucose-nonfermenting rods is 18. In my laboratory, most commonly encountered gram-negative rods are identified by the Vitek within 4 to 7 hours.

Once the GNI card has been incubating for sufficient time to allow for identification, the biochemical test results are matched to a data base termed the React File. This data base consists of a matrix of percent probabilities of positive tests for each biochemical and each organism in the GNI card data base. These probabilities were derived from GNI test results of representative strains of each organism in the data base. The results of biochemical tests are converted into positive or negative test probabilities for each taxon listed in the data base. After establishing the positive and negative test probabilities for each test, the absolute likelihood for each taxon in the data base is calculated. The two taxa with the highest absolute likelihood are listed as the first and second choice identifications. Normalized percent probabilities are calculated for the first and second choice identifications. This figure numerically expresses how well these choices are separated from the remaining taxa in the data base. Before final identification, the first-choice organism must pass a likelihood screen that has been established for each taxon in the data base to determine the overall likelihood that the identification is correct. If the absolute likelihood of the identification is smaller that the predetermined specified screen for that hour, the card is incubated until the next interval that identification may be attempted. Following this, the normalized percent probability is checked to determine whether it is greater than or equal to 90 percent. If this test fails, then the card is incubated and processed until the first-choice organism has passed the likelihood and the probability screens, at which point the final identification report is generated. If the absolute likelihood screen of the first choice identification is below the likelihood screen at the final hour of attempted identification, a final report of "Unidentified Organism" is rendered. A bionumber consisting of 10 digits (11 for nonfermenters) is printed on the final identification report that is derived from the GNI biochemical profile.

The 30 tests (31 for nonfermenters) are divided into groups of 3, from which each individual digit in the bionumber is obtained. The first test in each group of three has a numerical value of 4 if positive or 0 if negative; the second has a value of 2 if positive or 0 if negative; and the third a value of 1 or 0 in the same manner, the sum providing the bionumber digit.

Messages may appear on the final report explaining why an identification cannot be made or acting as a qualifying statement for the identification. Notes may be printed referring to supplemental information in the technical manual. The manual suggests appropriate additional biochemical tests, utilizing conventional media, to assist in final identification.

If there is a problem with the instrument during the incubation period, or a problem with identification, the technologist can read the reactions visually, construct a bionumber, type the results into the computer, and obtain a computer assist in arriving at a correct identification. The raw values and the percent changes over the incubation period are available to aid the technologist in troubleshooting the results. All data remain available to the operator as long as the card remains in the Reader/Incubator module.

Gram-Positive Identification. The GPI card consists of the same 30 wells that contain a peptone base as a growth control, bacitracin, optochin, novobiocin, and 26 biochemical substrates, including an arginine-negative control. Catalase, coagulase, and beta-hemolytic results are entered by marking specific areas of the card. A circular depression in the upper left of the card serves as the catalase mark, and the area designated on the card with a oval marking serves as the beta-hemolytic mark for catalase-negative organisms or as the coagulase mark for catalase-positive organisms. Absence of a mark indicates a negative reaction. The cards are read and the data processed in the manner as described for the GNI cards.

Yeast Identification. The yeast identification card (YBC) requires that incubation take place off-line in a 30°C incubator. After incubation, the card is inserted in the Reader/Incubator module and read once. Raw values are taken only once and stored in the Vitek computer until an interim or final report is generated. Once the raw values are recorded, the percent change in light transmission is calculated for the test wells, and each well is compared with a unique threshold for that well. The well is declared positive if the percent change for that well is greater than the threshold, and conversely declared negative if less. An interim report may be rendered with the notation to incubate an additional 24 hours at 30°C in the event that a final identification is not accomplished within the 24-hour period. A mark is made in the appropriate place on the card to record the additional 24-hour incubation, and additional reading is made by placing the card in the Reader/Incubator module. Analysis rules for a 48-hour incubation are used to determine the identification at this point. As with the other identification cards, special messages may appear, qualifying the identification or assisting in further testing.

Susceptibility Tests. These tests for gram-negative and gram-positive organisms are performed using the same Reader/Incubator modules. The data analysis is somewhat different from that used for identification and differs between these two categories of microorganisms.

The program that analyzes the data collected by the Reader is the same for any of the gram-negative susceptibility (GNS) cards. The analysis rules are applied per drug rather than on a set of rules for a particular card. The program contains the rules and coefficients needed for all the antimicrobials recognized by the system at the time of the software update. The configuration of the card is recognized by the card code stamped in bars on each card. The Reader measures the light passing through each well at each hour to a maximum of 15 hours. As the organism grows, the light transmission decreases and is expressed as percentages of the maximum reading. These percent changes represent a growth curve. When a preset threshold percent is reached in the positive control (PC) well, and the minimum hour of call for the organism identification is met, the type of growth curve and its slope are calculated for each well. The growth curve is made linear by converting the hourly percent changes into log values. The slope of the linear line is optimized to choose the log phase of the growth curve. The well slope is compared with the slope of the PC well and is expressed as a fraction of the PC well. This is termed a normalized slope. Well slopes range from 0 (indicating no growth) to 1 (indicating growth equal to the PC well). The normalized slopes are grouped according to the antimicrobial and added, producing a composite slope.

The composite slope for each antibiotic is used to calculate the organism's **MIC (minimal inhibitory concentration)** for that antimicrobial, using the following equations:

Doubling dilution value	Discrete value
$A_0 + A_1S + A_2S^2$	$A_0 - .585 + A_1S + A_2S^2$
MIC = 2	MIC = 2

where S is the composite slope and A_0, A_1, and A_2 are the coefficients for the particular organism/drug combination. These coefficients for each organism/drug combination were derived by plotting standard-method MIC values against composite slopes for a large number of strains of each organism group that represent MICs covering the range for the drug. Regression analysis is used to obtain the "best fit" line through the data points. The line represents growth characteristics of the test organism in the presence of the test antimicrobial and relates standard MIC values to growth in the card. The coefficients are numbers that describe the line as follows:

A_0 = The "Y" intercept or where the line crosses the MIC axis

A_1 = The slope of the line

A_2 = A correction factor (optional) for non-linearity

Using the equation, the coefficients are used to map a composite slope obtained by the instrument to its corresponding MIC value.

In gram-positive susceptibility (GPS) cards, different sets of coefficients for staphylococci, enterococci, and streptococci are used. Each group of organisms utilizes a set of three coefficients for each antimicrobial because of their growth characteristics. The coefficients for each organism/drug combination were derived by plotting standard method MIC values against composite slopes for a large number of strains of each organism group representing MICs covering the range for the drug. Regression analysis is used to obtain the "best fit" line through the data points. The line represents growth characteristics of the test organism in the presence of the test antimicrobial and relates standard MIC values to growth in the card. By using these unique coefficients more accurate MICs can be calculated.

Operating Procedures

Once an organism has been isolated, the appropriate test kit (card) is selected and identified with a specimen or culture number by writing in the embossed area of the card with a permanent fine-tipped marker (blue or black). The instrument automatically records this number. To inoculate the miniaturized card, a suspension of the test organism is made in sterile 0.45 percent saline in 12 × 75 mm. capped plastic culture tubes. The turbidity must be carefully adjusted according to a specific McFarland standard that is different for each card. The turbidity adjustment is especially critical for the susceptibility cards, and a small colorimeter is provided to aid in achieving the correct turbidity. The card is placed in a specially designed filling stand that holds the card and the tube containing the suspension. A transfer tube is inserted into the card and the card is placed so that the transfer tube extends down into the tube containing the suspension of the test organism. The filling stand containing ten kits is placed into the Filling Module/Sealing Unit, where a vacuum is drawn and then released, driving the inoculum into 30 test wells. After filling, the transfer tube is cut and sealed with the sealing unit. The cards are then placed in the Reader/Incubator module and the rest of the procedure is automated.

A print-out of the identifications and susceptibilities is rendered within as little as 4 hours to as long as 18 hours, with the majority being completed in 4 to 7 hours. The unit can be interfaced with a number of laboratory information systems; it is interfaced in my laboratory directly to a patient care system.

Data management software, termed the *Information Management System (IMS),* is available to enable the user to enter complete patient demographics either manually or by means of a bidirectional interface with many of the Laboratory Information Systems; to produce patient chartable results; and to provide epidemiologic data for use in treatment or infection control. Summaries of antibiotic susceptibilities (antibiograms) performed on isolates from the hospital are readily available from the IMS. IMS also has the capability of entering the results of other testing procedures, thus providing a system capable of total microbiology logging and reporting. This is especially useful for institutions that do not have a laboratory information system.

Advantages

The Fully Automated Bacteriology Identification Systems provide for hands-off identification and susceptibility testing of the most commonly encountered organisms in the clinical microbiology laboratory, often within 4 to 7 hours, enabling same-day reports. The manual work load is reduced, providing greater productivity, reduced labor costs, and reduced turn-around time. The reduced turn-around time provides for timely treatment and may result in earlier patient discharge, further reducing costs. The IMS provides the data necessary for accurate organism and susceptibility monitoring essential to infection control.

MicroScan, AutoScan, and TouchScan

MicroScan panels are available from Baxter Diagnostics, Inc., using conventional media, or as rapid panels. The conventional panels are read using a colorimetric technique.

MicroScan Rapid Panels provide identification of gram-negative and gram-positive bacteria in 2 hours and susceptibility results in as little as 3.5 hours up to 15 hours using the WalkAway-40 system or the WalkAway-96 system. As their name indicates, these two systems are fully automated. They utilize 96-well microtiter trays with a variety of antibiotics and biochemical substrates.

The rapid identification process is made possible by measuring fluorescence to detect the action of microbial enzymes on fluorescent-tagged substrates. Fluorescence is more sensitive to changes than colorimetry, enabling the tests to be completed more quickly. Fluorescent pH indicators are used to detect pH changes. Synthetic fluorogenic substrates are used that are composed of two parts, synthetic and metabolic. The action of microbial enzymes hydrolyzes the substrate, which frees the synthetic moiety enabling it to fluoresce, signaling bacterial activity.

The same technique is used in determining antimicrobial susceptibility. Wells containing the growth medium, fluorogenic substrate, and antimicrobial agents at various concentrations are incubated after inoculation with the test organism. The fluorescence in the test well is compared with that in the control well containing no antimicrobial agent. If a similar amount of growth occurs, then the organism is resistant, whereas less fluorescence, therefore less growth, indicates susceptibility. The end susceptibility test result is calculated when a predetermined "growth index" in the control well has been reached.

System Description

The WalkAway-40 system and the WalkAway-96 system process up to 40 or 96 Conventional or Rapid MicroScan panels automatically. Fiberoptics provide readings at multiple wavelengths and include initial and final readings for increased accuracy. The instruments contain a carousel with slots into which the panels are inserted after inoculation. The panels are incubated, reagents are automatically added at the appropriate time, and the results are sent to an IBM PS/2 computer with Data Management System (DMS) software. The software provides flexibility, allowing expansion for multiple-instrument capability. The DMS enables the user to retrieve data in a variety of formats, including antibiograms and hospital incidence and epidemiology reports.

The TouchSCAN-SR provides the user with a sonic digitizing pen to record visual interpretation of the reactions in conventional identification and susceptibility panels. This instrument can be used with the same computer and software just described.

A new software package, termed the pharmLINK, is available from Baxter Diagnostics, Inc. This software package links the pharmacy with the microbiology laboratory. The pharmacy can then review the reports or report summaries and recommend adjustments in therapy that are relevant in terms of cost and therapeutic efficacy.

Operating Procedures

Dehydrated panels can be quickly inoculated manually with a device termed the RENOK Rehydrator/Inoculator. A suspension of the test organism is prepared to the correct turbidity and poured into an inoculation tray. The RENOK device holds a sterile disposable inoculator with 96 tips matching the configuration of the panel. The inoculum is aspirated from the inoculation tray and then dispensed into the appropriate test panel. The panels are then either inserted into the WalkAway-40 system or the WalkAway-96 system or incubated and processed by means of the touchSCAN-SR.

Advantages

Many of the advantages of Vitek Systems are appropriate to the Microscan WalkAway-40 and the WalkAway-96: greater productivity, reduced labor costs and turnaround time, timely treatment, and earlier patient discharge.

UniScept and ALADIN

UniScept. Analytab Products offers the UniScept system with products designed for identification of gram-negative and gram-positive organisms. A wide range of organisms is covered, including fermenters, non-fermenters, *Neisseria* sp., anaerobes, and yeasts. The UniScept 20E and the UniScept 20GP are used for gram-negative and gram-positive identification, respectively, and are designed to attach to the susceptibility test panel. The system includes products designed to utilize a variety of susceptibility formats. These include the UniScept KB for routine testing and reporting in the standard (SIR) format, UniScept MIC for quantitative testing on a single 120-well panel, and the UniScept MICRO-MIC that enables users to add the latest susceptibility tests to their protocols. A variety of rapid or overnight tests may be chosen and combined by physically attaching test kits (designed to "snap" together). Results can be read manually, semiautomatically, or automatically. For manual reading, the UniScept Touch-reader is used, which allows for touchkey entry of results. The UniScept Autoreader, which requires manual placement of the test panels, employs multiple wavelength readings to ensure reproducibility and accuracy and automatically reads, interprets, and records data, which may be entered directly into the UniScept Dezine-er System. The UniScept Dezine-er system is a data management system that links various other hospital departments to the microbiology laboratory via a computer network. The system provides total microbiology data management, allowing entry of results of conventional testing, plus the mycology, mycobacteriology, and virology sections of the laboratory. Up to 30 stations can be linked, including the pharmacy, pathology laboratory, infection control, and hospital administration, with software designed to make the best use of microbiology data in each area.

ALADIN. The ALADIN is Analytab Product's fully automated instrument. The user needs only to place the inoculated susceptibility and/or identification panel in the incubator and the instrument does the rest.

The ALADIN has been designed to use a unique system for interpretation of the individual wells in the test panel. A video camera reads the entire area where the reaction occurs. Increased accuracy is claimed by the manufacturer over instruments that interpret reactions based on one detection point. Video pixels are interpreted by the image processor in this system, which has been designed to eliminate errors by interference from such things as pinpoint or dispersed growth patterns, very light growth, fading end-points, or scratches on the plastic of the test panel. All testing is controlled by software, enabling the use of any of the present UniScept test panels and the addition of test panels that may be developed in the future through software updates.

Use of a variety of test panels with different configurations and physical dimensions is made possible by a "universal" carrier within which the test panels are placed prior to insertion in the instrument. Once the carrier is placed in the instrument, a computer records its presence and directs the retrieval and reading of the panel. Automatic reagent addition, when required, is programmed with any of up to 20 different liquid reagents. When the results of identification and/or susceptibility testing are complete, the instrument can either automatically dispose of the test panels into autoclave bags or provide for manual retrieval for review.

Analytab Products provides a choice of three computer formats. The ALADIN *Stand Alone* provides the instrument for testing and reporting, plus an external AT/PC computer with software that includes databases, susceptibility programs, patient demographics, result storage, and antibiogram capability. The ALADIN *Mainframe/Lab Systems Interface* is designed for users who already have a laboratory information system (LIS); it provides the ability to directly interface to the existing system, enabling a bidirectional interface for up-loading daily test results, and down-loading demographics. The ALADIN *Microbiology Data System (MDS) Network* is designed for users who are linked to the Analytab Products MDS network. The UniScept Dezine-er System provides direct data retrieval from the ALADIN.

Advantages

The advantages of the ALADIN are similar to those listed for Vitek Systems and Microscan: greater productivity, reduced labor costs and turn-around time, timely treatment, and earlier patient discharge. In addition, the user may configure the test kits by use of the "snap-together" design.

Sensititre Microbiology Systems

The Sensititre Microbiology Systems, available from Radiometer America, Inc., is an instrument that provides bacterial identification and microdilution susceptibility capability. It is designed as a modular system, consisting of the Autoinoculator, the Autoreader, the SensiTouch, and the ARIS (Automated Reading/Incubating System). The computer module controls the readers and collects, stores, and analyzes data. In addition, the software provides for data management for patient reports and epidemiology surveys.

The Sensititre Microbiology Systems was the first to employ fluorogenic technology for identification and antimicrobial susceptibility. A nonfluorescent substrate is prepared by conjugating a fluorescent compound (a fluorophore) to the specific enzyme substrates with a bond that prevents fluorescence. This process is referred to as "quenching" the fluorophore. Bacterial growth results in the production of specific enzymes, causing cleavage of specific substrate-fluorophore bonds, releasing the fluo-

rophore and enabling it to fluoresce. The amount of fluorescence is proportional to the level of activity of the surface enzymes produced by the bacteria. This is an extremely sensitive analytical tool providing measurements as low as 10^{-11} to 10^{-13} mg/ml. The conventional biochemical tests have been modified to yield the fluorescent signal, which is then converted to a positive or negative result.

The user prepares the inoculum by suspending the test organism in demineralized water, matching a **0.5 McFarland turbidity standard.** Ten microliters are then transferred to 10 ml of Mueller-Hinton broth for a final density of 100,000 CFU/ml. The tube is fitted with a disposable dosing head to dispense the suspension to the microtiter plate utilizing an automatic inoculator, termed the *Autoinoculator.* Each tube of broth must be manually clamped into the pumping arm of the Autoinoculator. The appropriate volume is delivered by the Autoinoculator based on selection of one of a number of patterns available by keypad selection. Each gram-negative or gram-positive identification plate is designed to test three organisms using 32 biochemical and enzymatic tests that do not require reagent addition. Susceptibility plates are available for MIC or breakpoint concentration to antimicrobics for gram-negative, gram-positive, and urinary isolates. The plate is then sealed and incubated either in a standard 35° to 37°C incubator or placed into the ARIS module that provides on-line incubation and automatic reading. If the plate is incubated in a standard incubator, it must be loaded onto the Sensititre Autoreader for reading and interpretation. The ARIS module may be retrofitted to the Autoreader. The reader contains a fluorometer to measure the intensity levels of fluorescence, which are then transmitted to a microcomputer. The bacterial identification and/or susceptibility data bases are referenced, and the results are displayed, printed, and stored.

The data management program may be interfaced to a laboratory information system.

Sceptor

The Sceptor System (Becton-Dickinson) is available from Becton-Dickinson and consists of dehydrated panels for bacterial identification and/or susceptibility testing. Sceptor MIC Panels consist of an 84-well tray, with up to 83 wells containing antimicrobial reagents and one control well. The Sceptor MIC/ID and Breakpoint/ID panels contain antimicrobial agents and biochemical substrates in the 84-well configuration, each panel containing up to 59 wells with antimicrobial agents and up to 24 wells with biochemical substrates with one control well. A bacterial suspension in Sceptor broth medium is used for rehydration. Following incubation, the wells with the antimicrobics are checked for growth, while the biochemical substrates are checked for color change. The AutoSceptor may be used to read and record the results automatically for gram-positive MIC panels, gram-negative MIC, and MIC/ID panels. Other panels, including the Sceptor Anaerobe MIC and MIC/ID panels may be read on the Sceptor Reader/Recorder, an electromechanical device that reads and facilitates transcription of MIC values and biochemical data to the report form.

The Sceptor Automated Preparation Station provides automatic rehydration and inoculation of the panels. The Sceptor Data Management Center provides the data bases for bacterial identification and susceptibility testing, as well as providing a variety of patient, quality control, and epidemiologic report functions.

FUTURE TRENDS/NEW DEVELOPMENTS

The development of the computer has been crucial to the design of automated microbiology instruments. In fact, the development of Vitek Systems Fully Automated Bacteriology Systems had its beginnings in space exploration, which stimulated miniaturization and computerization. McDonnell Douglas originally undertook the development of a system to detect life on Mars. This instrument was the forerunner of the current system. A number of noncultural methodologies have been developed over the past decade, capable either of detecting the presence or identity of microorganisms in clinical specimens or of rapid, nongrowth-dependent identification of isolates. These techniques include the use of monoclonal antibodies, genetic probes, nucleic acid hybridization, and most recently, polymerase chain reaction. Polymerase chain reaction has, in fact, been made possible by the use of a microprocessor-controlled heating bath that supplies time- and temperature-controlled heating and cooling essential for management of the process.

Ultimately, automation of these technologically advanced processes will occur through use of precisely controlled instrumentation made possible by progress in the fields of robotics and computerization. The end-result of the merging of biologic technology with these two fields will be the ability to identify accurately, at the molecular level, the microorganisms involved in infectious disease, many of which are difficult or impossible to grow on lifeless media or in cell cultures, greatly enhancing diagnostic and treatment modalities.

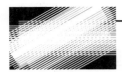

REVIEW QUESTIONS

Choose the one correct answer.

1. Microbial growth can be measured by incorporating into substrates which of the following labeled elements:

   a. ^{14}C
   b. ^{125}I
   c. ^{51}Cr
   d. None of the above

2. The atmosphere provided above the anaerobic culture medium used in the Bactec 460 system is:

   a. 50% CO_2 and nitrogen.
   b. 5% CO_2 and nitrogen.
   c. 5% CO_2 and air.
   d. CO_2.

3. The Bactec 660 measures microbial growth using:

   a. fluorimetry.
   b. bioluminescence.
   c. infra-red spectroscopy.
   d. turbidity.

4. The NHI and ANI Vitek cards contain substrates that are designed to react with:

   a. inducible enzymes.
   b. allosteric enzymes.
   c. preformed enzymes.
   d. none of the above.

5. Which of the following advantages pertain to automated microbiology instruments?

   a. Reduced turn-around time
   b. Reduced labor costs
   c. Greater productivity
   d. All of the above

REFERENCES

1. Barreau C, Wagener G: Characterization of *Leuconostoc lactis* strains from human sources. *J Clin Microbiol* 28:1728–1733, 1990.
2. Coovadia YM, Solwa Z, van den Ende J: Meningitis caused by vancomycin-resistant *Leuconostoc* sp. *J Clin Microbiol* 25:1784–1785, 1987.
3. Coovadia YM, Solwa Z, van den Ende J: Potential pathogenicity of *Leuconostoc*. *Lancet* 1:306, 1988.
4. Isenberg HD, Vellozzi EM, Shapiro J, Rubin LG: Clinical laboratory challenges in the recognition of *Leuconostoc* spp. *J Clin Microbiol* 26:479–483, 1988.
5. Long EG, Ebrahimzadeh A, White EH, Swisher B, Callaway CS: Alga associated with diarrhea in patients with acquired immunodeficiency syndrome and in travelers. *J Clin Microbiol* 28:1101–1104, 1990.

BIBLIOGRAPHY

Balows A, Hausler WJ Jr, Herrmann KL, Isenberg HD, Shadomy HJ (eds): *Manual of Clinical Microbiology.* Washington, DC, American Society for Microbiology, 1991.

Baron EJ, Finegold SM: *Bailey and Scott's Diagnostic Microbiology,* 8th edition. St. Louis, CV Mosby, 1990.

Brock TD, Madigan MT: *Biology of Microorganisms,* 5th edition. Englewood Cliffs, NJ, Prentice-Hall, 1988.

Chapter 11

IMMUNOCHEMISTRY ANALYZERS

VIVIEN A. SOO, MS, MT (ASCP)

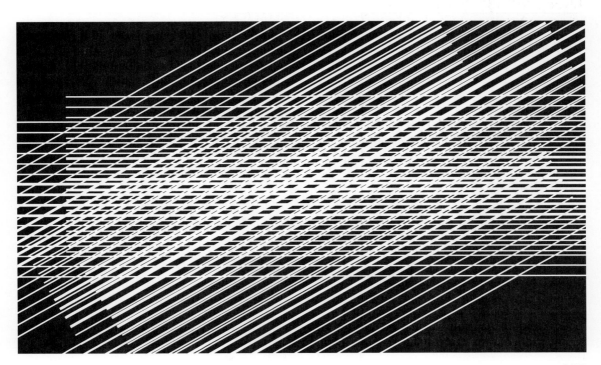

After studying this chapter, the student should be able to:

- Describe two nonlabeled immunoassay systems. Highlight their differences and their limitations.
- Describe the difference between the competitive and the noncompetitive immunoassays.
- Describe how the development of monoclonal antibody and the solid phase technology paves the way for automation in the field of immunoassay.
- Give examples of four labeled immunoassay systems and describe their detection methods.
- Describe an ideal automated immunochemistry analyzer for your laboratory. Give specific requirements.

KEY WORDS

Chemiluminescent reaction. A chemical reaction in which an unstable product is formed; when it reverts to its ground energy state, it releases energy in the form of visible light.

Competitive immunoassay. An antigen-antibody reaction in which labeled antigen and unlabeled antigen compete for limited antibody binding sites. The amount of bound labeled antigen is indirectly proportional to the concentration of the analyte.

Double antibody separation. The separation of the antigen-antibody complex from the free antigen is accomplished by adding a second antibody (antigammaglobulin) to form a larger precipitating complex.

Enzyme multiplied immunoassay technique (EMIT). A homogeneous enzyme immunoassay in which enzyme-labeled drug competes with free drug in the sample for antibody binding sites. When the enzyme-labeled drug is bound, the enzyme activity is blocked. The free enzyme-labeled drug is allowed to react with its substrates. The enzyme activity is directly proportional to the concentration of the drug in the sample.

Fluorescent polarization. When fluorescent molecules are excited with polarized light, they emit partially polarized light whose intensity is indirectly related to the degree of rotation of the molecules. Free molecules have a higher rate of rotation and emit lower intensity of light than bound molecules, which have a low rate of rotation and therefore emit higher intensity of light.

Fractional precipitation separation. Antigen-antibody complex can be precipitated by neutral salts, such as ammonium sulfite and ammonium sulfate, and organic solvents, such as ethanol.

Heterogeneous immunoassay. Immunoassay reaction in which a separation step is required to physically separate the bound label from the free label before measurement can be performed.

Homogeneous immunoassay. Immunoassay reaction in which no separation step is required by using labeled reagent whose activity is modulated by the binding reaction.

Immunoprecipitation. Certain serum proteins can form insoluble immunocomplexes in the presence of their specific antibody.

Luminometer. An instrument designed to measure a flash of light. It consists of a light-tight, temperature-regulated chamber and a sensitive light detector that is capable of measuring light in nanoseconds.

Noncompetitive immunoassay. Immunoassay reaction in which the antibody is labeled.

Polymer enhancement. Nonionic hydrophilic polymers, such as polyethyleneglycol (PEG) and dextran, are used to improve the speed and sensitivity of nephelometric reactions.

Radioimmunoassay (RIA). Immunoassay reaction in which the labeling molecule is a radioisotope such as ^{125}I.

Sandwich (two-site) immunoassay. Immunoassay reaction in which the molecule is first incubated with an antibody immobilized on a solid phase and then with a second labeled antibody directed at the second antigenic site on the molecule. Excess labeled antibody is removed by washing the solid phase, and the concentration of the analyte is directly proportional to the amount of bound label on the solid phase.

Solid phase separation. Antigen or antibody can be immobilized onto a solid phase surface, such as polymer beads, plastic tubes, glass fiber, filter paper, or magnetized particles. Separation of the bound from the free label can be achieved by centrifugation, decantation, simple washing, or the application of a magnetic field.

INTRODUCTION

For the last 30 years, immunoassays have played an increasingly important role in diagnostic medicine. Before the advent of immunoassays, the measurement of many important hormones was not possible except through lengthy, insensitive bioassays. Today immunoassay analytes include not only endocrine and fertility hormones but also many serum proteins, drugs for therapeutic monitoring, tumor markers, and various infectious agents as well.

Immunoassays can be broadly categorized as either labeled or nonlabeled. Nonlabeled assays do not need a label for measurement whereas labeled immunoassays need a labeled product for detection. Both assays require the use of a specific antibody (Ab) as a reagent and an appropriate detection system for the quantification of the analyte (Ag, antigen).

Nonlabeled immunoassays employ turbidimetry or nephelometry for the direct measurement of the antigen-antibody immunocomplex (AgAb). Currently, because of their limited sensitivity, these assays are mainly used for the measurement of serum proteins and drugs for therapeutic monitoring.

Labeled immunoassays, on the other hand, are more widely used in all areas of the clinical laboratory. The sensitivity of the labeled immunoassay is limited by the antigen-antibody affinity and the types of label used.

This chapter presents the principles behind various nonlabeled and labeled immunoassay systems and the analyzers based on these methodologies.

NONLABELED IMMUNOASSAYS

Immunoprecipitation Reaction

Serum proteins, such as immunoglobulins, complements, and acute phase proteins, as well as some coagulation proteins, can form insoluble immunocomplexes in the presence of their specific antibodies. These immunocomplexes can be measured directly without the aid of labels by turbidimetric or nephelometric methods, which are based on the light-scattering properties of immunocomplexes.

When an antigen and its specific antibody combine, an immunocomplex is formed. This association is noncovalent and follows the law of mass action:

$$Ag + Ab \rightarrow AgAb$$
$$K = \text{Association constant}$$

The strength of association of the AgAb complex depends on the affinity of the antibody for the antigen, as well as on other forces such as the Van der Waals bond, hydrogen bonding, and hydrophobic interactions. At constant antibody concentration, increasing the antigen concentration will favor the formation of AgAb complexes. The formation of immunocomplexes follows three stages of development during which detectable **immunoprecipitation** of the immunocomplexes occurs. At this stage, soluble immunocomplexes become insoluble and precipitate out of solution. Figure 11–1 shows the three stages of the immunoprecipitation reaction. In the zone of antibody excess, increasing antigen concentration results in increasing formation of immunocomplexes until a zone of maximum immunoprecipitation (zone of equivalence) is reached. At this point, further increase in antigen concentration will result in a decrease in precipitation (zone of antigen excess).

This phenomenon can be explained by the fact that most antibodies are bivalent and most antigens are multivalent. At the beginning of the reaction, more antibodies are available to bind to the antigens. Therefore, all antigenic sites on the antigens are bound by antibodies. Only simple AgAb complexes are formed, and precipitation is minimal in the zone of antibody excess. As the concentration of the antigen increases, antibody molecules are able to form lattice networks with the antigens, resulting in visible precipitation of larger complexes in the zone of maximum precipitation. Further increases in the antigen concentration result in a rearrangement of the binding sites in such a way that antibody molecules are prevented from forming the necessary lattice network for the precipitation reaction in the zone of antigen excess. Precipitation is again mini-

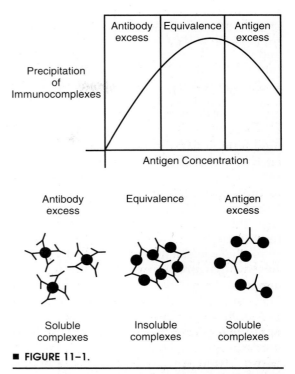

■ **FIGURE 11–1.**

Immunoprecipitation curve generated by adding increasing amounts of antigen to a solution of antibody and corresponding schematic diagram of antigen-antibody complexes in the different stages of the immunoprecipitation reaction.

mal in this region of the immunoprecipitation curve.

In the zone of antibody excess, the concentration of the antigen is directly proportional to the number of AgAb complexes formed. The amount of immunocomplexes can be measured by determining their light-scattering properties.

Light-Scattering Properties of Immunocomplexes

When light is directed at a solution of suspended particles, light is absorbed, scattered, reflected, and transmitted. The degree to which this happens depends on the wavelength of the incident light and the size and shape of the particles. Particles smaller than the wavelength of the incident light scatter light almost symmetrically. This is known as Rayleigh scatter. Most soluble serum proteins are small compared with the wavelength of visible light. They scatter light symmetrically and contribute to the background scatter noise level. Larger particles, whose sizes are approximately equal to but not larger than the incident wavelength, scatter light in a more forward direction; this is known as Rayleigh-Debye scatter. Particles whose sizes are much larger than the wavelength of the incident light scatter light predominantly in the forward direction, known as Mie scatter (Fig. 11–2). Most immunocomplexes in serum range in size from 250 to 1400 nm, which is near to or larger than the wavelengths used in most nephelometers. Therefore, nephelometers that measure scattered light at a more forward direction will give higher sensitivity. They will be less affected by interferences from endogenous proteins and lipid molecules.[1]

Measurement of Light Scatter

The measurement of light can be performed by turbidimetry or by nephelometry. Turbidimetry is the measurement of transmitted light after it has passed through the liquid solution containing suspended particles. It measures direct light transmission by a photodetector such as a photometer or spectrophotometer (Fig. 11–3). This method is often used to measure dense and visibly turbid samples. Its current application in the clinical immunoassay field is limited because of its lack of assay sensitivity.

Nephelometry is the measurement of light scatter at an angle to the incident light and not in the direct path of the transmitted light (Fig. 11–4). Most immunocomplexes

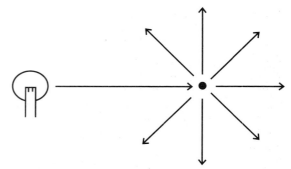

Small particle scatter (Rayleigh scatter)

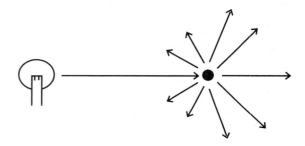

Larger particle scatter (Rayleigh-Debye scatter)

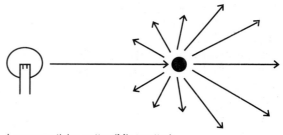

Larger particle scatter (Mie scatter)

■ **FIGURE 11–2.**

Effects of particle size on the scattering of incident light.

scatter light in the more forward angle, following the Rayleigh-Debye and Mie scattering patterns. Nephelometers capable of measuring light scatter at a more forward angle will give greater sensitivity. In most clinical laboratories, nephelometry is the method of choice for the determination of relatively abundant serum proteins.[1, 2]

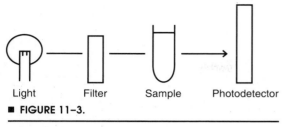

Light   Filter   Sample   Photodetector

■ **FIGURE 11–3.**

A simple photometer.

PRINCIPAL COMPONENTS IN NEPHELOMETRIC ASSAYS

Light Source

For the measurement of light scattered by a suspension of particles such as the AgAb complexes, a stable, high-intensity light source is required. Some of the commonly used light sources are a mercury arc at a wavelength of 357 nm, a tungsten-halogen lamp at 400 to 620 nm, lasers at 632 nm, and more recently, an infrared high-performance, light-emitting diode (LED) at 840 nm. The latter two light sources do not generate as much heat as the other light sources at similar intensities. Thus, they do not require cooling and are less likely to burn out prematurely.[1]

Angle of Detection

The angle at which the scattered light is measured is important in determining the sensitivity of the detection system. Most immunocomplexes measured in the clinical laboratories scattered light primarily in the forward direction (Rayleigh-Debye and Mie scatter). Sensitive photodetectors placed in the forward angles, therefore, will give higher sensitivity. Most commercial nephelometers utilize forward angles of 13 to 90 degrees.[1]

Antigen Excess Detection

In an immunoprecipitin reaction, it is important to use an antigen-antibody ratio on the side of antibody excess, as shown in Figure 11–5. In this region, there is a direct quantitative relationship between immunocomplex formation and the concentration of the antigen. At constant antibody concentration, light-scattering signals from the immunocomplexes can be plotted against increasing antigen concentration. The resultant curve is similar to the immunoprecipitation curve. As antigen concentration increases, the light-scattering signal increases until it reaches a region of maximum signal response S(max). Beyond this point, further increases in antigen concentrations will result in a diminished light-scattering response. Therefore, it is possible that two significantly different antigen concentrations (a and b) can give the same light-scattering response as seen in Figure 11–5. This is one of the inherent limitations of the nephelo-

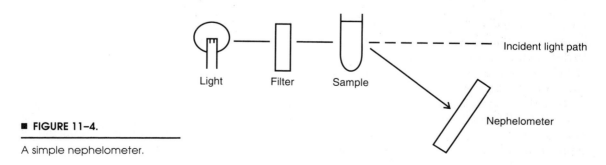

Light   Filter   Sample   Incident light path   Nephelometer

■ **FIGURE 11–4.**

A simple nephelometer.

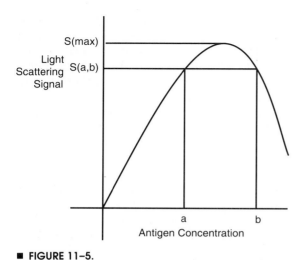

■ **FIGURE 11–5.**

Antigen excess curve. Effects of increasing antigen concentrations on the light-scattering response of immunocomplexes. Concentrations *a* and *b* have the same light-scattering signal responses.

metric assay procedure. However, most nephelometers in the clinical laboratories have a built-in capability to check for antigen excess. The Behring nephelometer has extended its assay ranges to minimize this potential problem.[3]

Polymer Enhancement

The use of a nonionic hydrophilic polymer such as polyethylene glycol (PEG) and dextran in a nephelometric reaction has greatly improved the speed and sensitivity of the assay procedure. In an immunologic reaction, these polymers compete for water molecules, decreasing their availability, thereby reducing the solubility of the AgAb complex formed. The net effect is an increase in the slope of the antibody excess side of the precipitin curve and a shift of the equilibrium point to a higher antigen concentration with a corresponding increase in the rate of reaction. One of the most commonly used poly-

mers in nephelometry is PEG 6000. With its introduction in nephelometry, reaction times in end-point assays have dramatically decreased from hours to minutes. It has increased the peak rate in kinetic assays by as much as tenfold.[4]

End-Point Versus Kinetic Assay

Nephelometric reaction can be determined by end-point or kinetic rate methods. End-point reaction measures light scattering when the AgAb reaction has reached equilibrium or steady state. It uses a single measurement of light scatter at a time when the rate of change is very small *(R)*, as shown in Figure 11–6. End-point reaction requires an incubation period (t1) before measurement is made. A serum blank reading *(B)* is sometimes necessary to correct for high background light-scattering signals caused by endogenous macromolecules in the serum. This problem may be minimized by using a high dilution of serum or by pre-

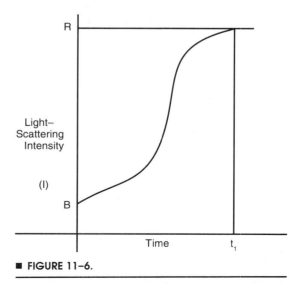

■ **FIGURE 11–6.**

The end-point, or equilibrium reaction, measures the light-scattering signal at steady state *(R)*.

treatment of the sample to remove interfering substances. The measured values are compared with a reference curve and converted to concentration units.

The kinetic, or rate, method monitors the rate of formation of light-scattering AgAb complexes. The concentration of the analyte is determined by measuring the rate of change of light scattered during the initial phases of the AgAb reaction. No incubation step is involved. A serum blank is not required, since background scatter constitutes a constant background signal and has no effect on the rate measurement. Measured kinetic values are compared with corresponding values on a reference curve and converted to concentration units.[1, 2]

INSTRUMENTATION

Beckman Array Nephelometer

The Beckman Array is a highly microprocessor-controlled, kinetic nephelometer that measures serum protein and therapeutic drug levels in the serum. It uses a tungsten-halogen lamp with a bandwidth of 400 to 620 nm. The wide bandwidth is advantageous because light-scatter signals from a heterogeneous mixture of sizes of immunocomplexes are averaged. Scattered light is detected at a forward angle of 70 degrees. The assay sensitivity is 1 μg/ml. Beckman provides all assay reagents. Calibration data and other reagent characteristics are supplied with each reagent kit in the form of microprocessor cards. Calibration data can be entered into the instrument by inserting the microprocessor card. Only a single-point calibration is performed to standardize the instrument to run the assay. The microprocessor analyzes the data and reports the concentration of the unknown in a variety of assay modes.

For assay samples that have the potential to be in the antigen excess region, e.g., IgM, the automatic antigen excess check mode can be used. In this mode, a small amount of calibrator is added to the reaction mixture and reassayed. If the reaction causes an increased response, the reaction is in antibody excess and the initial assay result is valid. On the other hand, if the reaction mixture produces no additional response after the addition of the calibrator, the reaction is in antigen excess, and the sample is automatically rerun at a higher dilution. The limitation of this mode of operation is that the assay time will be prolonged. Only 15 to 30 samples can be run in an hour.[5, 6]

Behring Nephelometer

The Behring nephelometer is a fully automated instrument that measures serum proteins. It utilizes a high-performance, light-emitting diode as a light source at 840 nm, and it measures light scattered in the forward direction from an angle ranging from 13 to 24 degrees. This light signal is converted to an electrical signal by a sensitive photodiode. The scattered-light intensity is directly proportional to the concentration of the immunocomplex measured. The light signal response is compared with values from a reference curve previously stored in the memory of the computer terminal and converted to concentration units.

Behring primarily uses a fixed-time method for the measurement of serum proteins. The fixed-time method makes two sequential scattered-light measurements. One measurement is taken at 10 seconds after initiation of the reaction (t1), and the other one is made at 6 minutes (t2) (Fig. 11–7). The difference in scattered-light intensity between these two points is converted to concentration units by comparing its values with reference curve values previously stored in the analyzer. A calibration curve

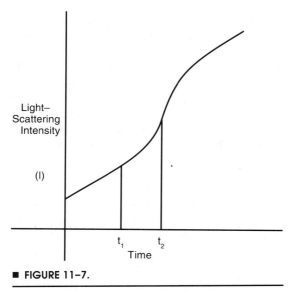

■ FIGURE 11–7.

Fixed-time reaction measures the light-scattering signal at two fixed-time intervals (t1, t2).

can be run with 4 to 8 standard concentrations. It is stable for up to 7 days and can be stored in the memory of the computer terminal. Alternatively, single-point calibration may be performed by using predetermined assay parameters that are included in the Behring Reagent kits.

The Behring nephelometer does not require antigen excess detection. The manufacturer claims that the extended measuring range of the assay will cover the extreme increases in concentration up to the maximum soluble concentration in the serum.[3]

LABELED IMMUNOASSAYS

One of the earliest labeled immunoassay was the the **radioimmunoassay (RIA).** The label used was ^{125}I, which is still one of the most widely used radiolabels. It was first developed by Yalow and Berson in 1959.[7] Its application in hormone assay constituted a major breakthrough in the field of

endocrinology. The main advantages of radiolabel are high sensitivity (10^{-12} gm/ml) and resistance to interferences in the assay environment. Despite these advantages, RIA has its limitations. Short reagent shelf-life, requirement for a separation step, a licensing requirement, and the high cost of waste disposal have hampered its widespread use. Attempts are being made to replace RIA with alternative nonradiolabeled immunoassays. Some of the more promising labels include enzymes, fluorescent molecules, and chemoluminescent precursors.

Competitive Immunoassays

Most of the early immunoassays employ labeled antigens in their assay design. They are known as **competitive immunoassays.** In these reactions, a labeled antigen (Ag*) and an unlabeled antigen (Ag) compete for limited antibody binding sites. The bound, labeled antigen (AgAb) and the free labeled antigen are separated and the amount of labeled bound antigen (Ag*Ab) is determined. The concentration of analyte (Ag) is indirectly proportional to the concentration of the labeled bound antigen.

$$Ab + Ag^* + Ag \rightarrow$$
$$AgAb + Ag^*Ab + Ag^*$$

Noncompetitive Immunoassays

In the late 1960s, Miles and Hale described a novel labeling technique by which they were able to label antibodies.[8] The introduction of labeled antibody technology, as well as the introduction of the hybridoma monoclonal antibody production technology by Kohler and Milstein in 1975, greatly expanded the scope of labeled antibody immunoassay.[9, 10] The availability of an unlimited supply of purified specific antibodies at relatively low cost makes it feasible to develop immunoassays using excess labeled antibodies, or **noncompetitive immunoassays.**

In this reaction, the antibody is present in excess and carries the labeling molecule. The amount of bound label (AgAb*) is directly proportional to the concentration of the analyte (Ag) in the sample. The unreacted labeled antibody (Ab*) is removed by the addition of excess analyte coupled to a solid phase and centrifugation. The bound label in the supernatant is then removed for measurement.

$$Ab^* + Ag \rightarrow AgAb^* + Ab^*$$

This assay is also known as a one-site assay, because only one antigenic site is involved in the reaction, as opposed to the two-site assay in which the two antigenic sites on the analyte are bound to two specific antibodies. This reaction is also known as the **"sandwich" immunoassay.**

Two-site or Sandwich Immunoassays

For analytes large enough to have two distinct antigenic sites, the two-site assay offers increased specificity and sensitivity. This assay employs two antibodies. The first antibody is coupled to a solid phase. The analyte binds to the first antibody. A second labeled antibody recognizing the second binding site on the analyte is added. The bound label coupled to the solid phase is washed to remove any unbound free labeled antibodies. No centrifugation step is required, and the bound label can be measured directly. The concentration of the analyte is directly proportional to the bound label.[11]

Homogeneous Immunoassays

Most immunoassays require a separation method for the physical separation of the bound label from the free label. These are known as **heterogeneous immunoassays**. The requirement for a separation step presents a major technical challenge for the development of an automated immunoassay system. In 1972, Rubinstein and associates developed a new immunochemical procedure that they termed **homogeneous,** in which no separation step is required.[12] This uses labeled reagents whose activities are modulated by the binding reaction. This development led to the first commercial production of the homogeneous immunoassay system, known as the **enzyme multiplied immunoassay technique (EMIT),** by SYVA Company. It is a competitive immunoassay in which enzyme-labeled drugs compete with free drugs in the sample for antibody binding sites. When bound by antibody specific for the drug, the enzyme activity of the enzyme-labeled drug is blocked. If the unlabeled drug is present in the sample, it competes with the enzyme-labeled drug for binding sites on the antibodies and displaces enzyme-labeled drug into the reaction mixture. The free enzyme-labeled drug is allowed to react with the enzyme substrate present (glucose-6-phosphate and nicotinamide-adenine dinucleotide, NAD). The enzyme activity is measured as the rate of conversion of the coenzyme NAD to NADH (reduced form), in absorbance units at 340 nm.

$$Ag + Ab + Ag^*e \rightarrow AgAb + Ag^*eAb + Ag^*e$$
$$\text{G-6-phosphate} \rightarrow \text{6-gluconate}$$
$$\text{NAD} \curvearrowright \text{NADH}$$

where e = G-6-phosphate dehydrogenase.

Since EMIT, other homogeneous assays have been developed and automated. The Abbott TDX is an example of a homogeneous immunoassay based on the principle of **fluorescent polarization.** Because of its assay design, homogeneous immunoassay systems have been used mainly in the determination of haptens, such as therapeutic drugs and nonprotein hormones, at concentrations measured in the microgram per milliliter levels. However, efforts are being made to develop systems with lower detection limits and easy automation.

COMPONENTS IN THE IMMUNOASSAY SYSTEM

Analytes

In the clinical laboratory, most analytes measured by immunoassay procedures are components found in the serum or plasma, ranging in concentrations from picogram per milliliter to milligram per milliliter. Analytes that elicit an immune response (production of specific antibody) when injected into an animal are called antigens. Smaller analytes that require carrier molecules to become immunogenic are called haptens. Some of the more commonly encountered

analytes measured by immunoassay procedures are listed in Table 11–1.

Antibody

Antibodies are the most important components of the immunoassay system. They ultimately determine the specificity and sensitivity of the assay procedure. Generally, antibodies demonstrate two characteristics, specificity and affinity. *Specificity* represents the degree of uniqueness of the antigen-antibody reaction and the freedom from interference from other reactants. *Affinity* is a measure of the tightness of the antigen-antibody binding defined by K, the association constant.

Polyclonal Antibodies

Before the development of monoclonal antibody technology, antisera were obtained

TABLE 11–1. ANALYTES MEASURED BY IMMUNOASSAY

SPECIFIC PROTEINS	THERAPEUTIC DRUGS	REPRODUCTIVE HORMONES
Albumin	Amikacin	Chorionic gonadotropin (hCG)
Alpha$_1$-acid glycoprotein	Carbamazepine	Estradiol
Alpha$_1$-antitrypsin	Digoxin	Luteinizing hormone (LH)
Alpha$_2$-macroglobulin	Gentamicin	Follicle-stimulating hormone (FSH)
Antithrombin III	Lidocaine	Prolactin
Apolipoprotein A1	Phenobarbital	Progesterone
Apolipoprotein B	Phenytoin	**TUMOR MARKERS**
Ceruloplasmin	Primidone	Chorionic embryo antigen (CEA)
Complement C3	Procainamide	Alpha-fetoprotein (AFP)
Complement C4	N-acetyl procainamide	Prostate-specific antigen (PSA)
C-reactive protein	Quinidine	CA-50
Fibrinogen	Theophylline	**CARDIAC ISOENZYME**
Fibronectin	Tobramycin	CK-MB
Haptoglobin	Valproic acid	**MISCELLANEOUS**
Immunoglobulin A	**THYROID HORMONES**	Ferritin
Immunoglobulin G	Triiodothyroxine (T3)	Cortisol
Immunoglobulin M	Thyroxine (T4)	
Kappa light chain	Thyroid-stimulating hormone (TSH)	
Lambda light chain	Free T4 (FT4)	
microAlbumin	Free T3 (FT3)	
Plasminogen		
Properdin factor B		
Prothrombin		
Rheumatoid factor		
Transferrin		

by immunizing an animal (rabbit or sheep) with the purified antigen. After the required immunization schedule, the animal was bled regularly to obtain polyclonal antisera that contained antibodies directed at different antigenic determinants on the antigen molecule. For most diagnostic immunoassays, no purification procedures are required. In competitive immunoassays and methods dependent on immunoprecipitation, polyclonal antibodies have often been used in the form of diluted crude serum. These procedures depend only on the function and not the chemical purity of the antibody reagent. However, if an antibody of higher specificity is required, the polyclonal antisera will have to undergo further purification by means of affinity chromatography. In general, polyclonal antibodies are characterized as having high affinity and general specificity.

One obvious disadvantage in using polyclonal antibodies is their limited availability. The amount of serum obtained during any one bleed is limited. The life-span of the animal producing the antisera is also limited. When the animal dies, the antisera will no longer be available. Furthermore, purification of polyclonal antibodies can be costly and tedious.

Monoclonal Antibodies

In 1975, Kohler and Milstein developed the hybridoma technology for mass production of monoclonal antibodies. This discovery made a tremendous impact on the development and design of immunoassay chemistry.[9, 13] The production of monoclonal antibodies is not technically difficult, but it is tedious and time consuming. However, once the cell line producing the monoclonal antibodies has been established, an unlimited supply of the monoclonal antibodies is guaranteed as long as the cell line is maintained.

In this procedure, Kohler and Milstein immunized animals (rats or mice) with a purified antigen. Antibody-producing spleen cells from the animal were removed and fused with myeloma cells (cells in continuous culture). They found that the hybrid cells secreted antibodies that have the specificity characteristic of the parent spleen cells but in the quantity typical of the myeloma cells. These hybrid cells were screened for their ability to produce antibodies of the required specificity and affinity. The screening procedure for the selection of hybridoma cell line–producing antibodies is of critical importance. Once the desired hybridoma cell line has been identified, it can be maintained in continuous cell culture. Monoclonal antibodies produced can be harvested from the culture fluid. The supply of monoclonal antibodies is essentially limitless. Figure 11–8 illustrates the stages of the production of monoclonal antibodies.[14]

With the availability of an unlimited supply of relatively pure specific antibodies, noncompetitive, two-site immunoassays that were at one time too impractical and costly to perform are being developed. Furthermore, the availability of an unlimited supply of well-defined and well-characterized antibodies makes possible the standardization of immunoassay systems around the world.

Monoclonal antibodies generally do not individually form a precipitation lattice with most analytes, which makes them unsuitable for immunoassays based on immunoprecipitation, e.g., nephelometric methods. Also, monoclonal antibodies generally have lower affinities than their polyclonal counterparts. Despite these limitations, the use of monoclonal antibodies in immunoassays accounts for greater than 50 percent of all new assays developed since 1980.[15]

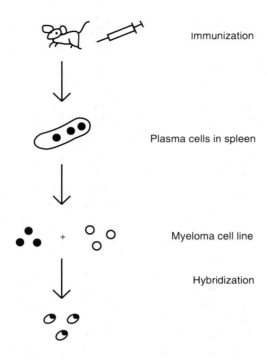

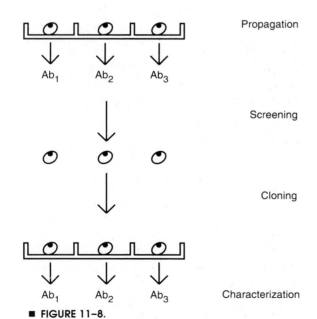

■ FIGURE 11–8.

The different stages of monoclonal antibody production.

Separation Methods

Most competitive immunoassay procedures require a method for the separation of the bound label from the unbound label. The ideal separation method should have the following characteristics:

- Rapid and complete separation
- Reproducible results
- Technically simple and inexpensive
- Not be subject to nonspecific interferences
- Easily automated

Recent advances in **solid phase separation** technology have demonstrated that this method may be the one of choice for most immunoassay systems.[16] Table 11–2 lists some of the more commonly used separation methodologies in immunoassay procedures.

Labels

The selection of a suitable labeling substance depends on the following properties:

1. High specific activity, defined as the number of detectable events/unit time for each labeling molecule.
2. Ease in labeling.
3. End-point signal easily and efficiently detected.
4. End-point signal not subject to interferences.

Table 11–3 lists some of the most commonly used nonisotopic labels and their method of detection.

Enzyme Labels

The use of enzyme labels in immunoassay design has gained increasing acceptance. They have long shelf-lives and are more sta-

TABLE 11–2. SEPARATION METHODS IN IMMUNOASSAYS

METHOD	SEPARATION TECHNIQUE
Fractional precipitation	Bound antibody-antigen complex is precipitated by neutral salts or organic solvents, e.g., PEG, ammonium sulfate, and ethanol. Separation is by centrifugation.
Double-antibody	Antibody-antigen bound complex is precipitated by a second antibody (anti-gammaglobulin), forming a larger precipitating complex. Separation is by centrifugation.
Solid-phase	Separation of the bound complex is achieved by adsorption of antibody or antigen to a solid phase, such as polymer beads, plastic tubes, glass-fiber filter paper, and magnetized particles, followed by centrifugation, decantation, simple washing, or the application of a magnetic field.

TABLE 11–3. NONISOTOPIC LABELS

SUBSTANCE	DETECTION METHOD
ENZYME	
Alkaline phosphatase	Colorimetric
	Fluorometric
	Chemiluminescent
β-D-Galactosidase	Colorimetric
	Fluorometric
Horseradish peroxidase	Colorimetric
	Fluorometric
	Chemiluminescent
LIGAND	
Avidin-biotin	Colorimetric
	Fluorometric
	Chemiluminescent
FLUORESCENT MOLECULES	
Fluorescein	Fluorometric
Europium chelates (Eu3+)	Time-resolved fluorometric
CHEMILUMINESCENT MOLECULES	
Isoluminol derivatives	Chemiluminescent
Acridinium esters	Chemiluminescent

ble than radiolabels. Enzyme labels have relatively high specific activities because 1 molecule of enzyme can catalyze the conversion of many molecules of substrate to give amplified signal response. The most widely used enzyme label is horseradish peroxidase. This is followed by alkaline phosphatase, and β-D-galactosidase. Both horseradish peroxidase and alkaline phosphatase have relatively high specific activities. Their catalytic end-points are easily detected by colorimetric and fluorometric, as well as **chemiluminescent** methods. Currently, about 35 percent of the new assays developed use enzyme labels.[15, 17, 18] Furthermore, certain few homogeneous immunoassays have been developed using enzyme label technology, e.g., EMIT and fluorescent polarization.

Table 11–4 lists some of more common enzyme labels and their substrates.

Fluorescent Labels

Fluorescein. Fluorescent substances such as fluorescein isothiocyanate (FITC) have the potential to yield high specific activities. Each fluorescent-labeled molecule

TABLE 11–4. COMMON ENZYME LABELS

ENZYME	SUBSTRATE	END-POINT
Alkaline phosphatase	P-nitrophenyl phosphate	colorimetric
Horseradish peroxidase	5-Aminosalicylic acid	colorimetric
Horseradish peroxidase	Ortho-phenylene diamine	colorimetric
Glucose-6-P-dehydrogenase	NAD, NADH	340 nm
Alkaline phosphatase	4-Methylumbelliferyl phosphate	fluorometric
Horseradish peroxidase	Luminol	chemiluminescence

may be induced to yield many photons if excited by a high-intensity light of appropriate wavelength. When a fluorescent molecule is excited from its ground state to a higher electronic state that is extremely unstable, it loses much of its energy and relaxes to its ground state by emitting a photon of light (fluorescence) of a longer wavelength. The difference between the excitation wavelength and the emission wavelength is known as Stokes' shift. A wide Stokes' shift is usually more desirable, because the excitation and emission signals are well separated so that they will not complicate the end-point detection.

One major drawback using a fluorescent label such as fluorescein is background fluorescence generated by components in the assay system—biologic fluids, plastic support, and reagents. Figure 11–9 demonstrates the effects of interference from human serum. The emission spectrum of FITC is compared with the emission spectrum of human serum. There is substantial overlap above wavelength 500 nm. These effects limit the sensitivity of the fluorescent-labeled assays.

Another problem common in conventional fluorescent labeling is a narrow Stokes' shift. In FITC, there is an area of overlap above 500 nm, thereby increasing background fluorescence and decreasing assay sensitivity.[19, 20]

Lanthanide Chelates. In an attempt to minimize the effects of background fluorescence and the narrow Stokes' shift of the conventional fluorescent labels, europium chelates are sometimes used as labels. These fluorescent materials have a high specific activity, a large Stokes' shift, and an optimal emission and excitation wavelength (Fig. 11–9). They have the unique property of having a delayed period of fluorescence (microseconds), compared with the nanoseconds of fluorescence generated by conventional fluorescent labels. The advantage of the delayed fluorescence is that with properly designed instrumentation, the detection of this signal can be delayed until the majority of all the background fluorescence generated by endogenous interfering materials has completely decayed away. The fluorescent signal from the europium chelates can therefore be separated from the much faster fluorescence of the background noise. This increases the signal-to-noise ratio of the label and thus the sensitivity of the assay.[21]

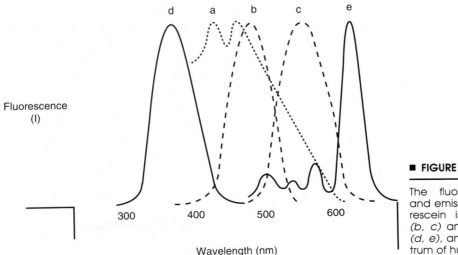

■ **FIGURE 11–9.**

The fluorescence excitation and emission spectrum of fluorescein isothiocyanate (FITC) (b, c) and europium chelate (d, e), and the emission spectrum of human serum (a).

Fluorescence (I)

300   400   500   600

Wavelength (nm)

Chemiluminescent Labels. Chemiluminescent labels are compounds that can undergo chemical reactions in which unstable products are formed. When this unstable product relaxes to its ground state, it releases energy in the form of visible light. The reaction is usually oxidative, involving oxygen and peroxide molecules. The emitted light can be measured by a **luminometer.** The light intensity is directly related to the concentration of the reactants. The sensitivity of detection is high, in the ranges of 10^{-12} to 10^{-15} gm/ml because light is detected against a completely dark background. Chemiluminescent labels are safe, easily available, and stable for years if properly stored. Some of the most common chemiluminescent labels used in immunoassays are luminol and its derivatives and acridinium esters.[22, 23]

Luminol and Derivatives

Luminol is a simple organic molecule. When luminol is oxidized by H_2O_2 in the presence of a catalyst (peroxidase), it yields an unstable 3-aminophthalate that emits light as it reverts to its ground state.

$$\text{Luminol} + 2\ H_2O_2 + OH^- \xrightarrow{\text{peroxidase}}$$
$$\text{3-aminophthalate} + \text{light}$$

However, the use of luminol labels in immunoassay has its limitations. Compounds such as luminol, when linked to protein or hapten, reduce light emission. This property limits the detection limit of these labels. Another problem with using luminol is the high reagent blank light emission. Contaminants in water used to prepare the buffer and the type of buffer used all contribute to a high level of background noise. These problems are partially alleviated by using peroxidase as the labeling enzyme and lu-

minol as its luminogenic substrate. This assay design is used in the Amerlite assays by Amersham.[24–26]

Acridinium Esters

Acridinium esters are triple-ringed organic molecules with an ester linkage to a "leaving group." Upon oxidation by H_2O_2 in an alkaline pH solution, this ester linkage is broken, leaving a highly excited molecule, N-methylacridone, and a leaving group. When the unstable N-methylacridone reverts to its ground state, it emits light. Unlike luminol, no catalyst is required for this reaction. In addition, since there is no catalyst molecule to complicate the reaction mixture, the reagent blank reading is greatly reduced, increasing assay sensitivity.

Though acridinium esters can be easily attached to protein molecules with minimal effect on their specific activity, coupling an acridinium ester to some haptens may result in products that are poorly chemiluminescent and have short shelf-lives. Another major problem associated with acridinium esters is the formation of "pseudobases," which effectively slows down the chemiluminescent reaction. To avoid this problem, acridinium esters are best assayed by preincubating at pH 5 to 7 and then rapidly increasing the pH by the addition of NaOH just before adding H_2O_2 reagent. This technique is used in the design of the ACS-180 immunochemistry analyzer manufactured by Ciba-Corning.[23, 27, 28] The pathways for the production of the unstable intermediate N-methylacridone and the pseudobases under alkaline and acid conditions are:

$$\text{Acridinium ester} \xrightarrow[OH^-]{H_2O_2} N\text{-methylacridone}$$
$$+ CO_2 + H_2O + \text{light}$$

$$\text{Acridinium ester} \xrightarrow{OH^-} \text{pseudobases}$$

DETECTOR SYSTEMS AND THEIR ANALYZERS

As the search for more sensitive nonisotopic labels continues, improvements are being made in the area of detector technology. Improved design and configuration of the detectors to maximize assay sensitivity are being attempted. Depending on the types of labels used, five major types of detector systems are commonly encountered in the clinical laboratory. They include:

Photometers (spectrophotometers)
Fluorometers
Fluorescent polarizers
Time-resolved fluorometers
Chemiluminometers

This section describes the different detector systems and the clinical immunochemistry analyzers that best represent them.

Photometers

Photometers and spectrophotometers measure light-absorbing compounds in enzyme immunoassays. Both measure the absorption of light by a solution at an appropriate wavelength. A photometer employs filters to select its wavelength, whereas a spectrophotometer isolates the desired wavelength by means of a prism or grating. The measured light intensity of the solution can be used to determine the concentration of the analyte in the solution. This relationship is defined by Beer's law:

$$A = \frac{I}{IO} = e^{-kcx}$$

This states that if light of intensity IO passes through a solution of thickness x and a concentration c of the absorbing molecules, some of the light will be absorbed, and that the light passing through the solution will be of lower intensity. The concentration of the light-absorbing analyte is linearly related to the amount of light absorbed. However, the detection limit of most photometers is in the microgram per milliliter range, falling short of the sensitivity for most hormones and other analytes in low serum concentrations.

Figure 11–10 illustrates the schematics of a simple photometer. Colorimetry is a term in this chapter referring to all methods by which light absorption determines the concentration of substances in a solution regardless of how the light measurement is made. The ES 300 and the Immuno I are examples of analyzers using colorimetry for the measurements of their analytes.

ES 300

ES 300 (Boehringer Mannheim) is a totally automated batch enzyme-immunoassay analyzer that performs up to 100 tests per hour and 12 different tests per sample. It employs "universal" streptavidin-coated tube technology in which the streptavidin molecule on the tube wall binds up to three antibody-labeled biotin molecules. ES 300 takes advantage of the strong interaction

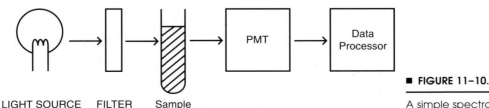

LIGHT SOURCE   FILTER   Sample

■ **FIGURE 11–10.**

A simple spectrophotometer.

between the streptavidin and the biotin molecules and the increased binding sites on the streptavidin molecule to increase its assay sensitivity and reproducibility. The ES 300 uses horseradish peroxidase as an enzyme label and a universal chromogenic substrate, ABT. Depending on assay design, either the antibody or the antigen is labeled with the enzyme. Both competitive and one-site or two-site immunoassay procedures are employed.

The analyzer has the following components: reagent rotor (12 test reagents), sample rotor (150 positions for sample, controls, and standards), multifunction arm, which has four arms on which the sample/reagent needle, wash needle, substrate/reagent needle, and photometer/mixer needle are located, incubator rotor, dispensing assembly, and the photometer at 422 nm. Data analysis, quality control, and system operation parameters are performed by a Hewlett Packard computer system.[29]

Technicon Immuno 1

The Immuno 1 analyzer (Miles Inc.) is an automated random access, high-throughput (120 tests/hour) enzyme immunoassay system. It employs alkaline phosphatase as an enzyme label and p-nitrophenyl-phosphate (PNPP) as its chromogenic substrate. The system can perform both homogeneous and heterogeneous assays. Both labeled antigens and labeled antibodies are used according to whether the competitive or the sandwich assay formats are used. Measurements are made by either colorimetry or turbidimetry. Separation of the bound complex from the free is achieved by using a universal magnetic particle reagent. Currently, the analyzer has a test menu of 22 analytes.

The Immuno 1 analyzer consists of five basic components: (1) a sample and reagent delivery system, (2) an incubation and separation system, (3) a detection system capable of colorimetric as well as turbidimetric measurements, (4) a data reduction system, and (5) a printer for patient reports.[30, 31]

Fluorometers

In a photometer, the amount of light absorbed by a sample is independent of the intensity of the incident light, whereas in a fluorometer, the intensity of the fluorescent emission is directly proportional to the intensity of the incident light and to the concentration of the fluorescent substance in the sample.

Three types of fluorometers are found in clinical analyzers: right angle, front surface, and straight through, depending on the the placement of the sample in relation to the excitation light source and the emission detector. The most commonly encountered is the right-angle fluorometer, in which light emission is detected at a right angle to the incident light. This arrangement is also used for the fluorescence polarization measurement. The front-surface fluorometers are designed for solid phase fluorescence detection, and the straight-through arrangement is not commonly used except in unusual circumstances.[32]

Figure 11–11 illustrates a typical right-angle fluorometer. It consists of a light source and a means to select the wavelength maximizing excitation of the sample. This may employ a monochromator, which is based on a diffraction grating or optical filter to isolate the appropriate wavelength for excitation of the sample. Light emission is detected by the photomultiplier tube at a right angle to the incident light. Most fluorometers have 10 to 100 times the sensitivity of an absorbance spectrophotometer. The detection limit for a conventional fluorometer is in the nanogram per milliliter to picogram per milliliter range. Examples of immunoassay analyzers that employ fluo-

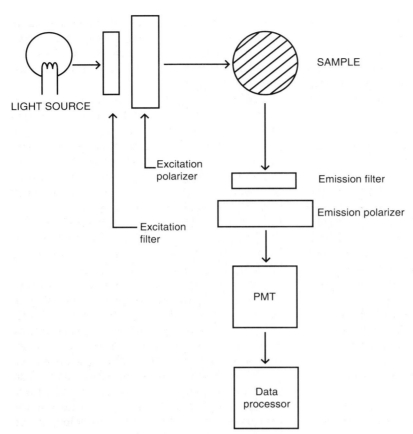

A right-angled fluorometer.

rometers for the measurement of their analytes are given next.

AIA-1200 Immunoassay System

The AIA-1200 analyzer (Tosoh Medics, Inc.) is a fully automated, random access, high-throughput (120 tests/hour) immunoassay system. The AIA-PACK test cup contains magnetized microbeads coated with antibodies to the analyte to be measured, as well as the enzyme alkaline phosphatase. The enzyme is either conjugated to a second antibody (sandwich assay) or to an antigen (competitive assay). The instrument currently has a test menu of 17 tests (thyroid and reproductive hormones, tumor markers, cardiac isoenzymes, and others). Its chemistry is based on an enzyme-labeled heterogeneous immunoassay, using alkaline phosphatase as the enzyme label and 4-methylumbelliferyl phosphate (4-MUP) as its fluorogenic substrate. Enzyme activity is measured by the rate of transformation of 4-MUP to a fluorescent compound, which is detected by a top-to-top fluorometer. Both competitive and one-site sandwich immunoassay procedures are used.[33]

Stratus IIntellect

The Stratus IIntellect (Baxter Scientific) is a batch immunoassay analyzer that has a sample capacity of up to 30 samples and provides the first test result in approximately 8 to 10 minutes. It uses radial partition immunoassay technology in which the antibody is immobilized on a small area of a glass-fiber filter paper (tab). After separation of the bound from the free labels by radial partition, a process by which the unbound fraction is washed to the periphery of the filter paper, enzyme activity is determined by a front-surface fluorometer. The enzyme label used is alkaline phosphatase, and its fluorogenic substrate is 4-methylumbelliferyl phosphate (4-MUP). Both competitive and sandwich assays, as well as sequential type assays, are used to measure both large and small molecules. Currently it has an impressive test menu of 30 analytes, including thyroid and fertility hormones, tumor markers, and therapeutic drugs.

The Stratus IIntellect system is composed of four basic components: (1) a carousel and tab magazine to hold up to 30 samples and tabs, (2) a fluid-dispensing system to dilute and deliver sample, conjugate, and substrate/wash reagents to the tab, (3) a front-surface fluorometer in which a mercury lamp provides the excitation light at 365 nm and an emission light wavelength of 450 nm, and (4) a computer system for data processing, storing, quality control, calibration parameters, and patient demographics, as well as providing files to assist operators with system functions.[34, 35]

Time-Resolved Fluorometer

In the time-resolved fluorometer, a fast light pulse is used to excite the fluorescent sample. The fluorescence emission is measured after a certain "time" has elapsed from the moment of excitation. The fluorescence decay time of europium lanthanides is in the order of 10 to 100 microseconds, whereas the decay time of most background nonspecific fluorescence in serum is about 10 nanoseconds. By delaying measurement of fluorescence until after most of the endogenous fluorescence has decayed away, i.e., after 100 microseconds, this instrument has the potential to be more sensitive than conventional fluorometers.[36–38]

Delfia. The Delfia immunoassay system (Pharmacia) is a semiautomated batch immunoassay analyzer based on the principle of time-resolved fluorometry, discussed previously. Depending on the analyte, the assay may be competitive, using a europium-labeled antigen, or a sandwich assay using a europium-labeled antibody. An enhancement solution is added to the bound complex to dissociate the europium ions from the labeled antibody or antigen molecules (Fig. 11–12).

The Delfia system consists of a workstation to facilitate sample setup. The assay is carried out on the antibody-coated 96-well strips, a dispensing unit to dispense buffer or tracer solutions automatically, a plate-shaker to allow optimal shaking speed for the reaction mixture, a platewash to wash away excess reagent adequately to minimize contamination, and finally a fluorometer that uses a xenon flash lamp and clock-pulse generator to control the time-resolved detection. Measurement takes 1 second per sample. The unit can plot standard curves and calculate results. An external computer using the FiaCalc software can provide data processing and quality control functions.[39]

Polarization Fluorometer

When fluorescent molecules in solution are excited with polarized light, they emit partially polarized fluorescence. The intensity of this polarized light is related to the degree of rotation of the molecules. Small molecules, such as those of the unbound analyte, have higher rates of rotation than does bound analyte. Increased rotation (unbound analyte) decreases the intensity of polarized light, whereas decreased rotation

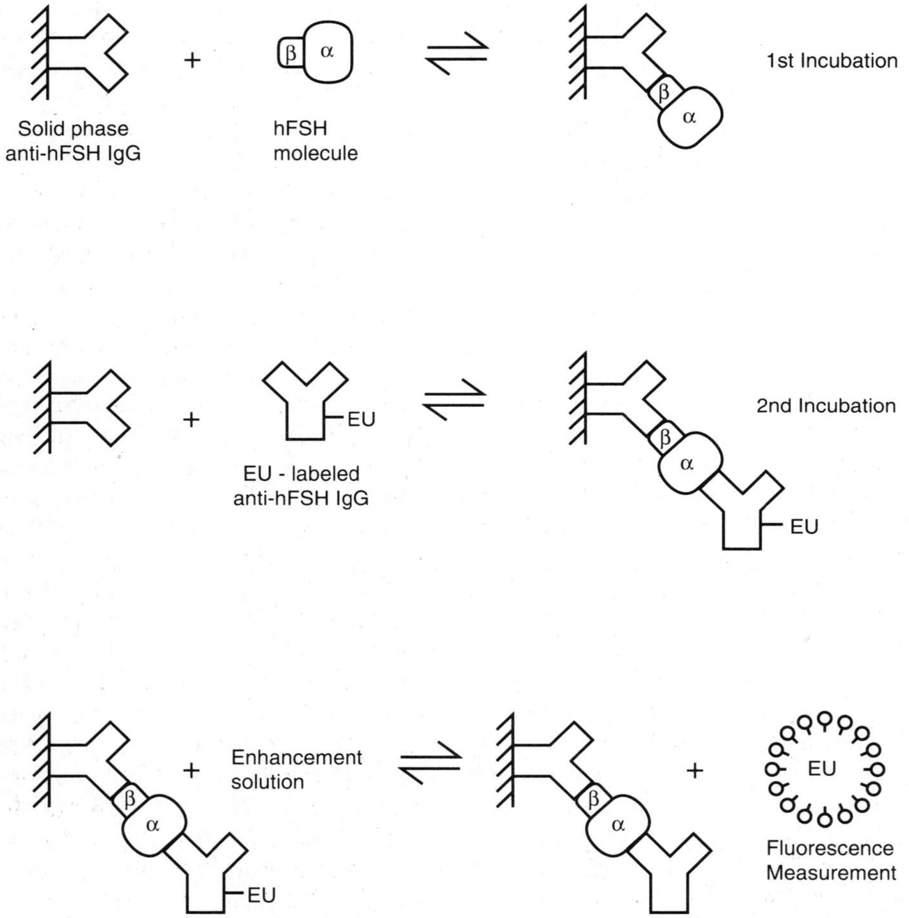

■ **FIGURE 11–12.**

Principles of dissociation-enhanced lanthanide fluoroimmunoassay (Delfia).

(bound analyte) tends to increase polarized light intensity. This polarized light intensity is directly related to the concentration of the analytes. Since no separation step is required to separate the bound from the unbound, the fluorescence polarization immunoassay is categorized as a homogeneous immunoassay. The limitation to this methodology is that it is only suitable for the measurement of small analytes, such as therapeutic drugs and some peptide hormones.[32, 40]

IMx. The Abbott IMx (Abbott Labs) is an automated batch immunoassay analyzer that combines the microparticle capture enzyme immunoassay technique (MEIA) for high molecular weight analytes, with the fluorescent polarization immunoassay technique for hapten assay.

The MEIA technology has two unique features. One is the use of microparticles as solid phase, which provides greater surface area than conventional coated tubes or polystyrene beads. Second, it uses glass-fiber matrix to separate the bound microparticle from the unbound and to serve as a mechanical support for the microparticle during optical measurement of the reactants.

Both competitive and sandwich assays are run on the analyzer. The label used is alkaline phosphatase, and the fluorogenic substrate is 4-MUP. Fluorescence is detected on the surface of the glass-fiber matrix by means of a front-surface fluorometer with an excitation wavelength of 365 nm and an emission wavelength of 448 nm. The other detector system is a polarization fluorometer based on the fluorescent polarization immunoassay (FPIA) procedure described previously. By combining both MEIA and FPIA methodologies, a wide range of analytes can be detected. Currently, the IMx has a menu of 25 tests, including endocrine and fertility hormones, hepatitis antibodies, tumor markers, infectious disease agents, cardiac isoenzymes, and therapeutic drugs.[41, 42]

Chemiluminometers

Chemiluminometers are instruments that are capable of measuring a flash of light. Unlike spectrophotometers or fluorometers, in which measured absorbance or fluorescence is accumulated in the reaction cuvet, measured light is transient in a chemiluminescent reaction. Figure 11–13 contrasts the measurement of chemiluminescence to that of absorbance and fluorescence reactions.

A chemiluminometer consists of the following components: (1) a light-tight, temperature-regulated reaction chamber, (2) a device that can introduce and mix reagents rapidly and efficiently, (3) a sensitive detector that has fast response time (1 ns to 1 μs), and (4) a data-processing device to plot and print data.[43] Figure 11–14 is a schematic illustration of a basic luminometer. Amerlite and the ACS-180 are examples of

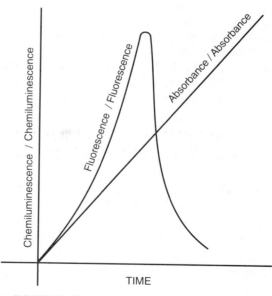

■ **FIGURE 11–13.**

Comparison between measurements of chemiluminescence and absorbance and fluorescence reactions.

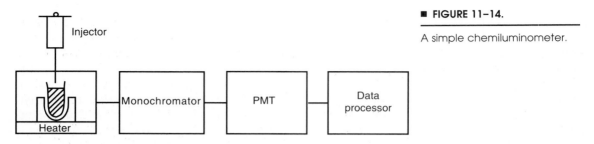

immunoassay analyzers that use lumino-meters for their assays.

Amerlite

Amerlite (Amersham Inc.) is a semiauto-mated batch immunoassay system that em-ploys horseradish peroxidase as an enzyme label to catalyze a chemiluminescent reac-tion using luminol as a chemiluminescent substrate. An enhancer is used in the reac-tion to increase light intensity and to pro-long light emission so that measurement can be made 2 to 20 minutes after the addi-tion of the substrate and the enhancer. Cur-rently it has a test menu of 17 analytes.

The Amerlite system includes a worksta-tion to facilitate the addition of samples and reagents to the antibody-coated well strips, a shaker/incubator for the incubation steps, an automatic washer to wash off the un-bound label, and the luminometer, which is a microprocessor-controlled luminescence reader and data reduction system.[24]

ACS-180 The ACS-180 (Ciba-Corning) is a fully automated, random access, high throughput (180 tests/hour) chemilumines-cent immunoassay system. The label used is an acridinium ester. Depending on the ana-lyte to be measured, either labeled antigen (competitive) or labeled antibody (sandwich) assays are performed. The reactants are im-mobilized on antibody-labeled magnetic par-ticles. Separation of the bound from the free label is achieved by means of stationary magnets mounted on the process track. The

reaction mixture is washed and acidified to reduce pseudobase formation. The reaction mixture is placed in front of the detector, where H_2O_2 and NaOH are then added and mixed to activate the chemiluminescent re-action. Light emission is measured by the photomultiplier tube, and the analyte con-centration is calculated from a stored stan-dard curve. The time to the first test result is 15 minutes.

The ACS-180 analyzer system consists of the following components: (1) a cuvet feeder, which holds as many as 200 reaction cu-vettes and sends them down the process track every 20 seconds as needed, (2) a sam-ple transport system, which can accommo-date up to 60 samples, (3) a reagent trans-port system, which provides carrier for 26 reagent bottles for 13 assays, (4) a barcode reader, which provides positive patient iden-tification and reagent information, (5) a fluid delivery system, which consists of four digital diluters for the delivery of the correct volume of samples and reagents for each as-say, (6) a thermal system, which maintains a temperature of 37°C for the reaction mix-ture, (7) a magnetic separation and wash system, which is designed to remove the un-bound and immobilizes the bound particle on the back wall of the cuvet by magnets, where they are washed and the H_2O_2 oxidiz-ing reagent is added, (8) a luminometer, which is housed in a light-tight chamber with six wells, with a photomultiplier tube (PMT) mounted in front of the third well and an injection port above this well that delivers the NaOH basic reagent to trigger the chemiluminescent reaction; light emission is detected by the PMT, and (9) a built-in computer system with its own disc drive, CRT display, and keyboard to provide data analysis and quality control functions, patient reports, and other system functions to facilitate user operation.[28]

EVALUATION OF IMMUNOCHEMISTRY ANALYZERS

Table 11–5 lists some of the performance characteristics of automated and semiautomated immunoassay analyzers recently introduced into the market.

To evaluate an analyzer for use in the clinical laboratories, three basic requirements must be met.

- The properties of the immunoassay reagents must meet the sensitivity, specificity, and stability requirements of the assays performed in the laboratory.
- The analyzer must provide instrument specifications, such as sample throughput, turn-around time, and stat capability, satisfactory to the clinical needs of the institution.
- The cost of the instrument and the reagents, including consumables, must be within the operating budget of the laboratory.

Properties of Immunoassay Binding Reagents

Specificity

Assay specificity is influenced by two factors. One is the presence of interfering substances that will cross-react with the antibody reagent. The other factor is the presence of environmental factors and substances, such as pH, temperature, and ionic strength of the solution, that may influence the kinetics of the antigen-antibody reaction.

Assay specificity can be improved by using an antibody reagent with a high specificity, such as monoclonal antibodies. The use of monoclonal antibodies minimizes the potential of cross-reactivity with other structurally similar substances. Alternatively, a two-site or sandwich assay system may be used in the assay design in which the analyte is recognized by two different specific antibodies directed at two distinct antigenic sites on the analyte.

Dependent on the assay design, some assays are more susceptible to the influences exerted by the assay environment, such as pH, temperature, presence of salt and urea, than other assays. In the competitive immunoassays, environmental effects can affect the equilibrium constant of the binding reaction, whereas in the noncompetitive immunoassay in which antibody reagent is in excess, the law of mass action favors the binding reaction. The effects of the environment are minimal.

Sensitivity

Assay sensitivity, or detection limit, in an immunoassay system depends on the assay design, the specific activity of the label, the affinity of the antibody, and the sensitivity of the detection system. In both competitive and noncompetitive immunoassays, the maximum sensitivity attainable depends on the affinity of the antibody. The higher the antibody affinity, the more efficiently the antibody binds with trace amounts of analyte molecules, thereby increasing the sensitivity of the assay system. By design, however, noncompetitive immunoassay employing excess antibody reagent offers greater assay sensitivity than competitive immunoassay using antibody of identical af-

TABLE 11–5. PERFORMANCE FEATURES OF IMMUNOCHEMISTRY ANALYZERS

	BMD ES-300	MILES IMMUNO-1	CIBA-CORN. ACS-180	TOSOH AIA-1200	ABBOTT IMx	BAXTER STRATUS II	AMERSHAM AMERLITE	PHARMACIA DELFIA	BEHRING NEPHELOM.	BECKMAN ARRAY-360
ANALYZER TYPE	Automated random access	Automated random access	Automated random access	Automated random access	Automated batch	Automated batch	Semi-automated	Semi-automated	Automated random access	Automated random access
CHEMISTRY LABEL/ SUBSTRATE	EIA Streptavidin/ biotin AP/ABT	EIA AP/PNPP	CLA Acridinium esters/H_2O_2	EIA AP/4-MUP	MEIA/FRIA AP/4-MUP	EIA AP/4-MUP	Enhanced CLA HRP/Luminol	Time-resolved fluorom. Europium chelate	Accel. equilibrium neph.	Rate nephelometry
ANALYTES	15	22	25	17	23	30	17	29	20	14
THROUGHPUT TEST/HOUR	100	120	180	120	MEIA 24–40 min FRIA 48/hr	30–40	384/90 min	NA	225	40–80
CALIBRATION STABILITY	2 weeks	30 days	1 week	30 days	2 weeks	2 weeks	Calib. required	Calib. required	1 week	2 weeks
TEST CAPACITY	12	24	13	21	20/24	1	NA	1	14	20
SAMPLE CAPACITY	160	78	60	100	24	30	96	96	45	40
SAMPLE VOLUME μl	5–200 μl	2–50 μl	10–20 μl	10–100 μl	150 μl/50 μl	200 μl	50 μl	25 μl	80–150 μl	7–20 μl
INCUBATION TIME	45–225 min	5–32 min	7.5 min	40 min	30–40 min	8 min	15–60 min	150 min	6 min	Rate
PATIENT I.D.	Keyboard entry	Keyboard or barcode	Barcode	Keyboard entry	Keyboard entry	Keyboard entry	None	None	Barcode	Keyboard entry
QC PROGRAM	Yes	Yes	Yes	Yes	No	Yes	Yes	Yes	Yes	Yes
STAT CAPABILITY	NR	Yes	Yes	Yes	No	Yes	NR	NR	Yes	Yes
DETECTION LIMITS	ng/ml	ng/ml	ng/ml	ng/ml	ng/ml	ng/ml	ng/ml	pg/ml	μg/ml	μg/ml
DETECTION SYSTEM	Photometer at 422 nm	Photometer at 405–450 nm	Chemilum. at 430 nm	Fluorom. Exc: 325–385 nm Emis. 440–500 nm	Fluorom. w/ polarizer Exc: 365 nm Emis: 448 nm	Fluorom. Exc: 365 nm Emis: 450 nm	Chemilum.	Time-resolved fluorom. Exc: 340 nm Emis: 613 nm	Nephelom. 13–24° angle	Nephelom. 70° angle

AP, Alkaline phosphatase; CLA, Chemiluminescent assay; EIA, Enzyme immunoassay; FPIA, Fluorescent polarization immunoassay; HRP, Horseradish peroxidase; MEIA, Microparticle enzyme immunoassay; 4-MUP, 4-Methylumbelliferyl phosphate; PNPP, p-Nitrophenyl phosphate; NR, Not recommended; Exc. Excitation; Emis, Emission; Chemilum., Chemiluminometer; Fluorom., Fluorometer; Nephelom., Nephelometer.

finity. The assay sensitivity is limited only by the minimum number of labeled antibody molecules bound to the analyte that can be distinguished from the background noise level. Increased sensitivity can be achieved by using labels with high specific activity and minimum background noise level. This can be accomplished by using enzyme labels with substrates that produce fluorescent or chemiluminescent products, which can be measured by a time-resolved fluorometer or a luminometer, respectively. Both the fluorometer and the luminometer are capable of measuring analytes down to 10^{-15} gm/ml, contrasted to 10^{-9} gm/ml with the best spectrophotometer.

Reagent Stability

Lack of reagent stability is one of the limitations of the radioimmunoassay system. The half-life of ^{125}I is only 60 days. The average shelf-life of radioimmunoassay kits is about 1 to 3 months. Most nonisotopic reagents have shelf-lives of 6 months or longer if they are properly stored. Some of the reagents for chemiluminescent immunoassays have shelf-lives of more than a year.

Properties of the Instruments

Table 11–5 lists some of the operational features of several automated and semiautomated clinical immunoassay analyzers that are on the market today. Dependent on analyzer type, some instruments are more suited for the small hospital laboratory, whereas others are designed for high volume commercial laboratories.

A random access analyzer is an instrument capable of performing single or multiple tests on the same sample, whereas a batch analyzer performs the same test on all the samples presented to it. Batch analyzers such as the Stratus IIntellect and the Abbott IMx can process only a limited number of samples per analysis: 30 and 24, respectively. Random access analyzers such as the BMD ES-300 and the Tosoh AIA-2000 can process over 100 samples per analysis.

The sample throughput is the maximum number of samples or tests the analyzer can process in an hour. In general, high throughput instruments are desirable in a laboratory where high test volumes are anticipated. High throughput does not equate with fast turn-around time.

The turn-around time is the minimum time required to obtain a result after the initial sampling of the specimen. It is dependent on the assay types. Assays that require long incubation steps would require long turn-around times. For most random access analyzers, when multiple tests are requested on the same sample, the test with longest incubation steps will determine the turn-around time for that sample's results.

Tests that require fast turn-around time include serum hCG levels to rule out ectopic pregnancies, serum estradiol levels for ovulation induction procedures, and serum cardiac CK-MB isoenzyme levels for the diagnosis of myocardial infarction. However, not all assays require fast turn-around time. For example, assays for vitamin and some serum protein levels usually do not require same-day turn-around time.

Many clinical situations justify STAT test results. Instruments that are capable of performing STAT testing usually have a short turn-around time for their assays and the versatility to allow interruption of the sample processing.

The detection limit of the instrument is determined by the detector system used in the analyzer. It is usually measured as the concentration of the analyte corresponding to the mean plus 2.5 standard deviations of the response in the absence of the analyte (blank). In general, detector systems based on nephelometric and photometric measurements are less sensitive than either the fluorometer or the luminometer. With improved detector design, some of the time-resolved fluorometers and the luminometers have the potential to measure analytes at fentogram per milliliter level, 10^{-15} gm/ml, achieving even greater sensitivity than radioimmunoassay methods.

Other features of the analyzer that are desirable in the selection of a laboratory immunoassay instrument include calibration curve stability and the ability to identify patient samples using barcoding. Today, most automated analyzers are equipped with a microcomputer to facilitate data processing and system control functions. With the aid of a sophisticated computer system, a few analyzers can identify patient samples, perform appropriate tests, calculate results using stored calibration information, and generate a full report with minimal user intervention.

Cost of Instrumentation

In the instrument selection process, the cost of producing a patient test result is a major consideration. It consists of instrument cost (capital equipment depreciation, lease, or reagent rental costs); cost of reagents and consumables (including quality control and calibration materials); labor costs, which take into consideration technologist time spent processing the sample; preparation and maintenance of the instrumentation; and the cost of a service contract if the instrument is purchased.

SUMMARY

Immunoassays are powerful diagnostic tools in the clinical laboratory. They are analytical methods that make use of the highly specific and sensitive immunologic reactions for the measurement of a wide range of analytes. Recent improvements in the production of unlimited supplies of monoclonal antibodies of well-defined specificity, and the use of nonisotopic labels with high specific activities, have increased the specificity and sensitivity of the immunoassay methodologies. Further refinement in solid phase technology and the development of new assay designs and formulations have made it feasible for the production of automated systems. Currently, over 50 analytes are measured by immunoassay methods, often at detection limits measured at the picogram per milliliter level.

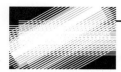

REVIEW QUESTIONS

Choose the best answer. One or all of the answers can be correct.

1. A nephelometric immunoassay is an example of a(n)

   a. competitive immunoassay.
   b. homogeneous immunoassay.
   c. heterogeneous immunoassay.
   d. immunoprecipitation reaction.

2. Which of the following statements applies to nephelometric immunoassay analyzers?

   a. Analyzer of choice for the measurement of serum proteins.
   b. Measurement of light scatter at an angle to the incident light.
   c. Measurement of direct transmitted light.
   d. Use polymer enhancement to increase sensitivity.

3. Noncompetitive immunoassay has the following characteristics:

   a. Uses labeled antigen as a reagent.
   b. Uses labeled antibody as a reagent.
   c. The amount of bound label is directly proportional to the concentration of the analyte.
   d. The amount of bound label is indirectly proportional to the concentration of the analyte.

4. The enzyme multiplied immunoassay technique (EMIT) is an example of a(n)

   a. homogeneous immunoassay.
   b. competitive immunoassay.
   c. enzyme immunoassay.
   d. heterogeneous immunoassay.

5. Monoclonal antibody has the following characteristics:

   a. Supply is limited.
   b. High specificity.
   c. High affinity.
   d. Readily forms precipitation lattice with most analytes, making it suitable for nephelometric assay.

6. Lathanide chelates have the following advantages over the conventional fluorescent labels:

   a. High specific activity.
   b. Narrow Stokes' shift.
   c. Delayed period of fluorescence.
   d. Optimal emission and excitation wavelengths.

7. Amerlite immunoassay uses the following in its assay design:

   a. Uses luminol as a chemiluminescent label.
   b. Peroxidase is used as labeling enzyme and luminol as its substrate.
   c. Uses a luminometer to measure light emission.
   d. Uses an enhancer to increase light intensity and to prolong light emission.

8. The Stratus IIntellect is an example of a(n)

   a. batch analyzer.
   b. fluorescent polarization analyzer.
   c. analyzer that uses radial partition immunoassay technology in which antibody is immobilized on a small area of a glass fiber filter paper.
   d. analyzer that uses reagent cup containing magnetized microbeads coated with antibody to the analyte.

9. Fluorescent polarization immunoassay is based on the following principles:

   a. Fluorescent molecules when excited by polarized light emit partially polarized light.
   b. The intensity of polarized light is inversely related to the degree of rotation of the fluorescent molecules.
   c. Small molecules, such as the unbound analyte, have high rate of rotation and decreased polarized light intensity, whereas large molecules, such as the bound analyte, exhibit low rate of rotation and increased intensity of polarized light.
   d. In a competitive reaction, the concentration of the analyte is directly related to the polarized light intensity.

10. The ACS-180 analyzer

   a. is a high throughput chemiluminescent immunoassay analyzer.
   b. uses an acridinium ester as a label.
   c. has reactants that are immobilized on antibody-labeled magnetic particles.
   d. is able to reduce "pseudobase" production by acidification of the reaction mixture.

REFERENCES

1. Kusnetz J, Mansberg HP: Optical considerations: Nephelometry. *In* Ritchie RF (ed): *Automated Immunoanalysis;* Part I. New York, Marcel Dekker, 1978.
2. Whicher JT: Nephelometric methods. *In* Butt WR (ed): *Practical Immunoassay: The State of the Art.* New York, Marcel Dekker, 1984, pp 117–177.
3. *Behring Nephelometer Instruction Manual.* I. Basic Information. Marburg, Germany, 1987, Behringwerke AG Diagnostica, p 14.
4. Hellsing K: Enhancing effects of nonionic polymers on immunochemical reactions. *In* Ritchie RF (ed): *Automated Immunoanalysis,* Part I. New York, Marcel Dekker, 1978.
5. Alpert NL: Array protein system. *Clin Instr System* 11(1):1–8, 1990.
6. Schotters SB, McBride JH, Rodgersin DO, Higgins S, Pisa M: Determination of five protein analytes using the Beckman Array and Behring Nephelometer System. *J Clin Lab Anal* 2:108–111, 1988.
7. Yalow RS, Berson SA: Assay of plasma insulin in human subjects by immunological methods. *Nature* 184:1684, 1959.
8. Miles LE, Hales CN: Labelled antibodies and immunological system. *Nature* 219:186, 1968.
9. Kohler G, Milstein C: Continuous culture of fused cells secreting antibody of predefined specificity. *Nature (London)* 256:495, 1975.
10. Kemp HA, Woodhead JS: Labeled antibody immunoassays. *In* Butt WR (ed): *Practical Immunoassays.* New York, Marcel Dekker, 1984, pp 103–115.
11. Readhead C, Addison GM, Hales CN, Lehmann H: Immunoradiometric and 2-site assay of human follicle-stimulating hormone. *J Endocrinol* 59:313, 1973.
12. Rubinstein KE, Schneider RS, Ullman EF: "Homogeneous" enzyme immunoassay. A new immunochemical technique. *Biochem Biophys Res Comm* 47:846–851, 1972.
13. Ekins R, Jackson T: Non-isotopic immunoassay—an overview. *In* Bizollon A (ed): *Monoclonal Antibodies and New Trends in Immunoassays.* New York, Elsevier Science Publishers, 1984, pp 149–163.
14. Zola H, Brooks D: Techniques for the production and characterization of monoclonal hybridoma antibodies. *In* Hurrell JGR (ed): *Monoclonal Hybridoma Antibodies: Techniques and Application.* Boca Raton, Florida, CRC Press, 1982.
15. Gosling JP: A decade of development in immunoassay methodology. *Clin Chem* 36(8):1408–1427, 1990.
16. Catt K, Tregear GW: Solid-phase radioimmunoassay in AB-coated tubes. *Science* 158:1570, 1967.
17. Avrameas S: Coupling of enzymes to proteins with glutaraldehyde. Use of the conjugates for the detection of antigens and antibodies. *Immunochemistry* 6:43–52, 1969.

18. Wisdom GB: Enzyme immunoassay. *Clin Chem* 22:1243–1255, 1976.
19. Landon J, Kamel RS: Immunoassays employing reactants labelled with a fluorophore. *In* Voller A, Bidwell D (eds): *Immunoassays for the 80s*. Lancaster, England, MTP Press Limited, 1981, pp 91–112.
20. Soini E, Hemmilin I: Fluoroimmunoassay: Present status and key problems. *Clin Chem* 25:353–361, 1979.
21. Hemmila I, Dakubu S, Mukkala V, Siitari H, Lovgren T: Europium as label in time-resolved immunofluometric assays. *Anal Biochem* 137:335–343, 1984.
22. Weeks I, Behesti I, McCapra F, et al: Acridinium esters as high-specific-activity labels in immunoassays. *Clin Chem* 29:1474–1479, 1983.
23. Weeks I, Campbell AK, Woodhead JS: Immunoassays using chemiluminescent labels. *In* Butt WR (ed): *Practical Immunoassay*. New York, Marcel Dekker, 1984, pp 103–115.
24. Edwards JC: *Development of the Amerlite System*. Amersham, United Kingdom, Amersham International, 1986, pp 1–5.
25. Thorpe GHG, Kricka L, Moseley SB, Whitehead TP: Phenols as enhancers of the chemiluminescent horseradish peroxidase luminol–hydrogen peroxide reaction: Application in luminescence-monitored enzyme immunoassays. *Clin Chem* 31:1335–1341, 1985.
26. Whitehead TP, Thorp GHG, Carter TJN, Groucutt C, Kricka LJ: Enhanced luminescence procedure for sensitive determination of peroxidase-labelled conjugates in immunoassay. *Nature* 305:158–159, 1983.
27. Boland J, Carey G, Krodel E, et al: The CIBA-Corning ACS-180 Benchtop Immunoassay Analyzer. *Clin Chem* 36:1598–1601, 1990.
28. Dudley RF: The CIBA Corning ACS:180 Automated Immunoassay System. *J Clin Immunoassay* 14(2):77–82, 1991.
29. LaBrash B, Engelberth L, Duncan T: The Boehringer Mannheim ES 300 Immunoassay Analyzer. *J Clin Immunoassay* 14:108, 1991.
30. Schneider NE: Technicon Immuno I Automated Immunoassay System. *J Clin Immunoassay* 14:103–104, 1991.
31. Technicon Immuno I: Instrument Evaluation. Personal communication, 1992.
32. Li TM: Fluorescence polarization immunoassay. *In* Boguslaski E, Maggio ET, Nakamura RM (eds): *Clinical Immunochemistry; Principles of Methods and Application*. Boston, Little, Brown, 1984.
33. AIA-1200 Automated Immunoassay Analyzer. *Instrument Specification*. Tosoh Medics Inc, 1990.
34. Giegel JL, Brotherton MM, Cronin P, D'Aquino M, Evans S, Heller ZH, Knight WS, Krishnan K, Sheiman M: Radial partition immunoassay. *Clin Chem* 28(9):1894–1898, 1982.
35. Lifshitz MS, DeCresce R: Baxter Stratus II Immunoassay System. *Instrument Report* 3(8):1–8, 1990.
36. Lovgren T, Hemmila I, Pettersson K, Halonen P: Time-resolved fluorometry in immunoassay. *In* Collins WP (ed): *Alternative Immunoassays*. New York, John Wiley, 1985, pp 203–217.
37. Soini E: Pulsed light, time-resolved fluorometric immunoassay. *In* Bizollon A (ed): *Monoclonal Antibodies and New Trends in Immunoassays*. New York, Elsevier Science Publisher, 1984, pp 197–208.
38. Soini E, Lovgren T: Time-resolved fluoroimmunoassay. *In* Ngo TT (ed): *Nonisotopic Immunoassay*. New York, Plenum Press, 1988, pp 231–243.
39. Delfia: *Instrumentation System for the Performance of Time-Resolved Fluoroimmunoassays*. Pharmacia Diagnostic AB, 1990.
40. Folley ME, Stroupe SD, Schwenzer KS, et al: Fluorescence polarization immunoassay. III: An automated system for therapeutic drug determination. *Clin Chem* 27:1575–1579, 1981.
41. DeCresce RR, Lifshitz MS: The Abbott IMx. *Lab Med* 20:47–49, 1989.
42. Flore M, Mitchell J, Doan T, et al: The Abbott IMx Automated Benchtop Immunochemistry Analyzer System. *Clin Chem* 34(9):1726–1732, 1988.
43. Campbell K: *Chemiluminescence: Principles and Applications in Biology and Medicine*. Chichester, England, E. Horwood, 1988.

Chapter 12

FORENSIC INSTRUMENTAL APPLICATIONS

RICHARD O. PFAU, PhD, MT (ASCP)

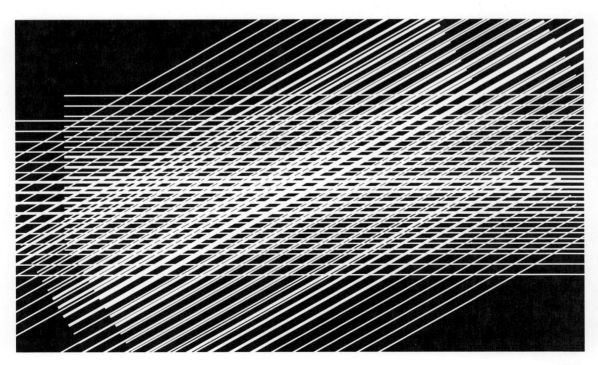

LEARNING OBJECTIVES

After studying this chapter, the student should be able to:

- Define what is meant by "physical evidence" and list at least four examples.
- Compare and contrast the analytical sensitivity and specificity of the following techniques: thin-layer chromatography, ultraviolet spectrophotometry, infrared spectrophotometry, and gas chromatography.
- Describe the DNA profile analysis technique and list the major steps involved in the performance of this investigative procedure.
- Define the term pyrolysis.
- Give the purpose and applications of neutron activation analysis and x-ray diffraction.
- Write the principle of microscopic polarization.

KEY WORDS

Alpha particle. A type of radiation, consisting of helium atoms minus their orbiting electrons, that is emitted by radioactive elements.

Beta particle. A type of radiation, composed of electrons, that is emitted by radioactive elements.

Birefringence. The difference between the two indices of refraction seen to exist among some crystalline materials.

Fingerprint. The ridge patterns of the fingers that have become a pillar of modern criminal identification.

Gamma rays. A form of high-energy electromagnetic radiation emitted by radioactive elements.

Microspectrophotometer. An analytical instrument, combining microscopy with spectrophotometry, that provides absorption spectra from trace quantities of evidence being observed microscopically.

Neutron activation analysis (NAA). The technique of bombarding specimens with neutrons and measuring the resultant gamma ray radioactivity.

PCR (polymerase chain reaction). Procedure by which hundreds of thousands of copies of a specific sequence of DNA are synthesized.

Pyrolysis. The decomposition of organic substances by heat.

RFLP (restriction fragment length polymorphism). Variation in DNA sequence that can be detected as a change in the length of the DNA fragments produced by a restriction enzyme.

Scanning electron microscope (SEM). An instrument that focuses a beam of electroms on a specimen and produces a highly magnified image upon a TV tube.

Spectrogram. A graph or photograph of a spectrum

Thermocouple. A thermoelectric device consisting of two dissimilar metals joined so that a potential difference generated between the points of contact is a measure of the temperature difference between the points.

X-ray diffraction. The technique of directing x-radiation at a crystal and studying the reflection patterns that are produced.

INTRODUCTION

The lateral mobility enjoyed by clinical laboratorians includes employment in forensic science laboratories.[1] A strong case can be made in favor of Medical Technology as a discipline that provides an academic background amenable to the analytic tasks found in the "Crime Lab."[2] What exactly is forensic science and what types of analyses are generally performed in those laboratories identified as forensic? *Forensic science* is the application of science to law, more especially to those criminal and civil laws that are enforced by police agencies in a criminal justice system. Physical evidence collected during the investigation of any crime comprises the specimens received by these laboratories. Before discussing the types of examinations and analyses utilized, a better understanding of physical evidence is needed.

The following definition is one provided by a federal judge in 1947; while it was written some 45 years ago, it remains valid by today's standards. "Wherever he steps, whatever he touches, whatever he leaves, even unconsciously, will serve as silent witness against him. Not only his fingerprints or his footprints, but his hair, the fibers from his clothes, the glass he breaks, the tool mark he leaves, the paint he scratches, the blood or semen he deposits or collects—all of these and more bear mute witness against him. This is evidence that does not forget. It is not confused by the excitement of the moment. It is not absent because human witnesses are, it is factual evidence, physical evidence cannot be wrong; it cannot perjure itself; it cannot be wholly absent, only its interpretation can err. Only human failure to find it, study and understand it, can diminish its value."[3]

Given this broad scope of types of specimen to be analyzed or examined, it becomes readily apparent that the methodologies employed in the forensic science laboratory are derived from a myriad of disciplines. As analytical techniques are purloined from a variety of other scientific endeavors, it necessarily follows that the instrumentation inherent to those techniques is incorporated into the modern Crime Lab. In many cases, the "borrowed" methodology must be modified, owing to the unique nature of physical evidence. Physical evidence is almost always contaminated upon receipt, and this problem is further exacerbated by the fact that the quantity received is an uncontrolled variable. Added to these are the problems of biologic specimens (i.e., blood and semen) deteriorating upon standing at room temperature, liquid items (i.e., flammables, accelerants, and alcoholic beverages) being lost to evaporation, and the legal requirements necessary to ensure that the analytical findings are acceptable.

This chapter provides a broad overview of the instrumentation commonly encountered in today's forensic science laboratory. The applications, while perhaps not as the manufacturer envisioned, are insightful, enterprising, and, in some cases, ingenious when physical evidence is the specimen being analyzed or examined.

SIGNIFICANCE OF PHYSICAL EVIDENCE

The examination/analysis of physical evidence is conducted for the purposes of corroboration or investigation. An analytical scheme that provides positive identification of the analyte by excluding all other substances is frequently required to corroborate arrests. Charges of possession of illicit drugs or driving while under the influence of alcohol are difficult, if not impossible, to sustain legally without physical evidence, properly analyzed, of the drug in question: crack, cocaine, alcohol, others. At other times these procedures may serve to confirm the investigator's suspicions that the material in question is in fact human blood, animal hair, window glass, automotive paint, and so on and not something totally unrelated to the matter at hand. Finally, these identification tests are useful to substantiate the information obtained from witnesses and victims pertaining to the events said to have occurred at a crime scene, such as gunpowder residue on the hands of a suspect alleged to have fired a weapon.

Those analytical procedures useful during the investigative effort are termed "comparison tests," and the findings speak to the "WHO" of the crime rather than the "WHAT." These tests, many of which do not result in a specific identification, comprise an analytical scheme being applied to two or more specimens that are thought to derive from a common origin. One or more of the items being tested or examined is of known origin, and the others are termed of questioned origin. The first consideration of the forensic scientist is, "Does this material (glass, paint, hair, blood, impression) possess a sufficient number of individual characteristics to be unique unto itself?" The characteristics may be physical or chemical in nature (or a combination), detected and measured in a scientifically acceptable manner.

The second significant consideration is, "Do these specimens (the known and the questioned) share a sufficient number of the aforementioned individual characteristics that it may be said, with a scientific certainty, that they come from a common source?" Without this affirmation, evidence items that can be associated only with a group are said to possess class characteristics. The ABO blood groups exemplify this type of evidence: identification of a blood stain as "human group A" does not identify the source of that stain. Even HLA typing, when performed in cases of questioned paternity, succeeds only in reducing the size of the group in which the alleged father is to be found. Such evidence is nonetheless quite valuable when it derives from items in the environment that demonstrate a significant diversity.

In some instances, class evidence links together other investigative findings, and in other cases, it provides a sheer weight of evidence when taken with other types of class evidence. The comparison or investigative tests are capable of:

- placing the suspect at the scene of the crime,
- placing the suspect in the company of the victim,
- placing the victim at the scene of the crime, or
- exonerating the suspect from ever having been in the company of the victim or at the crime scene.

Ultimately, the legal significance accorded physical evidence is left entirely to a jury of laypersons. As a rule, the results provided by the forensic scientist are given great weight and go far in overcoming doubts about guilt or innocence.

CLINICAL TECHNIQUES IN FORENSIC SCIENCE

In contemporary American Crime Labs, organic compounds make up the majority of the evidence submitted for analysis. The common drugs of abuse provide the major portion of the case load in full service laboratories; added to these organic substances are synthetic fibers from such common sources as clothing, carpets, draperies, and upholstery, to name a few. One invaluable tool necessary to the characterization and identification of organic substances is spectrophotometry, which includes ultraviolet, visible, and infrared applications. Properly used, spectrophotometric analyses require that relatively pure samples be employed. Because the concept of sample purity is all but nonexistent when applied to the physical evidence received for analysis, the first order of business is that of separating components and purifying those of relevance. "Street drugs," as an example, are commonly "cut" with a diluent (i.e., lactose, quinidine, maltose, and so on), the sole purpose of which is to increase the quantity of drug for sale. The illicit drug is the ingredient vital to sustaining the arrest, and, except for police intelligence uses, the excipient materials are of little interest. A variety of chromatographic techniques are used as methods of producing specimens suitable for spectrophotometric analysis.

Chromatography

Gas chromatography (GC), high-performance liquid chromatography (HPLC), and thin-layer chromatography (TLC) are the techniques found to be most suitable to the unique concerns of the forensic science laboratory. The chromatogram produced by the strip chart recorder of GC and HPLC instruments provides useful identifying characteristics of the materials being analyzed. The sensitivity of these instruments coupled with the incorporation of internal standards makes quantitation possible at the nanogram level. Figure 12–1 shows a GC instrument with a strip chart recorder.

Absolute identification of materials is not provided because, given the same chromatographic parameters, other substances may share a particular retention time. An adjunct to GC analysis frequently employed by forensic scientists is **pyrolysis**. Pyrolysis GC enables the analysis of solids (synthetic fibers, plastics, paint chips) by converting these materials (with heat at 500 to 1000°C) into gaseous components in a closed system leading to the column.

Although specific identification is not provided by the aforementioned processes, known and questioned exemplars can be analyzed and the resultant chromatograms then visually compared. In some instances, the chromatograms can be superimposed

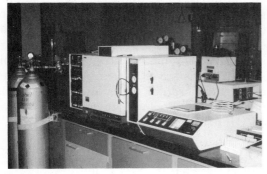

■ **FIGURE 12–1.**

A gas chromatography set-up with a strip chart recorder.

and seen to possess identical peak patterns, thus establishing common origin.

HPLC, which is equally sensitive and capable of providing quantitation, is most useful when the forensic scientist is confronted with heat-sensitive evidence, such as lysergic acid diethylamide (LSD) or some organic explosives, owing to the analysis being conducted at room temperature.

The retention peak patterns of high-performance liquid chromatograms produced by known materials also can be compared with the patterns resulting from the HPLC analysis of questioned specimens. Similarly, known and questioned chromatograms found to be identical at all points (superimposable) are considered to have derived from the same source. Depending upon the diversity of the material in question, such findings may be accorded substantial weight as evidence.

The third separation method routinely used by forensic scientists is TLC. This technique is frequently applied to drug evidence for tentative identification, as well as separation of the components for subsequent spectrophotometric analyses. Drugs, generally received in the laboratory as solids, are readily soluble in water in order to be pharmacologically effective. Glass plates thinly coated with a granular material (commonly aluminum oxide or silica gel) bound by plaster of Paris provide the solid phase, into which is incorporated a fluorescent dye. The questioned specimen is spotted on the TLC plate in series with known drugs. The liquid phase, driven by capillary action, is allowed to migrate 10 cm, whereupon the plate is removed from the chamber and permitted to dry. Ultraviolet light reveals dark spots against a fluorescent background. Those drug entities known to fluoresce are spotted on plates made without the aforementioned dye substance.

Visualization can also be accomplished by spraying the plate with a reagent known to cause a color reaction with the suspected drug(s). Tentative identification results when components of the questioned material share Rf (retention fraction) values and reactions in common with the known drugs. Additional separations can be performed (without chemical visualization) and pure components obtained by collecting the granular matrix material from the appropriate migration distance (Rf). Thin-layer chromatography is inexpensive, sensitive, and rapid and enables the simultaneous analysis of multiple unknowns composed of less than 100 μg of specimen. Figure 12–2 shows an example of a commercial TLC system designed to screen for drugs in body fluids.

Electrophoresis

Forensic serologists, faced with contaminated blood stains as opposed to liquid specimens obtained under aseptic conditions, have developed several techniques that provide an isoenzyme profile of the "donor." As a rule, forensic applications utilize an agar or starch gel coated onto a glass plate, with specimens of known blood stains being electrophoresed simultaneously with the questioned stains. As with the HLA analogy, the results serve only to identify the class to which the alleged donor belongs and NOT to

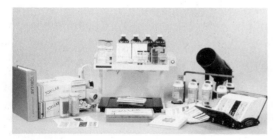

■ **FIGURE 12–2.**

A thin layer chromatography set-up for drug screening. (Courtesy of Toxi-Lab, Inc., Irvine, CA.)

identify the individual. DNA profile analysis represents the final arbiter in the identification of biologic stains and will be discussed in a separate section.

Spectral Techniques

Spectrophotometry, the mainstay of the clinical laboratorian, is similarly ensconced in the forensic science laboratory. Basically, different chemical substances possess different energy requirements and will absorb those photons of radiation having that corresponding frequency. The **spectrograms**, produced by all spectrophotometers, depict the UV, visible, and infrared (IR) radiations absorbed as a function of frequency, thus providing qualitative data relevant to identifying organic substances. Regardless of the type of radiation employed, the basic components are (1) a radiation source, (2) a frequency selector, (3) a sample holder, (4) a detector that will convert the radiation into an electrical signal, and (5) a recorder.

The type of desired radiation controls the selection of the source to be used. Ultraviolet (UV) usually involves a hydrogen or deuterium discharge lamp, an ordinary tungsten bulb is used for visible radiation, and infrared (IR) frequencies are provided by a heated rod containing rare earth oxides. Monochromatic frequencies are produced using colored glass filters (actually a range of wavelengths) and prisms or gratings in combination with a variable slit. Sample cells must be transparent to the radiation in use; therefore, quartz cells are used with UV, glass with visible, and sodium chloride or potassium bromide with IR radiation. Photoelectric tubes will detect UV and visible radiation, whereas **thermocouples**, or photomultipliers, are utilized to convert IR radiation to electrical signals.

The spectrograms produced by UV and visible radiation are quite simple, involving a few (1 to 5) broad absorption peaks, and they provide tentative identifications that can be confirmed by other procedures, e.g., TLC or GC. These bands of absorption are indicative of the entire molecule of the substance being analyzed, as opposed to the highly complex spectrograms that are the result of analyses employing IR frequencies (Figs. 12–3 and 12–4). The IR spectra differentiate between various intramolecular activities, such as bending or stretching bonds, as well as elemental combinations, such as CO or NH functional groups. The numerous peaks thus produced are quite distinctive and can be compared with commercially available catalogues of IR spectra and the questioned substance specifically identified.

The final arbiter more commonly used to identify drugs, whether received as solid dose forms or present in toxicologic samples (biologic fluids or tissue samples) is the *mass spectrometer (MS)* in combination with GC. The gas chromatograph serves to separate the material into components that are caused to flow directly into the spectrometer. There, within a high-vacuum chamber, the specimen molecules are bombarded with high-energy electrons, causing them to form extremely unstable ions. The fragments formed by the instant decomposition of these ions are caused to pass through a magnetic or electric field and become separated according to their masses (Fig. 12–5). Since no two substances produce the same pattern of fragmentation, a **fingerprint** of the sample is produced that serves to identify it specifically (Fig. 12–6). With the incorporation of a computer capable of recording, storing, searching, and comparing mass spectra with known spectra in memory, the GC/MS instrument provides speed, sensitivity, and accuracy of analysis. Technologic advances in microcircuitry have enabled the production of desk-top GC/MS instruments currently priced under $50,000 (Fig. 12–7).

Not unlike clinical laboratorians called upon to detect and identify elements such as chloride in urine or lead and iron in blood, forensic scientists perform similar analyses on physical evidence. The techniques employed make use of the phenomena that the elements will both absorb and emit light. *Emission spectroscopy, atomic absorption,* and *neutron activation* analyses are some of the analytical techniques currently to be found in contemporary Crime Labs. The first two techniques utilize the aforementioned phenomena resulting from natural elemental states and the third, neutron activation analysis, relies upon isotopic ele-

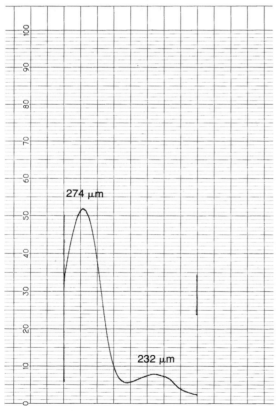

■ **FIGURE 12–3.**

An ultraviolet spectrogram.

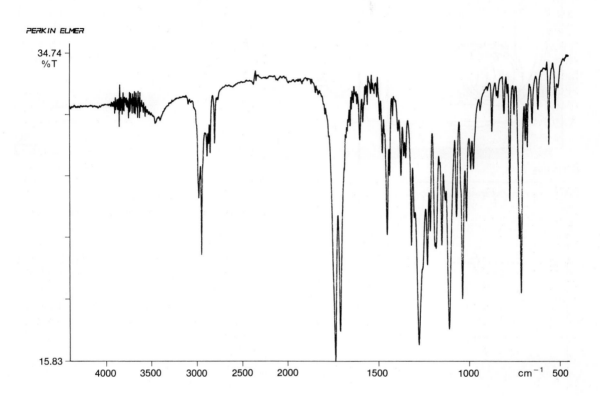

PERKIN ELMER

34.74
%T

15.83

4000   3500   3000   2500   2000   1500   1000   cm⁻¹ 500

91/03/06   14:17
CokeBase: 16 scans, 4.0cm−1
March 6, 1991

■ **FIGURE 12–4.**

An infrared spectrogram.

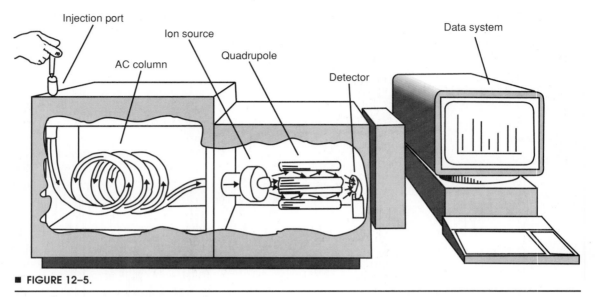

■ **FIGURE 12–5.**

Sketch of a mass spectrophotometer interior.

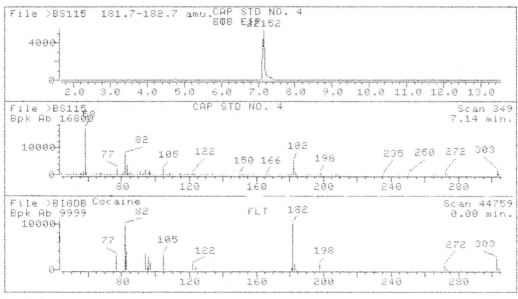

■ **FIGURE 12–6.**

A spectrogram (''fingerprint'') produced from a mass spectrophotometer.

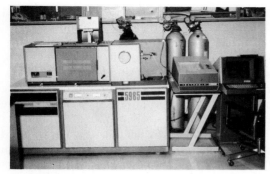

■ FIGURE 12–7.

A GC/mass spectrophotometer in operation.

mental states created during the analytical process.

Emission spectroscopy provides for specific identification by obtaining and recording the line spectra of the elements present in the specimen under analysis. In brief, specimens are placed between two carbon electrodes and vaporized with a direct current arc that excites the atoms of elements so that they emit select frequencies of light. A collimating lens causes the emitted light to be focused onto a prism, which disperses it into component frequencies. The frequencies thus dispersed are directed onto a photographic plate and recorded as line images.

Most materials contain numerous elements, and the resultant spectrum contains many lines identified by comparison with commercially available standard charts. More frequently the emission spectra of known and questioned exemplars are compared (matching line for line) as proof of a common source.

Recent advancements employ microscopically focused laser beams to vaporize the specimen; the vapors are then excited, collimated, dispersed, and so on. This technology is capable of detecting trace elements in 0.1 to 0.01 per cent concentrations. Emission spectroscopy was originally used extensively in the analysis of automotive paint chip evidence obtained during the investigation of hit-and-run (hit-skip) accidents. The advent of the acrylic paints currently used by automotive manufacturers has served to limit the forensic applications of emission spectroscopy.

Atomic absorption (AA) makes use of the fact that an atom vaporized but NOT excited will absorb many of the same frequencies that it emits when excited. With AA analysis, specimens are vaporized with an air-acetylene flame, through which is directed a beam of light. The light utilized is from a discharge tube constructed from the element of interest and therefore consisting of select frequencies. Samples containing the element will absorb this light, which is isolated, detected, and recorded on a strip chart recorder. The quantity of light absorbed is directly proportional to the concentration of the element under study.

Atomic absorption analysis, similar in principle to flame photometry, is fraught with inherent drawbacks. Since analyses are performed element by element, general unknowns are quite time consuming, and the numerous individual discharge lamps needed are cost-prohibitive. Although forensic scientists have not found wide application for AA, the technique is employed routinely to detect and quantify the elements bismuth and antimony. These elements are frequently obtained from the person (usually the hands) of individuals who have recently discharged firearms. Such information can be invaluable to the investigation of "crimes against persons," i.e., homicide and assault, as well as suicide.

NOT-SO-CLINICAL TECHNIQUES IN FORENSIC SCIENCE

Contemporary clinical laboratorians might be tempted to label as esoteric such methods as **neutron activation analysis (NAA)** and **X-ray diffraction**. These applications, borrowed from other realms of scientific endeavor, can be found in today's forensic science laboratory providing solutions to specific problems. The information gleaned by atomic absorption spectrophotometry and emission spectroscopy serves to identify various atoms by the existence of characteristic energy levels. NAA creates isotopes by activating the nuclei of atoms with neutron bombardment produced by a nuclear reactor. The spontaneous disintegration of unstable isotopes thus synthesized is accompanied by the emission of radiation.

This radioactive decay consists of three types of radiation: **alpha particles, beta particles**, and **gamma rays**. The characteristic energy value of the latter specifically identifies the parent element. The concentration of element in a specimen is directly proportional to the intensity of the gamma ray radiation produced. This off-beat technology is both a nondestructive and an extremely sensitive method (median detection sensitivity = 1 ng) of identifying and quantifying trace elements. This elegant technology is, however, generally cost-prohibitive, despite the capability of the simultaneous analysis for 20 to 30 elements.

X-ray diffraction, like the aforementioned methods of AA spectrophotometry, emission spectroscopy, and neutron activation analysis, which perform elemental analyses, brings the new dimension of detecting atomic arrangement. Applicable only to solid crystalline materials, which fortunately includes 95 per cent of all inorganic compounds, this method employs x-radiation to examine the lattice design of the crystal being analyzed. Stated simply, x-rays penetrating the crystal are partially reflected by its parallel planes. Upon leaving the crystal's planes, these beams combine with one another to form a series of light and dark bands. The pattern thus produced is unique for each compound, providing yet another "fingerprinting" technique. Useful to forensic scientists, owing to its nondestructive nature, x-ray diffraction lacks sensitivity (often failing to detect concentrations of less than 5 per cent) and is therefore considered suitable only for identifying the major constituents of a mixture.

Forensic laboratories, not usually blessed with a lavish annual budget, are often forced to forego these instrumental applications, using a more economical approach. In drug cases when quantitation is not needed, an analytical scheme might begin with (1) spot tests to rule out large classes, proceed to (2) TLC to identify tentatively a specific drug within the class not eliminated, and end with the little-remembered technique of (3) microcrystallography to confirm the presence of a specific drug.

Mindful of the "crystal garden" demonstration used in elementary school science instruction, microscopic crystallography makes use of the production of crystals, on a less grand scale, which require microscopy to be observed. Many of the illicit drugs received by the Crime Lab produce characteristic crystal forms in combination with various reagents. The most common reagents are halogenated precious metals: platinum, palladium, and gold with chlorine and bromine, but other less costly materials such as potassium permanganate find use in specific cases. The characteristic crystals thus formed (pennate quills and rosettes are among the more unusual) provide specific identification of the drug suspected to be present. While quantitation is not possible, the method is sensitive and provides specific identification of the drug suspected to be present. This technique is reminiscent of the crystal identifications requisite to the microscopic examinations performed upon urine specimens by clinical laboratorians.

Microscopy, no stranger to the clinical laboratory, finds many applications within the forensic science laboratory. Among those familiar to the clinically trained are stereoscopic microscopes, polarizing microscopes, and comparison microscopes. Undoubtedly the most versatile and, therefore, the most frequently used is the *stereoscopic microscope*. Much of the physical evidence examined in the forensic laboratory can be characterized using low magnifications ($10\times$ to $125\times$) to include items as diverse as paint chips, marijuana, gunpowder residues, and soil. Additionally, this type of microscope produces three-dimensional images and provides a large working distance (distance between the objective lens and the specimen), enabling the examination of large, bulky items of evidence. The forensic scientist has frequent occasion to examine tools, weapons, garments, and so on for the presence of trace evidence (hairs, fibers, glass, paint), and the great depth of focus and wide field of view make this instrument ideal.

The *polarizing microscope* consists of a compound microscope modified to include a polarizer and analyzer. Light passing through a polarizer is confined to a single plane of vibration and is said to be plane polarized. Used in microscopy, light is polarized, passed through a specimen, and then through a second polarizing lens called an analyzer en route to the eye piece. Light is observed when the polarizer and analyzer are parallel, and no light is observed when the two lenses are perpendicular to one another. Specimens that reorient the polarized light are readily distinguishable by the vivid colors and intensity contrasts observed. Obvious applications involve the study of materials that polarize light, particularly crystalline substances that are birefringent. **Birefringence** refers to the phenomenon seen when crystals split a beam of light into two component beams possessing different refractive indices. Under polarizing conditions, the resultant beams of birefringent substances are polarized at right angles to

each other. The refractive indices of these beams can be determined using standard liquids of known refractive index. This technique, originally developed for the study of minerals, is employed by forensic scientists to characterize those ubiquitous synthetic fibers (which, incidentally, are birefringent) encountered in contemporary America.

The frequent need of firearms examiners to observe specimens side-by-side brought about the introduction of the *comparison microscope*. This unique instrument is basically two compound microscopes united by a bridge incorporating mirrors and lenses, which joins two independent objective lenses into a single binocular unit. Matching the optical characteristics of the objective lenses ensures that the specimens (questioned and known bullets, cartridge casings, and so on) are viewed with equal magnification and identical distortion. Firearms impart striations upon the bullets that are fired from them; by simultaneously examining two bullets, the forensic scientist is able to determine whether or not the same gun barrel was involved (Fig. 12–8). Specialized microscope stages are available for the comparison of hairs and fibers.

With modern technology advancing at the speed of light, many innovations are being incorporated in the tool kit of today's forensic scientists. Two of these purloined techniques are the **microspectrophotometer** and the **scanning electron microscope (SEM)**. The microspectrophotometer is the product of combining the microscope with a computerized spectrophotometer. This instrument permits the analyst to view colored items (ink, paint, fibers) microscopically, direct a beam of light at the specimen, and plot an absorption spectrum indicating the exact wavelengths absorbed. Many times materials that appear to be similar when examined visually will demonstrate significantly different absorption spectra. Using infrared radiation with the micro-

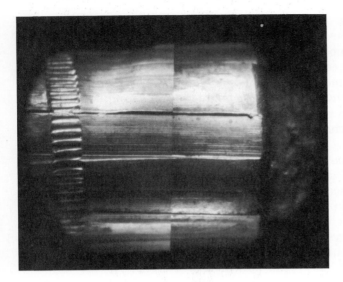

■ **FIGURE 12–8.**

A photomicrograph of two bullets, utilizing a comparison microscope.

spectrophotometer provides spectra that are unique to each chemical substance and has found forensic applications with fiber and paint evidence.

The development of SEM and its utilization is further evidence of today's technology being rapidly assimilated by the forensic science community. Termed *microscopy* by convention, SEM produces images that are displayed on a cathode-ray tube in the following manner. A primary beam of electrons from a hot tungsten filament is focused by means of electromagnets onto the surface of the specimen, causing the emission of electrons from the surface layer. By collecting the emitted electrons, an amplified signal is produced. When synchronized with the scanning of the primary beam, an image is produced of the specimen on the cathode-ray tube. Combining high magnification (up to 1 million times), high resolution, and great depth of focus (300 times that of optical systems), SEM produces images that appear almost stereoscopic. Additionally, elemental analysis can be performed by the marriage of SEM to an x-ray analyzer. X-rays, with characteristic energy values, are produced

by the bombardment with electrons and converted to electrical signals by means of a detector. The signals, sorted according to energy values, are displayed to provide an elemental distribution of the specimen being analyzed. This technique has been very successful in the positive identification of gunpowder particles that frequently contain the elements lead, antimony, and bismuth.

The recent emergence of methods for the analysis and comparison of DNA (deoxyribonucleic acid) by forensic science laboratories best exemplifies their propensity to adopt, adapt, and apply clinical techniques designed with an entirely different set of problems in mind. When faced with evidence consisting of biologic fluids, DNA profile analysis provides the forensic serologist with the ultimate means for the specific identification of individual human beings (Fig. 12–9). DNA, which is found in the nucleated cells of all life forms, is present in the tissues (hairs, fingernails, skin), and the biologic fluids (blood, semen, and stains thereof), which become evidence in crimes of violence. These substances are transferred from assailant to victim to crime scene and

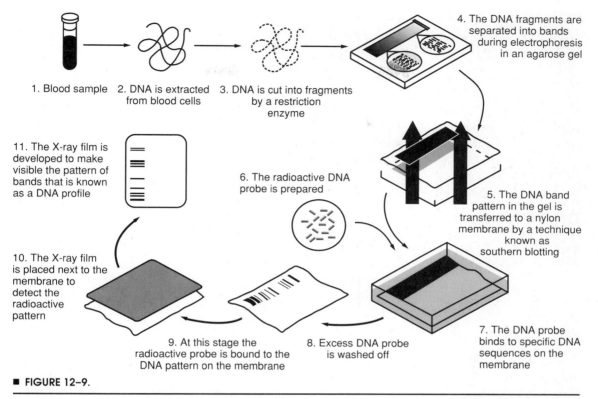

1. Blood sample
2. DNA is extracted from blood cells
3. DNA is cut into fragments by a restriction enzyme
4. The DNA fragments are separated into bands during electrophoresis in an agarose gel
5. The DNA band pattern in the gel is transferred to a nylon membrane by a technique known as southern blotting
6. The radioactive DNA probe is prepared
7. The DNA probe binds to specific DNA sequences on the membrane
8. Excess DNA probe is washed off
9. At this stage the radioactive probe is bound to the DNA pattern on the membrane
10. The X-ray film is placed next to the membrane to detect the radioactive pattern
11. The X-ray film is developed to make visible the pattern of bands that is known as a DNA profile

■ **FIGURE 12–9.**

The DNA analysis process. (Reprinted with permission from Chemical & Engineering News, November 20, 1989, 67(47), pp 18–30. Copyright 1989 American Chemical Society.)

vice versa, and DNA markers serve to ascribe their source(s) individually. The most valuable application of this method occurs with the analysis of rape evidence in which the semen present on vaginal swabs serves to place the person of the suspect within the person of the victim.

The **RFLP (restriction fragment length polymorphism)** methods currently used in forensic laboratories involve the following process or modifications thereof:

1. Known blood specimens are obtained from all involved individuals.
2. DNA is extracted from all specimens known and questioned.
3. DNA is cut into fragments by a specific restriction enzyme.
4. The fragments are separated by electrophoresis with an agarose gel.
5. Using the Southern blot technique,[4] the pattern of bands in the gel is transferred to a nylon membrane.
6. A radioactive DNA probe (complementary to the restriction enzyme) is caused to bind to specific sequences on the membrane.
7. Excess probe is washed off, and the membrane is placed on x-ray film and incubated at $-70°C$ for several weeks.
8. The film is developed to visualize the DNA pattern.

The patterns thus obtained are analyzed by densitometry, and migration distances (akin to the Rf values in TLC) are calculated.

Identical patterns are considered to have derived from the DNA of the same individual to the exclusion of ALL other inhabitants of the planet. The only exceptions are identical twins inasmuch as they arise from one zygote.

Another innovation being considered for use in forensic serology is **PCR (polymerase chain reaction)**. The question arises: "Will the courts regard this as the manufacture of evidence?"

ON THE HORIZON

Numerous court decisions rendered during the 1970s and 1980s have placed increasingly greater reliance on physical evidence and the results of its examination or analysis. Despite the concerted efforts of the law enforcement community, the incidence of reported crime does not appear to be diminishing. Forensic science laboratories provide viable employment opportunities, with job security, for individuals possessing the knowledge, skills, and abilities of clinical laboratorians. Both professions, forensic science and clinical laboratory science, consist of a blend of analytical techniques with those of microscopy and morphologic identifications. In 1988, a study conducted by my colleagues and me indicated that more than 5 per cent of forensic scientists then employed were educated as medical technologists.[5] With the exception of OSHA regulations, forensic science remains the last bastion of the baccalaureate degree scientist, working unfettered by the myriad of regulatory watchdog agencies that currently plague clinical laboratorians.

Forensic science will continue to monitor the applied research activities of all scientific disciplines, from agricultural chemistry to zoology, with an eye to "liberating" applicable methods and techniques. At this writing, DNA methodology appears to be enjoying great attention. Currently, the requirement of radioactive materials poses a great problem to the majority of the nation's nonfederal forensic science laboratories. Ongoing research activity seeks to eliminate the radioactive portion of the current method by substituting chemiluminescent techniques. The success of this endeavor would enable any laboratory, no matter how small or geographically remote, to perform DNA profile analyses.[6] Given their education and training, clinical laboratorians would constitute a reservoir of very desirable potential forensic serologists.[7]

In summation, a precedent is well established for the inclusion of clinical skills and knowledge within the forensic laboratory. The criminal activity reported by the media on a daily basis ensures the stability of the forensic science profession, and our rapidly advancing technology serves to guarantee an exciting future in the Crime Lab.

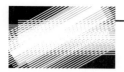

REVIEW QUESTIONS

Choose *all* answers that apply.

1. Which of the following may be sources of physical evidence?

a. The crime scene.
b. The person of the victim.
c. The person of the suspect.
d. All of the above.
e. None of the above.

2. Which of the following techniques provide specific identification?

a. Thin-layer chromatography.
b. Ultraviolet spectrophotometry.
c. Infrared spectrophotometry.
d. Gas chromatography.
e. Polarizing microscopy.

3. Neutron activation analysis enables the identification of elements by collecting and measuring the energy of emitting:

a. electrons.
b. neutrons.
c. beta particles.
d. protons.
e. gamma rays.

4. Which of the following statements is false?

a. The lens nearest the user's eye is called the ocular lens.
b. Light that is confined to a single plane of vibration is said to be polarized.
c. In a polarizing microscope, no light will penetrate when the polarizer and the analyzer are positioned parallel to each other.
d. The image produced by a compound microscope is called virtual.
e. Crystals commonly display birefringence.

5. The DNA ``Profile Analysis'' employs the following steps: (1) digestion with a restriction enzyme, (2) Southern blotting, (3) electrophoresis, (4) contact with x-ray film, and (5) hybridization with a radioactive probe. The proper sequence for these steps is:

a. 5,3,2,1,4
b. 1,3,2,5,4
c. 1,2,3,4,5
d. 5,1,2,3,4
e. 5,2,3,4,1

REFERENCES

1. Snyder JR, Pfau RO, Jeurick G, Banks J: Alternate sites for testing: Forensic sciences laboratories, penal institutions, and industry. *J Med Technol* 3(12):613–616, 1986.
2. Pfau RO: Medical technology: A viable source of criminalists. *J Forensic Sci Soc* 27(3):199–205, May/June, 1987.
3. Harris vs. United States, 331 U.S. 145, 1947.
4. Southern EM: Detection of specific sequences among DNA fragments separated by gel electrophoresis. *J Molec Biol* 98:503–517, 1975.
5. Pfau RO, Snyder JR, Rudmann SV, Scott JE: Employment of medical technologists in forensic science laboratories in the United States. *Lab Med* 22(1):40–44, Jan, 1991.
6. Wiedrauk DL: Molecular methods for virus detection. *Lab Med* 23(11):737–742, 1992.
7. Klosinski DD, Matta N, Hunter SI: Work force adaptations and future molecular pathology. *Lab Med* 23(11):747–751, 1992.

Chapter 13

LABORATORY INFORMATION SYSTEMS

KAREN M. ESCOLAS, MS, MT(ASCP)

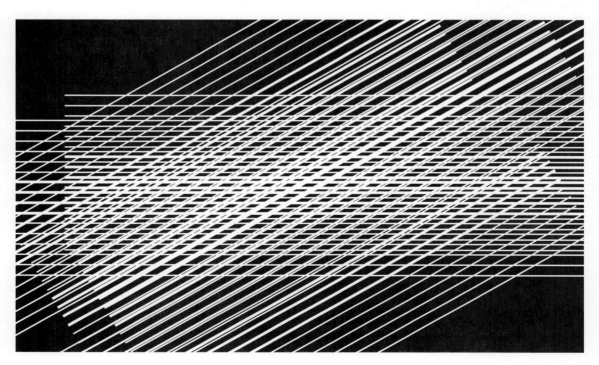

LEARNING OBJECTIVES

After studying this chapter, the student should be able to:

- Identify the major components of a laboratory information system.
- Define memory and describe the hardware devices involved in data storage.
- Describe the mechanisms by which input/output devices allow communication between the system and the users.
- Differentiate between a minicomputer LIS configuration and a microcomputer LIS configuration.
- Identify the major points of user interaction during routine operation of the laboratory information system.
- Outline the pathway of a specimen through the laboratory information system, from ordering the test to reporting the results.
- Describe the LIS features that make laboratory reports more readable and patient care thorough.
- Describe how barcode technology has improved the efficiency of the laboratory information system.

KEY WORDS

Barcode. A series of lines and spaces that vary in width to represent alphanumeric symbols. A bar code reader hits the code with a laser beam and interprets the light reflected into a computer readable form.

Cathode ray tube. A screen or monitor upon which computer data are displayed in the form of numbers, letters, and symbols that allow for communication between the user and the computer.

Database. A method for computerized storage of data that allows for quick and easy access of the information as well as simple insertion and deletion of data.

Hardware. The physical components containing all the electronics necessary for the operation of a computer system.

Hospital Information System (HIS). The computer system that stores the data and programs utilized in administrative hospital operations (billing, admitting, medical records, and so on).

Interface. The electrical connection that allows for communication (passage of data) between multiple computer systems (e.g., the LIS and automated instrumentation).

Laboratory Information System (LIS). The computer system that stores the data and programs utilized in laboratory operations (e.g., specimen accessioning, results processing).

Local area network (LAN). A connection of multiple computers within a localized area that allows for data and hardware and software components to be shared at more than one user terminal.

Modem. A specialized communication device that allows for multiple computers to exchange data over telephone lines.

Software. The programmed instructions that operate the computer system.

Terminal. The point at which the user may interact with the computer by entering or retrieving data. Usually consists of a monitor and a keyboard along with any other specialized input/output devices (modems, bar code scanners).

INTRODUCTION

The application of computer technology to clinical laboratory operations began in the 1960s. Prior to this time, the **"Laboratory Information System"** (LIS) consisted of a system of log books, worksheets, and patient slips that were manually prepared. In the late 1950s, the patient workload and associated clerical tasks increased because of the implementation of third party reimbursement. During the same time frame, the introduction of automated analyzers resulted in increased turnaround times for routine tests, again overloading the technologist with clerical tasks. The first attempts at a computerized LIS in the 1960s mainly were meant to automate these clerical tasks in the laboratory. At this time, hospital administrators were also establishing **Hospital Information Systems (HIS)** for tracking patient data and automating patient billing.

During the 1970's, the expanded capabilities of microprocessors resulted in fully functional, user-oriented computer systems in the laboratory. Similar advances in the HIS led to an interface that allowed information to be passed between the two systems, such as patient demographics from the HIS to the LIS or test results from the LIS to the HIS. In the 1980s, advances in both the hardware and software of the two systems expanded their interactive usability and led to improvements in both systems.[1]

The implementation of a LIS in the clinical laboratory should lead to improvement of the quality of patient care, increased productivity in the laboratory, and more efficient management of administrative and financial responsibilities. The quality of patient care is improved with the added efficiency of information sharing between the laboratory and the health care providers via the LIS. The productivity of the laboratory increases as formerly manual, time-consuming clerical tasks such as data transcription and report preparation become part of the LIS function. Computerization also reduces clerical error and allows for more complete tracking of patient information and testing data, thus improving the efficiency of resource management and the billing system.

LABORATORY INFORMATION SYSTEM COMPONENTS

A computer system consists of two elements: **hardware** and **software**. The hardware refers to those physical components containing all the electronics necessary for the system to function. The software is the programmed set of instructions that actually operates the system.

Hardware

All data used by the computer are stored in the *memory* of the system. The stored information is in the form of binary code, a combination of 0s and 1s expressed in powers of two. Each 0 or 1 represents a *bit* (binary digit) in the data bank, with a string of 8 bits forming a *byte*. Each alphanumeric character is represented by one byte of data in the computer's memory. The storage capabilities of computer memory devices are expressed as the number of bytes that can be held using the nomenclature defined in Table 13–1.

The *central processing unit (CPU)*, or *microprocessor*, executes the instructions of the software. Contained within the CPU is an *arithmetic-logic unit (ALU)* that performs all numerical computations called for by the software, and a *control unit (CU)* for coordination of all machine activities. The *main memory*, or *Random Access Memory (RAM)*, is the computer's primary memory located in the CPU. The system's set of instructions is held in RAM during computer operations and is usually erased when the machine is shut down. Another memory chip, the *Read Only Memory (ROM)*, contains a permanently accessible set of instructions that the computer uses to communicate with other devices.

Information needs to be stored in a more permanent location than the main memory—one that retains the data when power is lost. The information stored in this *secondary memory* also must be easily accessible to the user when needed. Typically, data are held by *discs* upon which magnetized bits may be deposited and erased on command. The bits are retrieved from or written onto

TABLE 13–1. TERMINOLOGY FOR EXPRESSING MEMORY CAPACITY

Bit	=	Binary digit (0 or 1)
Byte	=	8 bits or 1 character
Kilobyte (K or KB)	=	2^{10} or 1024 bytes
Megabyte (MB)	=	1000 K
Gigabyte (GB)	=	1000 MB
Terabyte (TB)	=	1000 GB

the disc by read/write heads located in the disc drive. Discs are considered random access or direct access storage media because information may be stored on or retrieved from any position on the disc, resulting in shortened data access times.

Hard discs are rigid magnetic platters that may be either internal, encased within the computer cabinet with the CPU and main memory, or external, connected to the cabinet by a cable. A hard disc typically can hold from 10 to 2000 or more megabytes of data that can be stored and retrieved at a faster rate than most other disc forms.

Floppy discs, also known as diskettes because of their relatively small capacity of 360 kilobytes to 2.8 megabytes, are made of flexible magnetic tape encased in a rigid, protective jacket. These diskettes are relatively inexpensive and convenient for transport of data between remote computers but hold much less information, have longer access times, and are more easily damaged than other storage forms.

Magnetic tape stores information in magnetized bits and is capable of holding many gigabytes of data; however, tape has the slowest access time of all storage media since the data must be accessed sequentially. Magnetic tape is available as reel-to-reel tapes and cartridge tape units and is used predominantly for backup of large amounts of stored data not requiring routine access.

Optical discs store information as holes burnt into an aluminum disc by a high-powered laser beam. A laser beam of lower power is then used to retrieve the data. The advantages of optical discs are the durability of the disc material and the storage capability. Each side of an optical disc is capable of storing 300 to 650 megabytes of data.

The remaining category of hardware is that of *Input/Output (I/O) devices*, components that allow the user to "communicate" with the computer system. Also referred to as *peripheral devices* because of their location external to the CPU, these components translate information between the computer and the laboratory technologist or a piece of laboratory instrumentation.

The most prominent I/O device is the *monitor*, or **cathode ray tube (CRT)**, the screen at the computer terminal that displays a mixture of words, numbers, and graphics. The monitor is predominantly an output device, producing a "soft copy" of the computer's contents in either monochrome or color display. The output ability is limited by size, since once the screen fills with information it must be partially erased to display additional data; thus the monitor is used primarily for interactive functions. The monitor also may be used for specialized input in conjunction with a *light pen* or the technology of a *touch screen*. A light pen utilizes a light-sensitive photoelectric cell to designate a desired position on the screen, a technique similar to drawing on the screen with a light. Touch-screen technology allows the user to choose a screen location by applying slight pressure on that area, an input method incorporated into a number of automated clinical analyzers.

The *keyboard* is the most commonly encountered input device associated with computers. The standard typewriter keys depicting letters, numbers, and punctuation marks allow alphanumeric input that is then translated to computer-usable code. The *function keys* are those keys labeled F1, F2, F3, and so forth. These keys are used to perform commands and are referred to as programmable keys, since the command performed depends upon the software instructions running the system at the time. The special-purpose keys on the keyboard are used for editing and performing functions and include keys such as the Ctrl (Control), Del (Delete), Ins (Insert), and Alt (Alternate) keys. Cursor-movement keys are marked with arrows and are used to move the *cursor*, the symbol that depicts where the next keystroke will be positioned, around the screen. The keyboard can be enhanced by the use of a *mouse*, a hand-held device connected by a cable to the computer. Movement of the mouse across a flat surface moves the cursor across the monitor screen. The cursor appears as an arrow on the screen; it must be pointed at the desired choice for the user to make a selection.

A variety of scanning devices also may be used in the laboratory for input of information. These devices use *optical character recognition (OCR)* to read printed material and convert it to computer-usable form. The *optical mark reader (OMR)* reads pencil marks on a sheet of paper, using a beam of high-intensity light that detects the number and location of the marks. The data are then converted into electrical signals for the computer's use. Similarly, *barcode readers* scan a series of lines and spaces of varying widths using a laser beam. Again, the data collected are converted into computer-usable electronic signals. Advances in barcode technology have led to widespread use of **barcodes** and barcode readers in conjunction with the LIS and computerized laboratory instruments for specimen identification and processing.

The *printer* is the main device for generation of hardcopy output, thus producing a permanent record of the data stored in the computer system. Characters, symbols, and graphics may be printed on paper by the printer. Dot-matrix printers print a line of text by serially printing dots to form characters. Character printers operate in typewriter fashion, printing each character individually. Line printers print text one line at a time, with each space in a line having its own set of characters on a drum or belt. Laser printers and thermal printers are also available that produce high-quality characters using laser beams and heat application to transfer images to paper.

Specialized I/O devices referred to as *data communications hardware* serve to transmit data between remote computer systems. This can be done only by using devices that are able to convert the signals sent by the computer into a form that can be transmitted over telecommunication equipment. Computers communicate using *digital* signals, which are a series of discrete electrical pulses. Conversely, people communicate using analog signals, which are continuous waves that vary in frequency and in amplitude to form the human "voice." Telephone lines are an analog transmitting device, therefore, the digital signal produced by the computer must be converted to an analog signal to be moved across the cables, a process referred to as *modulation*. When the signal reaches the computer at the other end of the cable, *demodulation* must then occur to convert the analog signal to its original digital form. The device responsible for this conversion is a **modem** (modulator/demodulator). In a similar way, computerized instruments used in the laboratory may be **interfaced** with the LIS to allow direct electronic communication between the instrument computer and the CPU of the system. Again, the type of signal transmitted may require further manipulation from analog to digital form to maintain a compatible data stream.

Software

The software, or *program*, is a sequence of detailed instructions necessary for the computer to function. To alter the format of a particular system, e.g., the LIS, the program must be changed. Three pathways are possible for each sequence of events in a program: (1) the program may simply proceed to the next sequential step; (2) the program may conditionally branch out to a step farther along in the program, such as "*if* this condition is met *then* proceed with a further step *or else* move on to an alternate step"; or (3) the program may cycle around on itself in a "loop," such as *"do* this series of steps *until* this condition is met," with all other parameters held constant and the one variable being the condition tested.

The *language* is the terminology or symbology used to write the program. The most basic or "low-level" languages are machine language and assembly language. *Machine language* is written in the numeric code of 0's and 1's that the computer operates in. *Assembly language* is a set of simple mnemonic codes or compact phrases and structures that must be converted to the numeric codes of machine language by an *assembler*. Most programs are written in "high-level" languages, which more closely resemble spoken language in their mnemonic codes. These languages must be converted back into machine language by a *compiler* or *interpreter* for the computer to operate. A compiler translates the entire program at once, whereas an interpreter translates each portion of the program as it is activated. Examples of high-level languages and their primary applications are listed in Table 13–2.

Database Storage

In older systems, data were stored in a file structure format that limited the ability to add new data to the files at a later time. In a file structure, the data for each file were entered into the computer and stored sequentially in the memory. For example, if each file represented a patient and each patient had a name, identification number, and date of birth as its data, the memory would hold this information in the following manner:

Name1,ID#1,DOB1; Name2,ID#2, DOB2; Name3,ID#3,DOB3,etc.

If a fourth parameter were to be added to each file, such as patient gender, the program would have to be rewritten to alter the file structure to allow for new data to be stored. This type of program is then "data-dependent." Presently, the use of a **database** program allows for a more flexible system that can easily adapt to the addition of new parameters. The database stores each piece of data in a logical order that allows for retrieving, changing, adding, and deleting the information without rewriting the entire program. Using the previous example, a database would store the information as depicted, with new parameters easily inserted into the structure for the third patient:

Name1	ID#1	DOB1	
Name2	ID#2	DOB2	
Name3	ID#3	DOB3	GENDER3

TABLE 13–2. HIGH-LEVEL LANGUAGES AND THEIR USAGE

LANGUAGE	FULL NAME	USAGE
FORTRAN	**Fo**rmula **Tra**nslator	technical and scientific applications
COBOL	**Co**mmon **B**usiness **O**riented **L**anguage	business applications
BASIC	**B**eginners' **A**ll-Purpose **S**ymbolic **I**nstruction **C**ode	simple language to teach programming interactively
Pascal	Named for 17th century mathematician Blaise **Pascal**	structured language to teach programming
MUMPS	**M**assachusetts **U**tility for **M**ultiple **P**rogramming **S**ystems	medical applications

A database structure is a "data-independent" program that is much better suited to the ever-changing environment of the clinical laboratory.[2]

LABORATORY INFORMATION SYSTEM CONFIGURATIONS

Early laboratory information systems were designed around small mainframe computer systems, or minicomputers. A minicomputer is a computer that is capable of supporting the processing requirements of many users. The system is set up as in Figure 13–1, with the main computer being housed separately from user **terminals** that consist of a monitor and a keyboard. Each terminal is considered a *dumb terminal*, one that cannot carry out any function without the main system, and is thus dependent on the capabilities of the minicomputer. Throughout the 1970s and early 1980s, clinical laboratory systems were almost exclusively planned as minicomputer systems.[3]

In the later 1980s, advances were made in the technology of microcomputers. A *microcomputer* is a computer with a microprocessor *chip* as its CPU that can be used by only one user at a time. Clinical laboratory systems use this technology by building a microprocessor *network*, a linkage of computers by communication cables and modem-like devices that allow users to share information, programs, and equipment through the use of communications hardware and software (Figure 13–2). In this type of system, the user terminal is a *smart terminal* that is capable of carrying out functions independently, using the main computer as a database source and as a link to devices such as printers. Connections can be made throughout a department, throughout an institution, or globally.

A **local area network (LAN)** is a con-

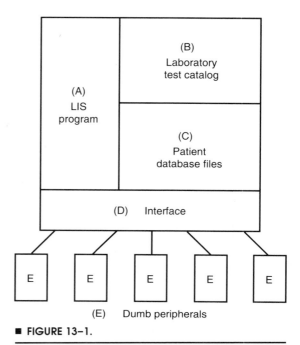

■ FIGURE 13–1.

A block diagram of a minicomputer-based LIS. One machine holds the LIS program instructions *(A)*, laboratory test catalog *(B)*, patient database, including cumulative and archive files *(C)*, and *(D)* an interface that connects the minicomputer to *(E)* dumb peripherals, including user terminals, printers, and laboratory instrumentation.

nection of a group of users within the same location that allows them to share printers, files, databases, disc storage, and other expensive peripheral devices. A microcomputer-based LIS is an example of a LAN. A *wide area network (WAN)* is a connection between users scattered over a large area, such as throughout a country or large institution, that allows electronic communication among users and the sharing of files, programs, and information. An example of a WAN is the connection of a remote LIS to a HIS for reporting laboratory results, such as a reference laboratory reporting to a hospital-based laboratory.

The source of software for a LIS is optional and depends upon the needs and re-

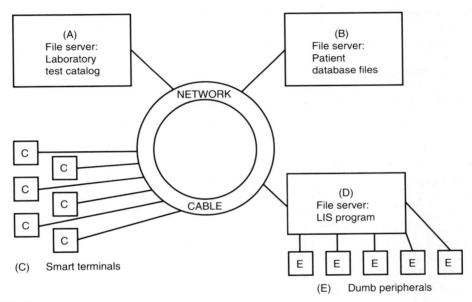

(A)
File server:
Laboratory
test catalog

(B)
File server:
Patient
database files

NETWORK

C

C

C

C

C

C

CABLE

(D)
File server:
LIS program

(C)   Smart terminals

E   E   E   E   E

(E)   Dumb peripherals

■ **FIGURE 13–2.**

A block diagram of an LIS network. A file server holding the Laboratory Test Catalog *(A)* and a file server holding the patient database *(B)* are connected by network cable to *(C)* smart terminals containing the LIS program instructions and *(D)* a server containing the LIS program instructions that operates the *(E)* dumb peripherals, including system printers and laboratory instrumentation.

sources of the laboratory in question. LIS software may be custom designed by a programming team, resulting in a system that meets the criteria of the laboratory exactly, but this is in most cases prohibitively expensive and time consuming. A LIS system is most often purchased from a vendor specializing in LIS design as either a software package or as a turnkey system that includes both hardware and software.

The four attributes necessary for a computer system to achieve the expected goals are described by Lincoln and Aller[1, 4] as flexibility, friendliness, transparency, and forgiveness. Flexibility refers to the computer's ability to conform to the needs of the users. No system will ever be able to meet all the laboratory's needs because of constraints in the hardware or software ability, but the major tasks should be accomplished without computer limitations. Friendliness refers to the quality of user interaction at the terminal. The computer should be configured for ease of use by the technologist in performing the tasks. Transparency refers to the ability of the user to master the computer system without having any previous knowledge of computer technology. The user should be able to carry out all tasks using commands that respond consistently and reliably to perform the desired function. Forgiveness relates to the ability of the user to make errors without suffering any type of lasting penalty. An example is the system that alerts the user with some type of harmless default, such as an error code, then allows for simple corrective action to remedy the error.

LABORATORY INFORMATION SYSTEM OPERATIONS

The LIS serves a vital function in the operation of a clinical laboratory. Specimen management, information processing, laboratory management, and administrative functions all may be facilitated by the use of a computer system. The LIS assists the technologist by performing those tasks that are time consuming and most prone to error when done manually. For the most part, these tasks are the clerical duties involved in processing patient specimens through the laboratory and maintaining patient files, but the quality and functioning of the clinical setting may also be improved by the computer's other capabilities.

System Security

The use of *access codes* for entry into the LIS limits the amount of information that is accessible to each individual user. The access codes are actually passwords known only to the user that have been assigned specific levels of authority within the laboratory. The higher the level of authority, the more information accessible to the user. This feature is meant to protect the confidentiality of the patient and the integrity of system information. To further enforce the system, if a user attempts to access any terminal illegally, such as not entering the correct password, the main system is alerted. If repeated attempts are made at the same terminal, the main system will shut down that terminal for a short time, preventing user access even when the correct password is entered.

User Assistance

Even in the "friendliest" system, the user will not always know what information is asked for at the cursor. A **Help** feature will guide the user through the system by explaining what type of information is requested at the cursor and what process takes place with the selection of each available application. An example of a typical online Help feature might be the entry of a "?" at the cursor, followed by a list of the data entries that would be acceptable to the system:

Patient Gender: ?
                   M—male
                   F—female
                   N—not provided

For explanations of available applications, the programmer might have one of the function keys, F1, F2, and so on, designated as the Help key. When the user highlighted the selection in question and then depressed the system's Help key, a detailed description of the action that would take place would appear on the screen. The incorporation of a Help feature is meant to guide the unfamiliar user through the system while training that user for future system interaction.

Function Selection

The format of the screens that appear on the monitor during program operation should be arranged in such a way that the user may easily read the choices available and select the desired function. The *menu* is a commonly used format that lists the options available to the user. The user moves the cursor to highlight the desired function and then depresses the "enter" key to select that function. The use of graphics in conjunction with the text may also make this selection process easier.

Touch screens and light pens eliminate the need to use the keyboard for selection since the desired function may be selected directly from the screen. The use of a mouse also bypasses the keyboard for selection of menu items and movement through the system. The major advantage of these technologies is the time saved in making selections, but the selection process is also simplified for the technologist.

Patient Information

When a patient enters a medical facility, certain data must be collected from the patient, such as name, date of admission, status (outpatient, inpatient, preadmission workup, or ambulatory surgical unit), location (room, bed, floor), date of birth, gender, and clinician. This information makes up the patient *demographics* and is necessary for tracking and storing all further data acquired on that patient. The demographics are collected at a terminal of the HIS using an input screen. Each piece of information is asked for by the item descriptor on the screen; the line following that descriptor is the *input field* where the information is entered into the system.

At the time of admission, the patient is assigned an *accession number* that is unique to that patient and will be used as an identification number for all future patient-hospital interactions. A *check digit* is a mechanism that allows the LIS to verify that an accession number entered is valid. Ideally, the individual entering data should verify that the name that is displayed once the accession number is entered matches the name of the patient for whom data are being entered. Transcription errors during entry of the accession number might cause data to be entered into a different patient file than the file intended. By having a check digit built into the system, entry of data into the wrong patient file is avoided. The check digit is the final digit of the accession number that is determined by mathematical manipulation of the actual accession number.

Below, is an example of the mathematics that might be used to determine the check digit of an accession number.[1]

DETERMINATION OF A CHECK DIGIT FOR SAMPLE ACCESSION NUMBER
123456:
1. Multiply every other digit from the right by 2:
$6 \times 2 = 12$ $4 \times 2 = 8$ $2 \times 2 = 4$
2. Add all the digits of the resulting products to all the remaining digits:
$(1 + 2 + 8 + 4) + (5 + 3 + 1) = 24$
3. Subtract the sum from the next highest multiple of 10:
$30 - 24 = 6$
The check digit then is the number 6, making the complete accession number either 123456-6 or 1234566.

This system will catch most transposition errors by recalculating the check digit each time the number is entered and comparing it with the original check digit.

The demographics outlined are those that are typically necessary for access by laboratory personnel to complete patient testing. A link, or *interface*, between the HIS and the LIS allows the demographics to be copied from the HIS database into the LIS database. The name and accession number will then be used to identify that patient in all laboratory proceedings. The age and gender are important for determination of appropriate reference ranges for the patient. The diagnosis may be added to help the technologist interpret abnormal results, and the clinician's name is necessary if the technologist must report a highly abnormal or life-threatening result.

Specimen Processing

Order entry is the origination point of a test request and subsequent need for a specimen. With the presence of computer terminals linked to the laboratory at nursing stations, the orders may be entered directly into the system either by the clinician or by a nurse transferring the orders from the patient chart. Each test is assigned a code number unique to that test, which is then used for ordering tests and for sorting specimens in the laboratory. The option is usually given to order individual tests (ex. test #2836 is a potassium level), groups of tests categorized by disease or organ specificity (ex. test #4502 is an electrolyte panel of sodium, potassium, chloride, and total carbon dioxide), or tests to be performed at timed intervals (ex. test #5613 is cardiac enzymes to be drawn every 8 hours). The assignment of a collection priority such as STAT, routine, or specific time, may also be done at the time of the order. The tests ordered are immediately transferred into a queue in the laboratory awaiting specimen collection. The system validates all tests ordered against other orders, thus avoiding duplicate tests and saving the patient from unnecessary venipuncture and expense.

Once the orders are entered into the computer and queued for specimen collection, the appropriate information also will be sent to an attached printer for *label generation*. The printer will generate enough labels for each specimen that must be collected. A typical label includes the patient's name, accession number, location, and space for the phlebotomist's initials and date and time of collection. This process reduces the clerical effort required of the phlebotomist and the chance of misidentification due to poorly or improperly labeled specimens.

Specimen collection is also more efficient with the use of a computerized system. The LIS collects all test orders in a queue, then organizes the orders by time and location to dispatch the phlebotomy team efficiently. An on-line LIS terminal at the nursing station may be used by the phlebotomist to inquire about any special collection instructions or specimen requirements. The status of the order from "pending" to "collected" may also be changed at any LIS terminal, thus removing the order from the queue. This system will maintain a file that tracks all orders left uncollected, thus avoiding the chance of orders being misplaced.

Following collection, the specimen is delivered into the appropriate section of the laboratory for testing. Upon entering the laboratory, an *accession number* is assigned to the specimen that is specific for that particular specimen and is used for laboratory tracking only. The purpose of this accession number is to inform the LIS that the specimen is in the laboratory and to provide a means for the laboratory staff to locate, identify, and follow the course of each specimen independently.

Using the accession number assigned by the LIS, the specimen is directed to a specific workstation in the laboratory, based on the tests ordered and the priority designated at the time of order entry. Depending upon the laboratory configuration, the LIS is designed to compile all tests ordered into groups, each group consisting of all tests performed at a particular workstation within the laboratory. Upon command, a printer produces a hardcopy in the form of a *worklist* for the technologist to follow at each workstation. The worklist consists of a list of the specimens to be tested at each workstation, organized by laboratory accession number. This results in more efficient planning of the day's work and also further reduces the incidence of tests ordered not being run, especially when a specimen is misplaced.

Results Processing

When test results are generated, the technologist then must enter those results into the LIS. The appropriate patient file may be accessed by entering the patient name, patient accession number, or specimen accession number into the LIS. The results may be entered as each individual test is completed or as a profile of tests are completed. Routinely, results will be entered into the LIS as a batched group of the same tests ordered on different patients. An exception would be STAT results entered on a single patient as the tests are completed. The technologist will either type the results into a LIS terminal or have the results sent directly to the LIS from the automated instrument. The information obtained by the testing process will be entered in result form or as raw data obtained from the assay that the LIS has been programmed to convert into results. The results entered into the LIS are placed into a temporary "buffer" file accessible only to laboratory personnel.

Before results can be released to the LIS database for reporting, a technologist must verify that the results in the system match the results obtained from the assay. This verification step is mandated by both the Joint Commission on Accreditation of Hospitals (JCAH) and the College of American Pathologists (CAP) for all laboratory results prior to their being made available outside the clinical laboratory.[5] During the verification process, any discrepancies that are found may be edited on-line in the LIS. Following verification, the results are finalized by the technologist, which allows the system to distinguish between the results that are done and those that are verified. The verified results are then sent from the buffer file to a cumulative file that is accessible outside the laboratory. This cumulative file allows for *patient inquiry* by persons that have access to the system. With the patient name or accession number, the user has direct access to patient information available in the LIS.

Although results are available on-line for inquiry, a hardcopy report is also generated for the clinician's use and for documentation in the patient's chart. Reports may be printed on command for specific patients or, at specified intervals, all results completed and verified since the last printout may be printed in batches. The reports must be formatted to include results in a manner that is interpretive for quick and easy analysis by the clinician. The generation of cumulative reports that include a series of results on a patient over a period of time also assists the clinician in interpretation and may be accompanied by charts that visualize the changes in laboratory values over time.

Certain areas of the hospital, such as the emergency department, operating room, intensive care unit, and recovery room, may have terminals at the bedside or printers in the ward for immediate access to all results that are finalized. Clinicians at off-site offices may also be linked by a modem to the LIS to receive reports directly from the laboratory.

System Flags

The use of flags to draw attention to abnormal results on both the terminal screens and printed reports aids in the logical interpretation of the results. All abnormal values can be either highlighted or accompanied by a "hi"/"lo" or "H"/"L" flag. If the monitor or printer is capable of color display, abnormal results may be displayed in a different color than those that are normal, e.g., normal results in black and abnormal results in red. Other variations include italicized abnormal results and asterisks (*) next to abnormal values.

Delta checks are flags that appear next to a current result to indicate an inconsistency with previous results. When a test is ordered repeatedly on the same patient, the system compares the current result with all previous results within a predetermined period of time: for example, potassium results during the last 48 hours. If any change that has occurred is considered significant when compared with a programmed "acceptable" change limit, the result will be flagged to notify the technologist. Such a drastic change could come from testing errors, such as using the wrong specimen or using the wrong proportion of reagent to specimen, or any type of instrument malfunction. It could also reflect a drastic change in the patient's condition, e.g., a significant drop in potassium, that requires immediate attention. In either case, by alerting the technologist the system tries to ensure that action will be taken to correct the result or to verify the result by repeat testing followed by communication to the appropriate caregiver.

Flags for abnormal values and delta checks may not be adequate measures to ensure that all critical or questionable results are acted upon. In some systems, an *alerting system* will also be in place to call attention to laboratory results that demand immediate action, such as an extremely low potassium level. Prior to implementation of this system, the pathologist and hospital staff would set definitions for life-threatening situations requiring immediate attention. These criteria would then be programmed into the system; each time results were completed in the laboratory system, the program would compare the results with the alert criteria. When a match was found, the system would then alert the attending personnel through some type of display at the nursing station computer terminal. The alert would also be activated in the laboratory for the technologist to verify that the results were received and acted upon.[6]

Reflex Testing

Additional tests may be automatically ordered by the LIS upon entry and verification of the results. The decision would be based upon predefined patient criteria in conjunction with the finding of certain results. This system of *reflex testing* saves the patient from additional venipuncture, since the specimen already in the laboratory could be used for the additional tests. The time required for the clinician to receive the results and order the additional tests also would be saved. An example of a reflexed test would be isoenzymes ordered automatically when very high total creatine kinase and lactate dehydrogenase are reported and the suspected diagnosis is myocardial infarction.

System Storage

The LIS database has three major files: the cumulative file, the archive file, and a laboratory test file. The cumulative file that holds all patient information in the LIS is limited in the amount of data that can be held. After the data have been on-line for a specified period of time, it is *archived* and placed in another file that is not immediately accessible. Information in the archive file may still be accessed, but the procedure is more involved than on-line inquiry. The laboratory test file holds all information regarding test parameters, instrument parameters, tests available, reference ranges, quality control, specimen requirements, and all other definitional laboratory information necessary for laboratory operation.

Quality Control

The LIS greatly simplifies the quality control system of the clinical laboratory. The quality control samples are processed using the same protocol as patient samples, with the controls being automatically scheduled and printed on the worklists generated for each workstation. The control results are entered and verified along with patient results; the control results are then put into a file specially designated for quality control. After a specified period of time, usually monthly, the control results are statistically evaluated. The LIS may be programmed to calculate the mean and standard deviation for each assay run in the laboratory, printing out a summary of all results obtained during the month, along with the calculated parameters and a Levy-Jennings chart for each assay. The use of the computer for quality control evaluation ensures more meaningful statistics and reduces the technologist's time necessary to perform the statistical manipulations.

Barcode Technology

Barcode symbology consists of a sequence of bars and spaces of varying width, each set representing a code of letters, numbers, and punctuation marks. This code is readable to a computer or instrument that converts the barcode to the series of alphanumeric characters it represents. Barcodes were standardized in the early 1980s, therefore codes used by different vendors and manufacturers will be compatible with the same barcode readers and computers. To read the barcode, a laser beam scanner must strike the code; the light reflected back is then interpreted by the computer. Barcode readers may be incorporated into hand-held wands that the technologist aims at the test tube label. Readers built into the instrumentation require only that the technologist place the test tube onto the instrument, which then aligns the tube and reads the code automatically. The ability of the barcode reader to read barcodes on curved surfaces makes this technology especially useful for specimen identification in the clinical laboratory.

Barcodes were first adapted to automated instrumentation for the identification of specimens directly on the analyzers. The specimen would enter the laboratory and a technologist would pour off aliquots for the various workstations. The technologist at the automated workstations would then have to sort all aliquots and assign each barcode. Currently, barcodes are commonly used for identification in all areas of the laboratory and thus are applied to the specimen upon accession, with the barcode acting as the laboratory accession number. Some systems also use barcodes for patient identification, including a barcode as the accession number on the patient's wristband at the time of admission. This allows for barcodes to be used at order entry, patient identification, and specimen processing, and for all clinical testing. For use with patient identification, the HIS and LIS must both read barcodes and be able to share the barcode information. Printers must also be available with barcode printing capabilities to print barcodes directly onto wrist bands and specimen labels.

The use of barcodes in the laboratory significantly reduces manual labor and error incidence while increasing productivity and improving the quality of patient care. Labor is reduced by elimination of manual entering and sorting at clinical workstations. A worklist is also unnecessary, as the instrument will identify each specimen by reading the barcode and match that identification to the LIS patient information when transferring results. Error is reduced because barcode readers misread 1 in 15,000 to 1 in 36 trillion characters, whereas a human being misreads approximately 1 in 300 characters.[7] The shortened turnaround time for laboratory tests reflects the ability of the barcode reader to read 12 characters in 0.3 to 2.0 seconds,[7] reducing the time necessary for specimen identification by approximately 30 per cent.[8]

Instrument Interface

Computerized instruments used in the clinical laboratory may be linked to the LIS through an interface that allows direct communication between the two systems. The transfer of demographics and other data from the LIS to the instrument is referred to as downloading. Data and results obtained by testing on the instrument are then transferred back to the LIS, the process of uploading. This connection between the two systems saves technologist time and also reduces transcription errors when information is read from one system and entered into the other. To avoid errors that occur during transmission of information between the two systems, particularly in the numbers obtained for results on the instrument, a *checksum* is used to verify the data sent from the instrument.[1] First, the data obtained are put through a built-in series of calculations by the instrument, and a final numerical value is obtained. All the data are then transmitted to the LIS. Following transmission, the same series of calculations are performed on the data, and the final numerical value is compared with the final value obtained on the instrument. If the two values do not match, the data are flagged with a transmission error, and the procedure is repeated until the transfer takes place without error. This computer verification eliminates the need for a technologist to verify large quantities of numerical results.

Communications

An *electronic mail (EMail)* system within the LIS allows for communications between users at the system terminals. Messages may be sent from user to user through the EMail system as an improvement of interdepartmental correspondence. During user log-in, a message will appear informing the user that there are new messages in the file directed at that user. That message will appear each time the user signs on until the messages are read and the system is commanded to erase the messages.

The LIS may also be used for communications as an electronic library of laboratory information for use by clinicians. Such a *test catalog* contains pertinent information for each test available in the laboratory, such as indications for ordering the test, specimen requirements, reference ranges, test interferences, methodologies, and so on. The same database is shared with the laboratory itself for actual specimen processing and result reporting.[9]

FUTURE TRENDS

Advances in computer technology have resulted in smaller-sized machines capable of powerful applications. This technology is being put into use in the clinical setting through portable LIS terminals available to the staff. The mobility of a hand-held terminal provides access to the LIS at the patient bedside by a technologist or other staff member. A barcode reader attached to the terminal is used to identify the patient, and the technologist could require the LIS to review tests ordered, verify specimen requirements, and identify any special instructions. A small printer attached to the terminal prints barcode labels for the specimens to be collected. After collection, the technologist changes the specimen status at the patient bedside, and the LIS automatically records the time, date, and identification of the technologist. Hand-held terminals are not widely used with laboratory systems at present because of the prohibitively high price of the hardware.

Computer technology will continue to play a vital role in the clinical laboratory by determining the capabilities of Laboratory Information Systems. The only clear prediction that can be made is that the LIS will become an even more powerful tool in the laboratory, influencing the development of automated instrumentation.

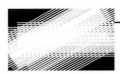

REVIEW QUESTIONS

Choose all the responses that are true.

1. Devices that fall into the category of input/output include:

   a. monitor.
   b. RAM.
   c. keyboard.
   d. CPU.
   e. printer.

2. Devices that fall into the category of secondary storage include:

   a. RAM.
   b. hard discs.
   c. floppy discs.
   d. modems.
   e. optical discs.

3. A simple system that may be programmed into a LIS to verify accession numbers is the:

   a. access code.
   b. check digit.
   c. delta check.
   d. system flag.

4. The system that may be programmed into a LIS that compares current results with previous results and alerts the technologist to any inconsistencies is the:

   a. checksum.
   b. check digit.
   c. delta check.
   d. reflex test.

5. The system that may be programmed into a LIS to verify data passed over an instrument interface is the:

   a. access code.
   b. check digit.
   c. checksum.
   d. delta check.

6. The use of barcodes for patient identification in the laboratory:

   a. greatly reduces transcription errors.
   b. shortens the time required for data entry.

REFERENCES

1. Aller RD, Elevitch FR: Hospital and laboratory information systems. *Clin Lab Med*, 1991.
2. Tietz NW: *Fundamentals of Clinical Chemistry*, 3rd edition. Philadelphia, WB Saunders, 1987.
3. Eggert AA, et al: Migrating a clinical Laboratory Information System between technologies. *J Med Systems* 15:379–389, 1991.
4. Aller RD, Elevitch FR: Computers in the clinical laboratory. *Clin Lab Med*, 1993.
5. Kaplan LA, Pesce AJ: *Clinical Chemistry: Theory, Analysis, and Correlation*, 2nd edition. St. Louis, CV Mosby, 1988.
6. Bradshaw KE, Gardner RM, Pryor TA: Development of a computerized laboratory alerting system. *Computers Biomed Res* 22:575–587, 1989.
7. Garza D, et al: Bar code technology in the clinical laboratory. *Clin Lab Sci* 4:23–25, 1991.
8. Tilzer LL, Jones RW: Use of bar code labels on collection tubes for specimen management in the clinical laboratory. *Arch Pathol Lab Med* 112:1200–1202, 1988.
9. Lazinger B, Steif J, Granit E: An online test catalog for clinical laboratories. *J Med Systems* 13:187–192, 1989.

BIBLIOGRAPHY

Bishop ML, Duben-Engelkirk JL, Fody EP: *Clinical Chemistry: Principles, Procedures, Correlations*, 2nd edition. Philadelphia, JB Lippincott, 1992.

Connelly DP: Embedding expert systems in Laboratory Information Systems. *Am J Clin Pathol* 94 (Suppl 1):S7–S14, 1990.

Eggert AA, Emmerich KA: Long-term data storage in a clinical Laboratory Information System. *J Med Systems* 13:347–353, 1989.

Friedman BA: The Laboratory Information System as a tool for implementing a strategic plan. *Am J Clin Pathol* 92 (Suppl 1):S38–S43, 1989.

Johnson LJ: Computer skills deemed necessary for entry level medical technologists. *Lab Med* 23:44–46, 1992.

Krieg AF, et al: *Clinical Laboratory Computerization.* Baltimore, University Park Press, 1971.

Lazinger B: A generalized laboratory software package—A prototype approach. *J Med Systems* 13:253–259, 1989.

Parvin CA, Hockett RD: Extending the capabilities of a laboratory computer system through cooperative processing. *J Med Systems* 11:359–365, 1987.

Robboy SJ, Trost R: Information in the clinical laboratory. *Ad Clin Chem* 27:269–301, 1989.

INTRODUCTION
ANALYTICAL SYSTEMS

A LOOK INTO THE FUTURE

Chapter 14

CHEMISTRY INSTRUMENTATION FOR THE SMALL OFFICE LABORATORY

HERBERT K. NAITO, PhD, MBA
YUN-SIK KWAK, MD, PhD

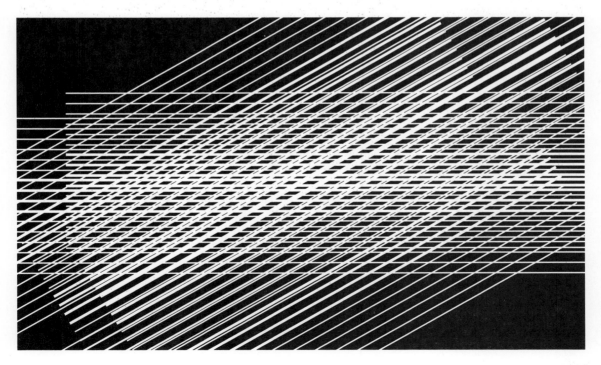

LEARNING OBJECTIVES

After studying this chapter, the student should be able to:

- List criteria to follow when selecting tabletop instrument systems.
- Identify advantages and disadvantages for the following tabletop analyzers: Seralyzer III, Reflotron, DT-60, Vision, Ready, and Analyst.
- Discuss the precision and accuracy of each analytical system.
- List instrument systems whose performance characteristics (precision and accuracy) are not dependent upon the technical skills and background of the operator.
- Discuss cost considerations for instrument acquisition and cost per test.

KEY WORDS

Accudata Glucose Test Station. A portable quality control management station used to assure reliability of glucose results at the patient's bedside.

AccuMeter. A small disposable cholesterol analyzer manufactured by ChemTrak, Sunnyvale, CA.

Analyst. A table-top chemistry profile analyzer manufactured by Dupont Corporation, Wilmington, DE.

DT-60/DTSC/DTE. A modular multichemistry table-top analyzer system manufactured by Eastman Kodak, Rochester, NY.

"Hot line." An emergency, 24-hour, manufacturer-manned troubleshooting phone line.

I-STAT. A hand-held microprocessor-controlled, ion-sensitive electrode, stat analyzer manufactured by I-Stat Corporation, Princeton, NJ.

One Touch II. A whole blood glucometer (Lifescan, Inc., Mountain View, CA).

POL (Physician Office Laboratory). A small laboratory that relies on smaller instrumentation.

Ready. Small table-top chemistry analyzer manufactured by Roche Diagnostic Systems, Montclair, NY.

Reflotron. A compact dry-reagent strip table-top analyzer manufactured by Boehringer-Manheim Corporation, Indianapolis, IN.

Seralyzer III. A table-top chemistry analyzer manufactured by Miles Laboratories, Elkhart, IN.

VISION. A table-top chemistry analyzer manufactured by Abbott Laboratories, Chicago, IL.

INTRODUCTION

Since the introduction of table-top or desk-top chemistry analyzers in the early 1980s, a new generation of compact instruments has emerged that are smaller, lighter, faster, and more user-friendly, with larger computer capabilities and test menus. They also are more reliable and accurate. There are now well over two dozen of these compact chemistry systems[1] that are being used for screening projects, wellness centers, bedside testing, other alternative-site testing (such as in emergency rooms, operating rooms, and outpatient clinics), and **physician office laboratories (POLs).** These newer-generation analyzers all have a general feature in common—they are far more automated and user-friendly than previous models.

Automation is the mechanization of steps in a test procedure, which generally include (a) specimen handling and delivery, (b) reagent handling and delivery, (c) mixing of sample and reagent(s), (d) incubation of the enzymatic reaction (25°, 30°, or 37°C), (e) measurement of the reaction, (f) calculation of the results, and (g) reporting and storage of the results.

Purchase of these instruments for the POL has grown rapidly because they are designed to:

- Provide rapid laboratory test results for patients on a single visit, which expedites diagnosis and treatment of patients. This is ultimately related to earlier treatment, greater convenience to the patient, and in most instances lower health care cost to the patient.
- Provide more convenient and effective means of monitoring the prognosis of a disease or the effectiveness of therapy.
- Increase efficiency of the physician's practice. When a test is sent to a reference laboratory, it takes an additional 14 minutes to retrieve the patient's chart, log the results in, and inform the patient by telephone of the laboratory results.
- Increase profitability for practitioners. Since the present third-party reimbursement system is based on *who* does the

test, in most instances it is to the advantage of the physician to do the test. When there is sufficient volume of tests, effective use of the CPT (Current Procedure Terminology) codes,* a cost-effective analytical system for the setting, and an efficiently run POL, additional revenues can be realized.

■ Enter new niches in the market place for increased profitability for manufacturers.

Manufacturers' data suggest that during the 1980s there was a substantial growth in the purchase of these small instruments for alternative-site testing (Fig. 14–1). In a national survey, slightly over half (52 per cent) of the 550 respondents indicated that alternative testing was being performed at their institution and that such testing had increased in the past 3 to 5 years.[2] In fact, 26 per cent stated that there was a significant increase, another 26 per cent indicated a slight increase, and only 10 per cent indicated a decrease in that activity. Also, 54 per cent indicated that they expected alternative-site testing to grow in the next 3 to 5 years. According to the survey data, STAT testing increased (44 per cent of the respondents) and 38 per cent felt that bedside/satellite testing was an effective solution to STAT testing. Those who did not feel that this was the case voiced concerns about the lack of quality control, the lack of expertise to operate the instruments, duplication of laboratory service, and less accurate instruments.

Forty-seven per cent of the respondents in the survey[2] stated that the physicians' office laboratories competed with their laboratory for test orders, suggesting that the POLs are a relatively large niche in the health care system. The large growth in this segment of the market during the 1980s has met some resistance by physicians because of the implementation of new regulatory laws based on the modification of the Clinical Laboratory Improvement Act (CLIA 1967). Until the laws are clarified and finalized, physicians who are interested in being involved with POLs will take a precautionary stand.

Although there are many choices of small chemistry analyzers, only a half dozen of the most popular analytical systems will be discussed in detail in this chapter. No one analyzer can be considered the "best"—they all have advantages and disadvantages. Thus, it is important to define the exact function of the compact analyzer in a specified environment. It could be a STAT laboratory that handles specimens for 75 glucose, 25 glycolated hemoglobin, and 12 phenytoin tests per day, with one registered medical technician, or a POL that does 18 admission panels (with 15 chemistries) and 4 drugs and 6 electrolytes per day with the help of three rotating persons (a nurse, receptionist, and physician) to do approximately 55 tests. Or it could be a screening event at the state fair, or a convention for which only cholesterol is tested with the help of volunteers with no previous laboratory experience. The volume of tests, the kind of analytes to be measured, the complexity of testing (organ profile panels, STAT, and so on), the technical skills and numbers of the operators, turnaround time requirements, fees per test, current reimbursement schedules, and the complexity, flexibility, reliability, and convenience features of the analytical system are just some of the important considerations when selecting a compact chemistry analyzer for alternative-site testing.

In general, the following considerations should be helpful when evaluating an instrument system:

---

*CPT is a systematic listing of descriptive terms and identifying codes for reporting medical services and procedures performed by physicians. The CPT codes are used mainly for the reporting of physician procedures and services under government and private health insurance programs for reimbursement purposes.

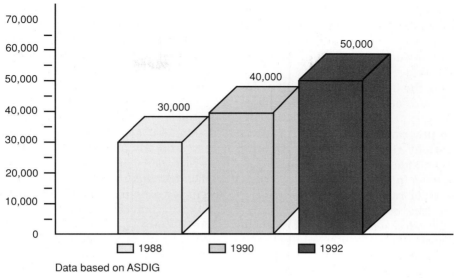

■ FIGURE 14–1.

Estimated growth of in-office testing based on the numbers of chemistry analyzers purchased between 1988 and 1992.

- Is it user-friendly, easy to operate?
- How much training is necessary to become competent as an operator of the instrument?
- How complex is the preventive maintenance program?
- How frequently must preventive maintenance be done?
- Is the calibration simple for each analyte?
- Is the need for recalibration frequent: every run, every week, every 3 months?
- Is switching from one test to another simple or even automatic by barcode identification?
- Is the within-day and day-to-day precision good, as in a 2 to 4 per cent (coefficient of variation (CV)?
- Has the manufacturer demonstrated accuracy with each test by doing parallel runs with a recognized or approved reference method?
- Is it compact, requiring little bench space?

- Is the throughput of test results fast enough for the needs of the laboratory?
- Is it a walkaway system or does the operator need to be present for most of the operation?
- How automated is the system?
- Does it identify the test (reagents) by barcode?
- Does it minimize critical manual measurements, e.g., specimen and reagent pipeting?
- Does it require specimen manipulation or dilution before analysis?
- Can it provide a hard copy of the results with the patient's name, identification number, date of analysis, chemistry results, reference ranges, name of operator?
- Can it identify a short or insufficient sample?
- Can it identify outdated reagents or reagents that have deteriorated and are unacceptable?

- Can it flag patient values that may be inaccurate because of excessive concentrations of known interfering substances in the specimen, such as bilirubin, hemoglobin, turbidity?
- Can it alert the operator that quality control values are outside the tolerance limits?
- Can it be programmed to prevent reporting of patient results when the quality control is outside of tolerance limits?
- Does it have a large test menu?
- Is it a batch or random-access system?
- What are the reagent storage requirements, i.e., freezer, refrigerator, room temperature? What about humidity?
- Do frozen or refrigerated items need to be brought to room temperature before analysis can proceed?
- What is the start-up time, that is, time from daily preparation of the instrument, reconstituting or preparing all reagents, controls, specimens, and calibration? Does it need a warm-up time?
- Do the calibrator and quality control materials have to be reconstituted with a specific volume of distilled water or diluent or are they ready to use without further manipulation?
- Is the shelf-life of the calibrator and quality control materials relatively long (1 to 2 months) to minimize frequent reconstitution (increase convenience and reduce labor and material cost)?
- What are the specimen requirements? Can it do whole blood, serum, and plasma? What is the minimum volume of specimens that it needs?
- Is the cost per test competitive, including the cost of reagents, calibrators, quality control materials, number of repeat analyses, hands-on labor? What is the cost of the " reportable test? "
- What is the cost of the instrument? How does it compare with a lease-option plan?

Is there a volume discount on reagents and other consumable supplies?
- Is it the least operator-dependent system?
- According to the new regulatory Test Complexity Model, in which category does it belong?

One of the major errors when selecting an instrument system is overemphasizing the cost. In many instances the initial cost may seem expensive, but certain added convenience features, its dependability, and being a highly automated, walkaway system may make it competitive with lower-priced systems. Usually, if a medical technologist, nurse, or physician operates the system, the most expensive component in the cost per test is not the instrument or consumable items but labor. Thus, the more automated and walkaway the analytical system, the better the cost per test.

Neglected areas when evaluating an instrument purchase are the cost of the service contract, negotiating discounts on consumables and the dependability of a technical or sales representative when technical assistance is needed. Manufacturers who have a commitment to quality and service should be selected. An expression of this commitment can be in the form of a dedicated **"hot line"** by which the manufacturer provides technical assistance around the clock 7 days a week, or in the form of frequent visits by the local sales representative. Manufacturers who provide their own quality assurance, quality control, or proficiency testing programs reinforce their commitment to excellence. One of the most reliable means of obtaining information on a manufacturer's product and sales and technical representatives is by communicating with the local hospital laboratory personnel (pathologists, clinical chemists, medical technologists). Their experience and expertise on this subject are invaluable. Their opinions on the manufacturer, the local sales representative, the analytical performance and dependability of the instrument/reagent system, and the company's commitment to quality and service should be regarded with high esteem during the decision-making process. Also, data on product evaluations in scientific journals can enlighten the fact-finding mission.

Another effective means of obtaining reliable information on a manufacturer's product is by obtaining a users' or clients' list and calling these people about their experiences. There is no substitute for obtaining hands-on experience; the system always should be field-tested for several days before purchase as in buying an automobile.

In evaluating the performance of the instruments discussed in the next section, the analyte of choice was cholesterol because it is the most frequently tested specimen in the POL, and because it has been used as a national "role model analyte" for the laboratory community in terms of analytical goals for precision and accuracy, which is 3.0 per cent CV or less for precision and 3.0 per cent or less from true value for accuracy. These guidelines were established by expert committees of the National Institutes of Health National Cholesterol Education Program, one of which was the Laboratory Standardization Panel.[3] The fact that the expert panel recognized the National Committee for Clinical Laboratory Standards National Reference System for Cholesterol, which includes the Abell-Kendall[4] reference method and the isotopic-dilution mass spectroscopy definitive method,[5] made it possible to develop such definitive guidelines. Today, the true value for cholesterol is established by either the reference method or the definitive method.

A key point to remember when evaluating accuracy is that one should always focus on an instrument system with the highest precision, because consistent accuracy is not possible with poor precision. With proper calibration, most systems can deliver accurate cholesterol values, if imprecision is not an issue. In today's clinical and reference laboratories, long-term precision of 2 to 3 per cent CV is customary on most dependable, large automated chemistry analyzers. Many compact chemistry analyzers can achieve precision similar to the large analyzers. Carefully selected compact chemistry analyzers can provide reliable analytical data. The real challenge in alternative-site testing is finding instruments with ease of operation and nonoperator-dependent systems that require little knowledge, skill, and experience in the user yet provide reliable patient results in a timely fashion. Some of the more commonly used analyzers will be discussed in this chapter. Refer to Table 14–4 for a summary of these instrument systems.

ANALYTICAL SYSTEMS

Seralyzer III

Manufacturer. Ames Division, Miles Laboratories, Inc., Elkhart, Indiana; 1(800) 248-2637

Instrument. This dry chemistry analyzer (plastic strips with a dry reagent pad impregnated with reagents) measures the concentration of a particular analyte by reflectance spectrophotometry. The unit is 28 cm wide, 46 cm deep, and 14 cm high and weighs 10 kg (Fig. 14–2). It has a digital display screen, but no printout device is included. It has a port so that a printer can be hooked up to the instrument, for this is not provided by the manufacturer. The **Seralyzer** differs from the other desk-top analyzers in that it has a hand-held, battery-operated pipeting step for *diluting* the specimen

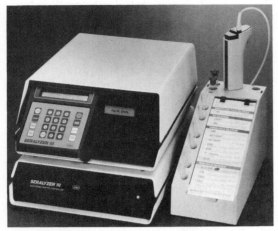

■ **FIGURE 14–2.**

Seralyzer III (Miles Laboratories, Elkhart, IN) with the automatic diluter (pipette) station.

(up to ninefold, depending on the chemistry) with water before applying the mixture to the dry reagent pad. The calibration is a two-level program in which the data for the calibration curve are stored for 2 weeks. However, weekly or biweekly calibration may be preferred to enhance the reliability of the analytical data.

For each analyte, a different test module that identifies the analytical parameters is inserted into the instrument, and the reflected signals are processed and converted into patient results with the appropriate units.

The Seralyzer III is considered a semiautomated system. However, it is not as automated as other systems: each specimen is loaded one at a time, which may be an issue if time and personnel are limited; in addition, one must consider the dilution step. Daily start-up time (which includes daily instrument preparation, warm-up time, calibration, reconstituting calibrators and quality control (QC) materials, preparing dilutions) is about 15 minutes. Hands-on time to perform one test is about 8 to 10 minutes.

The assay time is 1.5 to 4.5 minutes, depending on the analyte. The usual speed of the system is about 40 specimens per hour. The specimen-loading schedule of one sample at a time is not a convenient feature and is suited to small-volume laboratories.

Depending on the volume of daily tests done, the average cost per test is $1.00 to $3.00, which does not include labor, daily QC materials, any consumable materials (pipet tips, test tubes), or depreciation of the equipment. The instrument cost is $4,495.

Specimen. The minimum sample required is 100 μL of plasma or serum (added to 300 to 800 μL of water, depending on the test). It is not a whole-blood analyzer; thus, a centrifuge is required to process the specimen.

Analytical Performance. Most of the studies concerning the Seralyzer II and III[6–19] indicate that this system generally has a higher imprecision for various analytes when compared with other compact analyzers, particularly if the analyses were done by a non-laboratorian or medical technologist or technician with little technical background and skills; the problems are magnified if personnel rotate. Bills and associates reported a mean between-run CV on two levels of commercial QC materials and one patient specimen (on 5 successive days) of 3.0 per cent for glucose, 6.3 per cent for uric acid, 4.0 per cent for potassium, and 7.6 per cent for cholesterol.[19] These CVs can be considered relatively high when compared with the VISION, DT-60, and Gemstar, which were also evaluated by four certified clinical laboratory scientists.

The study of Nanji and colleagues demonstrates the greater imprecision and inaccuracy of this system with nontechnical personnel operating it.[17] Comparing results of various analytes obtained by the nontechnologists, which exceeded 5 per cent from the values obtained by the trained medical technologists, the Seralyzer was found to

TABLE 14–1. PRECISION STUDIES USING CHOLESTEROL FOR FIVE COMPACT CHEMISTRY ANALYZERS (mg/dL)*

ANALYZER	NUMBER OF ANALYSES	DAY-TO-DAY		
		LOW POOL	MID POOL	HIGH POOL
Seralyzer	20	99.5 ± 5.5 (5.53%)†	201.5 ± 9.4 (4.66%)†	255.1 ± 11.4 (4.50%)†
Reflotron	15	105.1 ± 3.5 (3.37%)	178.9 ± 6.5 (3.62%)	227.8 ± 10.4 (3.73%)
Ready	20		212.3 ± 6.8 (3.20%)	243.0 ± 10.3 (4.20%)
DT-60	15	97.4 ± 2.5 (2.58%)	130.1 ± 4.8 (3.66%)	294.6 ± 6.9 (2.35%)
Vision	20		136.0 ± 2.8 (2.05%)	242.0 ± 4.9 (2.00%)

*Mean ± 1 standard deviation.
†Coefficient of variance, %.

have the least desirable accuracy performance (41 per cent). Results for the VISION were 6 per cent, the DT-60, 28 per cent, and the Reflotron, 17 per cent. The extra specimen-pipeting step, the specimen-diluting step, and the sample application step can contribute significantly to this problem, especially with a sample-to-water ratio of 1:8 in the specimen-dilution step.

The study of David and associates on long-term precision for total cholesterol is, perhaps, an example of maximal performance of five analytical systems under ideal laboratory conditions (Tables 14–1 and 14–2).[18] The Seralyzer III was compared with four other commonly used chemistry analyzers, which were all operated by a highly trained medical technologist (Fig. 14–3); the Seralyzer III precision was 4.9 per cent CV, which represented the average of three

TABLE 14–2. ACCURACY STUDIES FOR FIVE COMPACT CHEMISTRY ANALYZERS USING CHOLESTEROL MEASUREMENTS (mg/dL)*

ANALYZER	N	r†	REGRESSION LINE	P VALUE	BIAS (%)
Seralyzer	99	0.990	Y = 0.93× + 8.0	0.0001	−3.6
Reflotron	96	0.989	Y = 0.99× − 11.6	0.0001	−6.0
Ready	34	0.950	Y = 1.023 − 5.5	0.0001	−0.4
DT-60	108	0.994	Y = 1.006× − 2.5	0.0001	−0.3
VISION	100	0.992	Y = 0.967× + 9.5	0.0001	+0.5

*Comparing fresh patient specimens that were compared with a CDC standardized method traceable to the Abell-Kendall reference method.[4]
†Correlation coefficient.

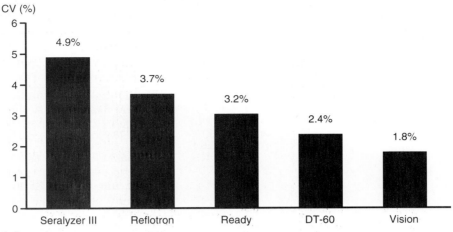

■ **FIGURE 14–3.**

A graphic representation of the average long-term precision of serum cholesterol measurements at three concentrations, using the Seralyzer III, Reflotron, Ready, DT-60, and VISION. (From David JA, Mooney CR, Naito HK: Comparison of physician office analyzers for cholesterol analysis in screening centers. *Clin Chem* 33(6):898, 1987.)

(high, medium, low) pools of QC materials analyzed over a 5-day period. Because the Seralyzer's performance is dependent on the technical skills of the operator, less than desirable results can occur if training is inadequate or if the trained operator is not being careful with the analytical steps. Thus, the fewer the steps, the less sample and reagent manipulation and pipeting, and the more automated the instrument, the better the analytical precision and accuracy.

The evaluation of the Seralyzer III for accuracy indicates that 99 fresh patient sera (covering a concentration range of 80 to 425 mg/dL) had a correlation coefficient (r) of 0.99, with a linear regression of $Y = 0.93 \times + 80$,[18] which means that the Seralyzer's values are lower than the cholesterol reference method values by about 3 per cent (Fig. 14–4). Similar findings were published by Lott and colleagues, who indicate an average precision (of two QC pools) of 4.1 per cent CV and a linear regression line of $Y = 0.966 \times + 3.5$ for 122 patient specimens analyzed in duplicate, which indicates about a 2 per cent overall bias.[9]

Test Menu. Bilirubin, cholesterol, creatinine, glucose, triglycerides, urea nitrogen, uric acid, potassium, aspartate aminotransferase (AST), alanine aminotransferase (ALT), lactate dehydrogenase (LD), creatine kinase (CK), carbamazepine, phenobarbital, phenytoin, theophylline, hemoglobin, digoxin, high-density lipoprotein cholesterol (HDL-C).

Desirable Features. Relatively fast analyzer (average 40 tests per hour); lightweight, portable; large test menu; relatively user-friendly (prompts on LCD); dry reagent strips stored at room temperature; reasonable cost per test (but labor-intensive); and low initial investment on instrument.

Less Desirable Features. Extra steps required for diluent pipeting, specimen pipeting, specimen application; very technique-dependent; precision and accuracy slightly less reliable than other systems; longer start-up time; more hands-on time; cannot use whole blood; frequent calibration (once a week) to achieve desired reliability; specimen loading one at a time; no multiple tests at one time; no patient identification

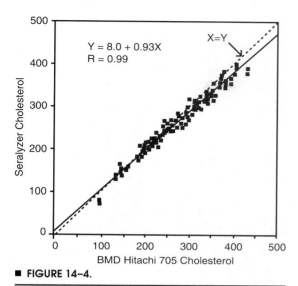

$Y = 8.0 + 0.93X$
$R = 0.99$

X=Y

■ **FIGURE 14–4.**

Linear regression curve illustrating the comparison of serum cholesterol measurements on the Seralyzer III (Miles Laboratories, Inc., Elkhart, IN) with a CDC-standardized method, the BMC/Hitachi 705 cholesterol method.

system or barcoding capabilities to facilitate test identification; not as automated as most systems; printout device not standard equipment.

Other Comments. This instrument is better suited for a POL or alternative site that does not intend to do a large amount of testing. Adequate training is paramount for good results; especially critical is the pipeting step for specimen dilution, which tends to be one of the major factors that leads to variability in analytical results. Because it is more labor-intensive, adequate staff planning is essential.

Reflotron

Manufacturer. Boehringer-Mannheim Corporation, Indianapolis, Indiana; (317) 845-2468.

Instrument. This dry chemistry analyzer has plastic strips with a glass-fiber pad to separate red blood cells from plasma, which then reacts with dry reagents impregnated in the strip; the developed color is read by reflectance spectrophotometry. The results appear on a display screen; thus, there is no printer (i.e., no hard copy). The instrument is small and compact, weighing 6 kg; it is 29 cm wide, 35 cm deep, and 19 cm high (Fig. 14–5). **Reflotron** is a semiautomated system; however, like the Seralyzer, it is less automated than other desk-top systems, e.g., each specimen is loaded one at a time and each specimen is analyzed one at a time, which may be an issue in a high-volume laboratory. Daily start-up time of the instrument is rapid, about 1 minute. The instrument assay time is 1 to 3 minutes, depending on the analyte that is being measured. Thus, it takes about 4 to 5 minutes to obtain a patient result (after QC materials have been run). The usual throughput of the system is about 20 specimens per hour, which makes it one of the slower systems on the market; this may not be an important issue if the POL does not have a large volume of patient specimens.

The system is calibrated before shipment from the manufacturer and does not need further regular recalibration, unless the instrument is dropped, severely bumped, or the QC values are not within acceptable limits (unrelated to reagents or QC materials). The optics system, however, must be checked every 2 weeks, which is an additional expense feature and a preventive maintenance requirement.

Depending on the quantity of tests performed, the average cost per test is about $1.60 to $3.00 (not including labor, QC materials, optics-checking test strips, and instrument depreciation). The cost of the instrument is $5,295.

Specimen. The minimum sample required is 30 μL of plasma, serum, or whole blood. Accuracy depends on obtaining a complete fill of the 30-μL capillary tube without bubbles. Ideally, the specimens should be

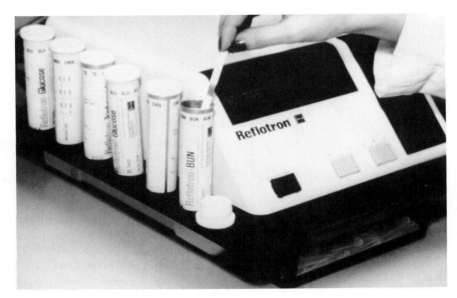

■ **FIGURE 14–5.**

The Reflotron (Boehringer-Mannheim Corporation, Indianapolis), shown with the dry reagent strip being removed from the canister containing a drying agent to insure elimination of moisture interference during measurement.

analyzed within 3 minutes, because even though the capillary tubes are heparin-coated, occasionally clotting occurs within the tubes to cause a "short" sample.

Analytical Performance. Most of the comparative studies on various compact chemistry analyzers indicate that the precision is between 3 and 5 per cent CV, depending on the analyte. It is a little less precise than the Kodak DT-60 or Abbott VISION systems.[17–27] The study of David and associates[18] on day-to-day precision of the Reflotron found the total cholesterol measurement to be 3.7 per cent CV, which was better than the Seralyzer but not as good as the Kodak, Roche, or Abbott analytical systems.

The accuracy studies on 99 fresh patient specimens indicate that there is relatively good comparison with the reference cholesterol method (Fig. 14–6). The correlation coefficient was 0.989 with a linear regression line of $Y = 0.990 \times -11.6$. Thus, the Reflotron can be considered accurate in the hands of a well-trained medical technologist with good laboratory skills. Kaufman and colleagues showed cholesterol measurement precision between 96 pairs of patient specimens to be 2.0 per cent for the VISION, 2.5 per cent for the DT-60, 2.6 per cent for the DuPont Analyst, 10.2 per cent for the Seralyzer, and 13.3 per cent for the Reflotron.[27] Their accuracy studies suggest that the bias was 0.8 per cent for the VISION, 1.4 per cent for the DT-60, 5.2 per cent for the Reflotron, 9.7 per cent for the Seralyzer, and 10.4 per cent for the Analyst. They concluded that the operation of the Reflotron is an operator- and instrument-dependent system. Rohac and Rohac demonstrated that the performance improved with additional training.[23] Gubata and Lefebvre reported considerable lot-to-lot variation of the Reflotron cholesterol reagent strips from the

■ **FIGURE 14–6.**

Linear regression curve illustrating the comparison of serum cholesterol measurements of fresh patient specimens on the Reflotron with a CDC-standardized method, the BMC/Hitachi 705 cholesterol method.

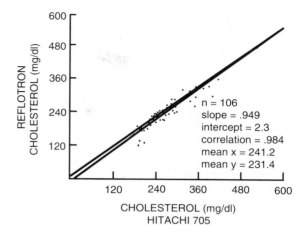

n = 106
slope = .949
intercept = 2.3
correlation = .984
mean x = 241.2
mean y = 231.4

manufacturer, which may be a contributing source of error.[28]

Test Menu. Amylase, bilirubin, cholesterol, creatinine, CK, hemoglobin, HDL-C, gamma-glutamyl transferase (GGT), potassium, AST, ALT, triglycerides, urea nitrogen, uric acid.

Desirable Features. User-friendly; compact and lightweight; requires little preventive maintenance; dry reagent strips stored at room temperature; large test menu; low initial investment on instrument; whole blood chemistries; quick start-up time; recalibration not generally required; barcode on each reagent strip to reset instrument automatically to each test chemistry.

Less Desirable Features. Relatively slow system (20 tests per hour); no printout device for reporting of results (thus, no hard copy and no walkaway system); cost of checking the optical system ($3.00/week or $150/yr); recalibration cannot be done on site readily by the operator; reagent strips susceptible to moisture uptake (causing bias results); QC materials need to be reconstituted with 10.0 mL of distilled water, short stability of QC materials; somewhat technique-dependent; precision and accuracy of results of some of the tests could be improved.

Other Comments. This system is very easy to learn to operate and would be ideal to use where there are multiple operators. The specimen collection by capillary tubes is a critical step and is dependent on good technical skills and training of the user. This system is best suited for smaller offices or alternative-site testing without a large volume of specimens. The manufacturer recently updated the Reflotron with the Reflotron Plus (Fig. 14–7), which has many sig-

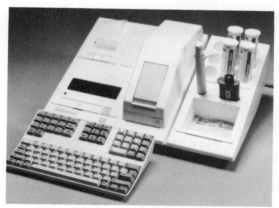

■ **FIGURE 14–7.**

The Reflotron Plus (Boehringer-Mannheim Corporation, Indianapolis), showing the addition of the keyboard and built-in printer.

nificant improvements, such as the addition of a printer. It has a full keyboard to enter patient data (age, gender, lipid and lipoprotein results, blood pressure, smoking, diabetes, and left ventricular hypertrophy status) to obtain a Heart Health (cardiac risk) Assessment, and to edit data and information to show patients how the risk of coronary heart disease can be lowered by compliance with treatment recommendations. The cost of the Reflotron Plus is $5,795.

The manufacturer has also recently introduced the ProAct Cholesterol System, which is a small, dedicated, hand-held dry chemistry cholesterol analyzer. It can be operated on four 1.5-volt AA batteries or by the use of a 110-volt AC adapter. The instrument has a serial port, which allows connection to a printer. The cost of the ProAct Cholesterol System is $995, and the cost per test is $2.

Kodak DT-60/DTSC/DTE

Manufacturer. Eastman Kodak Company, Rochester, New York; 1(800) 445-6325, ext 434.

Instrument. This instrument system is based on the famous Kodak film technology, in which the dry chemistry works with multilayer film impregnated with reagents, which are encased in a 1-inch-square plastic holder (Fig. 14–8). There are three modules (Fig. 14–9):

1. The DT-60, which does colorimetric endpoint chemistries; the signal is read by reflectance spectrophotometry,
2. The DTSC, which does the special chemistries by kinetic-rate colorimetric assays read by reflectance spectrophotometry,
3. The DTE, which measures electrolytes by potentiometric methods.

A motor-driven manual pipet is used to dispense the specimen onto the slide, followed

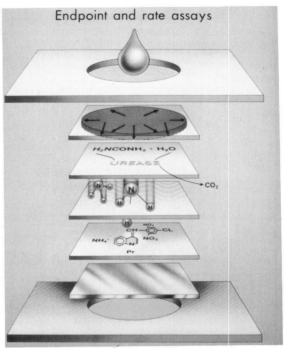

Endpoint and rate assays

■ **FIGURE 14–8.**

The Ektachem (Eastman Kodak Company, Rochester, NY), a layered, dry-slide technology used in over 30 chemistries.

by an incubation period of 40 seconds to several minutes, depending on the analyte being measured. The values are displayed on the screen, and a hard copy is provided by a built-in printer. The daily start-up time (which includes daily preparation of the instrument and reconstituting of the reagents and controls to be in a "ready" state for analysis) is about 35 minutes, which is one of the longer times of the instruments compared. Most of that time (20 minutes) is for instrument warm-up (to raise the incubation temperature to appropriate levels for the different chemistry reactions). Since the reagents and control materials are stored in the refrigerator, they should be brought to room temperature (20 to 30 minutes, depending upon whether stored in the freezer

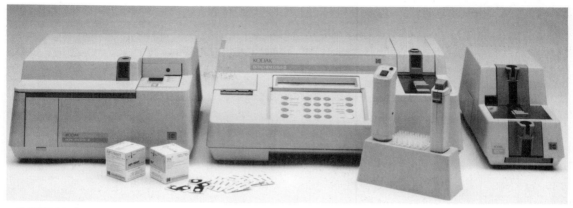

■ **FIGURE 14–9.**

Ektachem DT system (Eastman Kodak Company, Rochester, NY). Left to right: DTSC module for special chemistries, DT-60 analyzer for routine chemistries, and DTE module for electrolyte tests with battery-operated, handheld pipette in the foreground.

or refrigerator and on the room temperature). Forgetting to do either warm-up will cause a delay in the start-up time. Because the Kodak system is a random-access system with barcoded slides for test identification, multiple different test combinations do not significantly lengthen the start-up time or assay time.

The usual throughput for the **DT-60, DTSC,** and **DTE** is about 65, 20, and 15 tests/hour, respectively. The assay time of the DT-60 chemistries averages about 5 minutes, of the DTSC chemistries 3 to 5 minutes (depending on the concentration), and of the DTE chemistries around 3 minutes. Specimen-loading is up to six slides at a time for the DT-60 chemistries and only one at a time for the DTSC and DTE. The DT-60 is 48 cm wide, 35 cm deep, and 17 cm high and weighs 11.6 kg. The DTSC is 34 cm wide, 34 cm deep, and 17 cm high and weighs 7.7 kg. The DTE is 15 cm wide, 35 cm deep, and 17 cm high and weighs 3.7 kg.

The cost per test (only reagent cost) is $1.45 to $2.75 for the DT-60 chemistries, $1.50 to $4.05 for the DTSC chemistries, and $1.75 for the DTE chemistries. The modules cost $5,500 for the DT-60, $3,300 for the DTSC, and $3,200 for the DTE, which totals $12,000 for the entire analytical system. The modular concept is designed to tailor the system to the needs of the customer without overbuying and to allow expansion of the system as the workload and testing increase.

Analytical Performance. Most of the published studies on this analytical system indicate that it is very accurate and precise with most of the chemistries.[17, 18, 24, 27, 29–32] As an example, the day-to-day precision over a 5-day period for total cholesterol on the DT-60 averaged 2.4 per cent CV for the high, medium, and low concentration QC materials analyzed.[18] The accuracy study on 108 fresh patient sera indicated a correlation coefficient of 0.994, with a linear regression line of $Y = 1.006X - 2.5$. Figure 14–10 demonstrates the excellent correlation of the Kodak method to the Abell-Kendall cholesterol reference method.[4] However, it should be emphasized that in that study, a well-trained, highly skilled medical technologist performed the assays. Nanji and associates demonstrated that the average preci-

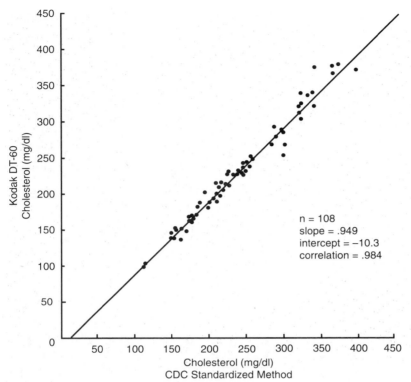

n = 108
slope = .949
intercept = −10.3
correlation = .984

■ **FIGURE 14–10.**

Linear-regression curve illustrating the comparison of serum cholesterol measurements of fresh patient specimens on the DT-60 and CDC standardized method, BMC/Hitachi 705 cholesterol method.

sion on the DT-60 was 8.2 ± 11.5 per cent CV on different chemistries done by 27 nontechnologists, which included nurses, physicians, and medical students.[17] The registered medical technologist had a mean precision of 4.2 ± 5.9 per cent CV for the same analytes, suggesting that, like the Seralyzer (8.0 ± 4.75 per cent CV versus 4.9 ± 1.4 per cent CV) and to a lesser extent the Reflotron (4.3 ± 1.6 per cent CV versus 3.2 ± 1.3 per cent CV), the DT-60's performance is technique dependent and thus influenced by the skills and training of the operator. Unlike the Abbott VISION (1.9 ± 0.4 per cent CV versus 2.0 ± 0.4 per cent CV), the Kodak system is better suited for laboratorians than nonlaboratorians, unless extensive training is part of the routine protocol.

As expected, as the imprecision went up,

the inaccuracies of results also went up. The number of test results by the nontechnologists that exceeded the test results of the trained registered medical technologist by 10 per cent or greater were 27 per cent by the Seralyzer, 19.3 per cent by the DT-60, 3.4 per cent by the Reflotron, and 0 per cent by the VISION. The study of Belsey and colleagues demonstrates the importance of considering the intended operators of the instrument when purchasing a compact chemistry analyzer for POLs.[30, 31] This study found that the precision and accuracy of testing were worse with the family medicine residents, a licensed practical nurse, and a secretary, compared with results of the registered medical technologist. As an example, the average precision of glucose for the four nonlaboratorians was 13.7 per cent CV, compared with 1.3 per cent for the medical technologist. Belsey and colleagues concluded that the combination of imprecision and inaccuracy of the glucose test on the DT-60 used by the nonlaboratorians could result in different patient management decisions than those based on the comparison method.

Test Menu

DT-60. Glucose, urea nitrogen, uric acid, cholesterol, amylase, HDL-C, total protein, triglycerides, magnesium, total bilirubin, creatinine, ammonia, hemoglobin, phosphorus, lactic acid.

DTSC. LD, AST, ALT, CK, CK-MB, GGT, alkaline phosphatase, calcium, creatinine, theophylline, albumin, lipase, cholinesterase.

DTE. Sodium, potassium, chloride, carbon dioxide.

Desirable Features. The tests on the DT-60 are fast, but the special chemistries and electrolytes are slow; the DT-60 is compact and lightweight (25 lb), but the whole group collectively weighs 51 lb; the DT-60 has six incubator slots; it has a printer (thus, a walkaway system) for patient results with identification number; reliable data can be obtained with a well-trained person; recalibration can be performed on-site.

Less Desirable Features. Cannot do whole blood; the pipeting step is critical; slides need to be brought to room temperature; slides taken out of the wrapper earlier than 15 minutes before analysis causes bias results; the instrument needs 20 to 30 minutes of start-up (warm-up) time; reagents need to be brought to room temperature; QC and calibration materials need to be reconstituted with distilled water; short shelf-life of calibration and QC materials (1 to 7 days when refrigerated); slides in the wrapper are unstable at room temperature beyond 48 hours (refrigeration needed), slides out of the wrapper are not reliable after 15 min-

utes; recalibration system is more complicated; some tests are expensive.

Other Comments. This system can be used in larger-sized POLs if the DT-60 module only is being used. The DTSC and DTE modules may not be rapid enough if a large volume of testing is required. This instrument system has the capabilities of delivering excellent laboratory data, comparable to the clinical or reference laboratory. However, it is more sophisticated (and thus, more complex) than other table-top analyzers, which requires attention to details in the training sessions. If more than one user operates the instrument, consistency can be achieved by thorough, standardized training of everyone. The sample pipeting step is critical and has the potential of causing errors; e.g., pushing the button of the hand-held pipet causes aspiration of the specimen, followed by a soft beep to alert the operator to remove the pipet and wipe the tip after the second beep. If the pipet tip is still in the specimen tube after the second beep, a 20 per cent positive bias will occur because of the 2 μL of specimen that was aspirated instead of air. The barcode system makes this a batch as well as a multiple-test selective analyzer. Kodak's toll-free technical hotline for customer service is excellent.

VISION

Manufacturer. Abbott Laboratories, Abbott Park, Illinois; 1(800) 323-9100.

Instrument. The **VISION** chemistries are based on conventional wet reagents; however, this is a very sophisticated system[33] and the reagents are packaged in an innovative multichambered test cartridge (Fig. 14–11). In this cartridge, an aliquot of the specimen is mixed with the reagents through a series of automatic cartridge rotations during the centrifugation process. Whole blood can be used because during the

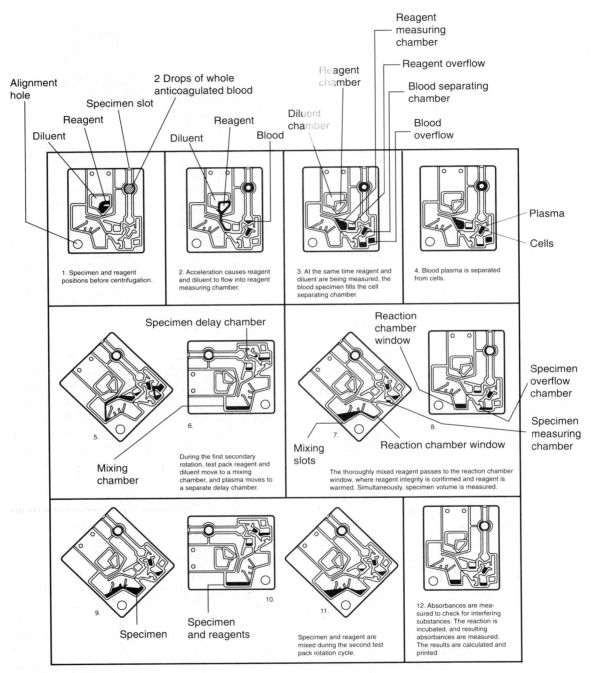

■ **FIGURE 14-11.**

VISION (Abbott Laboratories, Abbott Park, IL) multichambered test cartridge, containing wet reagents to measure a specific analyte (n = 28). (Reproduction of *Details of Fluid Movement Inside the TestPack and Vision Instrument Photo* has been granted with approval of Abbott Laboratories, all rights reserved by Abbott Laboratories.)

centrifugation process the red blood cells are separated from the plasma. The absorbance reading of the various chemistries are converted to concentration units of the measured analyte, and a built-in printout device provides a hard copy with the patient's identification number and result(s).

The system is fully automated; there are only three basic steps: (a) add the specimen to the cartridge, (b) place the cartridge into one of the ten holders in the instrument, and (c) press the "Start" button. There are no critical pipeting steps. The barcoded cartridges identify the test to be done. The system is both a random-access and batch analyzer. Thus, the assay time for doing one test or ten tests of the same analyte or ten different analytes in the same run is the same; the average time is about 11 minutes. The daily instrument warm-up time is short, less than 1 minute. Although the cartridges, calibrator, and control materials are stored in the refrigerator, warm-up time is not an issue because a sophisticated, built-in thermal device will bring the specimen, reagents, and calibrator to the proper incubation temperature for the enzymatic reactions of the various wet chemistries. The average assay time is about 11 minutes, and the average test turnaround time is 60 specimens per hour.

The VISION instrument utilizes a three-level calibration program, which is good for 3 months or until the control material fails. The system is 53 cm wide, 53 cm deep, and 43 cm high and weighs 32 kg (Fig. 14–12). The cost per test (reagent cost only) is $1.75 to $6.25 for the more esoteric drug testing. The cost of the instrument is $17,495. However, since it is a fully automated, walkaway system with little hands-on time, the labor cost is reduced. According to Bills and colleagues,[19] the total cost (which includes amortizing the initial instrument cost over 5 years, service, labor at $10.00/hour, reagent and other consumables), based on running 20 assays per day, 22 days per month, is

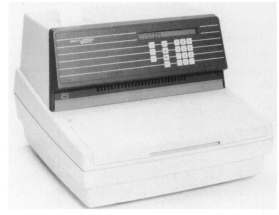

■ **FIGURE 14–12.**

VISION Analyzer (Abbott Laboratories, Abbott Park, IL), showing built-in printer and visual display screen. (Reproduction of *Details of Fluid Movement Inside the TestPack and Vision Instrument Photo* has been granted with approval of Abbott Laboratories, all rights reserved by Abbott Laboratories.)

$3.30, compared with $2.99 for the Kodak DT-60 and $3.10 for the Ames Seralyzer.

This is a good illustration of the importance of examining all components when considering total cost per test and not just the initial cost of instrumentation. As the volume of testing increases, the cost per test will decrease on semiautomated and fully automated systems. Labor can be a significant factor in the cost per test when one considers the hands-on time necessary to do the test and the level of technical skill required. The salary of a medical technologist, physician's assistant, or registered nurse versus a laboratory aide, receptionist, or nurse's aide could make a large difference in the cost per test. Also, in evaluating operator's time, Bills and colleagues[19] found the Seralyzer, DT-60, and Gemstar to have a significantly higher requirement than that of the VISION. Finally, the issue of convenience is an underestimated factor when selecting a chemistry instrument. The only person who truly examines that factor in detail is the operator. The Abbott VISION

System has ease of use, simplicity, reliability, and convenience.

Specimen. Forty-two microliters of whole blood, serum, or plasma can be used. The reagent cartridge has two modes for specimen addition: a slot to slide the capillary specimen into the cartridge and a well so that 2 to 3 drops of specimen can be added. During the centrifugation process only an aliquot will be processed for use with the reagent mixture. Thus, it is not critical to get the whole blood exactly to the 42-µL mark or the exact amount of specimen added to the well. If sample volume is insufficient, the patient's results will not appear; instead there will be a comment, "Low."

Analytical Performance. Published reports on the analytical performance of the Abbott VISION System are consistent;[17-21, 27, 33-35] the system is precise and accurate. When compared with other compact chemistry instruments, it usually always has the lowest per cent CVs for within-day, within-run, and day-to-day or overall precision, and the results are not influenced by the technical skills and background of the operator. When compared with reference methods, the biases are usually minimal. As an ex-

ample, the study of David and associates reported an average bias for three QC pools for total cholesterol measurement of 1.8 per cent CV.[18] When 100 fresh patient specimens were compared with the Abell-Kendall reference cholesterol method,[4] the correlation coefficient was 0.992, with a linear regression line of $Y = 0.967X + 9.5$, which suggests good agreement with the true value with a bias of only 0.5 per cent (Fig. 14–13).

Burke and Fischer[20] demonstrated an average overall precision for three levels of cholesterol (using CAP-certified reference materials analyzed in triplicate for 5 days) of 1.0 ± 0.3 per cent CV, which is better than most large chemistry analyzers costing hundreds of thousands of dollars. Their accuracy study indicated that the relation of the VISION to the CDC standardized reference method was $Y = 1.06X + 0.03$ with a total bias of 3.9 per cent, which seems somewhat high when compared with most studies.[17-21, 27, 33-35]

Abbott Laboratories has an ongoing Quality Commitment Program incorporating an external proficiency testing program for their USA Abbott VISION System custom-

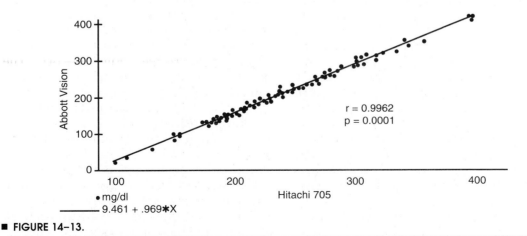

■ FIGURE 14–13.

Linear regression curve illustrating the comparison of serum cholesterol measurements of fresh patient specimens on the VISION and a CDC-standardized method, the BMC/Hitachi 705 cholesterol method.

ers. Each quarter the manufacturer sends out two survey pools with target values assigned by the cholesterol reference method. In one of their surveys, VISION users obtained a mean cholesterol value of 241.1 mg/dL and 100.6 mg/dL, respectively for Sample 1A and 1B, with CDC target values of 238.8 mg/dL and 99.6 mg/dL, respectively. Thus, the overall bias on cholesterol measurement was about 0.5 per cent, a figure similar to the data of David and associates.[18]

Test Menu. Albumin, alkaline phosphatase, amylase, C-reactive protein (CRP), calcium, cholesterol, CK, creatinine, GGT, glucose, glycated hemoglobin, hemoglobin, HDL-C, low-density lipoprotein cholesterol (LDL-C) by calculation, LD, phenytoin, potassium, prothrombin time, AST, ALT, T_4, theophylline, total bilirubin, total protein, triglycerides, urea nitrogen, uric acid, whole-blood HDL-C.

Desirable Features. Very user-friendly and easy instrument to operate; fast analyzer; uses whole blood, serum, or plasma; relatively small sample requirement; has dual method of loading a specimen; virtually no warm-up or start-up time; reagents, controls, and calibrators do not have to be brought to room temperature to begin assay; results not technique-dependent; low maintenance; calibrators and QC materials are already reconstituted and ready to use, have a long shelf-life, and are supplied by the manufacturer at no charge; excellent precision and accuracy; printout system will flag inadequate sample addition or sample with interfering substances (hemoglobin, turbidity, bilirubin) that are elevated enough to cause analytical bias in patient results; monitors reagent integrity in each cartridge and will flag results if reagent has deteriorated; is very easy and convenient to run multiple different chemistries in a single analytical run; a fully automated and walkaway system.

Less Desirable Features. Relatively large and heavy; cost is high (but is a true walkaway system—saving on the most expensive component, labor), some tests are relatively expensive.

Other Comments. This system is ideally suited for both small and large POLs, especially when there are multiple users and nonlaboratory operators. The multiple-test selective analyzer with barcoded cartridges makes batch, panel, and multiple testing very easy. Currently, it has the largest menu of tests; it also has other reporting options, such as customized operations (Cardiac Risk Assessment, health screening programs); automatic calculation of LDL and lipoprotein cholesterol ratios, enzyme conversion, expiration option, patient ID option, and lot option. Like Kodak, Abbott Laboratories has its own proficiency testing and QC programs. The toll-free technical 24-hour hotline is excellent.

Ready

Manufacturer. Roche Diagnostic Systems, Montclair, New Jersey; 1(800) 526-1247.

Instrument. The Roche Ready is a dry chemistry system in which plastic barcoded strips are impregnated with dry reagents and individually wrapped in foil to keep the strips moisture-free (Fig. 14–14). The **Ready** is a completely automated system in which the reagents are pipeted onto the reagent strips, and the colorimetric (end-point or kinetic) assays (at 37° C) are read by a dual wavelength reflectance spectrophotometer. The results are displayed on the screen, and the built-in thermal printer provides a hard copy of the patient's identification number and test results. The unit is compact and lightweight—45 cm wide, 35 cm deep, and 19 cm high, weighing 18 kg (Fig. 14–15). Daily start-up time is rapid, less than 1 minute; hands-on time to per-

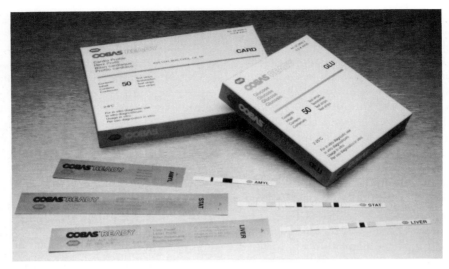

■ **FIGURE 14-14.**

Cobas Ready dry reagent strips (Roche Diagnostic Systems, Montclair, NJ) are individually wrapped to prevent moisture uptake.

form one test is about 1 minute. The automated pipeting and delivery system and barcoded reagent strips make this system especially convenient and simple to run, as either a random-access or batch analyzer.

The specimen-loading schedule is up to 12 tests on a single patient or as individual

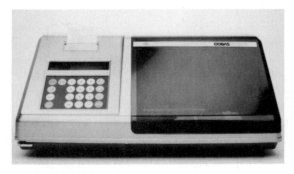

■ **FIGURE 14-15.**

The Ready system (Roche Diagnostic Systems, Montclair, NJ) showing a built-in printer and visual display screen.

tests (up to 6) on as many as six patients. The assay time is 3 to 5 minutes, depending on the chemistry, with printed results on 6 individual tests in about 6 minutes and printed results on a 12-test profile in about 11 minutes. The usual throughput is 60 tests per hour. The cost per test is between $2.25 and $2.50 per single test and $8.50 and $9.50 for six-test panels. The cost of the instrument is $15,995.

Specimen. Between 5 and 7 μL of serum or plasma is needed for the various chemistries. Since this is not a whole-blood chemistry analyzer like the Seralyzer and DT-60 systems, a centrifuge is required. The minimum volume of 20 μL of specimen is required for the sample tube from which the automated sampler aspirates the specimen to be delivered to the dry reagent strips.

Analytical Performance. Published data on this system are limited. Our evaluation (unpublished data) suggests that the day-to-day precision (n = 20 for 5 days) for two serum cholesterol concentrations averaged 3.2 per cent CV. In our accuracy study comparing 34 fresh patient cholesterol results to a standardized enzymatic method (traceable to a CDC standardized Abell-Kendall method), the correlation coefficient was 0.95 with a linear regression line of Y = 1.023× − 5.49, covering a concentration range of 69 to 329 mg/dL (Fig. 14–16). This suggests that the average bias is less than 1 per cent. More extensive studies are necessary to confirm this encouraging data. Okuda[36] had better precision: day-to-day precision for cholesterol at two concentrations averaged 1.5 per cent CV. For other analytes, Okuda obtained 1.6 per cent CV for glucose, 1.8 per cent for uric acid, 2.7 per cent for triglycerides, 2.2 per cent for BUN, 2.9 per cent for total protein, 2.2 per cent for albumin, 2.6 per cent for calcium, 3.2 per cent for AST, 2.7 per cent for ALT, 2.3 per cent for LDH, 3.3 per cent for CK, and 3.0 per cent for amylase. The comparison studies with their routine methods (using the Hitachi 726 and 736) demonstrate good correlation (between 0.924 and 0.995, depending on the chemistry).

Test Menu. Albumin, alkaline phospha-tase, amylase, calcium, cholesterol, CK, creatinine, glucose, GGT, HDL-C, LD, AST, ALT, total bilirubin, total protein, triglycerides, urea nitrogen, uric acid, cardiac profile (TC, BUN, TP, AST, CK, LD), liver profile (total bilirubin, TP, Alb, AST, ALT, LD), Profile I (total bilirubin, cholesterol, BUN, glucose, AST, ALT), Profile 2 (triglycerides, calcium, uric acid, total protein, albumin, LD), STAT profile (total bilirubin, BUN, AST, ALT, CK, LD).

Desirable Features. A fully automated system that automatically pipets specimens from sample cup to reagent strips; small and compact; very user-friendly; fast; good reagent stability (12 months); reagent strips barcoded for test identification and individually wrapped and stored at room temperature; calibration and QC materials provided at no extra charge; simple credit-card calibration (every 3 months); small sample requirement; provides reliable data.

Less Desirable Features. Presently this system has no drug or electrolyte tests available; 5-minute warm-up time; cost of instrument is relatively high.

Other Comments. This is a very simple,

■ **FIGURE 14–16.**

Linear regression curve illustrating the comparison of serum cholesterol measurements of fresh patient specimens on the Ready with a CDC-standardized cholesterol method, the Beckman Synchron CX7.

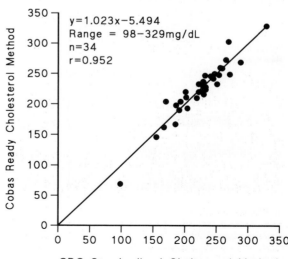

multitest chemistry analyzer that is suitable for both small and moderate-sized POLs. Its panel testing packages may be an attractive feature for some physicians.

Analyst

Manufacturer. Du Pont Company, Diagnostic Division, Wilmington, Delaware 19898; 1(800) ANALYST.

Instrument. The Du Pont **Analyst** is a prepackaged, dry chemistry system formatted into five rotor types (see Test Menu). Each rotor contains the reagent tablets and is barcoded to identify the tests. It takes less than a minute to aspirate/dilute the specimen (serum or plasma), dispense the specimen to the appropriate slot in the rotor, load the rotor, and start the instrument. After 10 minutes, the results are printed on a hard copy next to normal ranges. Thus, in this system there are no bottles to open, no reagents to dispense, and no reagent mixing. It is a very simple system to operate and, except for the pipet/dilution step, the results do not depend on the technical skills of the operator.

This walkaway system is light and compact; it weighs 18.9 kg and is 20.8 cm high, 27.9 cm deep, and 63.5 cm wide (Fig. 14–17). The cost of the instrument is $11,900. The cost of the reagents are $ 7.35 for CHEM-14, $ 5.48 for SELECT CHEMISTRIES, $ 8.98 for LIPID, $ 3.05 for glucose, and $ 8.45 for theophylline.

Specimen. This analytical system requires 90 µL of serum or plasma for the different panels. Because whole blood chemistries are not possible with this system, a centrifugation step is required to obtain serum or plasma.

Analytical Performance. There are few published data on this analytical system. Kaufman and coworkers reported that in a controlled laboratory environment, the Analyst showed proportional biases of around 10 per cent for total cholesterol, about − 11 per cent for HDL cholesterol, and from − 9.6 to 6.0 per cent for triglycerides, depending on the concentration. Precision studies indicated acceptability.[27]

Test Menu. The test menu is chosen from five different rotors. The CHEM-14 rotor has the following tests: glucose, BUN, cre-

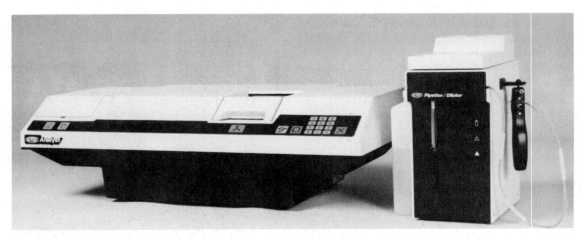

■ **FIGURE 14–17.**

Analyst (DuPont Company, Wilmington, DE) with Pipettor/Dilutor station.

atinine, BUN/creatinine ratio, uric acid, cholesterol, triglyceride, ALT, AST, total bilirubin, alkaline phosphatase, GGTP, calcium, total protein, and amylase. The SELECT chemistries rotor performs one, two, or three of the following tests: glucose, BUN, creatinine, uric acid, cholesterol, triglyceride, ALT, AST, total bilirubin, and alkaline phosphatase. The LIPID rotor has the following tests: cholesterol, triglyceride, VLDL cholesterol, HDL cholesterol, and calculated LDL cholesterol and total cholesterol/HDL cholesterol ratio. The glucose rotor can run up to two patient specimens on each rotor, but the theophylline rotor can run only one.

Desirable Features. Very user-friendly and easy instrument to operate; is not dependent on the technical skills of the operator; reagents can be stored at room temperature; low-maintenance system.

Less Desirable Features. Slow throughput: for the lipid panel, only six specimens per hour can be run; little flexibility: if only cholesterol test is needed, then one has the choice of using either the LIPID, CHEM-14, or SELECT rotors to choose from and the cost becomes an issue because of the wastage of reagents.

Other Comments. This system is more suitable in a laboratory with low volume and a minimal variety of test requirements. Since its introduction 5 years ago, no new test development has occurred; according to the manufacturer, none are planned for the immediate future.

A LOOK INTO THE FUTURE

As technologic advances are made, table-top analytical systems will become smaller, easier to use, faster, and more cost-effective and reliable. As an example, a couple of credit card–sized, noninstrument, disposable cholesterol analyzers are on the market today. One is the **AccuMeter** for cholesterol

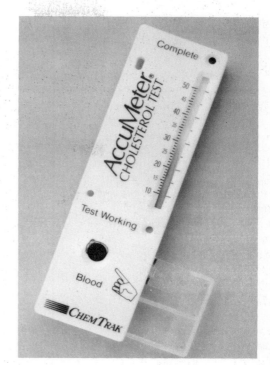

■ **FIGURE 14–18.**

AccuMeter cholesterol analyzer (ChemTrak, Sunnyvale, CA) a disposable, noninstrument, quantitative system.

measurement (Fig. 14–18), from ChemTrak (Sunnyvale, California). This system's technology is based on paper chromatography and a wicking reagent section, which allows the user to observe the capillary migration of the colored dye, which is proportional to the concentration of the cholesterol in the plasma (Fig. 14–19). This is a whole blood, dry chemistry system that automatically separates the plasma from the red blood cells, measures the precise sample volume, and produces precise and accurate quantitative results in about 15 minutes. The height of the purple bar is read directly from the inscribed millimeter ruler on the cassette, and the value is converted to milligrams per deciliter of cholesterol from a con-

Diagram A

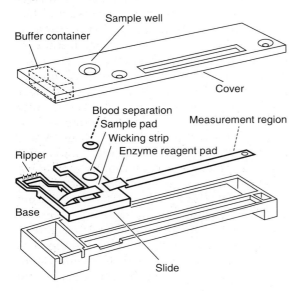

Diagram B

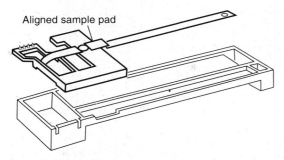

■ **FIGURE 14–19.**

The AccuMeter cassette (ChemTrak, Sunnyvale, CA).
A, The paper chromatography and wicking reagent
section; B, the sample pad in relation to the enzymatic reagent pad and measurement region containing the chromatographic strip.

version table. This is a user-friendly, single-
assay, disposable system that costs around
$10 per test.

Other similar types of hand-held chemistry systems are getting smaller, more user-
friendly, and more economical; a good example is the hand-held glucose meter being
used in hospital wards, outpatient clinics,
and homes. These systems can store up to
1000 patient data values, which can be
downloaded for review by the physician. The
quality control data also can be stored and
downloaded to be reviewed by laboratory
personnel. The reliability and analytical accuracy are excellent, mainly because they
are engineered to eliminate steps that lead
to imprecision and inaccuracies, like the
step after sample application that needs a
"wipe" step to remove the excess specimen
before the analytical process.

Our data on the **One Touch II** Blood Glucose Monitoring System (Fig. 14–20) from
Lifescan (Mountain View, California) indicate that the precision of the hospital version (compared with the home version) is

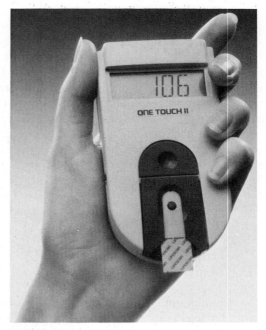

■ **FIGURE 14–20.**

One Touch II whole blood glucometer (Lifescan Inc.,
Mountain View, CA), which eliminates the procedural step of wiping excess specimens off the dry
reagent strip.

around 2 to 4 per cent CV, and the bias is less than 1.5 per cent from the reference method glucose values (unpublished data), which suggests high accuracy and precision. Glucose meters from other manufacturers, particularly earlier versions, are not as impressive analytically as the One Touch II, especially in the hands of a nonlaboratory-trained person. The One Touch II home-testing version can store up to 250 glucose results, which can be downloaded to a computer in the doctor's office. Figure 14–21 illustrates the sophistication of these new-generation glucose monitoring systems for hospital use; shown are the keyboard, CPU, printer assembly, and One Touch II Hospital Meter, which has additional software designed to meet the needs of the individual hospital's quality control program. The

LifeScan printer assembly and two new software programs (administrator disc and QC disc) allow the hospital quality assurance team new flexibility in designing, documenting, and ensuring compliance with a comprehensive QC program. The LifeScan administrator disc will allow changes to meet the hospital needs, in control ranges, units (mg/dL or mmol/L), printer assembly clock setting, date setting, and result mode (whole blood, plasma, or serum). When linked with the LifeScan printer assembly via the One Touch interface cable, the QC report disc will allow the generation of QC reports from the stored results, n = 210. The system has 249 ID numbers to monitor each operator using the system. Reports can be in the form of a summary report for all QC results, summary reports for each operator, trend

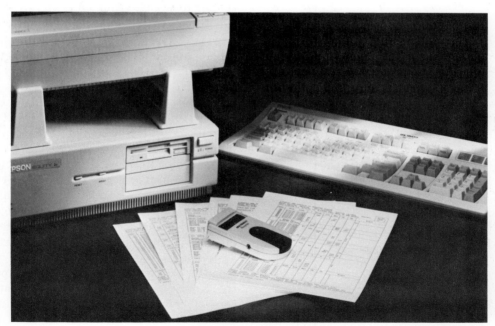

■ **FIGURE 14–21.**

One Touch II hospital meter (Lifescan Inc., Mountain View, CA), which includes the CPU, printer assembly, interface cable, and keyboard to allow the uploading of 210 QC results (from 249 operator IDs), for monitoring glucose testing.

graphs, and a linearity report that can be generated for the previous month, the current month, or the previous 30-day period.

The cost per test for these new-generation glucose meters is about 40 to 50 cents.

To assist health care professionals involved with monitoring patient test results, some manufacturers of glucose meters now have portable test stations available for bedside testing. Figure 14–22 shows the **AccuData Glucose Test Station** (GTS), from Boehringer-Mannheim Corporation, Indianapolis, that is designed to reduce or eliminate the manual record-keeping associated with the collection of both quality control and patient glucose test data. The GTS also can be customized to meet a specific hospital's needs for collecting, organizing and reporting this information. For example, this system can generate reports of specific patient data and perform various

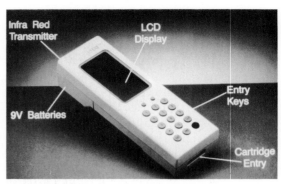

■ **FIGURE 14–23.**

i-STAT Portable Clinical Analyzer (i-STAT Corporation, Princeton, NJ), which uses disposable cartridges that can measure electrolytes, BUN, glucose, and hemoglobin.

quality control statistics, such as Levy-Jennings charts and linearity plots.

Finally, to illustrate the present state-of-the-art technology and what we can look forward to in the future is the recently introduced **i-STAT** Portable Clinical Analyzer. This hand-held, microprocessor-controlled instrument with liquid crystal display has a disposable multianalyte sensor array and self-calibration unit packaged into a single-use cartridge. The analyzer (Fig. 14–23) has a central data station (small laptop computer) with infrared communication for data transmission from multiple i-STAT analyzers. The first cartridge (Fig. 14–24) now available has the capabilities of analyzing sodium, potassium, chloride, glucose, urea nitrogen, hematocrit, and a calculated hemoglobin. This is an extremely user-friendly system that requires only 65 μL of whole blood, which is added to a capillary port in the cartridge. The analyzer automatically controls all functions from this point on, which includes self-calibration, fluid movements, continuous process control throughout each test with each cartridge, and analysis and reporting of the test results in about 10 minutes on a hard copy. The cost

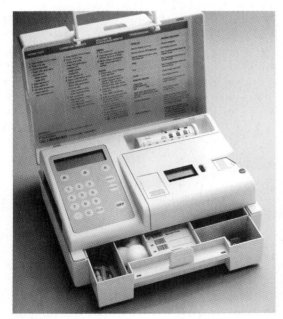

■ **FIGURE 14–22.**

The AccuData Glucose Test Station (GTS) (Boehringer-Mannheim Corporation, Indianapolis).

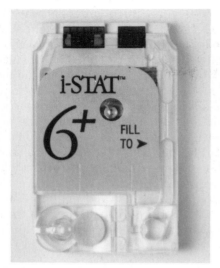

■ FIGURE 14–24.

A close-up view of the i-STAT cartridge (i-STAT Corporation, Princeton, NJ), which contains tiny ion-selective electrodes (ISEs) to measure the analytes.

of the i-STAT System is $3,000, and the cost of the cartridge is around $12. These types of portable systems will have great clinical applications in emergency departments, intensive care wards, trauma centers, ambulances, emergency care helicopters, and other crisis and acute care situations. We can expect to see more of these types of port-

able analytical systems going into the 21st century.

A look into the future also shows the need for standardization and addressing of preanalytical issues. We need standardization of methods to ensure accuracy of testing.[37–39] It is clear from proficiency testing surveys (Table 14–3) that interlaboratory and intralaboratory comparison can be enhanced. For example, the 1991 American Academy of Family Physicians Proficiency Testing (PT) Program indicates that the highest coefficient of variation for cholesterol measurement is with the Gemstar (8.7 per cent) and Seralyzer (6.7 per cent), and the lowest is with the VISION (4.5 per cent). The mean cholesterol value for that PT specimen (set L-21) was 309.8 by the CDC Abell-Kendall method.[4] Results were 279.4 ± 24.4 mg/dL (mean ± 1 SD) for the Gemstar peer group to 316.8 ± 18.2 mg/dL for the Analyst. This means that the range of submitted results was from about 230 to 353 mg/dL (at the 95 per cent confidence interval), which suggests that the accuracy of testing is compromised. Medical Centers of the Department of Veterans Affairs (174 clinical laboratories and outpatient clinics) have a standardization program establishing accuracy of testing in the nation's largest hospital system. Using fresh, unfrozen human

TABLE 14–3. PROFICIENCY TESTING PROGRAM OF AMERICAN ACADEMY OF FAMILY PHYSICIANS; 1991 EVALUATION REPORT—CHOLESTEROL*†

PEER GROUP	NO. LABS	MEAN (mg/dL)	SD (mg/dL)	CV (%)	LOW (mg/dL)	HIGH (mg/dL)
VISION	135	298.0	13.4	4.5	257	337
Seralyzer	33	293.5	19.6	6.7	265	347
Reflotron	43	290.3	16.5	5.7	244	324
Analyst	90	316.8	18.2	5.8	257	373
Gemstar	40	279.4	24.4	8.7	209	324
DT-60	137	315.1	16.2	5.2	271	379
All Multicon	317	300.7	20.4	6.8	234	363
CDC	—	309.8	1.8			

*Set AFP-H, Specimen L-21.
†HCFA acceptable limits = 271-331 mg/dl.

sera (six analyte concentration levels) sent by overnight mail, the instrument operator analyzes each specimen in duplicate each day for 3 days. The target values are assigned by established reference methods that are traceable to Serum Reference Materials from the National Institute of Standards and Technology. Each laboratory's data points (n = 36) are compared with the target values, using a computerized linear regression model, which determines overall precision and bias. The National Center for Laboratory Accuracy and Standardization at the Cleveland (Ohio) Veterans Administration Medical Center coordinates and monitors the standardization and certification of the laboratories in the VA medical centers and outpatient clinics. Standardization events throughout the nation will be increasingly more common as the focus on accuracy of testing intensifies.

The variability in patients' results is due not only to analytical variables but also to preanalytical variables,[40, 41] which also must be acknowledged when interpreting the laboratory results. Such preanalytical variables as age, gender, season, recent dietary and alcohol intake, body weight changes, acute exercise, recent trauma, viral and bacterial infections, and medication for other medical conditions need special attention, especially during long-term monitoring of the patient. A full understanding is necessary when the patient's values fluctuate, especially during therapy by dietary or pharmacologic means. In the future, laboratorians and clinicians must be more aware of both preanalytical and analytical issues that will lead to reliable patient results; whenever possible, every effort must be made to control these variables to ensure accurate patient test results.

SUMMARY

Compact chemistry analyzers (Table 14–4) have evolved over the decade into sophisticated, reliable analytical systems that are finding their way into many areas of health

TABLE 14–4. OFFICE CHEMISTRY ANALYZERS

INSTRUMENT	SAMPLE	INSTRUMENT COST (COST/TEST*)	TEST MENU	ADVANTAGES	DISADVANTAGES
Analyst DuPont Co., Diagnostic Division, Wilmington, DE 1-800-ANALYST	90 µl serum or plasma	$11,900 ($8.98 for LIPID PANEL, CHEM-14 PANEL $17.35, Select CHEM $15.48, glucose $3.05, Theophylline $8.45)	Offers five rotors: (1) LIPID PANEL, (TC, TG, VLDL-C, calculated LDL-C, HDL-C; TC/HDL-C ratio); (2) CHEM-14 (alkaline phosphatase, ALT, AST, amylase, BUN calcium, creatinine, BUN/creatinine ratio, GGT, TG, TC, total bilirubin, total protein, uric acid); (3) SELECT PANEL (1-3 of the following: alkaline phosphatase, ALT, AST, BUN, creatine, glucose, TG, TC, total bilirubin, uric acid); (4) glucose (two patients/rotor); (5) theophylline (one patient/rotor)	Easy to operate; walkaway system prints results next to normal ranges; except for pipet dilution step, accuracy does not depend on operator skills; reagents stored at 4° C; no bottles to open or reagents to dispense or mix; low maintenance; panel testing	Cannot use whole blood; slow throughput (six patients/hour for LIPID PANEL); little flexibility; no drugs or electrolytes

TABLE 14–4. OFFICE CHEMISTRY ANALYZERS *Continued*

INSTRUMENT	SAMPLE	INSTRUMENT COST (COST/TEST*)	TEST MENU	ADVANTAGES	DISADVANTAGES
DT-60 II Eastman Kodak Co. Rochester, NY 800-445-6325 ext. 434	10 μL plasma or serum for TC or TG, 50 μl for HDL-C	$5,500 ($1.45–2.75)	HDL-C, TC, TG; also ammonia, amylase, BUN, glucose, hemoglobin, magnesium, total bilirubin, total protein, phosphorus, uric acid; lactic acid	Modular, semiautomated, walkaway system with printer; throughput 65 tests/hr; can batch 6 tests; recalibration performed on-site; additional modules available to run special chemistries (DTSC) and electrolytes (DTE); excellent customer service hotline	Cannot use whole blood; 5–10 minute precipitation and centrifugation step for HDL-C; pipeting step critical; 20-minute start-up time; reagents must be run at room temperature; QC and calibration materials must be reconstituted; have short half life; reagents must be stored at 4° C; once reagent is taken out of foil, it must be used within 15 min; recalibration is not easy; need to watch pipeting step
DTSC II	5–7 μl serum	$3,300 ($1.50–4.05)	Albumin, alkaline phosphatase, ALT, calcium, cholinesterase, CK, CK-MB, creatinine, GGT, LD, lipase, theophylline	DTSC throughput is 20 tests/hr	
DTE		$3,200 ($1.75)	Carbon dioxide, chloride, potassium, sodium	DTE throughput is 15 tests/hr	
Ready Roche Diagnostic Systems, Monclair, NJ 800-526-1247	5–7 μl serum or plasma	$15,995 (2.25–2.50)	HDL-C, TG, TC; also albumin, alkaline phosphatase, ALT, amylase, AST, BUN, calcium, CK, creatinine, glucose, GGT, LD, total bilirubin, total protein, uric acid, and five profiles containing combinations of these tests	Fully automated; built-in thermal printer; start-up time less than 1 min; throughput 60 tests/hr; reagents stable for 12 months; barcoded at room temperature; QC and calibration materials free; simple credit card calibration every 3 months; small sample requirement; very easy to update; panel testing	Cannot use whole blood; no drug or electrolyte tests; relatively high cost of instrument

Table continued on following page

TABLE 14–4. OFFICE CHEMISTRY ANALYZERS *Continued*

INSTRUMENT	SAMPLE	INSTRUMENT COST (COST/TEST*)	TEST MENU	ADVANTAGES	DISADVANTAGES
Reflotron Boehringer-Mannheim Corporation, Indianapolis, IN 317-845-2468	30 μl plasma, serum, or whole blood	$5,295 ($1.60–3.00) $5,795 for Reflotron Plus	HDL-C, TG, TC; also ALT, AST, amylase, bilirubin, BUN, creatinine, CK, GGT, hemoglobin, potassium, uric acid	Uses whole blood; can do HDL without specimen preparation; little preventive maintenance; low initial cost; 1-min start-up time; automatic calibration; reagent strips automatically reset instrument to each test chemistry. Newly introduced Reflotron Plus offers printer, keyboard to enter patient data, Heart Health Assessment package, and ability to edit information and show patients how to lower coronary risk by complying with treatment; compact; lightweight; easy to operate	Throughput 20 tests/hr; no printer except with Reflotron Plus; reagent strips sensitive to humidity; $3/wk to maintain optical system; QC materials must be reconstituted with distilled water and have short stability time
Seralyzer Ames Division, Miles Laboratories, Elkhart, IN 800-248-2637	100 μl plasma or serum (added to 300–800 μl water)	$4,495 ($1.00–3.00)	HDL-C, TG, TC; also ALT, AST, bilirubin, BUN, carbamazepine, CK, creatinine, digoxin, glucose, hemoglobin, LD, phenobarbital, phenytoin, potassium, theophylline, uric acid	Throughput 40 tests/hr; large test menu; reagent strips stored at room temperature; low initial cost; large drug menu	Cannot use whole blood; 15-min start-up time; labor-intensive (extra steps for diluent and specimen pipeting; specimen application); accuracy dependent on operator technique; weekly calibration; specimens loaded one at a time; no barcoding or patient identification system; no printer (but does have printer port); poor electrolyte menu; pipeting is an added step

TABLE 14–4. OFFICE CHEMISTRY ANALYZERS *Continued*

INSTRUMENT	SAMPLE	INSTRUMENT COST (COST/TEST*)	TEST MENU	ADVANTAGES	DISADVANTAGES
VISION Abbott Laboratories, Abbott Park, IL 800-323-9100	42 µl plasma, serum, or whole blood	$17,495 ($1.75–6.25)	HDL-C, calculated LDL-C, TG, TC, whole blood HDL-C; also albumin, alkaline phosphatase, ALT, amylase, AST, BUN, calcium, CK, C-reactive protein, creatinine, GGT, glucose, glycolated hemoglobin, hemoglobin, LD, phenytoin, potassium, prothrombin time, theophylline, thyroxine, total bilirubin, total protein, uric acid	Uses whole blood; can do HDL from whole blood or from serum or plasma; offers Cardiac Risk Assessment package; fully automated walkaway system; virtually no start-up time; throughput 60 tests/hr; reagents, controls, and calibrators need not be at room temperature; controls and calibrators already reconstituted, have long shelf life, and are free; calibration good for 3 months; analyzer signals when sample volume is insufficient, sample contains interfering substances, or reagent has deteriorated; low maintenance; company offers proficiency testing, QC programs, and an excellent customer service hotline	Relatively large and heavy; high cost; some tests relatively expensive

Key: ALT, alanine aminotransferase; AST, aspartate aminotransferase; CK, creatine kinase; GGT, gammaglutamyl transferase; HDL-C, high-density lipoprotein cholesterol; LD, lactate dehydrogenase; LDL-C, low-density lipoprotein cholesterol; QC, quality control; TC, total cholesterol; TG, triglyceride; VLDL-C, very-low-density lipoprotein cholesterol.

*Calculated using cost of reagent only.

Adapted with permission from Gregory T: Office cholesterol testing. *Patient Care,* Issue 2/15/93.

care. This trend will continue, and these systems will evolve into smaller, easier to operate, more reliable cost-effective devices. Already about a half dozen hand-held non-instrument systems are dedicated to either glucose or cholesterol testing. They are the size of credit cards and take only a couple of drops of whole blood for analysis. These single-use, disposable systems appear to be reliable, but extensive evaluation is necessary to determine their clinical usefulness in the health care system. The present compact chemistry analyzers are reliable—some being more precise and accurate than others.

A key feature to success with these instruments is selecting the most affordable system that is as automated, user-friendly, and least dependent on the technical skills of the operator as possible, while providing the most reliable laboratory data technically feasible today. The bottom-line gain in use of these devices is providing greater convenience to the patient, enhancing the health care of patients, and advancing the practice of medicine.

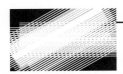

REVIEW QUESTIONS

Choose the best answer.

1. Identify the least important consideration for selecting a table-top analyzer:

   a. The amount of training necessary to become a competent operator.
   b. The manufacturer's technical information brochures.
   c. The degree of automation.
   d. The frequency of calibration.

2. Serum, plasma, or whole blood can be used as a specimen on which of the following instruments?

   a. Reflotron and Vision
   b. Vision and Analyst
   c. DT-60 and Analyst
   d. Ready and Reflotron

3. Which of the following systems have large test menus?

   a. Analyst and Ready
   b. DT-60/DTSC/DTE and Vision
   c. Reflotron and DT60/DTSC/DTE
   d. Vision and Analyst

4. Which of the following systems have a relatively large test menu for therapeutic drug monitoring?

   a. DT60/DTSC/DT and Vision
   b. Vision and Seralyzer
   c. Seralyzer and Ready
   d. Reflotron and Analyst

5. The reliability (precision and accuracy) of analytical performance is not compromised by non-credentialed operators in which of the following table-top analyzers?

   a. Analyst and Seralyzer
   b. Ready and Vision
   c. DT-60 and Reflotron
   d. Vision and DT-60

REFERENCES

1. Naito HK: The status of office-based cholesterol testing and monitoring. The Official Newsletter of the Educational Program. Cholesterol and Coronary Disease . . . Reducing the Risk. 2(3):4–7, 1989.
2. Barman MR: Alternate-site testing: Mixed feelings about the inevitable. *Med Lab Obser* 22(12):22–29, 1990.
3. *Recommendations for Improving Cholesterol Measurement: A Report from the Laboratory Standardization Panel of the National Cholesterol Education Program.* Bethesda, MD, US Department of Health and Human Services, NIH Publication No. 90–2964, 1990.
4. Abell LL, Levy BB, Brodie RB, Kendall FE: Simplified method for the estimation of total cholesterol in serum and demonstration of its specificity. *J Biol Chem* 195:357–366, 1952.
5. Cohen A, Hertz HS, Mandel J, Paule RC, Schaffer R, Sniegoski LT, Sun T, Welch MJ, White VE: Total serum cholesterol by isotope dilution/mass spectrometry: A candidate reference method. *Clin Chem* 26:854–869, 1980.
6. Nanji AA, Poon R, Hinberg I: Quality of laboratory test results obtained by non-technical personnel in a decentralized setting. *Am J Clin Pathol* 89:797–801, 1988.
7. Brown S, Savory J, Wills MR: Clinical laboratory evaluation of Ames' Seralyzer reflectance photometer for total bilirubin and cholesterol. *Clin Chem* 29(5):844–846, 1983.
8. Croci D, Nespolo A, Tarenghi G: A dry reagent strip for quantifying carbamazepine evaluated. *Clin Chem* 34:388–392, 1988.
9. Lott JA, Miller IL, Crowley LE: Cholesterol assays in the Seralyzer instrument. *J Clin Lab Anal* 3:232–235, 1989.
10. Kroll MH, Olson D, Rawe M, King C, Hagengruber C, Elin RJ: Comparison of creatinine as determined with the Ames Seralyzer. *Clin Chem* 31:1900–1904, 1985.

11. Stevens JF, Newall RG: Application of reflectance spectroscopy to the estimation of uric acid, urea and glucose: An evaluation of the Ames Seralyzer. *J Clin Pathol* 36:9–13, 1983.

12. Nanji AA, Sincennes F, Poon R, Hinberg I: Evaluation of the Ames Seralyzer. *Clin Chem* 33:1255–1256, 1987.

13. Gibb I: Evaluation and assessment of new disposable strip for determination of plasma potassium concentration. *J Clin Pathol* 40:298–301, 1987.

14. Singh P, Lim DT, Enright T, de la Cruz RY, Noutois S, Lim AT Jr, Mariano R, Chakrin AL: Correlation between Seralyzer reflectance photometer theophylline assay and an Emit assay. *Ann Allergy* 59:176–178, 1987.

15. Von Schenck H, Treichi L, Tilling B, Olsson AG: Laboratory and field evaluation of true desktop instrument for assay of cholesterol and triglycerides. *Clin Chem* 33:1230–1232, 1987.

16. Gibb I, Barton JR, Adams PC, Pratt D, Dean CR, Tarbit IF: Rapid measurement of creatinine kinase activity in a coronary care unit using a portable bench top reflectance photometer. *Br Med J* 290:1381–1383, 1985.

17. Nanji AA, Poon R, Hinberg I: Desktop analysers: quality of results obtained by medical office personnel. *Can Med Assoc J* 138(6):1517–1520, 1988.

18. David JA, Mooney CR, Naito HK: Comparison of physician office analyzers for cholesterol analysis in screening centers. *Clin Chem* 33(6):898, 1987.

19. Bills JK, Schaefgen KE, Planter ML, Brien BC, Karni KR: Comparison of four chemistry analyzers for physician office and clinical laboratories. *Clin Lab Sci* 2(2):111–115, 1989.

20. Burke JJ II, Fischer PM: A clinician's guide to the office measurement of cholesterol. *JAMA* 259(23):3444–3448, 1988.

21. Warnick GR: Measurement of cholesterol, triglycerides, HDL using compact analysis systems. *Clin Lab Med* 9(1):61–88, 1989.

22. Roberts K: A dry chemistry analyzer. *Am Clin Prod Rev*, Feb 16, 1987.

23. Rohac M, Rohac FG: Evaluation of two dry reagent systems: Determination of glucose, cholesterol and triacylglycerols with the Reflotron and Kodak Ektachem DT-60 analyzer. *J Clin Chem Clin Biochem* 24:790–791, 1986.

24. Koch TR, Mehta U, Lee H, Aziz K, Temel S, Donlon JA, Sherwin R: Bias and precision of cholesterol analysis by physician's office analyzers. *Clin Chem* 33:2262–2267, 1987.

25. Katan MB, Kruyswijk Z: Fingerstick cholesterol testing with the "Reflotron." *Clin Chem* 34:1007, 1988.

26. Ng RH, Sparks KM, Statland BE: Direct measurement of high-density lipoprotein cholesterol by the Reflotron assay with no manual precipitation step. *Clin Chem* 37(3):435–437, 1991.

27. Kaufman HW, McNamara JR, Anderson KM, Wilson PWF, Schaefer, E: How reliably can compact chemistry analyzers measure lipids? *JAMA* 263(9):1245–1249, 1990.

28. Gubata R, Lefebvre RC: Comparison testing of lot to lot variance in the Reflotron dry reagent strip method of cholesterol measurement. *Clin Chem* 35:1098, 1989.

29. Hicks JM, Iosefsohn M: Hemoglobin, electrolytes, and other major clinical analytes as measured with a physician's office analyzer, the Kodak DT-60. *Clin Chem* 32:2201–2203, 1986.

30. Belsey R, Goitein RK, Baer DM: Evaluation of a laboratory system intended for use in physicians' offices. I. Reliability of results produced by trained laboratory technologists. *JAMA* 258(3):353–356, 1987.

31. Belsey R, Vandenbark M, Goitein RK, Baer DM: Evaluation of a laboratory system intended for use in physicians' offices. II. Reliability of results produced by health care workers without formal or professional laboratory training. *JAMA* 258(3): 357–361, 1987.

32. Greenland P, Levenkron JC, Radley MG, Baggs JG, Manchester RA, Bowley NL: Feasibility of large-scale cholesterol screening: Experience with a portable capillary-blood testing device. *Am J Public Health* 77:73–75, 1987.

33. Schultz SG, Holen JT, Donohue JP, Francoeur TA: Two-dimensional centrifugation for desk-top clinical chemistry. *Clin Chem* 31(9);1457–1463, 1985.

34. Stavljenic A, Vrkic N, Herak C, Kummar K, Topic E: Analytical performance of the VISION system evaluated. *Clin Chem* 33:1672–1673, 1987.

35. Toffaletti J: Small chemistry analyzers for physician's office testing: A survey. *Lab Management*, 37–41, June 1986.

36. Okuda K: A compact, automated, dry-reagent chemistry analyzer. *J Int Fed Clin Chem* 2(1):39–43, 1990.

37. Myers GL, Cooper GR, Winn CL, Smith SJ: The Centers for Disease Control–National Heart, Lung and Blood Institute Lipid Standardization Program. *Clin Lab Med* 9(1):105–135, 1989.

38. Naito HK: The need for accurate total cholesterol measurement: Recommended analytical goals, current state of reliability, and guidelines for better determinations. *Clin Lab Med* 9:37–60, 1989.

39. Naito HK, Kwak YS, Hartfiel JL, Park JK, Travers EM, Myers GL, Ross JW, Eckfeldt JH, Hartmann AE: Matrix effects on proficiency testing materials: Impact on accuracy of cholesterol measurement in laboratories in the nation's largest hospital system. *Arch Pathol Lab Med* 117:345–351, 1993.

40. Naito HK, Kwak YS: Accurate measurement of serum total cholesterol: The need for standardization. *J Am Coll Nutr* 11:8S–15S, 1992.

41. Naito HK: Cholesterol: How do we manage laboratory and patient health data? *In* Martin ML, Addison BV, Wagner WM, Essien JDK (eds): *Proceedings of the 1989 Institute on Critical Issues in Health Laboratory Practice: Improving the Quality of Health Management through Clinician and Laboratorian Teamwork*. Wilmington, DE, Du Pont Company, 1991, pp 78–84.

INTRODUCTION
Overview of Quality Assurance
ESTABLISHING AND MONITORING PERFORMANCE OF AN INSTRUMENTAL METHOD
Method Validation Procedure

Calibration

Precision

Accuracy

Reportable Range

Specificity and Sensitivity

Reference Range

Written Procedures
QUALITY ASSURANCE FOR INSTRUMENTS USED FOR PATIENT CARE
Quality Control

Proficiency Testing

Review of Patient Results

Chapter 15

INSTRUMENTATION SYSTEMS: RELIABILITY AND VALIDITY ISSUES

DAVID J. THORNTON, PHD, C(ASCP)
BERNADETTE L. THORNTON, MT(ASCP)

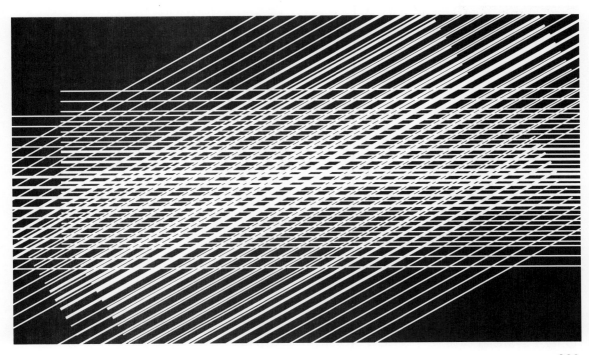

LEARNING OBJECTIVES

- Explain the relationship of quality assurance to quality control.
- Write procedures for preparing a quality assurance plan.
- Identify the steps required for validating a procedure prior to reporting patients.
- Use quality control and patient material to assure that a procedure is working.
- Utilize the Federal Register to understand the rules that must be followed for operating a laboratory.
- Calculate reference ranges, and explain how they are developed and how they are used.
- Describe proficiency testing and explain how it should be performed and interpreted.
- Perform linearity studies.

KEY WORDS

Accuracy. The ability of a method to produce a result close to the true result.

Analytical sensitivity. The lowest concentration that can be reported with a particular analytical method.

Analytical specificity. Ability of an assay to produce accurate results in the presence of possible interferences.

Bias. Observed result minus assigned value.

Calibration. The process of adjusting an instrument or test system to provide a known relationship between the analytical response and the concentration of analyte.

Calibration verification. The assay of calibration materials to confirm that a test system has remained stable throughout the reportable range.

Clinical decision concentration. The concentration at which a caregiver may act if the result is less than or greater than a certain value.

Clinical laboratory improvement amendment (CLIA). A federal law that regulates the performance of laboratory testing.

Clinical sensitivity. The percent of patients with a disease who have a positive test result.

Clinical specificity. The percent of patients who do not have a disease and do not have a positive result.

Coefficient of variation (CV). A statistic that describes the variability of results for a specimen assayed repeatedly, relative to the mean.

Delta checking. A procedure that compares a patient's previous result with the current result for a particular analyte.

Interference. The effect of a substance within the sample matrix on the analyte being analyzed.

Laboratory Information System (LIS). A computer system within the laboratory that stores patient information and results. The LIS may be interfaced (or linked) to analytical instruments for reporting of results and to a Hospital Information System for retrieval of laboratory results throughout the hospital.

Levy-Jennings charts. A quality control procedure that plots consecutive control results versus time on a graph.

Moderate and high complexity tests. CLIA has defined the complexity of clinical laboratory tests and classified them according to the difficulty in performing and interpreting the test. CLIA has determined who may perform these types of testing based on training, education, and experience.

NCCLS. National Committee for Clinical Laboratory Standards is a non-profit educational organization composed of laboratory professionals in industry, academia, and laboratorians. The committee produces protocols for operation of clinical laboratories.

Normal reference range. The range of values for a particular analyte, obtained from patients thought to be healthy. It is used to help determine whether a result from a patient may be abnormal compared with healthy patients. This range, however, does not define health. Some healthy patients may have results outside this range while patients with disease may have results within this range.

Panic value. A result that may indicate that a patient's life is in jeopardy and an immediate response may be required by a physician.

Postanalytical variation. Changes in patient results after analysis. This may be due to inaccurate calculations or to transcribing incorrect results.

Preanalytical variation. Changes in patients' results due to inappropriate specimen handling, test ordering, or specimen collection.

Precision. The ability of a method to repeat a result over numerous analyses. Good precision indicates that the results are reproducible, thus having a low standard deviation and coefficient of variation.

Proficiency testing. The testing of specimens whose concentrations are unknown to the participating laboratory. Results are returned to the specimen provider and the results are graded by comparing with results from all laboratories or reference laboratories. They are evaluated using criteria determined by either CLIA or the proficiency provider.

Quality assurance. A process that assures clinically useful results by monitoring procedures that affect the handling of patient samples, patient orders, patient reports, and other factors affecting the quality of patient results.

Quality control. A process that assures an accurate result of an analytical method.

Reference method. A method whose accuracy and precision is understood, which is used to validate methods used on a day-to-day basis. These procedures are usually very time consuming and are not appropriate for routine analyses.

Reference range. The range of values for a given analyte in a defined population. Usually used to guide the physician in detecting abnormal results. Reference range may depend on the population's age and sex.

Reportable range. The lowest and highest concentrations that can be reported without dilution or other treatment of the specimen.

Run. An interval within which the accuracy and precision of a testing system are expected to be stable, but it cannot be greater than 24 hours. For some methods, a run may be every time patients, calibrators, and controls are assayed, whereas other methods may define a run as once each day, or once each shift.

Standard deviation (SD). A statistic that describes how results vary about the mean when a specimen is assayed repetitively.

Standard deviation index (SDI). A number that describes the number of standard deviations away from the mean that a result is.

Target range. The range of results that are considered acceptable by the proficiency agency. Some of these target ranges are defined by CLIA.

Target value. The concentration of an analyte from a proficiency sample. This concentration is assumed to be the true concentration. The target value is based on the mean of all participants, or the mean established by reference methods.

Waivered tests. Tests that, according to CLIA, are either cleared by the FDA for home use, employ simple and accurate methodologies that have a negligible likelihood of erroneous results, or pose no reasonable risk of harm to the patient if performed incorrectly.

INTRODUCTION

Laboratorians use many types of instruments to provide clinical results to the clinician. These results are useful only if the instrumentation is properly used and maintained, the specimens properly collected, and results accurately reported. This chapter discusses what needs to be done when adding a new procedure to a laboratory's test menu; how to assure that a method continually produces accurate result, using quality control procedures; and steps to be taken to continually improve the services provided by the laboratory. Government regulations, as well as the rules of accrediting agencies, have had a major impact on the laboratory. Protocols to meet the requirements of these agencies will be stressed in this chapter.

Overview of Quality Assurance

The purpose of the clinical laboratory is to assay patient specimens and provide physicians with clinically useful results. The production of a clinically useful result depends on many factors, including handling of physician orders, collection of the specimen, turnaround time, accurate analysis, and timely physician notification[1] (Table 15–1). A **quality assurance** (QA) program monitors the laboratory's outcomes and subsequently helps laboratorians identify and correct problems that will improve patient care. Quality assurance is used to monitor pre- and postanalytical variation. **Preanalytical variation** would include improper specimen labeling and use of appropriate containers. **Postanalytical variation** would include improper reference range identifica-

TABLE 15–1. PROCEDURES THAT MAY AFFECT THE USEFULNESS
OF LABORATORY RESULTS

PROCEDURE	EXAMPLE
Transmission of orders	Orders are not received when needed
Timeliness of collection	A glucose tolerance test may be rendered useless if one of the specimens is not collected on time
Collection site	Specimens drawn above an intravenous (IV) site may be contaminated with IV fluid
Cleansing of collection site	Falsely elevated blood lead level may occur from contamination if the puncture site is not adequately cleansed
Specimen anticoagulant	Use of an EDTA tube for collection of a specimen for calcium assay will cause a falsely low result due to binding of calcium to EDTA
Specimen integrity	Wrong patient identification placed on tube would cause result to be wrongly interpreted
Accuracy of method	An inaccurate CKMB result may lead to an incorrect diagnosis of myocardial infarction in a patient
Specificity	Compounds other than the compound of interest, such as hemoglobin, lipids, drugs, may lower or raise the measured concentration of the analyte
Reporting of result in timely fashion	Long turnaround time, especially in an acute care laboratory, may delay patient treatment
Notification of panic result	Failure to report a panic result may delay appropriate treatment for the patient
Appropriate reference range	Babies often have potassium levels of between 5.5 and 6.5 mmol/L. Concentrations of this magnitude can be life threatening

tion, inaccurate recording of patient results (clerical errors), and slow reporting of results.

Quality control (QC) is a subpart of quality assurance.[2] Whereas quality assurance looks at the entire process of reporting a useful result to the physician, quality control monitors the analytical aspects of a method, verifying that results from a given method are accurate.

Most laboratorians continually strive to improve the quality of their department, but until recently many laboratorians have not formally documented these actions. Federal regulations (**Clinical Laboratory Improvement Amendment** of 1988 [CLIA])[3] and laboratory accrediting agencies (College of American Pathologists [CAP][4] and Joint Commission of Accreditation of Healthcare Organizations [JCAHO][5] require formally documented quality assurance plans. The Federal Register of February 28, 1992, con-

tains the final rule developed by the Department of Health and Human Services (DHHS): The laboratory must ". . . establish and follow written policies and procedures for a comprehensive quality control program, which is designed to monitor and evaluate the ongoing and overall quality of the total testing process (preanalytic, analytic, and postanalytic). The laboratory's quality assurance program must evaluate the effectiveness of its policies and procedures; identify and correct problems; assure the accurate, reliable, and prompt reporting of test results and assure the adequacy and competency of the staff. As necessary, the laboratory must revise policies and procedures based upon the results of these evaluations. . . All quality assurance activities must be documented (Subpart K, §493.1703)."[3]

The Federal Register for the CLIA regulations is fairly difficult to wade through. Pages 7137 and 7138 list the different sections of the rule. You can use this listing to help you find your way through all the material. Throughout this chapter, relevant sections within the CLIA rule will be preceded by the "§" symbol.

Ten activities performed by laboratories must be formally monitored, evaluated, and revised (when necessary) within a quality assurance program:

- Monitor and evaluate effectiveness of procedures and policies for handling patient specimens, orders and reports.
- Evaluate the remedial actions taken when quality control is unacceptable.
- Describe actions taken when proficiency testing is unsatisfactory.
- At least twice each year, define relationship between test results when an analyte concentration is measured on two different instrument systems.
- Set up procedures to identify and evaluate patient test results that appear inconsistent with patient's condition, diagnosis, age, sex, or other clinical results.
- Monitor employees for compliance with policies and procedures.
- Monitor procedures used for communication with clinical staff.
- Develop procedures to investigate complaints.
- Review quality assurance findings with laboratory staff.
- Document quality assurance records.

These activities are defined in CLIA Subpart P §493.1701–§493.1721.[3] After evaluation, if problems are found or if improvements can be made, revisions must be made in the procedures or remedial actions taken. Remember, "if it isn't documented, it wasn't done."[6]

The JCAHO has developed a ten-step quality assurance process that can be used at both the institutional and the clinical laboratory level for developing monitors of quality (Table 15–2).[7–10] The major purpose of this process is to improve quality and identify problems before patient care is affected. The first three steps give an overview of the structure of the organization, in this case the clinical chemistry laboratory. Step 1 describes the responsibilities of personnel within the chemistry laboratory and their function with regard to producing quality results and monitoring quality. Step 2 describes the procedures and protocols performed by chemistry laboratory personnel, including analytes assayed, times tests are offered, expected turnaround times for STAT and routine work, reference range reporting, and consultation. Step 3 describes the mission of the chemistry laboratory— those activities that have a major effect on the health and safety of the organization's clients. These activities may include proper labeling of specimens and requisitions, timely collection of specimens, accurate and timely analysis, and accurate reporting of results. The remaining seven steps focus on identifying problems and improving the services described in Steps 2 and 3.

The example of the Ten-Step JCAHO quality assurance process found in Table 15–2 is based on the need for notifying a physician, by phone, of patient results which are extremely abnormal (**panic values**). Panic values are results that must be communicated immediately to the physician so that an immediate decision on the care of the patient can be made, since the patient's life may be at immediate risk. A glucose determination of 25 mg/dL is an example of a panic value, for it indicates extreme hypoglycemia. In Step 4, identification of an indicator, technologists are instructed to enter panic results into the **Laboratory Information System (LIS)** and indicate who called, who was called, when they were called, and what results were called.

TABLE 15–2. QUALITY ASSURANCE PLAN: JCAHO TEN-STEP ACTION PLAN

STEP	DESCRIPTION: A MODEL	EXAMPLE
1. Assign responsibility	Describes the areas of responsibilities for laboratory staff	Director—Responsible for direction, coordination, and evaluation of QA activities Supervisor—Responsible for planning, implementation, and evaluation of QA activities Bench Technologist—Responsible for collection and documentation of data
2. Delineate scope of care	Describes the services provided by the laboratory to support patient care	The chemistry laboratory offers routine chemistry testing 24 hours/day, with turnaround time less than 2 hours for most tests STAT testing is available for electrolytes, BUN, calcium, creatinine, with turnaround time less than 1 hour STAT testing for blood gases is available with turnaround time of less than 15 minutes.
3. Identify important aspects of care	Describes the procedures and activities provided by the laboratory that have the greatest effect on the safety and health of patients	Perform accurate analyses in a timely fashion Obtain specimens safely, in a timely manner, and assure positive patient identification Ensure results are reported to the physician in a timely manner
4. Identify indicators and appropriate clinical criteria	Determines the laboratory activities that can be improved or corrected. An indicator is a well-defined, objective variable, used to monitor quality	The laboratory needs to make sure that all critical results are called to the caregiver. We will identify critical results and request that the technologists call these results and obtain the name of the person who received the results. The Laboratory Information System will print a report identifying all patient results in critical ranges
5. Establish thresholds for evaluation	Whenever a threshold is exceeded, the indicator needs to be evaluated	100% of all critical values must be called and documented
6. Monitor by collecting and organizing indicator data	Determine the information needed and the best format for review	Obtain daily report of all critical results, documentation of calling, and verifying technologist. Place in order of patient medical record number and sample number
7. Evaluate patient care support	What trends are noted and can be improved	Note technologists who do not routinely call panic values, and also note times when panic values are not called. Modify panic values if clinically reasonable
8. Take action to improve care or correct problems	Self-explanatory	Meet with technologists and develop an educational program for training new technologists
9. Assess the effectiveness of actions	Continue to monitor to make sure thresholds are not being exceeded	Continue to monitor the number of undocumented critical values
10. Communicate relevant information	Determine who should receive the QA results	Communicate with laboratory staff concerning the success of the quality assurance project and thank them for their cooperation. Inform laboratory administration of the success.

One criterion for success is that 100 percent of all panic values are called and documented in the LIS (Step 5). To monitor this activity, the LIS generates a daily report of all panic values and information input into the LIS regarding the calling of the panic value. The chemistry supervisor reviews this report daily (Step 6) to determine who may be neglecting to document calling results and which tests have an inordinate number of panic values (Step 7). Actions taken (Step 8) after review of these results may include having the supervisor retrain technologists who do not follow policy and the director modifying panic values if clinically reasonable. For instance, at Children's Hospital, Columbus, Ohio we discovered that a cholesterol level of 350 mg/dL was considered a panic value. This resulted in outpatient physicians being called at night. Although this cholesterol level is quite high, it is not imminently life threatening, and we determined that a panic value for cholesterol was not appropriate.

We continue to monitor panic results on a daily basis. To date we have seen an improvement in the delivery of care since results are being called (Step 9). The information from this study was communicated to the chemistry staff and to the quality assurance committee of the laboratory.

Several other monitors that can be used within the laboratory are

- turnaround time for STAT testing
- development of procedures for performing bedside glucose monitoring
- determination of why drug levels are being ordered when the previous three results were "no drug detected"
- determination of which patient units and phlebotomists are hemolyzing specimens
- review of reference range for lipase when a large number of specimens have elevated lipase but normal amylase results

- determination of shipping parameters for blood lead determinations
- review of panic values being telephoned

Quality assurance monitors may be long-term or short-term. Continuous (long-term) monitoring of the reporting of panic values ensures that technologists are following proper procedures. An example of a short-term study is the determination of the appropriateness of our lipase **reference range**. A physician at our hospital noted a significant number of inpatients and outpatients with plasma lipase activities three to four times the upper end of the **normal reference range** while amylase results were well within the amylase reference range. In most patients with pancreatitis the amylase and lipase levels are both increased. This observation raised the question of whether our reported lipase reference range adequately reflected the reference range of the hospital's population. A review of medical records from 20 patients indicated that the majority of these patients had some type of gastrointestinal disorder. We verified the lipase reference range by obtaining leftover plasma from specimens collected for blood lead screening and assaying the plasma for lipase and amylase. Since blood specimens from children being screened for blood lead are usually from children being seen for well-child checkups, the samples were assumed to be from healthy children. The results from these specimens fell within the lipase reference range previously determined. This brief QA study indicated that the reference range for lipase was appropriate, and that in some patients with gastrointestinal disease lipase results may be high while amylase results may be normal.

The College of American Pathologists (CAP) has developed a program called Q-Probes. These are quality assurance monitors developed by the CAP and distributed throughout the country. One example of a Q-Probe was Postanalytical QA: Hypercalcemia.[11] The purpose of this Q-Probe was to determine physician follow-up when an elevated calcium level was obtained. Over a 4-month period, a maximum of 20 different patients with elevated calcium results were evaluated. Participating laboratories reviewed each of the patients' medical records to determine (1) charting of result; (2) whether the result was noted by the physician; and (3) the types of follow-up tests performed, such as repeat calcium, ionized calcium, and parathyroid hormone. CAP collected the data and distributed a summary report. It was found that almost 99 percent (median = 100 percent) of the results had been properly charted, and that 85 percent (median) of the abnormal results had either been acted upon by ordering follow-up tests or were mentioned in the chart. It was suggested that laboratories improve the format of reports to make abnormal results more apparent. From our institution, we noted that the majority of abnormally high calcium levels came from patients receiving total parenteral nutrition. This report also allowed comparison between laboratories of reference range data and panic value data. Other Q-Probe studies have looked at turnaround times and reporting errors.

A good way to begin developing a quality assurance program is to develop a comprehensive Standard Operating Procedure Manual for the laboratory. This manual describes the processes occurring in the section other than the actual procedures used for analytical testing of the specimen. Sections of this manual include handling of mislabeled and unlabeled specimens, calling results, review of quality control and patient results, logging in specimens, staffing of critical areas, documentation of problems, maintenance procedures for common equipment such as centrifuges and refrigerators, and cleaning of the laboratory.

ESTABLISHING AND MONITORING PERFORMANCE OF AN INSTRUMENTAL METHOD

The Quality Assurance Plan monitors all aspects of the laboratory's role in patient care. Quality control, as stated previously, is a subpart of quality assurance and monitors the analytical aspects of patient testing. The laboratory must determine, verify, and monitor the accuracy and precision of methods over time. CLIA 88, Final Rule Subpart K §493.1201[3] states, "The laboratory must establish and follow written quality control procedures for monitoring and evaluating the quality of the analytical testing process to assure the accuracy and reliability of patient test results and reports." Suggested items in the Quality Control Plan are:

- Procedure format
- Method validation procedures
- Equipment maintenance and function checks
- Calibration
- Calibration verification
- Reference range verification
- Quality control procedures
- Remedial actions
- Maintenance of records
- Proficiency testing

The laboratory is free to develop criteria for assuring a test's reliability, but these criteria must be written and followed. The criteria cannot be too loose, since the laboratory must be able to pass proficiency testing.

Method Validation Procedure

One of the first things to do when developing a new procedure for routine use is to determine how the procedure is classified under CLIA. CLIA has three classifications for laboratory tests: waivered, moderate complexity, and high complexity. Based on how a specific test is classified, only certain persons within the laboratory may perform an analysis, and the verification of the method may be different. **Waivered tests** are those methods cleared by the FDA for home use, that employ methodologies unlikely to render erroneous results, or that pose no reasonable risk of harm to a patient if the test is incorrectly performed (§493.15).[3] The **moderate and high complexity tests** are categorized by how difficult the testing is and the need for the technologist to provide interpretation using criteria from §493.17. In most of the moderate complexity tests, pipetting is performed automatically by the instrument, no operator intervention is required during operation, and any manual procedures have limited steps. An example of moderate complexity testing is glucose on the DuPont ACA or Beckman Synchron. High complexity tests are usually manual, with multiple steps required in the analysis, or they require some type of operator action during the analysis. A high complexity test is high density lipoprotein (HDL) by a precipitation method, since a preliminary pipetting step must be done prior to analysis on a moderately complex instrument.

The first part of assuring an accurate and reliable result is to determine various characteristics of the method being added to the laboratory's repertoire. In most cases the manufacturer will have performed the majority of testing so that the method can be marketed. The performance characteristics that must be determined prior to offering a new test, as listed by CLIA (§493.1213) include accuracy, precision, analytical sensitivity, analytical specificity, reportable range, reference range, calibration procedures, and control procedures.[3] If a method is developed in-house, a manufacturer's method is modified, or the procedure has not been cleared by the FDA, then the laboratory must verify or establish all the foregoing characteristics. For methods that have been approved by the FDA as meeting the general requirements of quality control, the accuracy, precision, reportable range, and **reference ranges** of the manufacturer must be verified. Verification suggests that an extensive evaluation of each of these characteristics need not be performed, but they do need to be checked. There are no "golden rules" for verifying a manufacturer's claims, and CLIA does not indicate the procedures that need to be done. These must be developed within each laboratory and documented.

Calibration

When adopting an instrumental method, first become familiar with the manufacturer's procedure and follow it as closely as possible. Usually the first part of an analysis, after reagent preparation, is calibration of the instrument. **Calibration** is a process in which the response of the instrument is associated with the concentration of analyte. By plotting the output of the instrument (absorbance, freezing point, radioactive counts, potential difference) against the concentration of analyte in a reference solution, one can develop a calibration curve, which may be linear or nonlinear. Patient samples are then analyzed, the instrument response plotted on the calibration curve, and the patient concentration interpolated from the curve. Most instrumental methods do not require manual plotting of calibration curves, since the instrument performs these calculations internally.

The concentration of analyte in the reference solutions must be accurately known.

The concentrations can be determined by either preparing a *standard* by weighing the analyte and adding it to a known amount of solvent (water), or by determining the concentration of a *calibrator* by measuring the amount of analyte in a solution (urine, serum) using a reference method. With many methods the effects of other constituents in solution (such as serum) may affect the analysis because of "matrix effects." For example, a serum sample with 100 mg/dL glucose would react differently than an aqueous standard containing the same concentration of glucose on methods using dry-chemical technology because of the large amount of protein in the serum. For these instruments a serum calibrator must be used whose concentration has been determined by another method of known accuracy. Since serum samples contain endogenous glucose, the addition of pure analyte would not be helpful, since the initial concentration of glucose in the serum is unknown. Standard and calibrator are often used interchangeably. Standard connotes reference material prepared by weighing pure analyte and adding it to an appropriate solvent for analysis. Calibrator connotes a reference material whose concentration is determined by assay with a reference method.

Depending upon an instrument's stability, the instrument may need to be calibrated every 30 minutes (blood gases), from every time an analytical run is made (batch analyzers) to every 6 months (various multianalyte analyzers). The laboratory must follow the manufacturer's requirements for frequency of calibration.

Calibration verification is a process in which the calibration of the instrument is checked on a periodic basis. CLIA defines calibration verification as ". . . assaying of calibration materials in the same manner as patients to confirm that the calibration of the instrument, kit, or test system has remained stable throughout the laboratory's reportable range for test results (§493.1217)."[1] Verification may be done by assaying calibration material on the instrument as samples of unknown concentration (such as patient samples), and determining whether the results obtained are equivalent to the label value of the calibrator. Again, CLIA does not say how good is good enough, so it is the laboratory's responsibility to define the acceptability of a calibration verification procedure. Each analyte may have its own limits of acceptability, but these limits must be defined. One may also use materials whose concentrations are known, from the instrument manufacturer, material obtained from other manufacturers, or prepared in house with spiked serums. Laessig and associates give good descriptions of the process of calibration verification.[12]

Calibration or calibration verification must be performed, according to CLIA, at least once every 6 months; after a major preventive maintenance or repair; when controls suggest an unusual trend; when the manufacturer requires it; and when new lots of reagent are obtained unless it can be shown that patient and control results are not adversely affected.

Precision

After determining how to run the procedure and how to perform a calibration, the next step in method validation is to begin to determine the precision of the method. The **precision** of a method describes how closely repetitive measurements of a specimen repeat; it is expressed as both the standard deviation and the coefficient of variation.[13-16] The **standard deviation (SD)** describes the distribution of these repetitive measurements about the mean of those measurements, the mean being the average of the repetitive measurements. For example, if one measured the glucose concentration of a specimen 40 times, the same result would not be obtained with every analysis. This could be due to differences in pipeting, noise in the optical system, noise in the electrical system, temperature, and a host of other factors. A mean glucose of 250 mg/dL and a standard deviation (SD) of 6 mg/dL indicates that $\cong$ 68 percent of the results were within the range 250 ± 6 (244 to 256). Twice the standard deviation (2 SD) indicates that $\cong$ 95 percent of the specimen results fall within ± 2 SD (in this case, 250 ± 12 or 238 to 262). The higher the standard deviation, the more the results are spread out from the mean and the less precise the method.

The **coefficient of variation (CV)** describes the standard deviation relative to its mean (i.e., SD · 100/mean), so that one may more easily compare precision over the analytical range of an assay. The CV in the foregoing example is 2.4 percent. With a particular assay the CVs at various concentrations tend to remain similar, since at increased concentrations the standard deviation also increases. However, one must be careful when interpreting CVs if the concentration is low, since division by a low concentration results in a large CV. Many calculators and computer programs can calculate the standard deviation and the mean. One must be careful, however, to calculate the sample standard deviation as opposed to the population standard deviation. If a program calculates the population standard deviation, multiply this result by $n/(n-1)$, where n is the number of replicates measured.

The total precision of an assay is composed of within-run, between-run, and between-day precision. A **run**, as defined by CLIA (§493.1218)[3] is "an interval within which the accuracy and precision of a testing system is expected to be stable, but cannot be greater than 24 hours." Therefore a run is dependent upon the individual method. For instance, with the Abbott VP system, a run consists of no more than 30 specimens, including standards, patients, and controls, since standards and controls have to be run with every group of patients. With a DuPont ACA system, a run may be defined as once each shift, since controls are run at the beginning and end of the shift. The within-run, between-run, and between-day precisions are determined by calculating the standard deviations of a control assayed several times during an analytical run, several times during the day, and over a period of several days, respectively. Two NCCLS documents describe methods for determining precision.[13, 14]

Accuracy

Accuracy is how close a result is to the "true result." A method may be very precise but may give an inaccurate result. One of the challenges in laboratory medicine is to determine the true result. Different matrices found in clinical specimens make determination of the true result very difficult. Enzyme activity, in particular, is dependent upon the substrates, cofactors, and temperatures used in the analysis. To determine the accuracy of a method, one may use specimens whose concentrations are accurately known, or one may compare results with a method known to be accurate. Specimens whose concentrations are accurately known may be obtained from the National Institute of Science and Technology (NIST), formerly the National Bureau of Standards. The concentrations of analytes in these specimens have been determined by rigorous analytical methods that are unsuitable for routine use due to the labor, time, and equipment resources needed to perform the analyses.

Another source of specimens having well-defined concentrations are Survey Validated

Reference Materials available from the CAP. These products are extra samples of survey material that had been sent to several thousand laboratories for analysis. Studies have shown that the mean results obtained from these surveys are very close to the concentrations determined by reference methods. The expense of these materials, and their limited range of concentrations, makes their use for routine instrument calibration expensive. However, they can be used when developing a method to check that the routine calibration materials are acceptable, and they may be used on a monthly or quarterly basis to check results of routine standardization and controls.

Besides using accurately known reference standards to confirm a method's accuracy, a new method may be compared with an alternative method. A **reference method** is a method whose precision and accuracy are well described when the exact procedure is followed.[16] However, not all analytes have reference methods, and of those analytes that do, most laboratories do not have the resources to perform this type of testing, since these methods are time consuming and may require equipment not readily available in the laboratory. It is often left up to the manufacturer to compare their method with an acceptable reference method.

Even though the manufacturer of a method has compared its results with a reference method, the laboratory must validate that the method works appropriately. If a new procedure is replacing or supplementing the current procedure, then one may assay patient specimens using both procedures.[15–17] If, however, the procedure is new, one may have to split specimens with a reference laboratory; that is, save some specimen for analysis with the new procedure and send the remaining specimen to the reference laboratory. One caveat in splitting specimens is that extra specimen for comparison testing may not be able to be drawn without the patient's informed consent. The institution's Human Subjects Committee should be consulted before doing this type of comparison. Depending upon an institution's policies, for example, if 3 mL of blood is routinely drawn for test XYZ but test XYZ requires only 0.1 mL of blood, then the remaining blood may be used for comparison studies without patient consent. If, however, the current method requires 2 mL of blood and the new method also requires 2 mL, 4 mL may not be drawn from the patient unless the patient provides written informed consent, or unless the Human Subjects Committee grants permission.

Also be aware that strict patient confidentiality must be maintained when performing these studies. For example, listings of results should not carry any patient identifiers, such as medical record numbers or patient names. Only the primary investigator within the institution should be able to cross-reference results and names.

An alternative means of obtaining specimens for method comparison studies is from reference laboratories. Many reference laboratories are willing to send leftover samples from specimens they have already assayed for comparison of results.

There are no hard and fast rules for determining whether method comparisons are acceptable. The comparative method should be firmly established by consistently having acceptable results on proficiency surveys or be a documented reference method. Quality goals should be determined prior to the comparison. Both CAP[15] and NCCLS[17] suggest comparing at least 40 specimens, assayed in duplicate on both instruments. Specimen concentrations should span the analytical range of the method, with about one third of the specimens being in each of the ranges (low, mid, and high).

How does one determine whether the accuracy and precision are adequate? For those analytes for which CLIA has developed proficiency standards, the precision and accuracy must be at least as good as CLIA criteria. Ehrmeyer and associates recommend that a method's SD be one third the allowable CLIA SD.[18] For instance, the acceptable CLIA criteria for a total calcium result is "target value" plus or minus 1.0 mg/dL. The method should be able to have a between-day standard deviation of less than 0.33 mg/dL. This is assuming that there is no significant bias between methods. The **bias** is the difference between results from the reference method and results from the method under investigation. This criterion was developed to increase the chances of passing **proficiency testing**.

Reportable Range

The **reportable range** is the range of concentrations that may be reported to the clinician without the need for further treatments such as dilution. The manufacturer usually determines this range, but according to CLIA the range must be validated. To determine the reportable range, one plots the expected result versus the reported result of a series of known samples (calibration material) (Fig. 15–1). If this plot maintains linearity through the manufacturer's reportable range, then the manufacturer's range may be used. If the plot deviates from linearity, then further study is needed to determine where the assay begins to deviate from linearity. Judgment of linearity is best done visually. This linearity of "expected" versus "reported" concentrations must not be confused with the analytical response of a method. For instance, most radioimmunoassay methods have a nonlinear response when concentration is plotted against radioactive counts per minute (Fig. 15–2); however, if a specimen is diluted by one half, it is expected that the reported concentration would be one half its expected concentration

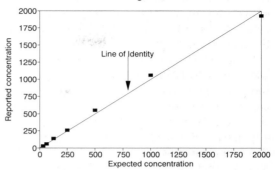

17-Hydroxyprogesterone by RIA
ng/dL

■ **FIGURE 15–1.**

Standards assayed as patient samples to check method linearity and to verify the method's reportable range. Expected results versus measured results.

even though the actual radioactive counts may be actually three to four times higher.

Linearity should be determined with at least three and preferably five evenly distributed points.[19] There are several ways to create linearly related specimens to determine the reportable range of an assay, including addition of high concentration analyte to specimens with low concentration

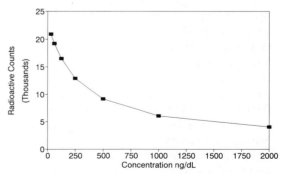

17-Hydroxyprogesterone by RIA

■ **FIGURE 15–2.**

Instrumental response to standards of known concentration.

(spiking), over- and underdilution of lyophilized control material and mixing specimens with high and low concentrations, or use of linearity specimens prepared by a manufacturer. Since manufacturers go through this process of determining a method's linearity, they can and should act as advisors to their customers in setting up a linearity study.

Spiking is a process in which a high concentration of a particular analyte is added to a specimen. The specimen should have a low concentration of the analyte of interest. The spiking process will increase the volume of the specimen by about 10 percent. The increase in volume should be no more than 20 percent, and the final increase in volume of the specimen should be the same for all spiked solutions (Table 15–3). One also may underdilute and overdilute calibrators or controls. With some instrument systems, underdilution or overdilution may cause problems owing to large changes in the sample matrix. Determining the upper limits of linearity is usually simple since addition of analyte can usually be easily done. However, determination of the lower limit of the reportable range is difficult for those analytes that have endogenous analyte (see *analytical sensitivity* in the next section). For glucose, a possible tactic is to allow the specimen to stand overnight without being separated from the blood cells. The glucose is slowly metabolized over time until no glucose is available. One also may be on the lookout for specimens that have low concentrations of an analyte.

Specificity and Sensitivity

The **analytical specificity** of a procedure is its ability to give an accurate result in the presence of numerous other compounds. These interfering compounds may be drugs, food products, in vivo compounds, or compounds added to blood after collection (Table 15–4). For example, if a specimen is hemolyzed, the hemolysis may interfere with the analysis of bilirubin in some methods. Common interfering agents that decrease the specificity of some methods include hemolysis, bilirubin, and lipids. Besides these, compounds similar in structure may interfere. For example, ion-selective electrodes for ionized calcium must not react in the presence of magnesium, sodium, potassium, or other metals when these metals are within physiologic concentrations. Assays for albumin should react minimally to high concentrations of other proteins, and procedures for glucose should not react with other sugars such as mannitol. NCCLS Document EP7-P provides guidelines for performing **interference** testing.[20]

The **analytical sensitivity** of an assay describes the ability of the assay to measure low concentrations of an analyte and is probably best described as the detection limit. Within CLIA there is no precise definition of analytical sensitivity. To determine the detection limit, assay a specimen that has either no analyte or a low concentration of analyte approximately 20 times over several runs. Determine the mean and standard deviation. Multiply the standard deviation by 2. This result becomes the detection limit for the assay, and results obtained that are less than this value should be reported as "less than" the detection limit. The detection limit of a blood lead assay, for example, was determined by measuring a patient sample 20 times over 10 runs. The mean was 2.5 μg/dL, with an SD of 0.8. Twice the SD, or the detection limit, is 1.6. Thus when a patient result of 1.0 μg/dL is obtained, it should be reported as "less than 1.6 μg/dL."[16, 21]

One must be careful not to confuse the analytical sensitivity and specificity of a test with its **clinical sensitivity** and **specificity**.[22] Clinical sensitivity gives the probability of a positive result when a patient has a

TABLE 15-3. PREPARATION OF LINEARITY SPECIMENS

SPIKING
1. Obtain primary specimen with glucose concentration less than 50 mg/dL
2. Determine upper concentration to be tested—600 mg/dL
3. Determine percent the primary specimen will be diluted by the spiking solution—10%
4. Determine concentration of the spiking solution. Upper concentration/percent diluted = 600/0.10 = 6000 mg/dL
5. Prepare spiking solution—dissolve 6 g of glucose in 100 mL of saline
6. Prepare working spiking solutions:

SOLUTION #	mL SPIKING SOLUTION	mL SALINE	FINAL CONCENTRATION
1	1.00	0.00	600 mg/dL
2	0.75	0.25	450 mg/dL
3	0.50	0.50	300 mg/dL
4	0.25	0.75	150 mg/dL
5	0.00	1.00	0 mg/dL

7. Pipet 0.1 mL of each of the spiking solutions into 1 mL of the primary specimen and assay each specimen, preferably in duplicate
8. Plot the final concentrations on the x-axis versus the reported result on the y-axis. Connect the points with straight lines and visually inspect for linearity
9. Note: The final concentrations shown above did not take into account the original glucose concentration of the specimen nor the dilution of the specimen with 0.1 mL of spiking solution. Since these are constants throughout the spiking solutions, they do not need to be corrected for, as we are looking only for linearity of the method

OVER- AND UNDERDILUTION OF CONTROLS
1. The high control is a dry lyophilized specimen normally diluted to 3 mL (0.003 L) with buffer, has an enzyme acitivity of 800 U/L
2. Dilute lyophilized high control with 2 mL (0.002 L) of buffer. This will result in a final concentration of 1200 U/L
Equations for determining concentration when underdiluted:

   800 U/L × 0.003 L/bottle = 2.4 U/bottle
   2.4 U/bottle × bottle/0.002 L = 1200 U/L

3. The low control is a dry lyophilized specimen normally diluted to 3 mL (0.003 L) with buffer, has an enzyme activity of 95 U/L

4. Dilute lyophilized low control with 5 mL (0.005 L) of buffer

   95 U/L × 0.003 L/bottle = 0.285 U/bottle
   0.285 U/bottle × bottle/0.005 L = 57 U/L

5. Mix various aliquots of the under- and overdiluted controls:

   1 part 1200 U/L + 1 part 57 U/L = 629 U/L
   3 parts 1200 U/L + 1 part 57 U/L = 914 U/L
   1 part 1200 U/L + 3 parts 57 U/L = 343 U/L

6. Assay each of the admixtures and each of the overdiluted and underdiluted controls
7. Plot the final enzyme activity against the calculated concentrations. Observe for linearity

TABLE 15–4. EXAMPLES OF INTERFERING SUBSTANCES

TYPE OF INTERFERANT	ANALYTE	METHOD
Bananas	Vanillylmandelic acid	Pisano
Hemolysis	Bilirubin	Jendrassik-Grof
EDTA	Calcium, magnesium	Wet chemical
Ascorbic acid	Oxalate	Enzymatic
Lipemia	Alanine aminotransferase	Enzymatic

particular disease. Clinical specificity is the probability of a negative test result when a patient does not have a particular disease. For example, a patient suffering from a myocardial infarction (heart attack) will have an elevated total creatine kinase (CK) level. This enzyme test is therefore very sensitive. However, patients who have had major muscle trauma, such as after an automobile accident, or muscle-wasting diseases will also have an elevated CK, making the CK test nonspecific—that is, diseases other than a myocardial infarction can result in an elevated CK level.

Reference Range

The laboratory must either develop or validate **reference ranges** for its procedures. A reference range describes the range of concentrations for a particular analyte in a defined group of individuals.[23–25] Usually the defined group consists of healthy individuals, described in the past as "normals." The reference range is used by clinicians to compare results from their patients with healthy persons to help them determine a diagnosis. Reference ranges may be found in manufacturers' literature, journal articles, and textbooks. Reference ranges described in journals and textbooks may not be appropriate, since they may have been developed on different instruments and methods. This

is especially true for enzymes, since different methods use different substrates, temperatures, and reaction sequences. In Tietz, two different reference ranges are given for lactate dehydrogenase in adults: 45 to 90 U/L for a lactate-to-pyruvate reaction and 150 to 320 U/L for a pyruvate-to-lactate reaction.[26] Immunoassays also can be different between assays because of differences in calibration materials.

When results between new and old instruments are shown to be equivalent, the old reference range probably can be used with the new method, but this must be validated. CLIA[3] and CAP[4] require that reference ranges be validated. However, CLIA provides no rules for developing reference ranges, so the laboratory is empowered to determine these ranges. The laboratory, however, must have a written procedure for developing and validating reference ranges.

Reference ranges usually are developed from specimens of "healthy people," usually ambulatory ones. How can one get samples from healthy people? From volunteers, from personnel within the laboratory; some places use medical students, and some places may use health fairs at which patients are screened for cholesterol and glucose levels; remaining blood could be used for development of normal ranges. Check with the Human Subjects Committee of your institution regarding informed consent prior to collecting these samples.

Reference ranges may be different for different ages (e.g., alkaline phosphatase), sex (e.g., creatinine clearance), time of collection (e.g., cortisol), time since last meal (e.g., triglyceride), smoking (e.g., carbon monoxide), or methods (e.g., lactate dehydrogenase). The defined group may be healthy individuals, hospitalized patients, individuals attending a health fair, and so on. When determining who should be used as representative of a reference population, criteria for exclusion of patients must be determined and may include prescription drug use, abuse of drugs, recent illness, fasting or nonfasting, and so on. Exclusion criteria should be based on the analyte being assayed and the population of interest.

NCCLS suggests that the reference population should resemble the patient population for which the test will be used but that clinic or hospitalized patients should not be used to help determine reference ranges unless absolutely necessary.[24] The NCCLS proposed guideline suggests that at least 120 subjects be tested to determine a reference range based on the findings of Reed and associates.[25] This guideline uses nonparametric statistics to determine the range within which 95 percent of the reference samples fall—that is, between the 2.5 and 97.5 percentiles, with a confidence of 90 percent. The use of mean plus or minus 2 standard deviations (gaussian statistics) is not appropriate for determination of reference ranges for most analytes.[25] When performing a reference range study, the sampling and instrumental methods must be the same as would be done for patients.

The subject of validation of reference ranges was not approached in the NCCLS document, although they do address "transference" of reference ranges. If two assays within the same laboratory are found to give equivalent results, then the reference interval can be transferred from one method to the other. If methods do not give equivalent results, then either the instruments must be adjusted to give equivalent results or two different reference ranges must be reported.

If a laboratory wants to transfer (validate) a reference range prepared at another laboratory or by the manufacturer, it should use approximately 60 reference individuals and compare these results with the other laboratory's results, using guidelines in the NCCLS document. If it can be shown that there are no significant differences between the reference intervals, then the reference range provided by the second laboratory can be used.

A patient's result that falls within a reference range of "healthy individuals" does not necessarily indicate good health. Cholesterol is a good example. The Lipid Research Clinics Program Epidemiology Committee reported reference values for total cholesterol of 150 to 260 mg/dL for supposedly healthy men between the ages of 40 and 45 years obtained from the North American population.[27] The ideal range for a healthy individual, however, is in the range of 130 to 190 mg/dL.[28] The American population as a whole has cholesterol concentrations that are too high. Some reference ranges are suggested by governmental agencies; in particular, the reference range for blood lead in children has been set at less than 10 μg/dL.[29] It is therefore important that all methods for lead analysis are equivalent. Equivalency of blood lead methods is determined by analysis of proficiency samples.

Laessig and associates[6] suggest obtaining 10 to 20 samples from normal subjects to validate reference ranges and compare these results with the manufacturer's range. If most of the results are within the specified range, they suggest that this validates the reference range. This shortened process could also be done for reference ranges from books and other literature.

Written Procedures

The Quality Control Plan should describe the format of how procedures are written and reviewed. The **National Committee for Clinical Laboratory Standards (NCCLS)** has developed guidelines for writing a laboratory procedure.[30] In fact, CAP inspection guidelines require that this document be available within the laboratory. Procedures must be reviewed at least yearly, according to CAP and CLIA guidelines. Table 15–5 lists items that must be included in the procedure, although the actual format is up to the individual laboratory. With multianalyte instruments such as the Ektachem or DuPont ACA, only one procedure needs to be written for the overall operation of the instrument. Separate procedures for each analyte may cross-reference this overall procedure.

After determining the accuracy, precision, sensitivity, specificity, reportable range, calibration procedures, and reference range and having developed a written procedure, the personnel who will be performing the assay must be trained. Employees who can perform this testing must be identified per CLIA testing categories. To help make training easier, a training guide for each instrument should be developed. This guide should outline the steps the trainee must perform to become proficient on the analyzer. Steps should include:

1. Read laboratory procedure
2. General overview of instrument by instructor
3. Perform preventive maintenance
4. Perform calibration
5. Perform controls and patient samples that have already been assayed
6. Understand how results are reported and identify panic values

After everybody is trained and has had a chance to assay a few practice samples, the instrument is ready to be placed on line to report patient results. Keep documentation of all the persons trained to operate the instrument and of all the validation procedures used to indicate that use of the instrument is appropriate for patient care.

TABLE 15–5. COMPONENTS OF A CLINICAL LABORATORY PROCEDURE ACCORDING TO CLIA

READILY AVAILABLE AND FOLLOWED:
- Include the following when applicable to the test procedure:
  Requirements for specimen collection, processing, and storage
  Step-by-step performance of procedure, including test calculations and interpretation
  Preparation of reagents, controls, standards, and other necessary materials
  Calibration and calibration verification procedures
  Reportable range for patient test results
  Control procedures
  Remedial action when calibration or control results are unacceptable
  Limitations of melthodologies (including interfering substances)
  Reference ranges
  Imminent life-threatening laboratory results (panic values)
  Actions taken when a laboratory method becomes inoperable
- Procedures must be approved, signed, and dated by the director
- Procedures must be reapproved, signed, and dated when the directorship changes
- Each change in a procedure must be approved, signed, and dated by the current director of the laboratory
- The laboratory must indicate the date of initial use and discontinuance of a procedure

ADDITIONAL CAP REQUIREMENTS
- Describe the clinical aspects of the procedure
- Describe the theoretical and analytical aspects of the method
- All procedures must be kept for a minimum of 2 years after being discontinued
- Clinical reason for the method

QUALITY ASSURANCE FOR INSTRUMENTS USED FOR PATIENT CARE

Now that the instrument is reporting patient results, the laboratory must assure itself that the instrument is working properly. This is done by assaying quality control material with each run, by participating in proficiency surveys, and by reviewing patient results.

Quality Control

Performing analyses on quality control material is used to help assure that the method is working properly. Quality control material should have chemical and physical properties as close as possible to patient samples and should be handled in the same manner as are patients. QC material may be purchased in various forms, including lyophilized serum that must be reconstituted with either water or special buffers, frozen or liquid. The concentrations of these controls should be close to the clinical decision levels but also have a wide spread. For glucose, controls should be around 60 mg/dL and 200 to 300 mg/dL. Of course these concentrations are dependent upon the availability of material. Quality control procedures that must be followed for CLIA are:

- Perform quality control at least once every 24 hours or as recommended by the manufacturer.
- Perform a positive and negative control for qualitative tests.
- Perform at least two controls for quantitative tests.
- If quality control and calibration materials are not available, there must be an alternative mechanism for assuring valid test results.

- Treat control specimens in the same manner as patients whenever possible.
- Determine the mean and standard deviation for each lot of quality control material by repetitive testing.

If an assayed material is used, the laboratory may use the target values provided by the manufacturer, as long as these values correspond to the method being used and the values are verified.

If an unassayed material is used, the laboratory must establish over time the mean and standard deviation by concurrent testing with materials that already have determined statistical parameters.

Special quality control rules for blood gas instruments are:

- Calibrate or verify calibration with a frequency recommended by the manufacturer.
- Test at least one quality control sample every 8 hours.
- Assay a high and low control at least once each day.
- Perform a calibration or control whenever patients are tested unless the instrument automatically verifies calibration every 30 minutes.

Once each run, at least two quality control samples must be assayed. Results of quality control should be reviewed immediately after being assayed by the technologist, on a daily and weekly basis by the supervisor, and on a monthly basis by the director and supervisor of the laboratory area.

The immediate QC review by the technologist is done to determine whether patient results can be reported. Definite policies must be established to guide the technologist as to whether results are acceptable and whether patient results can be reported.

One example of a procedure to follow when the QC results are found to be unacceptable would be to follow the steps below and document all findings on a problem log:

1. Repeat analysis of controls.
2. Check lot number of the reagent(s).
3. Make sure correct calibration is entered.
4. Check previous controls and determine whether there is a trend in results.
5. Assay controls on another analyzer.
6. Contact key operator and discuss problem.
7. Recalibrate.
8. Contact manufacturer.

Of course, these guidelines may be different for different assays or instruments.

Daily, the supervisor should review quality control results to make sure the instrument operators are properly reviewing the QC and that they are not reporting results when instrumentation is not in control. Weekly, the supervisor can check to determine whether instrumentation is beginning to give "noisy" results (loss of precision), or whether results are shifting. This type of review is most easily done using **Levy-Jennings charts** (Fig. 15–3). A Levy-Jennings chart is produced by plotting the date on one axis (usually the x-axis) and quality control results on a second axis (y-axis). One line is passed through the mean while other lines are passed through 1 and 2 standard deviations above and below the mean. Quality control results are plotted daily so that re-

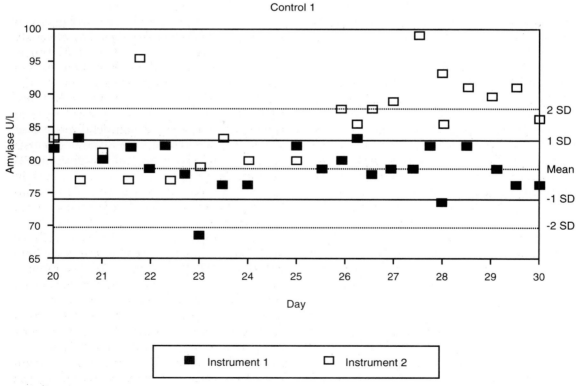

■ **FIGURE 15–3.**

Levy-Jennings plot.

sults can be viewed over time. If results are jumping above and below the mean, the procedure may be noisy. If the results start to move slowly in one direction, a trend in the results is indicated. An abrupt change in results indicates a shift. Noisy results may be caused by improper reconstitution of quality control material, electronic noise, and various other problems.

A trend in results may indicate numerous changes in the instrument system, including instrument temperatures, light filters becoming dirty, membranes needing change, or problems with a sampling system. A shift in results may result from changes in lot numbers of reagents or controls. Many other factors may cause these changes in quality control; they need to be investigated and the results of the investigation documented. Figure 15–3 indicates that while instrument 1 was operating within control, there was a large jump in the control values for instrument 2 on day 26. Since the same control was being assayed on each instrument, these results indicated a problem with instrument number 2 and not a problem with the control material.

Monthly, the results should again be reviewed by review of the Levy-Jennings charts and by review of the control's mean and standard deviation. This monthly review may indicate a need to change the mean and standard deviation. When and if this change is needed, it must be done carefully, with documented reasons for the change, such as new lots of reagents or controls, or major repair to the instrument.

Unfortunately, there are no hard and fast rules for determining acceptable quality control ranges.[31] For some instruments, the control results within a lot are so tight that when a new lot of reagent is obtained, there can be a shift in the control results. This shift may not be clinically significant but analytically may be quite significant. Some laboratories use the actual mean and standard deviation calculated from several runs of the control using reagent from a single lot. A more practical approach may be to review the standard deviations of controls having similar values over numerous lots of reagent. This combined SD would then be used regardless of the reagent lot. When a new lot of reagent is obtained, the control is assayed several times and the mean compared with the mean of the previous lot. If the difference is within 1 SD, then no changes need to be made. If the difference is greater than 1 SD, further investigation is needed. When changing between reagent lots, it is also a good idea to run patient samples on both lots to assure that patient results are not affected. Even if there are control changes, there may not be any changes in patients because of the matrix effects inherent in control material.

When a new lot of quality control material arrives, it should be assayed simultaneously with the current control, at least 20 times, over a period of 20 days. For some assays this may be quite unreasonable due to the small number of assays performed. In those cases, the control can be assayed several times on an analytical run. The mean and SD of the control is calculated. The SD should be compared with the combined SD of several lots of the control with means in the vicinity of the new control. If this combined SD is reasonable, it can be used with the new mean.

Westgard and associates[31] have developed a number of quality control rules to help determine whether results are acceptable; Laessig and associates[6] have developed some changes to these rules that may be helpful. One does not even need to use a strict calculated standard deviation to come up with a quality control range.[33] The range may be based on CLIA criteria, as mentioned earlier, or it may be based on the medical usefulness.

Besides following quality control on each

individual instrument, twice each year the laboratory needs to check that different instruments, using the same or different methodologies, are reporting equivalent results (§493.1709).[3] This can be done by duplicate sampling of patient specimens and by ongoing review of quality control when the same quality control material is being used on the different instruments.

Proficiency Testing

Proficiency surveys consist of samples sent to a number of laboratories for analysis. The concentrations of analytes or the identity of organisms in the specimens are unknown to the participants. Results from each laboratory are returned to the provider, who collates the data and determines whether a participating laboratory has acceptable results.

The first report of clinical laboratory **proficiency testing** was in 1947 by Belk and Sunderman, who reported on a study in which they sent solutions containing known amounts of glucose, sodium, chloride, protein, urea nitrogen, calcium, albumin, and hemoglobin to 59 laboratories.[34] Results from this first proficiency survey were not good. Glucose results reported for an aqueous solution having a weighed-in concentration of 375 mg of glucose/dL had results ranging from less than 100mg/dL to greater than 600 mg/dL.

After this initial survey, interlaboratory surveys improved considerably. The focus of the proficiency survey was to provide laboratories a voluntary means to compare their results with those of their peers and to allow these laboratories to find and correct problems.[35] Reports of inaccurate laboratory data causing serious injury to patients led to the Clinical Laboratories Improvement Act of 1967 in which proficiency testing was used to determine whether a laboratory would be reimbursed by Medicare. Participation in some type of proficiency testing became mandatory for a number of laboratories.

CLIA 1988 has mandated (§493.801) that all laboratories must participate successfully in an approved proficiency survey.[3] CLIA describes the procedures for performing proficiency testing:

- All laboratories performing moderately or highly complex testing must participate in proficiency testing.
- If a laboratory performs testing that does not have proficiency testing requirements listed in the Federal Register, they must have a system for verifying accuracy and reliability at least twice each year.
- Proficiency samples must be run within the routine patient workload, assayed by routine personnel, and assayed the same number of times as those of patients.
- Laboratories may not communicate with each other regarding proficiency samples until results have been reported. Laboratories with multiple testing sites must not communicate between sites regarding proficiency results until results have been reported.
- Proficiency samples cannot be sent to another laboratory for analysis.
- The laboratory must document the handling, preparation, processing, and each step in the analysis and reporting of results. Documents must be maintained at least 2 years.
- Proficiency testing is required for only the primary method used for patient testing during the proficiency testing event.
- The laboratory director and analyst performing proficiency testing must attest that the proficiency samples were integrated into the routine patient workload and routine laboratory methods were used.

The samples must be handled as nearly as possible to the laboratory's routine procedure for a patient specimen. If patient specimens are assayed only once, then the proficiency must also be assayed only once. If a result from a survey exceeds a limit when patient results are routinely repeated, then the proficiency sample may be repeated. The proficiency specimens are to be run by workers who routinely perform patient specimens. Personnel from one laboratory cannot exchange information with another laboratory regarding the proficiency samples until after the results are submitted. A laboratory also cannot send its survey material to a second laboratory and then report the results of the second laboratory. After analysis, the survey sample should be stored, if possible, to allow a repeat analysis if necessary after results have been returned. The laboratory must document and maintain records of who prepared, analyzed, and reported results from a proficiency study.

Before sending the survey to the proficiency survey provider, the laboratory director and all analysts must attest by signature that the procedures used to test the proficiency samples were as close as possible to the procedures used to test patients. Records of proficiency testing must be kept for a minimum of 2 years. It is a good idea to keep a photocopy of the result form sent in to the survey provider, along with all instrument printouts and copies of quality control from the day the specimens were assayed. Also, it is a good idea to have a second person review results to check for careless transcription errors. It also may be useful to send results by certified mail, return receipt requested, to prove that results were received by the provider. With the large number of results being handled by the proficiency provider, result forms could get lost. Also, keep a calendar that indicates dates surveys are to be shipped and start to look

for these surveys 2 to 3 days after this shipping date. If the material is not received within a reasonable time, you must contact the proficiency provider to obtain the samples.

CLIA has developed criteria for acceptable results for a large number of tests, although not all tests. Tests that do not have CLIA proficiency criteria may be evaluated using the provider's own criteria. If no proficiency surveys are available, the laboratory must develop a plan to determine its proficiency. This may entail sending several split specimens to another laboratory to confirm results.

After receiving results from a survey, review the results to make sure they were properly recorded by the provider, and contact the provider if any errors are found. The results should be reviewed by the director of the laboratory, the supervisor, and also the persons working in the area.

CLIA has developed criteria for proficiency survey providers to grade survey results (Table 15–6). Each analyte has a **target value** assigned by the survey provider. This target value may be the mean of results for all laboratories, excluding outliers, or may be the mean of results from a select group of reference laboratories. A result is considered unacceptable if the result is outside the range of the target value plus or minus a numeric criteria factor, known as

TABLE 15–6. EXAMPLES OF ACCEPTABLE PERFORMANCE OF PROFICIENCY TESTING USING CLIA CRITERIA

ANALYTE	CRITERIA FOR ACCEPTABLE PERFORMANCE
Albumin	Target value ± 10%
Amylase	Target value ± 30%
Glucose	Target value ± 6 mg/dL or ± 10% (greater)
Sodium	Target value ± 4 mmol/L

the **target range**. For example, if the mean for amylase from a CAP survey were 300 U/L, the target range would be 270 to 330, since the criteria factor is 10 percent. Proficiency reports grade results by determining the number of standard deviations a laboratory's result is from the target value. This **standard deviation index** (SDI) is calculated by subtracting the target value from the laboratory result and dividing this difference by the standard deviation of survey participants. For non-CLIA tests, SDIs less than 2.0 are acceptable.

If a result is unacceptable, the following steps should be taken:

1. Review a copy of the results to make sure they were transcribed properly
2. Make sure quality control was acceptable when the analysis was run
3. Repeat the analysis with leftover sample if available
4. Review calibration and instrumentation logs
5. Review protocol for handling samples
6. Check other results assayed at the same time on the same sample

For example, if all the results from a specimen were high for different analytes, this may indicate a problem in the reconstitution of the proficiency sample. Usually we can find a reasonable explanation for results being unacceptable.

After discovering reasons for a result being unacceptable, corrective actions must be taken and documented to assure that the problem does not recur.

Review of Patient Results

One of the best ways to review the quality of results is to review patient results in an organized manner. CLIA and CAP require ongoing review of patient results. Initial review should look for results that are obviously life-threatening or bizarre. Review includes looking at the previous result, or if one is not available, a repeat of the analysis, and checking of controls. If these checks are all right, then one should contact the patient's caregiver to make sure that the results are consistent with the patient's condition. In the case of results that may reflect life-threatening conditions, the results should be phoned to the caregiver, with the proviso that the testing will be repeated. In the medical record, the result should be labeled as being repeated, the result confirmed, and the call to the caregiver documented.

Some laboratory information systems allow comparison of previous results with current results of a patient by displaying both results simultaneously. Some systems go even further by performing **delta checks**: calculating differences in results and flagging results when differences are greater than certain criteria.[36] Delta checks are based on the observations that most analyte concentrations remain relatively constant over time. Large concentration changes may occur with major changes in a patient's condition. However, several other factors unrelated to the patient's condition may result in a failed delta check, including mislabeled specimens, instrumentation going out of calibration, or placing samples in the wrong position in a sampler tray. Performing delta checks helps identify these types of mistakes. Delta checks may be based on absolute differences (result [time 1]—result [time 2¢], or on percentage differences (result [time 1]—result [time 2])/(average of results [time 1] and [time 2]). Table 15–7 lists delta check criteria for several analytes. Delta checks may not be useful for all analytes, such as blood gases and glucose in critically ill patients, since these results can

TABLE 15–7. DELTA CHECK EXAMPLES

ANALYTE	RESULT	FAILED DELTA
Sodium	All results	≥6.0 mmol/L
Aspartate	0–30 U/L	100%
transaminase (AST)	30–60 U/L	60%
	60–480 U/L	50%
	>480 U/L	60%
Creatinine	0–0.7 mg/dL	100%
	0.8–1.3 mg/dL	60%
	1.4–10.4 mg/dL	50%
	>10.5 mg/dL	60%
Calcium		≥0.6 mg/dL
Glucose	None	

CALCULATIONS FOR PERCENTAGE DELTAS
For an acceptable delta check, the new result must be within the range calculated by the following equation:
First result ± (First result × percent delta)
Example: First AST result = 155
        Second AST result = 225
        Failed delta is ≥ 50% of first result
The acceptable delta range can be calculated:
High cutoff: 155 + (155×0.5) = 233
Low cutoff: 155 − (155×0.5) =   77
The second AST result of 225 passes the delta check.

CALCULATIONS FOR DIRECT DELTAS
Absolute value of (first result − second result) must be less than the cutoff.
Example: First sodium result = 139
        Second sodium result = 147
        Failed delta is ≥ 6.0
        j139 − 147 j = 8
The second result of 147 fails the delta check.

change rapidly with therapy or patient condition.

Patient data may also be used for long-term review of quality of results. Over a period of about 1 month, the mean and/or median of all patient results for a particular assay should be similar to those of previous months, particularly if a large sampling of data is collected. Large changes in the mean or median may indicate changes in the analytical method, indicating that the procedure should be looked at more closely for possible problems.

SUMMARY

In this overview of reliability of instrumentation systems, we have shown that many details must be attended to before, during, and after performing a clinical laboratory test to assure that the final results are useful to the clinician. Quality assurance programs should be developed within each laboratory to determine where improvements can be made throughout the entire process of having a test ordered by a physician to the result being reported. Quality control is a subset of quality assurance which insures that an assay is capable of providing accurate and useful results.

An instrumental method must be validated by determining its precision, accuracy, specificity, sensitivity, and reference range. When determining quality control ranges for an assay, it is up to the laboratory to make sure the ranges are appropriate for good patient care and will allow acceptable results for proficiency surveys.

After an assay goes on-line, then continuous monitoring of the method must take place by performing controls, participating in proficiency studies, and reviewing patient results. When control results are not acceptable, the reason must be determined and the assay fixed if necessary, and the event documented.

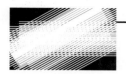

REVIEW QUESTIONS

Choose the best answer.

1. Which of the following would *not* be an example of preanalytic variation?

 a. Blood sample for calcium is collected in a EDTA tube.
 b. Fibrin material from sample clogs pipet tip.
 c. Child crying extensively during collection of blood gases.
 d. Specimen collected for glucose is left in phlebotomist's tray and not found for 2 hours after collection.

2. Which of the following *cannot* be done when performing proficiency testing?

 a. Send specimen to a reference laboratory.
 b. Assay specimen as a patient.
 c. Have director sign result form.
 d. Maintain records of how the sample was processed for 2 years.

3. To determine the accuracy of a method, one must

 a. Assay quality control material over several analytical runs.
 b. Assay standards having known concentrations.
 c. Assay samples that have been assayed by a method of known accuracy.
 d. Add known amounts of analyte to patient specimens.
 e. A or B or C or D.
 f. B or C or D.

4. When writing a procedure, which of the following does *not* need to be included?

 a. Author of procedure.
 b. Panic ranges.
 c. Method for developing quality control ranges.
 d. Reference ranges.
 e. Quality assurance monitors.
 f. Specimen storage requirements.

5. Quality assurance includes

 a. Quality control.
 b. Timely reporting of results.
 c. Timely collection of specimens.
 d. Making reports readable.
 e. B, C, and D above.
 f. All of the above.

6. Quality assurance programs are required by

 a. Clinical Laboratory Improvement Amendment of 1988.
 b. Joint Commission of the Accreditation of Healthcare Organizations.
 c. College of American Pathologists.
 d. All of the above.

7. When developing a new procedure that has not been modified from the manufacturer's instructions, which of the following must be done?

 a. Determine the sensitivity of the method.

b. Determine the interferences of the method.

c. Determine the frequency of calibration.

d. Verify the accuracy and precision of the method.

REFERENCES

1. Bachner P: Quality assurance of the analytic process: pre- and postanalytic variation. *Clin Lab Med* 6:613–623, 1983.
2. Diamond I: Quality assurance and/or quality control. *Arch Pathol Lab Med* 110:875–876 1986.
3. Clinical Laboratory Improvement Amendments of 1988; Final Rule. *Federal Register* 57:7001–7186, Feb 28, 1992.
4. College of American Pathologists: Laboratory accreditation program. *Inspection Checklist—Laboratory General*. Northfield, Illinois, 1992, pp 2–3.
5. Joint Commission on Accreditation of Healthcare Organizations: *Quality Assessment and Improvement*. Accreditation Manual for Hospitals, 1993, pp 139–144.
6. Laessig RH, Ehrmeyer SS, Lanphear BJ, Hassemer DJ: *A Poor Man's Guide to the New CLIA Rules: CLIA-88 and Procedure Manuals and Quality Control*. University of Wisconsin, 1992.
7. Clark GB: Quality assurance: An administrative means to a managerial end. Part I. *Clin Lab Management Rev* 7–15, 1990.
8. Clark GB: Quality assurance: An administrative means to a managerial end. Part II. *Clin Lab Management Rev* 224–252, 1990.
9. Clark GB: Quality assurance: An administrative means to a managerial end. Part III. *Clin Lab Management Rev* 463–475, 1991.
10. Westgard JO, Barry PL, Tomar RH: Implementing total quality management (TQM) in healthcare laboratories. *Clin Lab Management Rev* 353–370, 1991.
11. Cembrowski GS, Howanitz PJ: *Postanalytical QA: Hypercalcemia*. Q-Probes. College of American Pathologists, 1991.
12. Laessig RH, Ehrmeyer SS, Lanphear BJ, Hassemer DJ: *A Poor Man's Guide to the New CLIA Rules: Calibration*. University of Wisconsin, 1992.
13. National Committee for Clinical Laboratory Standards: *Evaluation of Precision Performance of Clinical Chemistry Devices*. EP5-T2. Villanova, Pennsylvania, NCCLS, 1992.
14. National Committee for Clinical Laboratory Standards: *Preliminary Evaluation of Clinical Chemis-*try Methods. EP10-T. Villanova, Pennsylvania, NCCLS, 1989.
15. College of American Pathologists: *Evaluation, Verification and Maintenance: Manual*, 4th edition. 1989.
16. Peters T, Westgard JO: Evaluation of methods. *In* Tietz NW (ed): *Textbook of Clinical Chemistry*, 3rd edition. Philadelphia, WB Saunders, 1986, pp 410–423.
17. National Committee for Clinical Laboratory Standards: *User Comparison of Quantitative Clinical Laboratory Methods Using Patient Samples*. EP9-P. Villanova, Pennsylvania, NCCLS, 1986.
18. Ehrmeyer SS, Laessig RH, Leinweber JE, Oryall JJ: 1990/Medicare/CLIA final rules for proficiency testing: Minimum intralaboratory performance characteristics (CV and bias) needed to pass. *Clin Chem* 36:1736–1740, 1990.
19. National Committee for Clinical Laboratory Standards: *Evaluation of the Linearity of Quantitative Analytical Methods*. EP6-P. Villanova, Pennsylvania, NCCLS, 1986.
20. National Committee for Clinical Laboratory Standards: *Interference Testing in Clinical Chemistry*. EP7-P. Villanova, Pennsylvania, NCCLS, 1986.
21. Willard HH, Merritt LL, Dean JA: Flame emission and atomic absorption spectrometry. *In Instrumental Methods of Analysis*, 5th edition. New York, D. Van Nostrand, 1974, p 378.
22. Galen RS, Peters T: Analytical goals and clinical relevance of laboratory procedures. *In* Tietz NW (ed): *Textbook of Clinical Chemistry*, 3rd edition. Philadelphia, WB Saunders, 1986, pp 387–409.
23. Solberg HE: Establishment and use of reference values. *In* Tietz NW (ed): *Textbook of Clinical Chemistry*, 3rd edition. Philadelphia, WB Saunders, 1986, pp 356–386.
24. National Committee for Clinical Laboratory Standards: *How to Define, Determine, and Utilize Reference Intervals in the Clinical Laboratory*. C28-P. Villanova, Pennsylvania, NCCLS, 1992.
25. Reed AH, Henry RJ, Mason WB: Influence of statistical method used on the resulting estimate of normal range. *Clin Chem* 17:275–284, 1971.
26. Moss DW, Henderson AR, Kachmar JF: Enzymes. *In* Tietz NW (ed): *Textbook of Clinical Chemistry*, 3rd edition. Philadelphia, WB Saunders, 1986, p 696.
27. Stein EA: Lipids, lipoproteins and apolipoproteins. *In* Tietz NW (ed): *Textbook of Clinical Chemistry*, 3rd edition. Philadelphia, WB Saunders, 1986, p 886.
28. Kannel WB: Cholesterol and risk of coronary heart disease and mortality in men. *Clin Chem* 34:B53–B59, 1988.
29. Rosen JF (Chair): *Preventing Lead Poisoning in Young Children—A Statement by the Centers for Disease Control*. Atlanta, US Department of Health and Human Services, 1991, pp 39–50.

30. National Committee for Clinical Laboratory Standards: *Clinical Laboratory Procedure Manuals; Approved Guideline.* GP2A. Villanova, Pennsylvania, NCCLS, 1991.
31. Westgard JO, Barry PL, Hunt MR, Groth T: A multi-rule Shewhart chart for quality control in clinical chemistry. *Clin Chem* 27:493–501, 1981.
32. National Committee for Clinical Laboratory Standards: *Internal Quality Control Testing: Principles and Definitions.* C24-A. Villanova, Pennsylvania, NCCLS, 1991.
33. Ehrmeyer SS, Laessig RH, Leinweber JE, Oryall JJ: 1990 Medicare final rules for proficiency testing: Minimum intralaboratory performance characteristics (CV and bias) needed to pass. *Clin Chem* 36:1736–1740, 1990.
34. Belk WP, Sunderman FW: A survey of the accuracy of chemical analyses in clinical laboratories. *Am J Clin Pathol* 17:853–861, 1947.
35. Laessig RH, Ehrmeyer SS: Proficiency testing programs—promises, progress, and problems: A 40-year perspective. *Arch Pathol Lab Med* 112:329–333, 1988.
36. Whitehurst P, Di Silvio TV, Boyadjian G: Evaluation of discrepancies in patient's results—an aspect of computer-assisted quality control. *Clin Chem* 21:87–92, 1975.

PREVENTIVE MAINTENANCE: DEFINITIONS AND TYPOLOGY
HISTORICAL ASPECTS
Why Preventive Maintenance?
The ``How to'' of Preventive Maintenance
REGULATORY ASPECTS
INSTRUMENT MAINTENANCE REQUIREMENTS OF VOLUNTARY ACCREDITING BODIES
Mandatory Instrument Maintenance
Some Deficiencies Cited During Regulatory Inspections
TROUBLESHOOTING
Process and Procedure
Selected Examples

Chapter 16

PREVENTIVE MAINTENANCE AND TROUBLESHOOTING

JOSEPH G. FINK, MD
SHESHADRI NARAYANAN, PhD

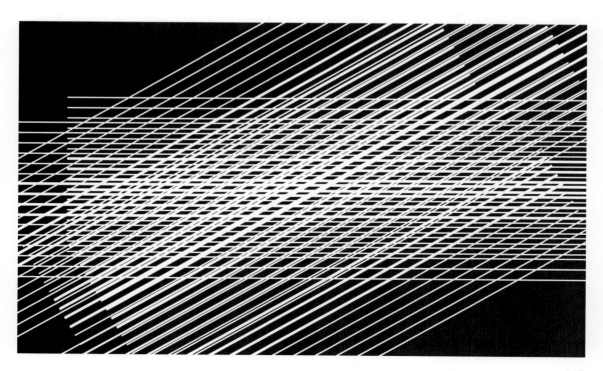

After studying this chapter, the student should be able to:

- Define preventive maintenance.
- Identify two examples of instrument verification routines.
- Describe the historical aspects of preventive maintenance in the clinical laboratory.
- List the essential elements in a PM program.
- List activities of performance checking.
- Describe outcomes of governmental regulations for instrument maintenance.

KEY WORDS

Function verification. Those activities that usually involve the checking of system operation.

Instrument maintenance. A two-component process: first, preventive maintenance per se, and second, troubleshooting and repair.

Performance verification. Activities designed to test and ensure that an instrument is working correctly and is properly calibrated.

Preventive maintenance. The scheduled inspection (of instruments or equipment) resulting in minor adjustment or repair to delay or avoid major repair and emergency or premature replacement.

Service contract. A contract with an outside vendor or the instrument manufacturer for maintenance and service of an instrument.

Troubleshooting. The process by which apparently unsatisfactory instrument performance is traced to root causes, which permits the correct solution to be applied to identified problems.

At this point in a book concerned with all facets of clinical laboratory instrumentation, the focus shifts to what is frequently perceived as an unpleasant aspect of the utilization of these devices, i.e., the responsibility for the user to assure that all laboratory equipment receives the attention it needs to preserve its usefulness and maximize its lifespan. This obligatory continuing care has come to be known, somewhat inaccurately, as preventive maintenance or PM. Despite the inexactness of this terminology (although the same may be said for quality control [QC]), it has served the useful purpose of consolidating under one label all those activities related to assuring the quality of the broad range of instruments and equipment on which the clinical laboratory depends.

This chapter deals with the twin topics of preventive maintenance and troubleshooting. The first section explores various aspects of preventive maintenance, beginning with definitions and clarifications of terminology. Next, a chronicle of the evolution of PM in the clinical laboratory is provided, followed by an examination of certain pragmatic aspects of PM that deserve emphasis. Finally, the increasingly important place of PM in regulatory compliance is explored and illustrated. The second section of the chapter deals with the subject of troubleshooting laboratory instrumentation and attempts to explain the special features of this form of **instrument maintenance.**

It seems natural and normal to me to make use of the small tool kits and instruction booklets supplied with each machine, and to keep it tuned and adjusted myself (p. 18).

R.M. PIRSIG[1]

PREVENTIVE MAINTENANCE: DEFINITIONS AND TYPOLOGY

It is well to appreciate that preventive maintenance may be used to describe both a *process* (def.: a systematic series of actions directed to some end; e.g., the process of making butter) and a *program* (a plan to be followed). Consequently, a variety of definitions of the term may be encountered. The process of PM will be examined first.

Beginning with dictionary meanings of the terms, *maintenance* is defined as the act of maintaining, in turn defined as keeping in good condition, well-preserved, operating and unimpaired, and, especially with regard to machinery, avoiding failure or decline in function. Prevention adds to the maintenance concept the notion of anticipating and effectively forestalling some future event.

When the two words are put together in clinical laboratory parlance, their meaning becomes, in the Centers for Disease Control (CDC) definition of 1973,[2] the "scheduled inspection [of instruments or equipment] resulting in minor adjustment or repair to delay or avoid major repair and emergency or premature replacement." Alternatively, Duckworth and associates[3] refer to preventive maintenance as the adjustment, care, and cleaning of laboratory equipment, whereas Eilers[4] speaks of PM as a regularly scheduled examination of all equipment involved in assay procedures before it breaks down, to assure that it is in proper functioning order. Stewart and Koepke[5] state that PM "involves the cleaning, adjustment, and scheduled replacement of parts to minimize the need for extensive repairs, reduce the amount of unexpected downtime, and extend the useful life of the instrument or piece of equipment." Finally, Garfield[6] holds that PM "includes specification checks, calibration, cleaning, lubricating, reconditioning, adjusting, and testing" of analytical equipment. Typical examples of preventive maintenance activities include the changing of pump tubing at regular intervals, changing membranes on electrodes in blood gas analyzers, cleaning sampling probes and lines, and changing motor brushes in a centrifuge.

The first caveat to be observed in this definitional analysis is to avoid confusing PM with a second type of maintenance, namely corrective, breakdown, or reparative maintenance, otherwise known simply as *repair*. In this form of maintenance, an instrument is restored to functioning or good condition, after damage or deterioration has occurred, by replacing a part, reworking a component, or putting together that which is broken.

From this distinction arises one of the more persuasive arguments in favor of PM, advanced by those originally advocating its adoption by clinical laboratories. They pointed out that the airline industry does not wait for an engine to give out in flight but routinely performs those prophylactic tasks known to industry as preventive maintenance, thereby avoiding the highly undesirable state of failure-in-operation. Thus, this argument ran, "Whether applied to precision laboratory equipment, giant manufacturing machines, or buildings and building systems, PM means planning ahead—scheduling certain inspection and maintenance functions that will prevent most breakdowns."[2]

As a corollary to this repair versus preventive maintenance distinction, another feature of the definition of PM is illuminated. Preventive maintenance is always a *scheduled* activity, and repair is *unscheduled*. Furthermore, PM as a scheduled activity must be part of the laboratory's routine, whereas repair is always routine-disruptive or nonroutine. To extend this train of thought, when an important laboratory instrument is down, repair becomes an emergency activity, whereas preventive maintenance never is. In fact, some components of PM may be advantageously scheduled for performance when the laboratory is not even in operation, so as to avoid interfering with the routine analytical workload.

Next, it must be appreciated that when preventive maintenance refers to a laboratory program, the term becomes somewhat of a misnomer. As alluded to earlier, PM is often used to describe a program of instrumental quality control, one which serves to complement the program of quality control for the analytical process (methodologic control). In this usage, PM takes on a larger meaning, one that would be better served if the more accurate term instrument maintenance (IM) were utilized. Instrument maintenance is in fact broader in scope than PM, involving as it does two components: preventive maintenance per se and troubleshooting and repair.

Additionally, since PM is widely used to refer to instrument quality control programs, the term is commonly understood to comprehend a quite different set of activities. The latter, which are only indirectly related to maintenance per se, constitute the verification component of an instrument control plan. Verification of laboratory instruments and equipment involves routine surveillance, involving observations and measurements of instruments' critical operating characteristics, in a process sometimes called performance monitoring (likewise abbreviated PM), but also known as performance confirmation, function checking, or confirmation checking. Examples of instrument verification routines include such activities as calibration or recalibration (def.: the comparison of a measurement standard or instrument of known accuracy with another standard or instrument, to detect, correlate, report, or eliminate by adjustment, any variation in the accuracy of the item being compared), temperature measurements of controlled-temperature devices, checks of linearity of photometric instruments, and checks on centrifuge speeds.

To summarize the foregoing analysis, PM programs, ideally, deserve to be called verification and maintenance (V&M) programs, but conventional usage has shown itself indifferent to such precision in language.

Finally, it is of some interest that PM has

come to be a key component of two different perceptions of laboratory operations, the technical and the managerial. In the technical sphere, PM is seen as an additional type of quality control, contributing to total quality control[4] or quality assurance. By contrast, in a management context, PM is a subset of equipment/instrument manage-ment, in which organizational niche it can be seen to be related to the managerial concerns of instrument acquisition and replacement. These differing but complementary viewpoints are diagramed in Figure 16–1. In confirmation of the new reality, the latest (1989) edition of the College of American Pathologists (CAP) *Laboratory Instrument*

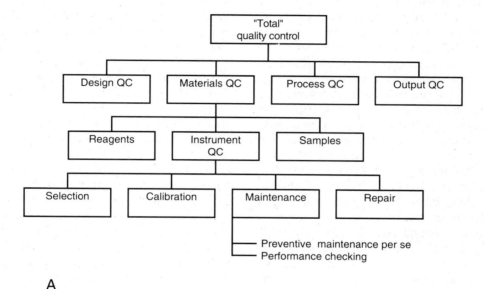

A

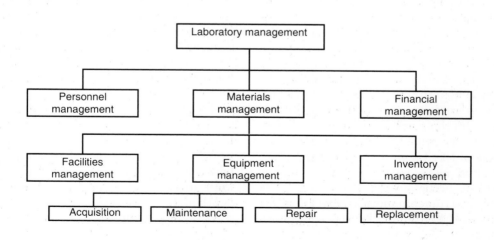

B

■ **FIGURE 16–1.**

Instrument maintenance in perspective. *A,* Technical perspective. *B,* Management perspective.

Evaluation Verification and Maintenance Manual "has been expanded to provide a broader view of instrument management by addressing subjects of financial analysis, instrument selection, and performance evaluation-validation."[7]

HISTORICAL ASPECTS

That there was a time when the function of laboratory instruments was taken for granted may seem impossible to contemporary clinical laboratory workers, accustomed as they are to carrying out PM tasks in their daily routines. However, it is less than 25 years since the phrase preventive maintenance made its debut in the literature of the clinical laboratory, and when it was first used it was in fact a cry for help.

Alpert, writing in 1981, describes how Veteran laboratories may smile wistfully in recalling how uncomplicated instruments were 25 years ago . . . . A buyer generally installed a device by plugging it in, and he learned to operate it by reading rudimentary instructions . . . . users generally made their own repairs and adjustments. In exceptional cases . . . he could phone the manufacturer for assistance . . . .[8]

This idyllic scenario began to change in the mid-1960s as clinical laboratory instrumentation underwent a revolution. There appeared on the market a new generation of laboratory equipment, ranging from mechanical pipets to multichannel analyzers, which was more complex than anything users were accustomed to. Practical problems of instrument choice and utilization were created by the availability of the new products.

In response to this challenge, a series of articles appeared in 1967 and 1968 in the *Bulletin of Pathology* of the American Society of Clinical Pathologists, in a column entitled "New Instruments." The intent of these articles was to share the practical experience of actual users with colleagues who had an interest in the acquisition of the new products. In the concluding article of this series (October 1968), Baer used the then-unfamiliar expression *preventive maintenance* for the first time, commenting as follows:

Relative to service and maintenance of instruments, it is apparent that, generally such provision is not altogether adequate. There is frequently a long delay between breakdown and repair of essential laboratory equipment. With few exceptions, instructions in the manufacturers' manuals concerning troubleshooting are inadequate . . . .

The laboratory director must attempt to protect himself against failure of instruments, and to ensure that their rapid repair can be counted upon. To realize those objectives, we suggest: 1) a program of preventive maintenance, including regular inspection of instruments and replacement of parts; . . .[9]

Underlining the concern of the laboratory community of this era with the lack of information resources, it may be noted that the College of American Pathologists had published in 1966 a small pamphlet entitled *A Suggested Guide for Manufacturers for Preparation of Manuals of Operation for Laboratory Instruments*. The *Guide* was intended to improve communications between instrument users and manufacturers, so that laboratory workers would secure enough information to enable them to keep their instruments operating without interruption. It made recommendations for the provision of manufacturers' information in such areas as initial operating checks, systems specifications, methods of checking, methods of isolation of instrument failure, and service.

The manufacturers proved responsive to these recommendations and the situation began to change. About this time, a new society, the Association for the Advancement of Medical Instrumentation (AAMI), was organized to enable manufacturers and users to cooperate in solving mutual problems. In 1970, a dozen laboratory instrument manufacturers collaborated in the publication of an article that provided composite PM guidelines for five classes of laboratory instruments, namely, centrifuges, colorimeters, flame photometers, pH meters, and spectrophotometers.[10]

Parenthetically, it may be noted that user-manufacturer cooperation which began at this point eventually led to the development, by the National Committee for Clinical Laboratory Standards (NCCLS), of two related documents. The first of these publications, *Development of User-Oriented Instrument Support Manuals* (1983), provided guidelines on the components, style, and forms that should be included in manufacturer-supplied instrument verification and maintenance manuals. The other, *Service of Clinical Laboratory Instruments* (1984), dealt with conditions of servicing and responsibilities of users and suppliers of clinical laboratory instruments.

Returning to our original chronology, just at this time (1969), Rand published a landmark article, "Practical spectrophotometric standards," which not only raised user consciousness about issues of calibration and standardization, but also detailed check-out procedures that had practical application.[11] Shortly thereafter (1971), Winstead's monograph, *Instrument Check Systems,* appeared.[12] It contained chapters devoted to autoanalyzers, densitometers, flame photometers, pH meters, and Coulter counters, in addition to one on spectrophotometers. For the first time the clinical laboratory community possessed a major information resource, which broadly addressed instrument maintenance theory and process.

In the same year (1971), Duckworth and Stevens[13] published the first of a series of articles that described their experience in establishing a systematic program of preventive maintenance. This was a major contribution, because it presented so clearly both program design principles and practical implementation steps, which other laboratories could easily follow in creating their own PM programs.

ELEMENTS OF TEN POINT PROGRAM OF INSTRUMENT MAINTENANCE

1. Equipment inventory
2. Service task definition
3. Task interval establishment
4. Personnel planning
5. Job assignments
6. Personnel training
7. Special equipment acquisition
8. Program implementation and control
9. Record-keeping documentation
10. Program surveillance

—Duckworth and Stevens, 1971

Subsequently, in 1973, the Centers for Disease Control (CDC) made available a chapter on preventive maintenance in its *Guide on Laboratory Administration,*[2] and, in 1974, the College of American Pathologists (CAP) brought out the first edition of its *Laboratory Instrument Maintenance* manual. The introductory section of the latter aptly captured the problem peculiar to that era when it said that it was concerned with "areas of quality control which are either neglected to some degree in the laboratory literature, or at least the information available is widely dispersed and difficult to assimilate and use in a practical day-to-day fashion."

It is important to note that, in this same

period, the clinical laboratory community awoke to a realization that a need existed for a revised and expanded approach to quality control. An awareness had developed that the statistical evaluation of the analytical process, i.e., methodologic QC, the conventional QC of the laboratory, was insufficient by itself to assure quality results. Topics such as the quality of laboratory water and the stability of the electrical supply intruded on the quality consciousness. A broader picture of total quality control as a means of achieving "quality assurance" consequently emerged, receiving conceptualization and popularization by Eilers.[4] In this expanded scheme of total quality control, preventive maintenance programs came to occupy a place of prominence. Accordingly, having attained both programmatic codification and conceptual legitimization, the preventive maintenance "movement" was well launched by 1975. PM practices were widely adopted in the ensuing 15 years, as the burgeoning literature on the subject attests.[14–25]

Yet another major change in the clinical laboratory environment can be identified as occurring throughout the 1970s and 1980s. Many clinical laboratory instruments became exceedingly complex in design and construction as they were transformed from the "basic" tools of an analytical workplace to the mechanized and automated leviathans of an assembly line. This phenomenon was accompanied and accelerated by the increased use of solid-state electronics in instruments. The net result was the presence in the laboratory of analytical test systems the use of which was exceedingly simple, requiring little scientific knowledge on the part of their nominal operators. At the same time, the sophistication of these machines made them correspondingly less intelligible to the custodial analyst, who was increasingly unable to contribute spontaneously to their maintenance, troubleshoot-

ing, and repair. As is frequently humorously stated by those involved, "It takes only a monkey to operate these machines when they're running well, but an electronic wizard or graduate engineer is required to diagnose and treat them when they fail." Consequently, in contrast to the situation that originally existed, in which the laboratory

OPERATOR'S MANUAL
TECHNICON DAX System
———————— SECTION 3 MAINTENANCE ————————

TITLE
  Introduction
  Daily Checks
  Daily Preoperation
  Daily During Operation
  Daily Postoperation
    Cleaning Reagent Nozzles
    Cleaning Dispense Points Along the Dilution Line
  Weekly
    Cleaning Sampler Wash Cups and Drain
    Cleaning Sampler/Reagent Waste Lines
  Monthly
    Checking System Water for Microbial Growth
    Cleaning Analyzer Module Wash Cups and Drain
    Cleaning Optical Read Station Prisms
    Cleaning ISE Wash Reservoir
    Cleaning Ceramic Syringes
  Every Two Months
    Washing the Cuvettes
    Replacing the Cuvette Wash Station Dryer Tips
    Replacing the Dilution Line Wash Station Dryer Tips
  Every 2000 Hours
    Replacing the Optics Lamp
  Every Three Months
    Servicing Reagent Filters
  Every Six Months
    Replacing the Water Tank Air Filter (NA only)
  Nonroutine Maintenance
    Cleaning the Dilution Line Wash Probe
    Cleaning the Check Valves
    Replacing a Sample Probe
    Cleaning Reagent Lines After a Method Change
    Replacing ISE Electrode
    Hydraulic Cleaning Procedure
    Replacing Stirring Bars
    Replacing Reagent/Sampler Syringes
    Replacing Cuvettes

■ **FIGURE 16–2.**

(From Technicon DAX System manual. Miles Inc., Tarrytown, NY.)

had to *discover* appropriate PM practices for its instruments, at the present time the clinical laboratory is almost totally dependent on the instrument manufacturer to specify the preventive maintenance required for a specific item of equipment. Examples of the type of PM program information currently provided for major laboratory instrumentation can be seen in Figures 16–2, 16–3 and 16–4. Figure 16–2 shows the table of contents of the maintenance section of the instrument operator's manual, Figure 16–3 is an example of the detailed instructions for performance of the required daily maintenance checks, and Figure 16–4 illustrates the type of record-keeping log sheet utilized.

PROCESS AND PROGRAM

Having presented a basic understanding of preventive maintenance and its evolution, we turn now to an examination of certain pragmatic aspects of the subject. This

TECHNICON DAX System Maintenance

DAILY CHECKS

Daily Preoperation

Perform the following task before operating the system:

WARNING—POTENTIAL BIOHAZARDOUS MATERIAL
Wastes containing human serum or plasma should be handled cautiously as a biohazardous material according to good laboratory practices. Wear glasses, gloves, and protective clothing.
The system wastes and any materials exposed to this waste should be handled at the Biosafety Level 2 as recommended for potentially infectious human serum or blood specimens in the Centers for Disease Control/National Institutes of Health manual ``Biosafety in Microbiological and Biomedical Laboratories,'' 1984.

1. Waste Lines. Verify that all waste lines are properly connected to the laboratory drain.
2. User Water Supply.
   a. Record the input and output pressures at the final filtration gauges. If the output pressure is less than 5 psi, replace the filter. The filter is user supplied. To replace the filter, shut off the water supply, pull off the old filter, and push on the new filter.
   b. Observe that the green indicator light on the tank is illuminated (NA only). If the light is not illuminated, call **TECHNICON**.
3. Degasser. Verify that the deionized water is supplied to the Degasser Module without leaks, and that the ``FULL'' LED on the Degasser Module is lit, indicating that a sufficient amount of degassed water is present in the tank. Also verify that the ``WATER ERR,'' and ``DEGASS ERR'' LEDs are not lit.
4. Visually inspect the following components for cleaniness. If needed, clean with DI water and lint-free cloth:
   Sampling probes and related tubes.
   Dispensing probes and related tubes.
   Reagent tubes and reagent nozzles.
5. Refrigerator and water bath temperatures: Check and record these temperatures.
6. Stirrers. Check each stirring section. If the stirrers are dirty, wipe with DI water and lint-free cloth. If any stirrer is bent, replace it (refer to Nonroutine Maintenance, page M-34).

■ **Figure 16–3.**

(From Technicon DAX System manual. Miles Inc., Tarrytown, NY.)

TECHNICON DAX™ System Maintenance Log

System Serial No. _____ Month _____ Year _____ Location _____

DAILY MAINTENANCE SCHEDULE

ACTIVITY	TIME	1	2	3	4	5	6	7	8	9	10	11	12	13	14	15	16	17	18	19	20	21	22	23	24	25	26	27	28	29	30	31
Before Operation Inspect all waste lines in drain.	1 min																															
Record DI water input pressure.	1 min																															
Record DI water output pressure.	1 min																															
Check Water Quality LED (NA only).	1 min																															
Check degasser FULL & RUN LEDs.	1 min																															
Clean/check nozzles, probes, tubes.	5 min																															
Record refrigerator temperature. **Modules A & B** **Modules C & D**	1 min																															
Record Water Temp. **D-Line** **Module A** **Module B** **Module C** **Module D**	1 min																															
Check all stirrers for straightness.	1 min																															
During Operation Check reagent delivery. **Module A**																																
Module B If nozzles are replaced, note **Module C** syringe number. **Module D**	5 min																															
After Operation Clean serum from analyzers/sampler.	5 min																															
Clean reagent nozzles.	5 min																															
OPERATOR'S INITIALS																																

WEEKLY MAINTENANCE SCHEDULE

ACTIVITY	TIME	1	2	3	4	5	6	7	8	9	10	11	12	13	14	15	16	17	18	19	20	21	22	23	24	25	26	27	28	29	30	31
Clean sampler wash cup and drain.	5 min																															
Clean waste lines. **Module A**	15 min																															
Module B	15 min																															
Module C	15 min																															
Module D	15 min																															
OPERATOR'S INITIALS																																

MONTHLY MAINTENANCE SCHEDULE

ACTIVITY	TIME	1	2	3	4	5	6	7	8	9	10	11	12	13	14	15	16	17	18	19	20	21	22	23	24	25	26	27	28	29	30	31
Check for microbial growth (pass/fail). **Sample Port 1** **Sample Port 2** **Sample Port 3**	2 min																															
Clean analyzer wash cup. **Module A**	5 min																															
Module B	5 min																															
Module C	5 min																															
Module D	5 min																															
Clean optics station prisms. **Module A**	10 min																															
Module B	10 min																															
Module C	10 min																															
Module D	10 min																															
Clean ISE wash reservoir.	5 min																															
Clean ceramic syringes. **Sampler**	15 min																															
Module A	5 min																															
Module B	5 min																															
Module C	5 min																															
Module D	5 min																															
Replace sampler waste syringes 21, 22, and 23, and ISE aspiration syringe(s)	10 min																															
Replace dryer tips. **D-Line**	5 min																															
OPERATOR'S INITIALS																																

BI-MONTHLY MAINTENANCE SCHEDULE

ACTIVITY	TIME	1	2	3	4	5	6	7	8	9	10	11	12	13	14	15	16	17	18	19	20	21	22	23	24	25	26	27	28	29	30	31
Replace dryer tips. **Module A**	10 min																															
Indicate line number (1-4) **Module B**	10 min																															
associated with replaced **Module C**	10 min																															
dryer tips. **Module D**	10 min																															
OPERATOR'S INITIALS																																

NONSCHEDULED OR CORRECTIVE MAINTENANCE

DATE	PERFORMED BY	REASON FOR MAINTENANCE	DESCRIPTION OF MAINTENANCE PERFORMED

■ **FIGURE 16–4.**

(From Technicon DAX System manual. Miles Inc., Tarrytown, NY.)

section will examine selected reported experience and enlightened comment but not attempt to restate program designs and process components, which are covered in detail in many of the references cited.[2, 7, 15, 23, 25–32]

Why Preventive Maintenance?

Although preventive maintenance has a basic plausibility, there may be occasions when formal justification for its adoption is required. This possibility is rendered remote by the strictures of CLIA '88 (see later), but occasionally even government mandates need to be rationalized. Indeed, as the CDC's 1973 guide on PM pointed out,[2] a PM program must be "sold," first to higher management, and then in a continuing effort to the personnel involved. To support that kind of sales pitch, the cornucopia of benefits expected to result from the adoption of PM is:

- Improved product quality
- Greater operator safety
- Fewer interruptions of production
- Decreased employee idle time
- Lower repair costs
- Avoidance of premature replacement
- Reduction of standby ("backup") equipment
- Identification of high maintenance costs
- Better spare parts control

Whether such benefits actually accrue from a PM program is the next question, and few published answers exist. In an early assessment of results, the Duckworth group[33] reported that instituting PM had reduced down time on blood gas equipment by at least 90 percent. In addition, payments to outside vendors for major repair work and troubleshooting had decreased "remarkably," from approximately $500 per month to less than $100. A decade later, Yapit recorded a 54 percent reduction in downtime

after the institution of a "comprehensive" PM program in her hematology department.[19] Still another report[21] claimed an annual savings of $70,000 in repairs and outside service charges when an in-house instrumentation technician was given responsibility for the maintenance of the 150 pieces of laboratory equipment used by a 450-bed hospital.

Another question relating to justification of PM relates to what might be characterized as its redundancy. Given the overall evaluation of process quality provided by conventional QC utilizing data from the assay of stable control materials, why is PM of instrumentation also required? With the current emphasis on eliminating unnecessary programs to reduce costs, would not the conventional QC program adequately monitor instrument performance?

One answer to this objection is that "good practice," in a total quality control framework, demands control of each contributory component of the analytical system (a position that is expressed in governmental laboratory regulations). However, a more persuasive answer to this challenge derives from a recollection of the dual nature of PM. Even as it is appreciated that the federal regulations (e.g., the HCFA Interpretive Guidelines to Section 493.1213(b)(1) of the CLIA '67—see later) explicitly recognize the usefulness of daily quality control samples serving as an instrument function check, there must follow the realization that function checks are only half of PM, and that actual maintenance (cleaning, adjusting, lubricating, changing replaceable items, and so on) needs to be performed if the goals of PM are fully to be met.

The purpose of performing routine PM on laboratory instrumentation is twofold:

(1) to forestall a failure in methodologic quality control, by preventing or identifying instrument malfunction before the quality of the analysis is affected, and

(2) to determine whether instrumentation

is the reason for any failure that does occur, from an examination of the details of PM observations that have been assiduously recorded.

The "How To" of Preventive Maintenance

Information Resources

Once convinced of the necessity for PM, how does the laboratory go about establishing the program? Sources of information to provide the answers to this question are now abundant and include such current texts of laboratory management as Becan-McBryde[31] and Snyder and Senhauser.[29] However, the previously noted 10-point program originated by Duckworth and colleagues[3] is rightfully recognized as the best set of instructions for a successful PM launch. This comprehensive plan of action is readily available, since it is included in the College of Pathologists (CAP) *Clinical Laboratory Improvement Manual.*[34] Additional planning guides for PM program implementation can be found in the articles by Warren,[17] Yeast,[35] Sohaney,[14] and Baldwin and Barasso,[24] and more recently in the chapter, "Quality Assurance and Instrument Maintenance," in the text by Stewart and Koepke.[5]

Essential Elements in a PM Program

All these guidelines for establishing a PM program generally agree on the fundamental considerations necessarily involved in such an undertaking. These may be stated to be:

(1) definition of the range of PM tasks that will be required, and the acquisition of any special measuring or calibrating devices that will be used;

(2) definition, likewise, of the frequency of the performance of the PM tasks;

(3) decisions regarding (and the designation of) the personnel who will carry out the PM assignments;

(4) performance of the planned activities, coupled with scrupulous documentation of what is done or observed; and

(5) careful managerial review and utilization of the information developed from PM activities.

These fundamental requirements of PM can be further condensed to "**three Ds,**"— the easily remembered admonition Define, Do, and Document.

The "Defining" Step: Value of CAP Instrument Manual. An additional CAP publication should be regarded as indispensable in the development of a PM program. Since the appearance of the first edition in 1974, the *Laboratory Instrument Evaluation Verification and Maintenance Manual*[7] has been the single best information resource in the PM subject area. Even today when, as has been pointed out, instrument manufacturers routinely provide users with detailed PM schemes for their complex analytical systems, the CAP *Manual* remains the major source of guidance for PM procedures applicable to basic laboratory equipment, as well as for much generally useful information.

The current (1989) edition[7] introduces a change in terminology regarding instrument verification processes that must be addressed. The *Manual's* authors, the CAP Instrument Maintenance Committee, now divide the verification process into function verification and performance verification.

Function verification is defined as "those activities that usually involve the checking of system operation." **Performance verification** encompasses "activities designed to test and ensure that an instrument is working correctly and is properly calibrated." The difference between these two forms of verification, if indeed one does exist, is not readily apparent from the definitions given. In one attempt to refine this uncertain distinction, the CAP *Manual* states that function verification "depends mostly on operating instructions in the operator's manual." Conversely, performance verification "is considerably more complicated. For many instruments, little or no guidance is provided in the operator's manual." Somewhat more usefully, however, the CAP Committee[36] also indicates that function verification is routinely performed at the start of each shift or run. Performance verification, on the other hand, is carried out relatively infrequently, using reference materials and special procedures to confirm the basic parameters of the instrument.

The distinction may best be clarified by examining examples of the two verification modes, as offered in the Stewart and Koepke text.[5] Function checking activities include the recording of temperatures, voltage readings, and background counts (as applicable) and instrument calibration, baseline or zero adjustment, and linearity adjustment. In contrast, performance checking comprises activities such as checking wavelength calibration of spectrophotometers using narrow bandpass filters at specific wavelengths, verifying thermometer accuracy with an NITS-referenced thermometer, establishing the accuracy of the analytical balance using NITS Class S weights, and checking linearity and precision in multichannel analyzers with the use of standard solutions.

Stewart and Koepke[5] make the additional important point:

Performance verification checks are not applicable to all laboratory instruments and equipment. The design of some instruments or the nature of the analyte being measured will make performance verification unnecessary or impossible. For example, there are no performance checks for centrifuges, water baths, or refrigerators.

Samples of verification and maintenance guidelines from the CAP *Manual* are given here:

GUIDELINE FOR VERIFICATION AND MAINTENANCE: THERMOMETERS

Function Verification
- Inspect
- Check accuracy of thermometer

Instrument Maintenance
- Clean

GUIDELINE FOR VERIFICATION AND MAINTENANCE: MICROSCOPES

Performance Verification
- Check light alignment
- Check visualization of slide material

Function Verification
- Adjust condenser height
- Center circular image of field diaphragm
- Adjust field diaphragm aperture
- Adjust condenser diaphragm aperture
- Check optical system for damage
- Check optical system for cleanliness
- Check fine and coarse adjustments
- Check condenser fork
- Check mechanical stage
- Check interpupillary distance
- Check slide fingers

Instrument Maintenance
- Cover instrument when not in use
- Thoroughly dust optical surfaces
- Thoroughly clean optical surfaces
- Thoroughly clean external surface
- Clean and lubricate slide ways and gears
- Complete general overhaul

GUIDELINE FOR VERIFICATION AND MAINTENANCE: BLOOD GAS AND pH ANALYZERS

Performance Verification
- Run quality control specimens, or buffer checks

Function Verification
- Check automatic calibrations for drift and reproducibility
- Check special calibrations for zero points and sensitivity
- Check barometric pressure against external mercury barometer (optional)

Instrument Maintenance
- Check water level in humidifier
- Change pH electrode membrane
- Check KCl level
- Check level of calibration solutions
- Check level of rinse and buffers
- Check gas pressures
- Check printer paper supplies
- Empty waste container
- Clean electrode ports, follow cleaning procedure specified by manufacturer
- Clean pH measuring
- Check KCl in pH reference electrode
- Examine dust and air filters
- Change pCO_2 and pO_2 electrode membranes, replace electrolyte and degas electrodes
- Lubricate printer, oil bearings (if needed)
- Service check-up

The first two are chosen to show the PM program for items of basic laboratory equipment, the thermometer and the microscope, whereas the last is representative of a ge-neric instrument class. Note in the first box, as Stewart and Koepke indicated, there exists no performance verification steps for a thermometer. The middle box, which deals with PM for the common laboratory microscope, may hold some surprises for those who could not have imagined such a plethora of PM tasks required by so uncomplicated and sturdy an item. In contrast, the PM program components outlined for the blood gas/pH instrument (bottom box) are hardly more numerous than those called for in the microscope outline, but the tasks identified are operationally more complex. It should also be noted that, contrary to what has been indicated, the performance versus function verification distinction based on frequency of task scheduling fails to be followed consistently. For example, observe that what is indicated to be a performance verification for the blood gas analyzer, i.e., running quality control specimens, obviously must be done each day of use. Similarly, checking "visualization of slide material" for the microscope's performance verification is hardly an activity that would not be performed every day. Consequently, it is possible that the distinction between function and performance checks that pervades the CAP *Manual*'s approach may be no more than an ignis fatuus.

The "Doing" Step: Overcoming Obstacles in Performing Preventive Maintenance

When and How Frequently Should PM Be Done? An answer to this question will obviously be device specific, with the manufacturer's recommendations being the major guidance. In addition, regulatory agencies may be quite explicit regarding the minimum frequency of PM activities that they expect to be performed (see the Regulatory section later).

The CDC *Guide*[2] helpfully observes that "one piece of equipment may have several frequencies for servicing, such as once daily for cleaning, once weekly for adjustment, once monthly for functional inspections, and once yearly for overhaul."

It can be taken for granted, however, that some form of PM, whether maintenance or verification, will be required on every day of instrument use, even if this amounts to no more than an observation or cleaning. And, in addition to periodic scheduled function checking, verification procedures are required when an instrument is first received in the laboratory, after repairs or adjustments, and whenever doubts concerning performance arise during use.

Who Will Do the Work Involved? Lorimor and Collins assert that "the most difficult factor in preventive maintenance is motivating technologists to do it."[31] Yeast commented, in a similar vein, that the low spot on the totem pole of the laboratory work assignments tends to be occupied by the unglamorous tasks of preventive maintenance.[35] Hence, we review here some of the relevant principles that can assist in handling the "personnel problem" of PM.

Shuffstall and Hemmaplardh express particularly well the conventional managerial principles for this sphere of operations: "In general, it is advisable to hold supervisory personnel accountable for maintenance and repair of all equipment assigned to their areas. Delegation of specific maintenance duties can then be made in accordance with the degree of difficulty and recommendations of the manufacturer."[30]

Making correct decisions regarding the duties to be delegated requires that the hierarchical nature of PM activities be taken into account. Even when a maintenance **service contract** with an outside vendor or the instrument manufacturer exists, all laboratory personnel continue to have some degree of responsibility for routine PM activities. Further, it is a grave error to foster the illusion that the existence of an in-house "maintenance" department, or the employment of an instrument technician, lifts the PM burden from laboratory workers. The early CDC document[2] pointed out:

PM is not strictly a maintenance responsibility. It is everybody's job. Equipment users and all employees coming into contact with equipment should be encouraged to report conditions that appear unusual; for example, strange equipment noises or vibrations, leaks, and frayed wires or cords.

Duckworth and associates were the first to define a stratified arrangement of four well-defined PM activity levels, intended to clarify differing degrees of responsibility for PM functions within and outside the laboratory.[3, 13, 33] Most other writers who have examined this aspect of PM also recommend a stratified activity approach.[15, 23, 29, 30, 37] The activity level scheme is based on the recognition that PM tasks range from the trivial and banal to the extremely difficult and complex. In that perspective, low-level activities are assigned to line laboratory workers, such as routine daily calibration, cleaning, maintenance, and simple troubleshooting, while at the other end of the scale complicated problems are handled by manufacturers' representatives (not sales people!), who are expected to perform major troubleshooting and repair work. In this context, the discussion by Stewart and Koepke of the considerations related to choice of various service contracts is particularly helpful.[5] The point should not be overlooked, however, that the existence of a service contract does not eliminate the responsibility of the laboratory to perform other routine maintenance that is not included in the PM contract.

The "Documenting" Step: Handling the Paper Work. As the cliché has it, no job is done until the paperwork is completed. PM demands the utilization of some form of a log for every piece of laboratory equipment, in which the records of maintenance and verification activities are recorded. At the same time, there has to be some organized scheme for assuring that performance of the planned maintenance activities takes place. These twin requirements can pose major paperwork difficulties for a PM program unless they are effectively handled. Keeping track of PM in the front end of the system (what has to be done and when = *scheduling*), as well as in its back end (the records of work performed = *record-keeping*), is often the most trouble-ridden aspect of the program.

Many differing schemes for addressing the documentation requirement of PM have been published, with their very number attesting to the intractability of the problem.[3, 18, 20, 22, 24, 29, 35, 38] More recent suggestions for contending with PM scheduling and record-keeping describe the use of microcomputers.[39] It is clear that the documentation dilemma is related to the most basic organizational aspects of PM. Hence, it would seem useful to enumerate and clarify the types of documents required in PM, since the absence of any of these items may impair the program fatally:

1) a form that identifies each instrument by such features as its name, manufacturer, model number, serial number, inventory number, and acquisition date (the **inventory record card**);

2) a list of the tasks to be performed, and with what frequency (the PM schedule);

3) a set of step-by-step instructions for carrying out each of the PM tasks that have been scheduled (PM methods or procedures, or PM standard operating procedures [PM SOPs]), and,

4) a record sheet of suitable format to facilitate the listing of PM work that has been completed (PM record sheet).

To sum up, documentation in PM involves written materials describing the instruments involved, the tasks scheduled to be performed, the methods involved in the performance, and the ultimate record that the tasks have been completed as scheduled.

REGULATORY ASPECTS

A program of preventive maintenance for clinical laboratory instruments is currently required by all voluntary laboratory accrediting agencies, as well as the various governmental regulators. Among the former are the College of American Pathologists (CAP), the American Association of Blood Banks (AABB), and the Joint Commission on the Accreditation of Healthcare Organizations (JCAHO). Government regulators include the Health Care Financing Administration (HCFA) and the Food and Drug Administration (FDA) at the national level and various state and local programs, such as those of the Departments of Health of New York State and New York City.

INSTRUMENT MAINTENANCE REQUIREMENTS OF VOLUNTARY ACCREDITING BODIES

The approach taken by the CAP's Inspection and Accreditation Program will be used to illustrate the requirements of the voluntary agencies in the area of instrument maintenance. The CAP Commission on Laboratory Accreditation's Standard IV, Quality Control, is the source of the instrument maintenance requirement, although it is not explicitly enunciated in the Standard itself. The Standard simply states, "Each pathology service shall have a quality control system that demonstrates the reliability and medical usefulness of laboratory tests." Insofar as preventive maintenance is involved in Standard IV, the Interpretation section of the Standard then elaborates as follows: "A laboratory quality control system shall contain the following components: ... (4) An instrument maintenance program which monitors and demonstrates the proper calibration and function of equipment/instruments; ..." (CAP Standards for Laboratory Accreditation, 1988 edition).[34]

The Standard's requirements are then spelled out in multiple questions in the **checklists** used in the course of the actual inspection, and the following questions are representative (as found in the clinical chemistry section, 1989–1990 edition):

Question No.   Category: Instrument Maintenance

03.0540 Is there a schedule or system AVAILABLE AT THE INSTRUMENT for the regular checking of the critical operating characteristics for all instruments in use?

03.0560 Are instructions for instrument check systems written (i.e., manufacturer's manual or written system prepared by the laboratory)?

03.0570 Are functions checks documented by the TECHNICAL OPERATOR in a convenient manner to detect trends or malfunctions?

03.0580 Are tolerance limits for acceptable function written for specific instruments wherever appropriate?

03.0590 Are instructions provided for minor troubleshooting and repairs of instruments (such as manufacturer's service manual)?

03.0600 Are records maintained AT each instrument to document all repairs and service procedures?

03.0610 Are RECENT instrument maintenance, service, and repair records (or copies) immediately available to and usable by the technical staff operating the equipment?

Category: Automatic Pipets

03.0520 Are pipets checked for accuracy of calibration before being placed in service (gravimetric, colorimetric, or other verification procedure)?

03.0530 Are pipets checked for accuracy and reproducibility at regular intervals?

Category: Temperature Dependent Equipment

Are temperatures checked and recorded daily (or when used) for the following types of equipment:

03.0620 Water baths?

03.0630 Dry baths?

03.0640 Automated Clinical Chemistry components (water baths, dialyzers, heating baths)?

03.0650 Incubators and ovens (where temperature control is necessary for a procedure)?

03.0660 Refrigerators and freezers?

03.0670 Have acceptable ranges been defined for all temperature dependent equipment?

Category: Thermometers

03.0710 Is an appropriate thermometric standard device of known accuracy available (NIST certified or guaranteed by manufacturer to meet NIST Standards)?

03.0720 Are all non-certified thermometers in use checked against an appropriate thermometric standard device before being placed in service?

Category: Centrifuges

03.0730 Are all centrifuges in the Clinical Chemistry laboratory clean and properly maintained (check lining for dried blood and other residue)?

03.0740 Is there a written protocol for maintenance of all centrifuges (i.e., cleaning, changing brushes, etc.)?

03.0750 Are the operating speeds of all centrifuges checked periodically as needed for the intended use and when it can be performed safely?

Additional similar questions in the checklist for clinical chemistry address the maintenance of such equipment as analytical balances, colorimeters and spectrophotometers, flame photometers, atomic absorption spectrophotometers, blood gas and pH instruments, multiple analysis automated instruments and systems, and electrophoresis apparatus. The effect of this avalanche of questions on laboratory operations can only be described as overwhelming.

Mandatory Instrument Maintenance

The approach taken by governmental regulators to compelling instrument maintenance generally resembles that seen in the CAP Laboratory Accreditation program. A progressive elaboration of detail is seen, paralleling that seen in the CAP's flow: i.e., from Standard to Interpretation to checklist.

For example, the quality control regulations written by the Centers for Disease Control (CDC) to implement the (Federal) Clinical Laboratory Improvement Act of 1967 (CLIA '67) required interstate laboratories to assure that "all equipment is in good working order, routinely checked and precise in terms of calibration." In 1979, this mandate was extended to hospital-based laboratories participating in Medicare. More recently, a new law, known as CLIA '88, was passed by Congress, replacing the earlier legislation. The regulations implementing the latter law were released in "final" version on February 28, 1992,[40] and the section

of these regulations (Section 493.1215 of Title 42 of the Code of Federal Regulations; 42 CFR 493.1215) dealing with instrument maintenance is presented in Figure 16–5. The outstanding feature of the new regulations is that laboratories must follow the procedures for maintenance defined by the manufacturer of the instruments (which require prior approval by the FDA). Should the laboratory modify the manufacturer's procedure, or use a procedure of its own devising, an additional burden will be incurred. The laboratory will then have to engage in a validation process for the instrument maintenance procedure adopted, i.e., demonstrate that the modified or alternative procedures are adequate to ensure "equipment, instrument, and test system performance necessary for accurate and reliable test results. . . ."[40]

An additional example of Federal regulations dealing with instrument maintenance, in this instance related to the FDA's authority to regulate blood banks, can be found in 21 CFR 606.60. Here the regulations begin by stating, "Equipment used in the collection, processing . . . and distribution of blood and blood components shall be maintained in a clean and orderly manner and . . . observed, standardized and calibrated on a regularly scheduled basis. . . ." The next paragraph then specifies the frequency with which performance checks and calibration are to be carried out, as may be seen in Table 16–1.

Deficiencies Cited During Regulatory Inspections

Deficiencies in instrument maintenance, whether of written procedure, actual performance, or documentation thereof, now constitute a substantial proportion of all compliance failures encountered during both government and voluntary accredita-

42 CFR Part 493

Clinical Laboratory Improvement Amendments of 1988;

Final Rules and Notice   (Feb 28, 1992)

sect 493.1215 Standard; Equipment maintenance and function checks

The laboratory must perform equipment maintenance and function checks that include electronic, mechanical and operational checks necessary for the proper test performance and test result reporting of equipment, instruments and test systems to assure accurate and reliable test results and reports.

(a) *Maintenance of equipment, instruments, and test systems.*
   (1) For manufacturers' equipment, instruments or test systems cleared by the FDA as meeting the CLIA requirements for general quality control, the laboratory must—
      (i) Perform maintenance as defined by the manufacturer and with at least the frequency specified by the manufacturer; and
      (ii) Document all maintenance performed.
   (2) For equipment, instruments, or test systems not cleared by the FDA as meeting the CLIA requirements for general quality control, or equipment, instruments, or test systems that have been modified or developed in-house, the laboratory must—
      (i) Establish a maintenance protocol that ensures equipment, instrument, and test system performance necessary for accurate and reliable test results and test result reporting;
      (ii) Perform maintenance with at least the frequency specified in paragraph (a)(2)(i) of this section; and
      (iii) Document all maintenance performed.

(b) *Function checks of equipment, instruments, and test systems.*
   (1) For manufacturers' equipment, instruments, or test systems cleared by the FDA as meeting the CLIA requirements for general quality control, the laboratory must—
      (i) Perform function checks as defined by the manufacturer and with at least the frequency specified by the manufacturer; and
      (ii) Document all function checks performed.
   (2) For equipment, instruments, or test systems not cleared by the FDA as meeting the CLIA requirements for general quality control, or equipment, instruments, or test systems that have been modified or developed in-house, the laboratory must—
      (i) Define a function check protocol that ensures equipment, instrument, and test system performance necessary for accurate and reliable test results and test result reporting;
      (ii) Perform function checks, including background or baseline checks specified in paragraph (b)(2)(i) of this section. Function checks must be within the laboratory's established limits before patient testing is conducted; and
      (iii) Document all function checks performed.

■ **FIGURE 16–5.**

A section of the federal regulations governing instrument maintenance in clinical laboratories.

TABLE 16–1. FEDERAL REGULATIONS FOR BLOOD BANK EQUIPMENT

EQUIPMENT	PERFORMANCE CHECK	FREQUENCY	FREQUENCY OF CALIBRATION
Temperature recorder	Compare against thermometer	Daily	As necessary
Refrigerated centrifuge	Observe speed and temperature	Each day of use	do
Hematocrit centrifuge			Standardize before initial use, after repairs or adjustments, and annually. Timer every 3 mo
General lab centrifuge			Tachometer every 6 mo
Automated blood-typing machine	Observe controls for correct results	Each day of use	
Hemoglobinometer	Standardize against cyanmethemoglobin standard	do	
Refractometer	Standardize against distilled water	do	
Blood container scale	Standardize against container of known weight	do	As necessary
Water bath	Observe temperature	do	do
Rh view box	do	do	do
Autoclave	do	Each time of use	do
Serologic rotators	Observe controls for correct results	Each day of use	Speed as necessary
Laboratory thermometers			Before initial use
Electronic thermometers			Monthly
Vacuum blood agitator	Observe weight of the first container of blood filled for correct results	Each day of use	Standardize with container of known mass or volume before initial use, and after repairs or adjustments

tion inspections. Since it is always easier to learn from the misfortunes of others, we conclude with a representative sampling of this type of compliance failure. All the examples are taken from records of FDA inspections of blood banks within the past 2 years.

item: "There is no written procedure for the daily quality control checks of laboratory equipment such as heating blocks, water baths, or incubators."

item: "Temperature readings were not recorded for the refrigerator and freezer on the following 19 separate days: . . . ."

item: "No procedure for maintenance of the microhematocrit centrifuges, and no record of maintenance is kept."

item: "No procedure exists to monitor the accuracy of the [brand name] autopipettor. This instrument identifies each sample by its bar code after pipetting. . . . No verification is conducted to assure all bar codes were read correctly and the correct results were assigned to each unit."

item: "The manufacturer's required daily calibration of the [automated hematology instrument] . . . has not been performed properly in that: (a) The calibration is not performed as per the detailed instructions included in the manual. . . . (c) Documentation of the steps is not recorded as per the manufacturer's instructions."

item: "[automated pipettor] technical manual requires tip threshold calibration to be performed when replacing tip nozzle, tubing syringe, or syringe plunger. No tip threshold (calibration) was performed on [four cited days]."

item: "The procedure for Quality Assurance of RPR rotators requires a quarterly test of the diameter of rotation but there is no record of the test being done since [date six months earlier]."

item: "The donor blood unit scale lacks an assay of the certification for the daily 500 gm wt used to calibrate the scales."

It cannot be concluded from this unrepresentative sampling of FDA inspection experience that one particular type of PM omission is predominant. Hence, it is not possible to validate the view expressed in the CAP *Manual* that verification activities "receive more attention and are a greater significance to inspectors, than details of instrument maintenance." It is, however, very interesting to reflect on the implications of the statement, "Whether or not a gear was oiled or a tubing replaced is of less concern than the qualified verification that an instrument meets its functional specifications."[7]

In summary, the message in the regulatory sphere is quite clear: Instrument maintenance will be scrutinized closely by laboratory inspectors, whether from the governmental or the voluntary sector. Consequently, whatever other reasons may exist for adopting a PM program, laboratories are well advised to comply completely with the instrument maintenance regulations or risk the loss of licensure or certification.

TROUBLESHOOTING

The carefully organized planning and implementation involved in the laboratory's PM program must be complemented by another planned-for activity, which takes place in the event of instrument malfunction or breakdown. Myhre captures the inevitability of the latter experience when he states, "Although the average machine of any type is quite tolerant of neglect, eventually it will fail, and seemingly it always does so when its use is most vital."[28] At such a dread moment, it becomes necessary to have in place some plan for troubleshooting, the type of laboratory activity evoked by instrument performance failure.

Not everyone understands what a completely rational process this is, this maintenance of a motorcycle. They think it's some kind of a "knack" or some kind of "affinity for machines" in operation. They are right, but the knack is almost purely a process of reason, and most of the troubles are caused by what old time radio men called a "short between the earphones," failures to use the head properly. A motorcycle functions entirely in accordance with the laws of reason, and a study of the art of motorcycle maintenance is really a miniature study of the art of rationality itself . . . (p. 98).

R.M. PIRSIG[1]

Process and Procedure

Troubleshooting, in the context of clinical laboratory instrumentation, is generally understood to comprehend the activities involved in defining and locating trouble (i.e., malfunctions), thereby making possible appropriate repairs in machinery and technical equipment. Put another way, troubleshooting is the process by which apparently unsatisfactory instrument performance is traced (much as the electronic technician traces circuits) down to root causes, which permits the correct solution to be applied to identified problems.

The importance of troubleshooting in an overall program of instrumental quality is almost axiomatic. However, the actual steps involved in the troubleshooting process are not easy to describe, and certainly are not as susceptible to formulaic prescription as are the components of a preventive maintenance program. The literature devoted to methods of troubleshooting is thus meager by comparison with the literature of clinical laboratory PM, with the notable exception of a continuing column dedicated to the pitfalls of chromatography in the journal LC.GC (published monthly by Aster Publishing Corporation).

The following general remarks are intended to summarize the more important aspects of clinical laboratory equipment troubleshooting, emphasizing how it differs from and complements preventive maintenance.

1. Troubleshooting had a well-defined existence in all laboratories before preventive maintenance was ever formally conceived and inaugurated. (Beginning with the Industrial Revolution, importance has always been placed on the existence of the "artful" master mechanic, who could coax dead or dying equipment back to life.)

2. Troubleshooting occurs as a natural and automatic transition of operator attention and activity, whenever an instrumental malfunction is detected or suspected. The detection may occur because of some signal recognized during instrument operation, such as escape from statistical quality control, total output failure, or even the occurrence of a sound unfamiliar to the bench technician. It may also be evoked when the function checking component of the preventive maintenance program identifies some aberration or deterioration in critical operating characteristics. (By now, it should be clearly understood that one of the major contributions PM record-keeping can make to the laboratory is to facilitate trouble-shooting at the critical moments when instrument failure has occurred[41.])

3. General (as opposed to instrument-specific) troubleshooting guidelines tend to consist, at best, of a series of insightful admonitions and reassuring statements or, at worst, of an array of platitudes. Thus, the reader encounters maxims such as, "The best-kept secret of any successful trouble-shooter is an intimate awareness of how an instrument runs when there is no trouble,"[41] and, "Remember the first of the 'Five Rules of Thumb' for troubleshooting: Change just one thing at a time."[42] Johnson provides a set of diagnostic questions for instrument troubleshooting.[43] The instrument maintenance chapter of the Stewart and Koepke text[5] also offers a representative assemblage of such generalizations:

GUIDELINES FOR TROUBLESHOOTING THE MALFUNCTIONING INSTRUMENT

1. Don't panic. Keep calm and you will think more clearly.
2. Define the problem. Don't make assumptions about what is wrong.
3. Try to think if there is any past experience that might shed light on what the problem may be and how it might be solved.
4. Try the simplest approach to solve the problem. Usually simple problems are the most common ones.
5. Replace good parts for bad.
6. When these simple solutions fail, ask for help from a supervisor or contact the manufacturer for information (p. 117).

---

4. Instrument-specific troubleshooting, whether provided by manufacturers' instru-

ment manuals or developed by the laboratory itself, are likely to be either frankly algorithmic or written in the form of "if . . . then" conditional propositions. An example of the latter, relating to a familiar malfunction of the microhematocrit centrifuge, is adapted from Larsen and associates:[16]

If:
Hematocrit tubes frequently "spin out" (lose their contents during centrifugation)—
Then:
a) Check rubber lining cushion to see whether it is punctured with through-and-through holes. (Occasional shifting of the rubber cushion should be part of preventive maintenance.)
b) Check to see whether hematocrit tubes are being properly plugged with sealing clay. (Make certain that the surface of the clay is flat and that the hematocrit tube is being inserted vertically, so that the inner aspect of the clay plug will be flat and perpendicular to the tube.)
c) Check to see that the clay-sealed ends of the hematocrit tubes are touching the rubber cushion, when loading the centrifuge head.

5. It is important to distinguish the essential initial stage of the troubleshooting process, i.e., finding the source of the trouble, from the subsequent reparative steps that may be required when the cause of the problem is identified. It must be understood that troubleshooting is a form of problem-solving, in which substitution of known good for possibly defective parts to identify the actual faulty component constitutes the experiment undertaken to prove or disprove hypothesis of causation. Indeed, as already indicated, instrument repair may be quite beyond the capabilities of the laboratory, either because of the complexity of the instrument involved, the lack of available parts on-site, or the lack of skills in the employees of the laboratory or the parent institution.

Accordingly, the fundamental aphorism of troubleshooting may be stated as: The major problem in resolving a problem is identifying the problem.

6. Part of the planning for the troubleshooting process must deal with the question, likewise encountered in PM planning, of who will be responsible for troubleshooting activities. Marxsen, after acknowledging that preventive maintenance must be every laboratory technologist's concern and responsibility, has humorously described the type of individual best suited to handle troubleshooting and repair (a combination he calls "meatball maintenance"):[44]

Meatball maintenance can only be handled by people with an instinctive feel for machines . . . Every lab needs a few techs who conceal grease-monkey desires beneath their high-strung professional exteriors: those techs who are only comfortable when they have a screwdriver or pliers within reach at all times, and who wait eagerly each month for their Popular Mechanics *to arrive. . . .*

This, like all caricatures, tends to exaggerate some feature of the subject—here, the alleged "instinctive" talent for machines possessed by the prototypical laboratory troubleshooter. In so doing, however, the caricature obscures the actual strategies and tactics used in successful troubleshooting and, additionally, devalues the essentially highly logical nature of the process itself.

7. Consequently, to better bring out the methodology and rationale that are the real basis of the troubleshooting enterprise, re-

sort is made to the description of the process formulated by Pirsig:[1]

... if the cycle goes over a bump and the engine misfires, and then goes over another bump and the engine misfires, and then goes over another bump and the engine misfires, and then goes over another bump and the engine misfires, and then goes over a long smooth stretch of road and there is no misfiring, and then goes over a fourth bump and the engine misfires again, one can logically conclude that the misfiring is caused by the bumps. That is induction: reasoning from particular experiences to general truths.

Deductive inferences do the reverse. They start with general knowledge and predict a specific observation. For example, if, from reading the hierarchy of facts about the machine, the mechanic knows the horn of the cycle is powered exclusively by electricity from the battery, then he can logically infer that if the battery is dead the horn will not work. That is deduction.

Solution of problems too complicated for common sense to solve is achieved by long strings of mixed inductive and deductive inferences that weave back and forth between the observed machine and the mental hierarchy of the machine found in the manuals. The correct program for this interweaving is formalized as scientific method.

... There's no fault isolation problem in motorcycle maintenance that can stand up to it. When you've hit a really tough one, tried everything, racked your brain and nothing works, ... you crank up the formal scientific method.

For this you keep a lab notebook. Everything gets written down, formally, so that you know at all times where you are, where you've been, where you're going and where you want to get. In scientific work and electronics technology this is necessary because otherwise the problems get so complex you get lost in them ... Sometimes just the act of writing down the problems straightens out your head as to what they really are. ...

In Part One of formal scientific method, which is the statement of the problem, the main skill is in stating absolutely no more than you are positive you know. It is much better to enter a statement "Solve Problem: Why doesn't cycle work?" which sounds dumb but is correct, then it is to enter a statement "Solve Problem: What is wrong with the electrical system?" when you don't absolutely know the trouble is in the electrical system. What you should state is "Solve Problem: What is wrong with the cycle?" and then state as the first entry of Part Two: "Hypothesis Number One: The trouble is in the electrical system." You think of as many hypotheses as you can, then you design experiments to test them to see which are true and which are false. ...

... By asking the right questions and choosing the right tests and drawing the right conclusions, the mechanic works his way down the echelons of the motorcycle hierarchy until he has found the exact specific cause or causes of the engine failure, and then he changes them so that they no longer cause the failure (pp. 107–111).

Selected Examples

Published examples of successful troubleshooting that document the methodology of the process, i.e., the stepwise reasoning and experimentation resorted to, are not readily available. This situation is largely due to the ephemeral nature of most instrument troubleshooting challenges. In most cases, once normal operations have been restored, there is little concern for preserving the details of the incident for their instructional value. However, the following two incident reports serve to bring out some practical applications of the troubleshooting principles already discussed.

An instructive example of how preventive maintenance records contribute to the troubleshooting process can be found in teaching case No. 2 in the chapter "Monitoring Quality Control" in the Becan-McBride *Textbook of Clinical Laboratory Supervision*.[31] Here, supervisory review of PM data revealed a pronounced downward trend in potentiometer settings for both the sodium and potassium channels of an automated multichannel instrument, occurring over a period of 2 weeks. Troubleshooting checks isolated the problem to the lithium detector, and replacement of this component brought the potentiometer readings back to normal levels. (Additional details of the troubleshooting tactics utilized may be found in the reference.)

Another example of successful instrumental troubleshooting can be found in Whitehead's *Quality Control in Clinical Chemistry* (pp. 69, 75, 76), this one arising from equipment malfunction in the preanalytical stage.[45] This incident involved two different out-of-control situations for the same analyte. In the first, an interlaboratory comparison of patient results, it was noted that one laboratory clearly recorded serum potassium results higher than those of any other participating institution. An explanation for this could not be found until a second unusual phenomenon was observed. As shown in Figure 16–6, the laboratory obtaining the high patient potassium results, by plotting the daily mean of patients' potassium values over a period of several weeks, was able to establish that, almost invariably, low mean values were obtained on Saturday mornings. Upon investigation it was shown that the Saturday results were probably correct,

and that results on weekdays were probably too high. Whitehead relates, almost triumphantly:

The fault was eventually traced to a centrifuge that was overheating, raising the temperature of blood during centrifugation and driving potassium out of the cells into the serum. On a Saturday morning, when technicians wanted to save time in the spinning process, so that they could get away for their half-day break, the blood was not left in the centrifuge for as long as on weekdays, thus the lower serum potassium values.

SUMMARY

Preventive maintenance (PM) is a useful, if inaccurate, way of describing a program of instrumental quality control. It is now a well-established mode of laboratory quality assurance. In actuality, PM requires activities of two different sorts: prophylactic maintenance per se and performance monitoring (which is understood to involve both calibration and checks of critical operating characteristics).

The essential elements of a preventive maintenance program are (1) a series of tasks to be performed; (2) a schedule of when these actions are to be carried out; (3) the designation of personnel responsible for the activities; and (4) a record-keeping process that documents the performance of the activities according to schedule. In the 25 years that have elapsed since its introduction into the clinical laboratory, PM has undergone an operational transformation. It has evolved from an intimidating figure-it-out-for-yourself activity to one that has become both highly routine and at the same time almost totally prescribed by instrument manufacturers. Currently, stemming

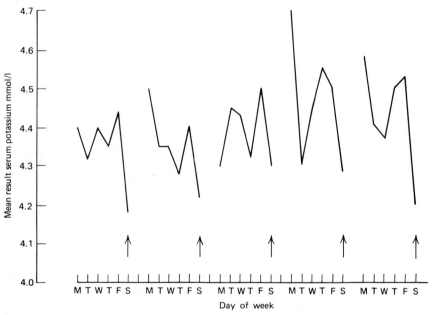

■ **FIGURE 16–6.**

Mean of patients' potassium results over a period of several weeks. Note the low values that were recorded on Saturday morning. For explanation, see text. (From Whitehead TP: *Quality Control in Clinical Chemistry.* New York, Churchill Livingstone; 1977.)

from the mandates of the CLIA '88 regulations, as well as because of the increasing complexity of the instruments themselves, the major source of PM routines for any specific laboratory instrument must be the instrument manual supplied by the manufacturer.

PM has come to be increasingly emphasized by regulatory authorities and is a favorite target in accreditation/licensing inspections.

Troubleshooting (and repair) is the necessary "other side of the coin" to preventive maintenance in a comprehensive instrument quality assurance system. Troubleshooting is far less routine and requires considerably greater creativity than preventive maintenance. It is best understood as involving an applied "scientific method" in its combination of hypothesizing and experimentation to detect and resolve instrument failure.

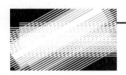

REVIEW QUESTIONS

1. Preventive maintenance is best described as

   a. scheduled maintenance.
   b. unscheduled maintenance.
   c. corrective maintenance.
   d. reparative maintenance.

2. The phrase "preventive maintenance" is

   a. generally a new phrase.
   b. less than 25 years old.
   c. more than 25 years old.
   d. less than 10 years old.

3. The best set of instructions for a successful PM launch is that of

   a. Lehmann.
   b. Warren.

   c. Yeast.
   d. Duckworth.

4. The "three D's" of PM are all of the following, *except*

   a. do.
   b. decide.
   c. define.
   d. document.

5. All of the following are essential elements of a preventive maintenance program, *except*

   a. a series of tasks to be performed.
   b. a schedule of when these actions are to be carried out.
   c. the designation of personnel responsible for the activities.
   d. a list of all activities prior to PM.

REFERENCES

1. Pirsig RM: *Zen and the Art of Motorcycle Maintenance.* New York, William Morrow, 1974.
2. Centers for Disease Control (CDC): *Guide on Laboratory Administration*; VIII Maintenance; Preventive Maintenance (PM)—Equipment. Atlanta, CDC Laboratory Consultation Office, 1973; pp 100–124.
3. Duckworth JK, et al: Preventive maintenance in the clinical laboratory. *Pathologist* [Bull CAP] 27(6):205–213, 1973.
4. Eilers RJ: Quality assurance in health care: Mission, goals, activities. *Clin Chem* 21:1357–1367, 1975.
5. Stewart CE, Koepke JA: Quality assurance and instrument maintenance. *In Basic Quality Assurance Practices for Clinical Laboratories.* Philadelphia, Lippincott, 1987, Chapter 19.
6. Garfield FM: *Quality Assurance Principles for Analytical Laboratories.* Arlington, VA, Association of Official Analytical Chemists, 1991, pp 40–44.
7. College of American Pathologists: *Laboratory Instrument Evaluation Verification and Maintenance Manual.* Northfield, IL, 1989.
8. Alpert NL: Lab and instrument manufacturer: A unique partnership. *MLO* 13(4):137–144, 1981.
9. Baer DM: Repair and maintenance of instruments. *Bull Pathol* [ASCP] 9(10):196–197, 1968.
10. Preventive maintenance in the laboratory. *Lab Management* 8(6):32–41, 1970.
11. Rand RN: Practical spectrophotometric standards. *Clin Chem* 15:839, 1969.
12. Winstead M: *Instrument Check Systems.* Philadelphia, Lea & Febiger, 1971.
13. Duckworth JK, Stevens MV: A design for preventive maintenance. *MLO* 3(6):34–37, 1971.
14. Sohaney JL: A quality control maintenance program for the clinical laboratory. *Lab Med* 2(10):23–25, 1972.
15. Hobbs WD: Equipment maintenance and repair. *In* Lundberg GD (ed): *Managing the Patient-Focused Laboratory.* Oradell, NJ, Medical Economics Publishing Company, 1975.
16. Larsen RC, et al: Equipment maintenance—A valuable asset to all laboratories. *Lab Med* 10(4):230–233, 1979.
17. Warren Brenda L: Instrument maintenance: A guide to optimum performance. *MLO* 10(7):55–69, 1978.
18. Yapit MK, Bredlinger BA: How to avoid maintenance muffs and misses. *MLO* 9(12):95–97, 1977.
19. Yapit MK: Keeping your instruments happy. *MLO* 15(11):32–39, 1983.
20. Crisafulli C: An uncomplicated system for preventive maintenance. *Lab Med* 7(11):23–28, 1976.
21. Beckman S: An instrument tech can save you money. *MLO* 10(12):43–50, 1978.
22. McDonald CW: Keeping track of preventive maintenance. *MLO* 12(3):77–84, 1980.
23. Wilcox KR, et al: Laboratory management. *In* Inhorn SL (ed): *Quality Assurance Practices for Health Laboratories.* Washington, DC, American Public Health Association, 1978, pp 56–77.
24. Baldwin M, Barasso C: The development and operation of an efficient laboratory preventive maintenance program. *Am J Med Technol* 45:216–218, 1979.
25. Veterans Administration: *Preventive Maintenance Guides for Selected Hospital Equipment.* Vol 1: Clinical Laboratory (VA-G-29/1). Springfield, VA, National Technical Information Service, 1973.
26. Dharan M: Quality control of laboratory instruments and equipment. *In Total Quality Control in the Clinical Laboratory.* St. Louis, Mosby, 1977, Chapter 11.
27. Ottaviano PJ, Disalvo AF: Equipment maintenance. *In Quality Control in the Clinical Laboratory.* Baltimore, University Park Press, 1977, Chapter 4.
28. Myhre BQ: Quality control of blood bank equipment. *In Quality Control in Blood Banking.* New York, Wiley, 1974, Chapter 2.
29. Thompson J, Leubbert PP: Concepts of preventive maintenance for laboratory instrumentation. *In* Snyder JR, Senhauser DA (eds): *Administration and Supervision in Laboratory Medicine,* 2nd ed. Philadelphia, Lippincott, 1989, Chapter 19.
30. Shuffstall RM, Hemmaplardh B: The care of equipment and laboratory safety. *In The Hospital Laboratory; Modern Concepts of Management, Operations, and Finance.* St Louis, Mosby, 1979, Chapter 9.
31. Lorimor KK, Collins FL: Monitoring quality control in the clinical laboratory. *In* Becan-McBride K (ed): *Textbook of Clinical Laboratory Supervision.* New York, Appleton-Century-Crofts, 1982, pp 189–204.
32. Baron EJ: Instrument maintenance and quality control. *In* Isenberg HD (ed): *Clinical Microbiology Procedures Handbook.* Washington, DC, American Society for Microbiology, 1992, Chapter 12.
33. Duckworth JK, Stevens MV: A preventive maintenance plan that really works. *MLO* 4(5):25–28, 1972.
34. College of American Pathologists, Commission on Laboratory Accreditation: *Clinical Laboratory Improvement Manual* (2 vols). Northfield, IL, 1990.
35. Yeast JL: Being systematic about preventive maintenance. *MLO* 14(7):41–48, 1982.
36. College of American Pathologists, Instrument Maintenance Committee: Instrument quality assurance for test result quality and laboratory operation. *Pathologist* 34(3):139–141, 1980.
37. Bender JL: Guidelines for laboratory administration—Part I. *MLO* 16(6):53–58, 1984.

38. Jaglinski K: A flexible reminder system for preventive maintenance. *MLO* 8(5):79–86, 1976.
39. Corcoran LG: Reliable instrument maintenance with a PC. *MLO* 23(1):77–79, 1991.
40. Clinical Laboratory Improvement Amendments of 1988 (CLIA-88); *Final Rules and Notice* (42 CFR 493). Federal Register, Vol 57, No 40; Feb 28, 1992 (57 FR 7002).
41. Pesek PA: Acquiring basic instrument troubleshooting skills. *MLO* 15(7):129–132, 1983.
42. Dolan JW: LC troubleshooting: LC problem guide. *LC-GC* 10(7):508–514, 1992.
43. Johnson JE: 'This Machine Isn't Working'—a set of diagnostic questions for instrument troubleshooting. *MLO* 18(8):77–81, 1986.
44. Marxsen B: Take care of your machines, and they'll take care of you. *MLO* 8(11):54–55, 1976.
45. Whitehead TP: *Quality Control in Clinical Chemistry*. New York, Wiley, 1977.

INTRODUCTION
WORKFLOW ANALYSIS
Facility Characteristics
Preanalytical Workflow
Analytical Workflow
Postanalytical Workflow

Chapter 17

IMPROVING LABORATORY EFFICIENCY THROUGH WORKFLOW ANALYSIS

CRAIG LEHMANN, PhD, CC(NRCC)
ALAN LEIKEN, PhD

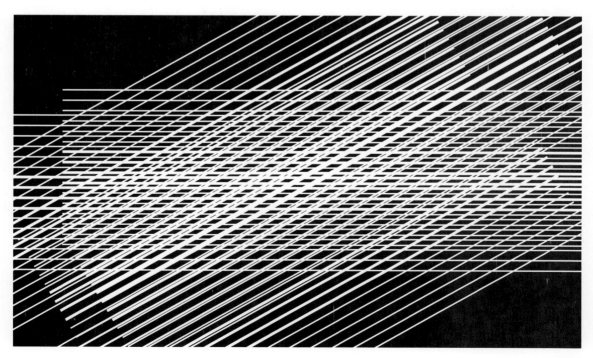

LEARNING OBJECTIVES

After studying this chapter the student should be able to:

- Define terms used in workflow analysis.
- Describe the differences between preanalytical, analytical, and post-analytical.
- Define cost per reportable.
- List the primary features found in most data management packages.
- Identify the major workstations found in a clinical chemistry laboratory.
- Describe the importance of turnaround time.
- Define the term *analytical throughput.*
- List five sample-handling features available on technology.
- List three reagent-handling features available on technology.
- Describe the advantages of sample barcodes.

KEY WORDS

Analytical. All functions performed at an instrument to produce a test result.

Analytical throughput. The maximum number of tests or samples an instrument can perform in 1 hour.

Autodilution. Dilutes samples automatically when assays are out of linear range.

Barcode. A line-coded label that identifies sample.

Cost per reportable. All direct costs directly related to producing a patient test result.

Data management. The data management features that can be found on a particular analyzer (i.e., quality control programs).

Downtime. When an instrument is not in operation.

Host computer. A facilities primary computer in which all data are collected and stored.

On-Board Stability. The lifespan of a reagent once placed on an instrument.

Postanalytical. All functions performed after analyzer results to get test results back to a physician.

Preanalytical. All functions performed prior to instrument.

Sample splitting. The sharing of a sample between multiple workstations.

Test menu. A list of tests any one instrument can perform.

Turnaround time. The time it takes for a laboratory to process a test.

Workflow analysis. The monitoring of all functions from the time a test is requested to results reported.

INTRODUCTION

Prior to the 1980s, laboratories were viewed by hospital administrators as revenue producers. However, because of the inflationary cycle of health care spending, the government began changing the financial structure of the health care industry, which eventually changed the laboratory into a major cost center. The legislation that was responsible for this change is the Tax Equity and Fiscal Responsibilities Act (TEFRA) along with the Prospective Payment System implemented by the Reagan Administration in the early 1980s. Based on this legislation, the reimbursement for hospital in-patients was set by a diagnosis-related group (DRG). Each diagnosis-related group (e.g., myocardial infarction) has a set dollar reimbursement regardless of how often ancillary services are used. For example, if a patient was admitted to the hospital with a possible myocardial infarction, the reimbursement would be the same whether a physician ordered 6 or 30 cardiac panels over the patient's stay. This financial change was followed by a shortage of qualified medical technologists. The combination of the two encouraged many laboratory administrators to begin to evaluate and improve the operation and efficiency of their laboratories.

In an effort to respond to the financial and personnel situation, yet at the same time still function and produce the high quality of services to which the medical community has grown accustomed, laboratory administrators focused on four primary areas: labor, revenue, costs, and technology. To respond to the shortage of qualified medical technologists, many laboratories have implemented recruitment outreach programs with incentives. For example, paid tuition is offered to medical technology students in return for a stated number of years of employment after graduation. Others have implemented on-the-job training for biology and chemistry majors with bachelor's degrees.

Since outpatient testing has not yet been affected by DRGs, in an effort to generate additional revenue the number of outpatient services and outreach programs (e.g., soliciting testing from physicians' offices) has been increased or programs started anew by many laboratories.

To decrease operational costs and possibly alleviate some of the labor shortages, many administrators have taken advantage of the newer technology. Many of the newer analyzers allow the laboratory to consolidate some of its workstations. For example, many of the newer routine analyzers have expanded menus to include therapeutic and thyroid testing. Consolidation of workstations has turned out to be one of the primary ingredients in dealing with labor shortages and costs. A more detailed discussion of this topic will follow in this chapter.

WORKFLOW ANALYSIS

The first step in evaluating staffing changes, revenue-producing programs, cost reduction programs, and technology changes for a clinical laboratory is the performance of a **workflow analysis.** Workflow analysis is the documentation and analysis of a laboratory's operation.

As demonstrated in Figure 17–1, the analysis begins with the physician's request for laboratory tests and ends with the physician's interpretation of the test results. This is a tedious task but should be the

Physician's Request for Laboratory Tests

Test requisition granted   A

Sample collection
                                  B
Sample transport

Laboratory Specimen Receiving

Sample processing
                                  C
Sample destination

Analyzer Entry

Test results
                                  D
Data verification

Data Transport

Physician's interpretation   E

■ **FIGURE 17–1.**

Workflow analysis.

basis on which all personnel, revenue enhancement programs, cost reduction programs, and technology decisions are made. To better understand the details involved in performing workflow analysis, the process has been separated into five major categories, shown as A through E in Figure 17–1. Each of these categories has to be assessed in its present operation as well as in any future operation.

Workflow analysis usually begins with the facility's characteristics (Fig. 17–2). However, before the process begins, the primary question of what is hoped to be accomplished by workflow analysis has to be answered. Many facilities perform workflow analysis for one or more of the following reasons:

■ The facility is planning an outreach program.
■ The laboratory is trying to reduce labor and operating costs.

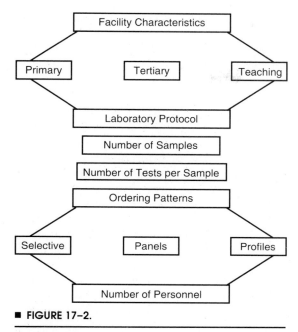

■ **FIGURE 17–2.**

Characteristics of a facility.

- The laboratory is trying to cope with the labor shortage.
- The laboratory is trying to improve turnaround time and efficiency.

Once the expected goals of the workflow analysis have been established, the process usually begins by outlining the facility's characteristics.

Facility Characteristics

Many of the characteristics outlined in Figure 17–2 can begin to predetermine or limit changes in technology, personnel, and so on automatically. For example, is the facility a primary, tertiary, or teaching hospital? This characteristic can predetermine the level of personnel and types of technology a laboratory should acquire. Teaching hospitals have residents who tend to order

many and more elaborate tests than do attending physicians in a primary care facility. This characteristic would begin to predetermine the type of technology (e.g., expanded **test menu,** high throughput) that the facility should be considering. Teaching tertiary care facilities may need more technologists than technicians because of the more elaborate testing that would take place (e.g., lecithin/sphingomyelin ratios). Teaching and tertiary care facilities tend to have a greater number of STAT tests and off-hour testing, which, again, might predict types of technology and number of personnel.

In any facility, the protocol set by the laboratory can have an impact on turnaround time, testing volume, STATs, and so on. If the laboratory limits its STAT menu to electrolytes and a few other tests, there will be fewer tests. In turn, this will require fewer personnel and possibly a smaller analyzer, especially for off-hours. On the other hand, if the laboratory offers a more expanded STAT menu that might include creatinine kinase and lactate dehydrogenase isoenzymes, the laboratory would need additional and possibly a higher level of personnel.

Laboratories should never make protocol changes without first trying to evaluate their impact. An excellent example of this was published in *Clinical Laboratory Science.** Here a facility decided to restrict the medical staff's ability to order a 20-chemistry profile. The laboratory set protocol that permitted physicians only one 20-chemistry profile for each patient at the time of admission. The medical staff was told by the pathologist that large numbers of tests on one requisition would be brought to his attention and that he would want an explanation for the order. It was hoped that this protocol would make the medical staff more reluc-

---

*Lehmann CA, Leiken AM, Fass J: *Clin Lab Sci* 1:305–307, 1988.

tant to order the large chemistry profile and that the laboratory would see a decrease in the number of tests performed.

The workflow analysis revealed that the medical staff did restrict the number of tests per requisition. The analysis also revealed that the laboratory samples to chemistry increased by 50 percent: many physicians, still wanting their 20 chemistries, ordered a group of tests in the A.M. and another group of tests in the P.M., with a total average per person of 18. Because of this protocol change, the laboratory was performing 50 percent more venipunctures in chemistry. This resulted in increased costs for venipunctures (phlebotomist, clerical and professional labor). Although the analysis did not measure the impact on patients' length of stay, it should be a concern for the facility. Not allowing the physician to order the perceived needed tests when necessary will only delay thought processes, keeping the patient in the bed longer. Under the present DRG system, it is far more beneficial to the hospital to keep the length of stay at a minimum.

Another report (unpublished) described a facility that removed the creatinine kinase isoenzymes test option from its medical staff on the weekend to save the cost of a weekend technologist. The laboratory saved $10,000 a year in personnel by this change in protocol. The impact of this protocol on the hospital was far more dramatic, as it increased the cardiac care unit (CCU) weekend stay by almost a day at a cost of $400 a day. The average monthly CCU weekend admission was 20 patients. Based on this, it is costing the hospital an additional $8,000 a month, or $96,000 a year. This loss far exceeds any cost savings gained by removing the weekend technologist. As demonstrated by these two cases, protocol changes can have a major impact on either the laboratory or the hospital. Because of this, it behooves the laboratory management to try

to measure the impact of the new protocol changes before implementing those changes.

Another preanalytical concern is the ordering patterns of the medical staff. Ordering patterns generally originate from previous experiences (i.e., as learned while a resident), the case mix, or design of requisition slips. To evaluate the ordering patterns of the medical staff, laboratory requisition slips have to be monitored on a daily basis. From this, one can derive whether medical staff is ordering large profiles (chem 20s), small organ-specific panels (liver panel), selective tests (1 to 5 tests per sample), or a combination of patterns. If the laboratory is trying to change the ordering patterns to improve its efficiency, workflow analysis should begin to document the average number of samples arriving at the laboratory per day and per shift and the types and number of tests requested for each sample. At the same time, the laboratory should document when the samples arrive. Are they arriving in small intervals throughout the day or are the majority arriving within a 2- to 3-hour period? Each of these factors influences the laboratory's labor, technology, and workstations. If a large number of samples with requests for a large variety of tests in a relatively short period of time are being received, the laboratory should be considering a high-throughput analyzer with a broad test menu. This type of analyzer would allow the laboratory to complete the majority of work in a relatively short period of time, keeping the turnaround time acceptable. Generally, such analyzers need qualified technologists to be available for troubleshooting and maintenance, which has an effect on personnel.

The last of the facility characteristics is the present number of workers, both technical and nontechnical, and whether or not the numbers are adequate. Questions regarding personnel should focus on how difficult it is to recruit clerks, phlebotomists, technicians, and technologists. What is the attrition rate for each? What is the general atmosphere of the laboratory? Are workers generally satisfied with their jobs? How well does the laboratory staff work together? Do they want changes in the laboratory? If an outreach program is being considered, are they in favor or do they see it as extra work? Keep in mind that the laboratory workers are the key to making any changes in the laboratory. Without their support, changes in technology or work distribution can create personnel and efficiency problems.

After facility characteristics are gathered and there is an understanding of the present operation, workflow analysis concentrates on three major areas of the laboratory: **preanalytical**, **analytical,** and **postanalytical.**

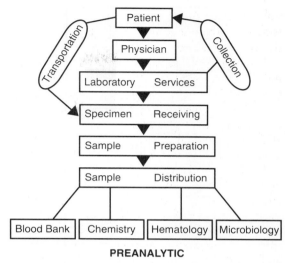

■ **FIGURE 17–3.**

Preanalytic workflow.

Preanalytical Workflow

The **preanalytical** portion of workflow, as demonstrated in Figure 17–3, is the documentation and evaluation of all procedures prior to analyzer (workstation) entry. Preanalytical can be divided into two segments, *prelaboratory* (requisition generation and phlebotomy) and *laboratory* (specimen-receiving).

Prelaboratory

The information gathered under Requisition Generation in Figure 17–4 is important not only for the laboratory but also for the physicians and nursing staff. For many physicians and nurses, this may be the only interaction they have with the laboratory. Therefore, many conclusions about laboratory services are conceived from this area.

Investigation of the prelaboratory area begins with interviewing users of the laboratory. Are they satisfied with test results,

turnaround time, test availability, sample collection, and requisition format? Is there communication among the medical staff, nursing staff, and laboratory? If there is not, plans should be implemented to establish this.

Requisition. Computers have been available to hospitals and laboratories for some time now. Yet, it is not uncommon to find laboratories that do not have a computer system or such luxuries as order entry from each service. If the laboratory does not have a laboratory computer system or is not communicating with its **host computer,** it is worthwhile to explore the financial outlay for such a system. At the same time, it is important to document the benefits of computerization. Computerization not only expedites the ordering process and decreases labor, it generally decreases turnaround time and errors. Computerization of the laboratory with the medical floors and the hospital's main computer can have one of the most significant impacts on clerical and professional laboratory labor.

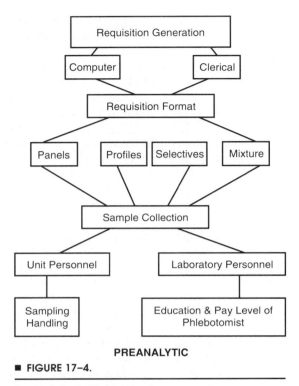

PREANALYTIC

■ **FIGURE 17–4.**

Preanalytic (prelaboratory).

Requisition Format. Whether the requisition slip is paper or electronic, its test presentation plays an intricate role in preanalytical workflow. If the format is not attuned to the medical staff's ordering practices, additional and needless tests can result. Cumbersome requisition formats tend to confuse the person doing the ordering. Keep in mind that, generally, the physician does not write the laboratory order—it is done by the nurse or clerk. Laboratory requisitions should display laboratory tests in a format that fits physicians' ordering patterns or case mix. The requisition should be designed to discourage needless testing. This can generally be accomplished in working with the medical staff.

When designing the requisition, the laboratory should keep in mind the present and future technology of the laboratory. The design of requisition profiles and panels should be based not only on case mix and physicians' requests but also on workstation technology. For example, to design a general 20-chemistry test profile when the primary routine analyzer can perform only 19 of the tests would create **sample splitting.** This forces the laboratory to split the sample so that the remaining test can be performed at another workstation, creating longer turnaround time, increased sample handling, and additional clerical activities. Many laboratories find that a general admission profile, with organ-specific panels and single test options, works best. Since physicians and case mix influence testing patterns, they warrant a close investigation by the workflow investigator.

Sample Collection. Sample collection for the laboratory has always been a difficult area. It is surprising to discover that sample collection is not always under the jurisdiction of the laboratory. Occasionally, all in-patient sample collecting is the responsibility of the nursing staff. Nevertheless, the sample collection process can expedite or hinder the workflow of a laboratory. Sample collection determines when the samples get to the laboratory, influences turnaround time, and to some extent influences technology choice (i.e., batch versus random access). Because of the potential impact on the laboratory's operation, the laboratory should have complete control. If this is not possible, than the operation should at least be under the supervision of the laboratory. The ideal situation is to have a phlebotomy team. Laboratory technicians and technologists are well qualified to perform such a task. However, the economic savings of using phlebotomists should be a primary consideration.

Laboratory

When the samples arrive at the laboratory (Fig. 17–5), sample identification, processing, and distribution take place. As with sample collection, this portion of preanalytical functions can also influence workflow dramatically.

Sample Arrival. The first step in evaluating this area is to document the time each sample arrives at the laboratory. At the same time, information should be collected on the number and types of tests requested for each of the samples. Through this information, one can begin to evaluate the needs of the laboratory. For example, the time of arrival, number of samples, and number of tests per sample will influence decisions about technology. Assume that 200 samples, of which 80 percent have requests for 12 routine chemistries, arrive at the laboratory between 7 and 10 A.M. This is an indication that the laboratory should have or should be considering a high-throughput analyzer. On the other hand, if the samples were arriving sporadically throughout the day with requests for an average of six tests per sample, then throughput would not be an issue.

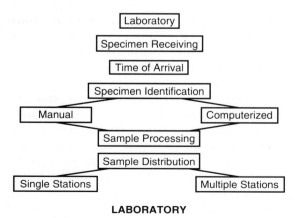

LABORATORY

■ **FIGURE 17–5.**

Preanalytical (laboratory).

This information becomes very important when designing workstations and choosing technology.

Specimen Identification. Specimen identification is limited unless the laboratory is computerized. Computerization along with **barcode** identification will reduce turn-around time, decrease ordering and identification errors, and cut down on the number of individuals needed to process the work. Under this type of system, samples are ordered electronically from each service. Based on these requests, the laboratory generates a worklist and barcodes for each sample drawn. The barcode is placed on the appropriate tubes and sent with the phlebotomist. The information in each of the barcodes includes the patient's name, identification number, and tests requested for each sample. When the samples arrive back at the laboratory, all the laboratory needs to do is check in and either distribute the sample directly to the workstation, or process the sample (centrifuge) and then distribute it to the appropriate workstation. Computerized laboratories most likely have or would be in the process of acquiring technology that is bidirectional. Bidirectional technology at workstations allows the barcoded samples to be placed directly on the analyzer. The analyzer, through the barcode, identifies both the patient and test requested. The role of the analyzer in both pre- and postanalytical information is discussed in detail in the data transport section of this chapter.

Workstations. Workstation evaluation is one of the most important aspects of workflow analysis. One of the primary goals in workstation evaluation is consolidation. The combining of two or more workstations into one can produce significant labor and cost savings, along with improved efficiency. Because today's analyzers offer high throughput and broad test menus, workstation consolidation is possible. Fewer analyzers in a laboratory can change the environment by improving workflow, reducing labor requirements, and decreasing the need to move samples from workstation to workstation. When samples need to be split in order to be sent to numerous workstations, the ability to expedite sample processing and distribution can be greatly hampered.

Of all the departments in the laboratory, the chemistry section has the greatest number of test requests. In addition, it is the most automated section of the laboratory and has the greatest possibility for workstation consolidation. As demonstrated in Figure 17–6, chemistry can be divided into four major areas: *drugs, routine, special,* and *stat testing,* with each having its own technologic needs.

Most hospital laboratories are experiencing increasing numbers of requests for therapeutic drug monitoring (TDM). To accommodate these requests, many laboratories have purchased or leased two or more ther-apeutic drug analyzers because of their low throughput. At the same time, many laboratories are being requested to perform drugs of abuse tests on urine (DAUs), which would require another analyzer, creating yet another workstation.

Routine workstations for moderate-sized hospitals consist either of two identical routine analyzers or one high-throughput analyzer. The hospital that purchases two identical systems generally does so in order to have a backup analyzer. Although this concept can be justified, it creates two workstations for routine chemistry.

Analyzers found in STAT workstations vary considerably. This is because STAT tests are determined by the laboratory and will vary based on hospital and medical staff needs. Whatever the STAT test menu, most laboratories have a separate analyzer that is used for STAT testing. It can be an analyzer utilized for routine and STAT testing during the day shift (i.e., one of the two identical analyzers in routine chemistry) and for STAT testing only on the second and third shifts. It can be a stand-alone analyzer that is only used for STATs when the menu is limited (i.e., electrolytes, urea nitrogen, glucose, amylase, and key enzymes). The other possibility is to use the primary routine analyzer for STATs. This last scenario can be accomplished only after careful evaluation of both STAT test requests and technology capabilities.

Special chemistry workstations can be single or multiple. Today, almost every laboratory performs some special chemistry tests. The availability of small analyzers that enable laboratories to perform such chemistries, such as thyroid function tests, isoenzymes, prostate specific antigens, and so on, has allowed laboratories to bring this type of testing in-house. For many laboratories, testing requests in this area are beginning to exceed the throughput of these small analyzers, thus requiring additional analyz-

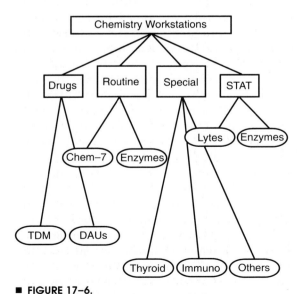

■ **FIGURE 17–6.**

Chemistry workstations.

ers. The increase is also placing higher demands on personnel (multiple workstations) and jeopardizing laboratory operating budgets (costs per reportable in this area are very high). Some instrument manufacturers are promising a high-throughput random access analyzer for this area. Such an analyzer would most assuredly assist facilities that have moderate-to-heavy requests for such testing. For those large facilities that have high-volume, special chemistry departments and use radioimmunoassays (RIAs) and other low-cost methods, a substantial increase in costs will be encountered when purchasing or leasing a new random access analyzer, because of high capital costs associated with cost per reportable. However, workflow analysis should be able to demonstrate cost savings by workstation consolidation, primarily in the area of personnel.

After all preanalytical data have been collected, workflow analysis concentrates on the possibility of workstation consolidation through technology replacement.

Analytical Workflow

Purpose—Throughput—Menu

Many of today's newer analyzers enable laboratories to consolidate workstations, that is, combine STAT and TDM operations.

As demonstrated in Figure 17–7, the purpose of the desired analyzer (workstation) will determine the needed throughput and test menu. On this basis, the laboratory can begin to narrow the type of technology needed (i.e., high- or low-throughput). Assume that laboratory administration is attempting to purchase a high-throughput analyzer that will enable combining the routine workstation with the STAT workstation. The workflow demonstrated that their busiest time was between 7 and 10 A.M. when 250 samples were received with an average request of nine tests per sample. If

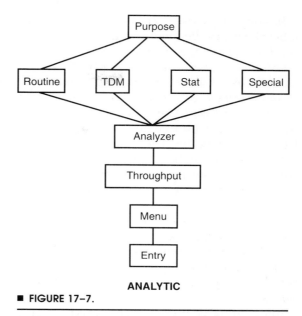

ANALYTIC

■ **FIGURE 17–7.**

Analyzer purpose and analytical features.

the goals of the laboratory are to complete this work by 11 A.M., the minimum throughput should be 750 tests per hour. In addition, the laboratory has to account for controls, interruption time for STATs, repeats, and future test growth. Based on these factors, the laboratory most likely should be considering an analyzer with a throughput of not less than 1000 tests per hour.

Each analyzer that is being considered has to meet the needs of both STAT and routine testing. Since STAT testing will occur sporadically throughout the day while routine testing is taking place, a number of questions arise, such as: How easy is it to interrupt a routine run for a STAT? How long does it take the analyzer to process the STAT request? How long does the STAT request delay routine work? The answers to these questions, along with throughput and test menu, further narrow the laboratory's choices. At this point the laboratory should begin to separate the remaining few analyzers by their features and determine how these features meet the immediate and future needs of the laboratory. The remaining list of questions generated should be analytical, nonanalytical, and regarding costs.

Additional analytical features to consider are described next.

Sample Requirements. How much sample will be aspirated to complete a single test and the largest profile? In addition, how much dead volume is needed? This is the excess volume of sample needed in each tube/cup. Dead volume can be as high as 300 μL. This is a serious consideration if the laboratory's population consists of large numbers of pediatric or geriatric patients. Large sample volumes are difficult to collect from these populations.

Many analyzers offer features that pertain to the sample. Some of these features are:

Direct tube sampling: Removes the need to pour off the sample into a cup.

Barcode reader: Automatically identifies patient and test.

Auto sampler: Feeds samples into the analyzer automatically.

Short sample detector: Alerts the operator to insufficient sample.

Clot detector: Alerts the operator to clot in the sampler probe.

Anticrash protector: Keeps the probe from crashing into the bottom or side of the sample tube.

No tube or cup detector: Identifies empty space on the sampler and moves sampler to the next location.

Ability to perform multiple reruns: Identifies the appropriate sample for a rerun.

Liquid volume sensor: Determines the liquid level of a sample tube.

Autodilution. Preferably, the analyzer will offer the ability to dilute samples automatically when assays are out of linear range. Analyzers offering a variety of dilutions are most convenient.

Linearity. Linearity ranges are important, especially if the analyzer of choice does not have an automatic dilution feature and the laboratory's population consists of patients out of linear range (e.g., diabetics).

Interferences. Most instruments either run a sample blank by a two-reagent system or have separate blank channels. Additionally, some analyzers can provide indices measurements which, when elevated due to lipemia, icterus, or hemolysis, dilute the sample.

Other analytical and nonanalytical features, as described in Figure 17–8, should also be considered when evaluating an analyzer.

Start-Up and Shut-Down Time. This can be excessive (over an hour) with some analyzers and requires a trained individual. Some of the newer analyzers have automatic start-up modes that do not require operator intervention.

Level of Laboratorian's Intervention. What are the requirements of the operator? How user-friendly is the analyzer? In a wet chemistry analyzer, how much reagent

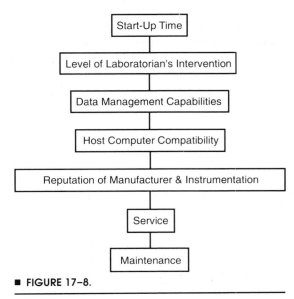

■ **FIGURE 17–8.**

Evaluating features of an analyzer.

preparation is required? The importance of these questions varies with the level of education of the analyzer's operator (i.e., medical technologist versus medical technician).

Host Computer and Data Management Capabilities. Options available with various analyzers include:

- Bidirectional system (two-way communication with host computer).
- Review and edit options.
- Patient file storage ability.
- Patient demographics.
- Quality control program (Westgard Rules).
- Cumulative patient reporting.
- CAP (College of American Pathologists) workload reporting.

Reputation of Manufacturer and Instrument. It is recommended that questions be asked regarding the reputation of the manufacturer and its product. For example, where is the manufacturer located? If it is overseas, are ample systems and parts available in this country? How long has the manufacturer been established and what is the track record?

What experiences have colleagues had with the manufacturer? Does any facility in the geographic region have the instrument, and what is its experience with this instrument? How long has the instrument been on the market? Analyzers that have been on the market for less than 2 years have not yet established track records.

Service. Service representatives can influence the degree of satisfaction or nonsatisfaction with an analyzer. If service representatives do not respond quickly, are less than competent, or otherwise unable to meet the needs of the client, the **downtime** and efficiency will be affected. Service response is critical if the laboratory has one primary analyzer with no back-up.

Maintenance. The amount of time required and the level of education of the operator affect the outcome of maintenance. If the maintenance is simple and requires little time, a technician with minimum experience will be sufficient to operate the analyzer. If the maintenance is time consuming and difficult, it is more appropriate to use a medical technologist or a technician well-trained in laboratory automation. Even though some laboratory administrators discourage the purchase of analyzers with excessive maintenance programs, many technologists enjoy this kind of interaction with the analyzer.

Instrument Selection

The final concerns with instrument selection are presented in Figure 17–9.

Reagents. The reagent monitoring features on some analyzers are excellent. Some analyzers allow the operator to place the reagent in any position in the storage area. Through barcode identification on the reagent container, the computer will identify the reagent and its location. Also, systems today can identify the lot number and the number of tests per container automatically. Such analyzers alert operators when reagents fall below a certain level (e.g., less than 100 tests). Analyzers use either dry or wet reagents; both have advantages and dis-

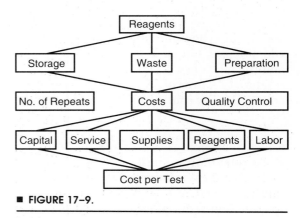

■ **FIGURE 17–9.**

Instrument cost factors.

advantages. For example, dry chemicals generally have longer shelf lives, require little to no preparation, and occupy less storage space. Wet chemicals require preparation but are considerably less expensive and offer a greater number of tests per package. Wet chemistry analyzers have a larger test menu than do dry analyzers. Preparation of wet reagents is not very difficult for today's laboratorians. Generally, all that is required is to add a vial of dry chemical or a volume of liquid chemical from one bottle to another. Laboratories with less than adequate workers could find this a problem. Dry chemistry analyzers claim to have little or no waste compared with wet chemistry analyzers. While this is generally true, this area requires close investigation because of the cost difference between dry and wet. The cost of the waste associated with wet chemistries might not be significant when compared with the cost of the more expensive dry reagents.

Repeats. Every analyzer has an efficiency rating (usually between 90 and 98 percent). The actual number of repeats for a particular laboratory is hard to predict. Variables such as case mix (e.g., patients out of linear range), compliance with preventive maintenance programs, as well as education and experience of operators, all affect the numbers of repeats. One possible way to assess repeats for a laboratory is to find a similar laboratory with comparable personnel and facility characteristics. Repeats not only add to costs but also decrease throughput and the efficiency of the laboratory.

Quality Control. Analyzers should have on-line quality control with the following options:

- Daily summaries of controls and tests
- Cumulative summaries of controls
- Daily and cumulative patient mean
- Quality control scattergrams, histograms with Westgard rules

Cost. The costs associated with reagents, number of repeats, and quality control are just a small portion of testing costs. To predict the true costs of a patient's reportable test (**cost per reportable**), all the variables presented in Figure 17–9 must be included. (A far more detailed description of costs associated with laboratory testing is presented in the following chapter.)

Capital. Analyzers can be acquired either through a purchase or through a lease/rental option (payments and interest spread out over a period of time). Either way, the costs have to be included in the cost of a patient reportable test. If the analyzer is on a lease/rental basis, more than likely the manufacturer has included the price in the cost per test. Remember, cost per test is not cost per patient reportable.

Service. Service is an important factor when choosing an analyzer as the laboratory cannot afford to have long downtimes. For this reason, inquiries about service satisfaction from other customers should be solicited.

As with capital costs, if the laboratory is going to acquire the analyzer with a lease/rental option, service costs are generally placed in the cost per test. If the analyzer is being purchased outright, then the rule-of-thumb is that the cost per service is about 10 percent of capital costs per year. This cost also has to be put in cost per patient reportable.

Supplies. Supplies—cups, paper, barcodes, and so on—are always extra. These also have to be placed in cost per reportable.

Reagent Costs. These vary, based on dry versus wet, type of test, priming requirements, and quality control protocol. When calculating costs per patient reportable, keep in mind that all these variables, along with the reagents needed to produce repeats, have to be added.

Many of the high throughput batch analyzers also require priming, which can consume small to large volumes of reagents. This factor becomes very important if the reagents are expensive (e.g., reagents for drugs of abuse).

Labor. This is an important factor in determining the appropriate type of analyzer. The match between the technical staff and analyzer can be as important as the compatibility of a cross-match. To place a technologist in front of an analyzer that requires only patient or test identification is not only a gross misuse of a qualified technologist, but also will offer no challenge to the technologist. Continued operation of this type of analyzer by the technologist will most likely result in job dissatisfaction. The same is true if an unqualified individual is placed in front of an analyzer that requires sophisticated interaction between operator and analyzer. Analyzers with sophisticated data management programs that require more elaborate preventive and routine maintenance programs should be used by technologists or well-trained technicians. Facilities that do not have a problem recruiting qualified technicians and technologists can take advantage of the high-throughput wet chemistry analyzers. Because of the needed compatibility between analyzer and operator, it is important to make sure that the designated operators of such analyzers are considered in the process of selecting instrumentation.

Postanalytical Workflow

The final phase of workflow analysis reviews the process of how the test data are sent back to the physician (Fig. 17–10). Whether the data are sent back electronically or manually (laboratory slip), the format can be helpful to physicians. A format that highlights abnormal information and puts it into a logical group (e.g., organ-specific panels) will help physicians assimilate

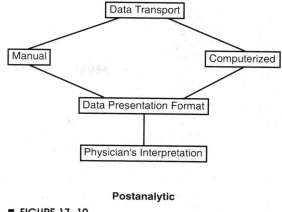

Postanalytic

■ **FIGURE 17–10.**

Data transport.

the data. Examples of grouping tests to help physicians use the laboratory more efficiently are presented in Table 17–1. These types of presentations for both ordering and receiving results of tests generally reduce excessive needless testing. To customize ordering and test data sheets, the laboratory should meet with the medical staff.

CASE STUDY

The appropriateness of using biochemical panels and profiles as an alternative to component testing in health care delivery has been debated by both researchers and clinicians over the past two decades. Although still unresolved, the introduction of federal regulations has created a new and greater concern. The Tax Equity and Fiscal Responsibility Act (TEFRA) passed in 1982, now referred to as Diagnosis-Related Groups (DRGs), attempts to reimburse hospitals by case and to set a limit for each case. This changes the hospital's present

TABLE 17–1. EXAMPLES OF TEST GROUPING

Cardiac Evaluation:	Chol, trig, HDL, LDL
Cardiac Injury Panel:	SGOT (AST), CK, LDH, CKMB
Hepatic Function Panel:	AST, ALT, LDH, alk phos, total bilirubin, total protein, GGT, albumin
Renal Panel:	Total protein, albumin, NA, K, Cl, CO_2, glucose, BUN, creatine clearance
Lipid Profile:	Chol, trig, HDL, LDL, VLDL, Chol/HDL ratio
Macrocytic Anemia Panel:	CBC, indices, reticulocyte, B_{12}, folate
Microcytic Anemia Panel:	CBC, indices, reticulocyte, iron, iron-binding capacity
Prostatic Panel:	Prostatic acid phos, PSA
Pancreatic Panel:	Amylase, lipase, glucose
Pulmonary Panel:	CO_2, Pco_2, pH, Po_2, O_2sat
General Health Screen:	Glucose, BUN, creatinine, NA, K, Ca, Cl, chol, t. prot, t. bilirubin, LD, AST, ALT, albumin, alk phos, uric acid, trig, GGT, CBC
Stat–Panel I:	NA, K, Cl, CO_2, glucose, BUN
Stat–Panel II:	NA, K, Cl, CO_2, glucose, BUN, CK, LD, AST
Stat–Panel III:	NA, K, Cl, CO_2, glucose, BUN, amylase

reimbursement system to one of prospective payment. This prospective payment system later included hospital-based physicians (eg, pathologists) by changing their reimbursement from the portion allocated for professional service rendered to that allocated for total hospital reimbursement.

As this prospective reimbursement system is implemented throughout the United States, hospital administrators and other fiscally concerned officials have focused on the laboratory in an effort to reduce costs. Special concern has been placed on the appropriateness of future investments in automated equipment. While the technologic advances made in laboratory automation have decreased the cost per test, overall laboratory costs have increased.[1-4] The initial cost savings in laboratory automation came about by labor reduction, but was soon offset by physicians increasing the number and variety of tests performed per patient. In fact, it has been demonstrated that as more highly automated tests became available, the demand for such tests became greater. These reports have demonstrated that 50 to 79% of all biochemical testing may be attributed to 20 highly automated tests.[5, 6] Because of this, physicians are being persuaded to reduce their use of these tests in the hope that test reduction would lead to cost containment. Although this concept may seem logical, it is neither easily implemented nor necessarily true.

While researchers have debated the relative merits and shortcomings of both types of ordering strategies (component or panels),[7-10] the authors have evaluated laboratory costs associated with physicians' use of component and panel chemistries. These two studies have focused on laboratory utilization at both a health care maintenance organization and an out-patient department of a community hospital.[11, 12] In both facilities the physicians were free to order component and panel chemistries. The outcome of the studies at both facilities demonstrated that the utilization of panel chemistries resulted in lower costs and fewer visits to the health care facility.

In today's cost containment climate, many hospitals have attempted to reduce laboratory costs by utilizing discrete analyzers rather than continuous flow profiling analyzers, and by urging physicians to decrease laboratory utilization. However, if physicians continue to order profiles or large quantities of tests at facilities that employ discrete analyzers, costs per test and time for completion of these tests will increase, thereby increasing the financial strain that hospitals have been trying to alleviate.

In order to determine whether physicians alter their use of laboratory services to take advantage of the cost-saving potential of discrete analyzers, the costs associated with ordering strategies were examined as a group of residents rotated through two institutions whose laboratories differ both in philosophy and automation requirement.

Patients and Methods

The present study was conducted at two teaching hospitals whose automated chemistry equipment and philosophy differed. Hospital "A" is a 250-bed tertiary care facility in suburban New York whose laboratory utilizes a Beckman Astra and a Boehringer Mannheim Hitachi for its biochemical assays. Physicians at this facility may order a 7 (Astra) or 16 (Hitachi) biochemical panel and components without restrictions as to time, day, or volume. Hospital "B" is a 340-bed primary care facility located within 20 miles of facility A, whose laboratory utilizes a Technicon SMAC 20 and SMA 6/60 for its biochemical assays. At this institution the medical staff is restricted as to what tests are available and when they may be ordered. The 6 or 20 biochemical panel is available between 8 A.M. and 5 P.M., Monday through Friday. At times other than those and during weekends, physicians may only order the 6 chemistry panel. The laboratory offered no unbundling of their 6 or 20 chemistry panel, nor were there any restrictions on the number of panels one could order.

As seen in Table 17–2 the 6 and 20 biochemical panel at facility B and the 7 and 16 biochemical panel at facility A are essentially the same. No other tests than those used in the panels were evaluated since the purpose of the study was to evaluate the impact of panels versus component chemistries in health care delivery.

Laboratory requests were monitored for 6 months, as the same group of internal medi-

TABLE 17–2. LABORATORY TEST GROUPINGS

	FACILITY A	FACILITY B
Large Panel	Albumin, alkaline phosphatase, phosphorus, direct bilirubin, total bilirubin, calcium, total protein, cholesterol, triglycerides, lactate dehydrogenase, uric acid, magnesium, gamma glutamyl transferase, aspartate aminotransferase, alanine aminotransferase, creatine kinase	Uric acid, sodium, calcium, potassium, chloride, total protein, bicarbonate, albumin, cholesterol, alkaline phosphatase, triglycerides, glucose, total bilirubin, aspartate aminotransferase, alanine aminotransferase, lactate dehydrogenase, creatinine, urea nitrogen, creatine kinase, phosphorus
Small panel	Glucose, urea nitrogen, sodium, potassium, chloride, bicarbonate, creatinine	Glucose, urea nitrogen, sodium, potassium, chloride, bicarbonate
Components	Any single test or combination of tests from large or small panels	—

From Lehmann CA, et al: The impact of technology on laboratory ordering strategies. *NY State J Med* 85:690–693, 1985. © Medical Society of the State of New York.

cine residents treated myocardial infarction, congestive heart failure, and airway passage blockage at facilities A and B. The number of panels and components of the panels were recorded to evaluate the effect of ordering strategies on laboratory utilization for each of the primary codes. These three primary codes were chosen because they gave the highest number of cases at both facilities.

In addition to the average number of panels and components of the panels associated with each primary code, the average per case cost for each laboratory was calculated.

Results

A comparison of the residents' use of laboratory services was made for three primary diagnostic codes at both facilities. For each diagnostic code the average length of stay, along with the average number of large panels (16 and 20 tests), small panels (6 to 7 tests), components, and laboratory costs, were calculated.

Patient demographics for both facilities were as follows:

- For myocardial infarction the mean age at facility A was 61 years (20% women, 80% men); the mean age at facility B was 60 years (100% men).
- For congestive heart failure the mean age at facility A was 67 years (45% women, 55% men); the mean age at facility B was 67 years (100% men).
- For airway passage blockage the mean age at facility A was 67 years (32% women, 68% men); the mean age at facility B was 68 years (100% men).

At both facilities, the patients' laboratory charges were not billed separately but were part of prospective payment.

The study first evaluated the residents' laboratory utilization in their treatment of myocardial infarction. As demonstrated in Table 17–3, the residents' utilization of laboratory services differed considerably depending on whether patients were treated at facility A or B. While the utilization of large panels was somewhat consistent at both facilities, there was almost a threefold increase in small panels at facility A compared with facility B. In addition to the small panel increase noted at facility A, the

TABLE 17–3. LABORATORY UTILIZATION: MYOCARDIAL INFARCTION

	FACILITY A	FACILITY B
Number of patients	N = 65	N = 65
Mean number of small panels	10.15 ± 8.89*	3.57 ± 4.74*
Mean number of large panels	7.81 ± 5.33	7.01 ± 6.58
Mean number of component chemistries	102.5 ± 79.81	—

*Statistically significant at P <0.05.
From Lehmann CA, et al: The impact of technology on laboratory ordering strategies. *NY State J Med* 85:690–693, 1985. © Medical Society of the State of New York.

residents utilized an average of 102 additional components.

Resident laboratory utilization in the care of congestive heart failure is seen in Table 17–4. Unlike with cases of myocardial infarction, the residents decreased their utilization of the large panel at facility A and maintained approximately the same use at facility B. For small panels, residents at facility A demonstrated a slight decrease while those at facility B had a slight increase. The component testing at facility A for congestive heart failure also demonstrated a small decrease (102 versus 86.07) when compared with component testing for myocardial infarction. For the third primary code—chronic airway obstruction—as seen in Table 17–5, laboratory utilization by the resi-

TABLE 17–4. LABORATORY UTILIZATION: CONGESTIVE HEART FAILURE

	FACILITY A	FACILITY B
Number of patients	N = 43	N = 96
Mean number of small panels	8.11 ± 7.06*	4.51 ± 5.02*
Mean number of large panels	3.46 ± 3.83*	6.72 ± 5.43*
Mean number of component chemistries	86.07 ± 75. 13	—

*Statistically significant at P <0.05.
From Lehmann CA, et al: The impact of technology on laboratory ordering strategies. *NY State J Med* 85:690–693, 1985. © Medical Society of the State of New York.

dents was consistent with that of congestive heart failure at both facilities. This is most likely attributed to the chronic implications of these two codes, compared with the acuteness of myocardial infarction. However, in all three codes at facility A residents utilized the small panel about twice as much as they did at facility B. As for the two chronic nature codes—heart failure and airway obstruction—at facility B residents utilized the large panel twice as often as they did at facility A.

Discussion

It is difficult to present convincing arguments for either ordering strategy at this time: the greater utilization of small panels at facility A or large panels at facility B. However, a more argumentative point is the utilization of components at facility A. As demonstrated in Figure 17–11, the utilization of components is practiced for all three primary codes. The availability of this service at facility A did not appear to reduce the utilization of panels by residents. In fact, there was a greater use of small panels. In the case of myocardial infarction patients at facility A, the residents not only tripled their use of small panels but also utilized an average of 102 compo-

TABLE 17–5. LABORATORY UTILIZATION: CHRONIC AIRWAY OBSTRUCTION

	FACILITY A	FACILITY B
Number of patients	N = 44	N = 40
Mean number of small panels	7.6 ± 9.53	4.6 ± 7.18
Mean number of large panels	3.61 ± 5.09*	6.5 ± 5.37*
Mean number of component chemistries	79.68 ± 96.61	—

*Statistically significant at P <0.05.
From Lehmann CA, et al: The impact of technology on laboratory ordering strategies. *NY State J Med* 85:690–693, 1985. © Medical Society of the State of New York.

nents. In 37 percent of the cases, physicians used 101 to 386 components. When the option of component testing was not available to the residents, as seen with facility B, there was no greater increase in the use of laboratory panels. The differences between the average number of panels at both facilities were tested for statistical significance using student t-tests; those that occurred with a probability of less than 5 percent were statistically significant.

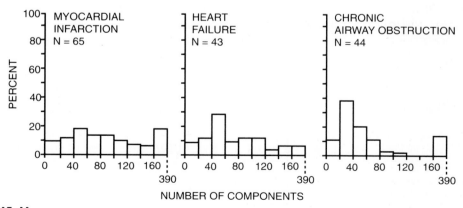

■ FIGURE 17–11.

Utilization of component testing for myocardial infarction, heart failure, and chronic airway obstruction. (From Lehmann CA, et al: The impact of technology on laboratory ordering strategies. *NY State J Med* 85:690–693, 1985. © Medical Society of the State of New York.)

Although the laboratory data were examined by type of case (myocardial infarction, heart failure, chronic airway obstruction), differences in the severity of the cases within each primary code could conceivably affect the results. To determine whether the severity of illness of patients treated at these two facilities differed, each case was examined for the average length of stay and average number of secondary codes. One might conjecture that the greater utilization of the laboratory noted at facility A could be due to the increased severity of cases treated at this facility. This study shows, however, that such is not the case. In fact, patients at facility B had more complications (3.38 versus 2.26) and a greater length of stay (14.08 versus 11.89 days) than those at facility A.

To evaluate the costs associated with the increased utilization of laboratory services, an average cost analysis for each primary code at each facility was performed. Table 17–6 demonstrates that laboratory utilization by residents at facility A is far more costly for all three primary codes than at facility B. In fact, even for those cases such as heart failure and airway obstruction at facility B, where there was greater utilization of larger panels, overall laboratory costs were less.

Previous studies have demonstrated

that equipment, sample volume, and number of tests per sample influence overall laboratory costs.[13,14] This is well demonstrated when the costs of panels and components at facility A are compared with those at facility B. The cost for a large panel was $3.68 and a small panel was $2.07 at facility A, while at facility B the cost was $2.35 for a large panel and $0.76 for the small panel. This difference in cost, along with greater utilization of the small panel, placed overall costs for panels at facility A much higher. While costs for the panels are much greater at facility A, it seems that the more costly fraction of the ordering strategy is with the use of components. As stated earlier, when the same group of residents is offered the option of ordering component chemistries, compared with ordering panels only, as seen with facility B, there appears to be no reduction in their use of panels. The high utilization of components by residents at facility A for all three primary codes is extremely costly as demonstrated by the following per case component costs: myocardial infarction, $26.65; airway blockage, $20.72; and heart failure, $22.38.

In addition to costs associated with the actual laboratory test, other factors that result from different ordering strategies must be considered, such as the productive time of technical, clerical, and aid staff. As demonstrated by the *Manual for Laboratory Workload Recording Methods*,[15] chemical analyzers that perform either one or a number of tests, such as the ASTRA and Hitachi used at facility A, receive a unit number for initial sample set-up plus a unit number per test. In contrast to facility A, simultaneous chemical analyzers, such as the SMA 6/60 and SMAC used at facility B, together receive only one unit number per specimen. A comparison of workload units for each in-

TABLE 17–6. LABORATORY COSTS PER CASE*

	FACILITY A	FACILITY B
Myocardial infarction	$76.40	$19.18
Congestive heart failure	$51.90	$19.21
Chronic airway obstruction	$49.73	$18.78

*Costs include reagents, supplies, service contracts, and capital equipment.
From Lehmann CA, et al: The impact of technology on laboratory ordering strategies. *NY State J Med* 85:690–693, 1985. © Medical Society of the State of New York.

stitution's equipment is as follows: the ASTRA used at facility A requires 2.1 units for each specimen set-up, along with an 0.1 additional unit for each test. The Hitachi requires 2.5 units for specimen set-up and an additional 0.2 unit for each test. However, the SMA 6/60 used at facility B has an overall value of 4.0, and the SMAC has a value of 2.5 units. Thus at facility A it requires 5.9 workload units for a large panel, compared with 2.5 workload units at facility B. Small panels at facility A require a total of 2.9 units, compared with 4.0 at facility B. In addition to panels, each time components were utilized at facility A, a workload unit for specimen preparation of 2.1 or 2.5 was required for each component, regardless of the number of components ordered. Since the bulk of the workload unit is in specimen set-up, especially in the small panel, the advantages of its components are questionable, especially since the small panel was utilized much more often at facility A.

The data demonstrate that residents utilize laboratory services far more often when at facility A compared with when they are at facility B. This pattern generated greater workload units and higher costs. If the choice of automation for facility A was to offer their physicians an al-ternative to panels and reduce the number of tests per case, this goal has not been accomplished. In fact, just the opposite has taken place as each primary code demonstrated increased testing. While each primary code had greater utilization of the small panel at facility A compared with facility B, the predominant factor was in the utilization by the residents of component testing. Since the same residents managed all three primary codes at facility B without component testing and demonstrated no greater utilization of the panel, the appropriateness of offering components is questionable. This is especially true for highly automated tests, since studies have demonstrated that component testing is cost-effective only if kept at a minimum.

SUMMARY

Selecting the appropriate technology to improve laboratory efficiency through workflow analysis is a most worthwhile endeavor. Successful evaluation and implementation can have a positive impact on the accuracy of test results, the speed at which they are achieved, monetary savings to the laboratory or hospital, and job satisfaction for laboratory employees.

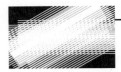

REVIEW QUESTIONS

Choose all the responses that are true.

1. When calculating costs per reportable, which of the following should *not* be included?

   a. Controls.
   b. Reagents.
   c. Laboratory administrative costs.
   d. Capital.

2. Which of the following best describes workflow analysis?

   a. Sample mapping.
   b. Amount of work needed to produce a test result.
   c. Documenting work in a laboratory.
   d. None of the above.

3. Which of the following statements are *not* true?

   a. Education of laboratory personnel should match sophistication of technology.
   b. Workflow analysis can be applied to any area of the laboratory.
   c. Workflow analysis measures productivity.
   d. Workstation consolidation is one of the primary goals of workflow.

4. Which term best describes the movement of one sample to multiple workstations?

   a. Multiple sample distribution.
   b. Sample sharing.
   c. Sample dilution.
   d. Sample splitting.

5. Of the following statements, which describes preanalytical workflow?

   a. The monitoring of all work required to collect and process a sample prior to placing it on an analyzer.
   b. All work required to process a test result.
   c. All work required to collect and process a sample to produce a test value.
   d. None of the above.

6. The collection of facility characteristics prior to doing workflow is:

   a. Very important.
   b. Important.
   c. Not very important.
   d. Not important at all.

7. Analytical throughput is best defined as:

   a. The number of tests or samples that can be performed on any given day.
   b. The maximum test or sample throughput per hour.
   c. The maximum number of tests per hour.
   d. The maximum number of tests per shift.

REFERENCES

1. Morrison JI, Tydeman J, Cassidy PA, Hardwick DF, Davies CT: Costs of clinical chemistry laboratory tests. *Lab Med* 14:567–570, 1983.

2. Tydeman J, Morrison JI, Cassidy PA, Hardwick DF: Analyzing the factors contributing to rising laboratory costs. *Arch Pathol Lab Med* 107:7–12, 1983.

3. Hardwick DF, Morrison JI, Tydeman J, Cassidy PA, Chase WH: Laboratory costs and utilization: A framework for analysis and policy design. *J Med Educ* 56:307–315, 1981.

4. Tydeman J, Morrison JI, Kasap D, Poulin M: The cost of laboratory technology: A framework for cost management. *Med Instrum* 17:79–83, 1983.

5. Morrison JI, Tydeman J, Cassidy PA, Hardwick DF: Automation and distribution of testing in the clinical laboratory. *J Med Technol* 1:132–137, 1984.

6. Stilwell JA: Costs of a clinical chemistry laboratory. *J Clin Pathol* 34:589–594, 1981.

7. Werner M, Altshuler CH: Utility of multiphasic biochemical screening and systematic laboratory investigations. *Clin Chem* 25:509–511, 1979.

8. Caceres C: By limiting the number of tests ordered and using automated panels, physicians can help the lab reduce unit costs from $250.00 to $7.00. *Lab World* 31:45–47, 1980.

9. Friedman G, Marshall G, Ahuja J, Siegelaub AB: Biochemical screening tests. *Arch Intern Med* 129:91–97, 1972.

10. Durbridge TC, Edwards F, Edwards RG, Atkinson M: Evaluation of benefits of screening tests done immediately on admission to hospital. *Clin Chem* 22:968–971, 1976.

11. Lehmann CA, Leiken AM: Influence on selective vs. panel chemistry tests on cost and diagnostic time. *Am J Med Technol* 48:833–836, 1982.

12. Lehmann CA, Leiken AM: Costs of ordering strategies. *J Lab Med* 15:759–760, 1984.

13. Weinstein MC, Pearlman LA: The implications of cost effectiveness analysis of medical technology. Washington, DC, Office of Technology Assessment, 1981.

14. Berkly Scientific Laboratories: *A Study of Automated Clinical Laboratory Systems.* DHEW Publ. No. (HSM)72–3004. Rockville, MD, US Dept of Health, Education and Welfare, 1971.

15. *Manual for Laboratory Workload Recording Methods.* College of American Pathologists, Skokie, IL, 1985.

INTRODUCTION
DETERMINING THE COST OF PRODUCING A LABORATORY TEST RESULT
FEATURES OF TECHNOLOGY THAT HAVE AN IMPACT ON COSTS
TECHNOLOGY AND THE LABORATORY'S GROWTH POTENTIAL
CASE STUDIES: COST SAVINGS VIA WORKSTATION CONSOLIDATION

Chapter 18

THE IMPACT OF INSTRUMENTATION ON LABORATORY COSTS

ALAN LEIKEN, PhD
CRAIG LEHMANN, PhD, CC (NRCC)

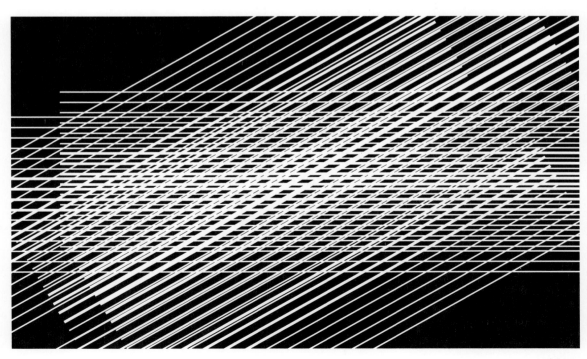

LEARNING OBJECTIVES

After studying this chapter, the student should be able to:

- Understand the concepts used to calculate costs associated with performing laboratory tests.
- Describe the difference between direct and indirect cost.
- Define and be able to utilize marginal cost analysis.
- Understand the importance of workstation consolidation.
- List the factors that influence variable costs.
- Identify the features and characteristics of instrumentation that have an impact on costs.

KEY WORDS

Capital acquisition. The purchase or lease/rental of clinical laboratory instrumentation.

Consumables. Disposable supplies used to produce test results.

Cost per reportable. All direct costs directly related to producing a patient test result.

Direct costs. Only those costs incurred as a direct result of producing a test result. Indirect costs, such as administrative costs, would not be included in this calculation.

DRGs (diagnosis-related groups). A prospective payment system used by Medicare to classify all hospitalized patients into one of 468 diagnosis-related groups. The hospital receives a fixed payment per DRG to cover operating costs.

Fixed costs. Costs that do not vary as test volume increases. Examples are rental payment, interest on debt, depreciation of plant and equipment, and wages of a skeleton staff that would be employed as long as the hospital stayed in business even if it produced nothing.

Lease. A contract that allows for the renting of instrumentation for a specified time under specified terms.

Marginal cost analysis. The additional cost incurred as output expands. It is cost associated with producing an additional patient test result.

Operational efficiency. Making the fullest utilization of available inputs. Alternatively, minimizing the use of inputs to produce the desired level of test results.

Price protection. An agreement whereby the vendor agrees to limit price increases by an agreed-upon amount during the term of the agreement.

Service contract. Contracts whereby the vendor agrees to supply maintenance and repair of instrumentation. A contract could cover response time and hours and days (e.g., including weekends) during which the services will be provided.

Variable costs. Costs that change as output (i.e., test volume) fluctuates.

Walkaway systems. Laboratory systems that allow the operator to walk away from the system after the system has been loaded with patient samples and test requests are entered.

Workstation consolidation. Reducing the number of laboratory instruments needed to meet testing demands.

INTRODUCTION

In the mid 1960s, the federal government introduced the Medicare program as a federally financed health insurance program for the elderly. The government agreed to reimburse hospitals for reasonable costs associated with providing care for eligible individuals. Private health insurance companies also agreed to reimburse hospitals for reasonable costs incurred in treating individuals covered by their health insurance plans. Laboratory tests, of course, were considered to be necessary in the diagnosis and treatment of these patients; costs associated with these tests were considered reasonable costs; therefore, these insurance plans could be billed or charged for the tests.

Although the hospital incurred a significant cost by providing laboratory services, revenue was generated to offset these costs because the hospital billed for these tests.

In fact, the laboratory made money for the hospital. It was not uncommon, for example, to find a laboratory charge of $150 for a routine 20 chemistry profile. This charge was many times greater than the cost of producing the test results, thereby enabling the laboratory to make money for the hospital by providing laboratory services for hospitalized patients.

This profit, the difference between charges and costs, was used to help the hospital provide services to individuals who were not covered by a third party insurance plan or were unable to pay for hospital care. Therefore, one can consider this excessive charge for laboratory tests as a subsidy to help the hospital provide free care. It was done with the knowledge and understanding of the third party insurance companies and the government.

Over the ensuing two decades, health care costs escalated quite rapidly—so much so that the federal government thought it necessary to stop reimbursing hospitals on the basis of reasonable costs. Instead, they decided to reimburse hospitals prospectively. That is, hospitals would be reimbursed on a predetermined basis, based on the diagnosis of the patient. The amount reimbursed is intended to reimburse the hospital for all costs, including laboratory costs, associated with providing the necessary care for the patient.

This reimbursement methodology, enacted as a result of the Tax Equity and Fiscal Responsibility Act (TEFRA) passed in the mid 1980s, is commonly referred to as diagnosis-related groups (DRGs). Upon a patient's discharge from the hospital, the physician attests to which one of the over 460 DRGs the patient should be assigned. The hospital then receives the reimbursement assigned to that group. This method is used nationally to reimburse hospitals for Medicare and Medicaid patients. The Medicaid program is a joint program between the federal government and the states and provides health insurance coverage for the indigent. In some states, such as New York, private health insurance companies, such as Blue Cross, also reimburse on the basis of the DRG system. In New York, therefore, the hospital laboratory, with regard to inpatients, is no longer generating any income for the hospital.

The laboratory, therefore, is now viewed as a major cost center of the hospital. Laboratorians have come under increasing pressure to provide the necessary quality and scope of diagnostic tests expected and demanded by the medical staff while attempting to minimize expenditures. For the first time, many laboratories have been given budgets. All the costs associated with providing laboratory services must be incurred within the budget given to the laboratory by hospital administration.

The federal government and the state governments find themselves facing huge budget deficits. One response has been to increase reimbursement rates at lower rates than the cost increases hospitals must deal with. As a result, laboratories have been under even more pressure to contain costs.

The task has been made more difficult because the shortage of qualified medical technologists has resulted in pressure to increase wages. Therefore, the laboratory management is faced with the conflicting goals of responding to increased demand for their services while staying within their ever-shrinking budgets, at a time when it is difficult to retain and attract qualified workers.

Although the situation described looks bleak, there are ways to accomplish the laboratory's goals while satisfying the hospital administration's goal of enhancing its financial position. The first step is to determine what it actually costs to produce a laboratory test result.

DETERMINING THE COST OF PRODUCING A LABORATORY TEST RESULT

To determine the cost of producing a test result, it is necessary to include all the direct costs to produce a reportable patient result. Before we proceed, it is necessary to define both **direct costs** and reportable patient results.

Direct cost refers to the costs of all the inputs directly related to producing a test result. For example, the cost of the technologist's time, the cost of the reagents, the equipment and its maintenance, and supplies are all necessary inputs directly related to producing a test result. These costs are influenced by the technology and therefore are relevant to our discussion. Indirect costs include such items as the cost of the buildings, maintaining space, and the cost of hospital administration. Such costs are constant regardless of the technology deployed.

The distinction between cost per test and **cost per reportable** patient result is an important one. Manufacturer claims of relatively low costs per tests may be misleading because they are only noting reagent costs. In calculating reagent costs, they may not be including reagent consumption, such as reagent waste, reagents used in priming the system if required, repeat tests, and quality control. Costs are therefore determined not only by the reagent cost per test but also by the amount of priming required by the analyzer, the number of repeat tests, and the quality control programs utilized. It has been our experience that for some analyzers, the technicians run many more controls than the number of controls recommended by the manufacturer, thereby increasing costs.

To illustrate this point, let's perform an operational cost analysis for a laboratory that is considering the purchase of a high-throughput routine chemistry analyzer on which it will produce 89,375 billable patient results per month. Let us first determine the total number of tests that must be processed in order to produce 89,375 patient results per month. The workload required to produce these patient results appears in Table 18–1.

The first column notes the tests to be performed on this analyzer; the second column notes the number of patient results to be produced each month. To produce these patient results, extra tests will need to be performed. These tests include controls and calibrators and a number of tests associated with repeats and the priming of the analyzer. When these tests are added to the number of patient test results, we obtain the total number of aspirations per month needed to produce the required patient results. In this example, without priming, a total of 103,108 tests are required to produce 89,375 patient results per month.

To determine the reagent costs to produce these tests, we need to determine the total number of reagent packages that will need to be purchased. Obviously, the smaller the package size, the less waste. However, generally speaking, reagents packaged in larger sizes have lower costs than reagents packaged in the smaller sizes. Analyzers that use dry systems have less reagent waste, but the cost per aspiration is generally higher for these systems. To determine the reagent requirements and the subsequent reagent costs, refer to Table 18–2.

The first column notes the tests to be performed. The next to last column notes the total aspirations per month required to produce the number of billable results noted in Table 18–1. The second column notes the number of tests per package. For example, albumin is packaged with 5,000 tests per package. A package of calcium has enough reagents to process 13,333 tests. The third

TABLE 18–1. OPERATIONAL COST ANALYSIS; WORKLOAD REQUIREMENTS*

METHOD	PATIENTS	QCs	Cals	RBLs	REPEATS AT 5%	PRIMES	TOTAL ASPIRATIONS/MON
Albumin	3,550	216	12	168	178	312	4,436
Alk phos	3,550	216	NA	168	178	480	4,592
ALT	1,775	216	NA	168	89	480	2,728
AST	3,550	216	NA	168	178	480	4,592
T bilirubin	3,600	216	12	168	180	480	4,656
Calcium	3,650	216	12	168	183	408	4,637
Chol	3,500	216	NA	168	175	336	4,407
CPK	3,700	216	12	168	185	480	4,749
Creat	6,500	216	12	168	325	408	7,629
Glucose	7,550	216	12	168	378	336	8,660
In phos	3,550	216	NA	168	178	480	4,604
LD	7,600	216	12	168	380	480	8,844
T protein	3,600	216	12	168	180	480	4,656
Trig	550	216	12	168	28	336	1,310
BUN	6,850	216	12	168	343	312	7,901
Uric acid	1,050	216	12	168	53	480	1,979
Chloride	6,900	216	168	168	345	312	7,953
CO_2	6,800	216	NA	168	340	480	8,172
Amylase	900	216	12	168	45	480	1,809
D bili	850	216	NA	168	43	480	1,769
GGT	700	216	12	168	35	480	1,599
Magnesium	1,500	216	24	168	75	480	2,451
Sodium	6,950	216	24	NA	348	NA	7,538
Potassium	650	216		NA	33	NA	923
TOTALS	89,375	5,184	384	3,696	4,469	9,480	112,588
Billable	89,375						
Total Tests (without priming)		103,108					

*Twenty-four days per month.

column notes the number of packages of each test required per month. The fourth column notes the list price per package, which when multiplied by the number of packages required per month produces the list cost per test per month. Vendors do discount their pricing, especially for high-volume accounts. This account will perform over 1 million tests per year. We therefore use a 24 percent discount off list pricing. The sixth column, therefore, notes the net cost per month. The last column notes the net cost per aspiration. Recall that this cost includes the cost per aspiration for reagents only. As we will see, the total cost per patient result will be higher.

We have so far determined that the monthly cost for reagents will be $4,725.70. To continue with our operational cost analysis, we now need to determine the monthly costs for supplies, including parts, miscellaneous fluids, and **consumables.** This information appears in Table 18–3.

Once again, we assume a 24 percent discount off list, and we determine that the monthly expenditure for parts will be $671.82. The monthly expenses for fluids and consumables is determined to be $1,408.93. These costs are added to the reagent costs determined in Table 18–2. The monthly costs for reagents and supplies is therefore determined to be $6,806.45. Recall

TABLE 18–2. OPERATIONAL COST ANALYSIS; REAGENT USAGE

METHOD	TESTS/ PKG	PKGS/ MON	UNIT LIST PRICE ($)	LIST/ MONTH ($)	NET/ MONTH ($)	TOTAL ASP/MON	NET COST/ ASP ($)
Albumin	5,000	1.0	118.75	118.75	90.25	4,436	0.020
Alk phos	16,000	0.5	500.00	267.86	203.57	4,592	0.044
ALT	8,000	0.4	194.00	69.29	52.66	2,728	0.019
AST	8,000	0.6	200.00	114.79	87.24	4,592	0.019
T bili	4,000	1.2	148.50	172.85	131.37	4,656	0.028
Calcium	13,333	0.5	280.00	150.00	114.00	4,637	0.025
Chol	11,429	0.4	628.60	242.40	184.22	4,407	0.042
CPK	8,000	1.5	805.00	1,207.50	917.70	4,749	0.193
Creat	6,667	1.1	230.00	263.20	200.03	7,629	0.026
Glucose	5,714	1.5	207.90	315.05	239.44	8,660	0.028
In phos	8,000	0.6	134.00	77.11	58.60	4,604	0.013
LDH	4,000	2.2	142.00	313.96	238.61	8,844	0.027
T protein	8,000	1.0	118.00	118.00	89.68	4,656	0.019
Trig	5,714	0.4	651.45	232.66	176.82	1,310	0.135
BUN	10,000	0.8	333.75	263.68	200.40	7,901	0.025
Uric acid	8,000	0.4	337.00	120.36	91.47	1,979	0.046
Cl (DCL)	1,250	6.4	55.00	349.93	265.95	7,953	0.033
CO$_2$ (int)	6,000	1.4	327.60	446.19	339.11	8,172	0.041
Amylase	8,000	0.4	2,376.00	848.57	644.91	1,809	0.357
D bili	4,000	1.1	148.50	159.11	120.92	1,769	0.068
GGT	8,000	0.5	433.00	231.96	176.29	1,599	0.110
Magnesium	4,000	0.6	220.00	134.81	102.45	2,451	0.042
Total/Month for Reagents				$6,218.02	$4,725.70	104,128	

that we needed to produce 89,375 patient results per month. Therefore, the cost for reagents and supplies per reportable patient test result is computed to be $.076. To continue with our assessment of the cost of operating this analyzer, exclusive of labor and indirect costs, we need to determine the cost per month for the capital and for the service of the analyzer.

When money was available for **capital acquisition** purposes, hospitals would purchase the analyzer. This money is now scarce, and hospitals must determine which capital acquisition projects have priority. Laboratories, therefore, find themselves competing for such funds with, for example, radiology. Laboratories, more often than not, find that the way to acquire new technology of this type is through a rental agreement. The laboratory agrees to rent or **lease** the system for a specified term, usually 60 months. At the end of the lease the laboratory has the option of buying the analyzer at a price determined at the beginning of the agreement. Typically, the laboratory will have the right to purchase the instrument at the end of the lease for 10 to 15 percent of the original net selling price.

The monthly rental cost is determined by spreading out the capital acquisition cost over the term of the lease. Of course, the finance charge is included in this calculation. The hospital has the option of allowing the instrumentation manufacturer to arrange the financing, or the hospital can use its own financing source. In this example, the monthly cost for acquiring this system, which is valued at approximately $300,000, is $6,824.

Service is provided free during the first year. In subsequent years, service needs to be purchased. We are therefore purchasing

TABLE 18–3. OPERATIONAL COST ANALYSIS; SUPPLIES

PARTS	PACKAGE	LIST (%)	USAGE/MON	COST/MON AT LIST ($)	COST/MON AT NET ($)
Drier tip, Ana	pkg/4	79.20	1.00	79.20	60.19
Check valve	piece	22.25	2.00	44.50	33.82
Drier tip, D-line	pkg/4	79.20	0.38	30.10	22.87
Source lamp	piece	269.50	0.66	177.87	135.18
Syringe, ISE	pkg/5	103.20	0.17	17.54	13.33
Syringe, reagent	pkg/5	16.05	3.30	52.97	40.25
Plunger, reagent	piece	29.20	16.50	481.80	366.17
Total/Month for Parts:				$883.98	$671.82

MISCELLANEOUS FLUIDS AND CONSUMABLES					
ISE electrode	piece	1,171.85	0.33	386.71	293.90
ISE buffer	1 × 1000	20.45	4.27	87.40	66.42
Mid conc cal	1 × 2000	37.95	2.37	90.11	68.48
Serum cal low	12 × 10	150.00	1.00	150.00	114.00
Serum cal high	12 × 10	150.00	1.00	150.00	114.00
Serum blank	1 × 2000	40.00	0.58	23.02	17.49
Acid detergent	1 × 250	20.00	0.20	4.00	3.04
Alkaline detergent	1 × 500	20.00	2.88	57.60	43.78
ISE detergent	10 × 12	200.00	0.50	100.00	76.00
Water bath additive	1 × 500	100.00	2.88	288.00	218.88
Sample cups	1000 pc	24.50	0.00	0.00	0.00
Paper (1 ply)	3400 shts	108.90	1.03	112.10	85.20
Printer ribbon	1 piece	84.00	1.00	84.00	63.84
Water sampler	pkg/24	102.00	0.13	13.26	10.08
Silicone oil	piece	20.25	0.25	5.06	3.85
Setpoint calib	12 × 3 ml	69.65	4.00	278.60	211.74
Setpoint diluent	2 × 2 ml	6.00	4.00	24.00	18.24
Total/Month for Fluids and Consumables:				$1,853.86	$1,408.93

4 years, or 48 months of services, but we are spreading the cost over 60 months. Annual **service contracts** generally cost approximately 10 percent of the purchase price. In this case, the annual service cost is approximated to be $27,500, and the monthly cost for service is computed to be $1,973. Therefore, the monthly cost is determined in Table 18–4.

Some instrumentation manufacturers will bill monthly for the system, the service, and the reagents and supplies. Some will offer the laboratory the option of being billed per test. All the aforementioned costs will be included in the cost per test billing program.

Whichever method is preferred by the lab-

oratory, another consideration is negotiating price increases over the life of the agreement. As we learned in the 1980s, prices can rise rapidly. Without negotiating a limit on such increases, costs 5 years from now can be substantially higher than the costs in the original agreement. This issue should be ad-

TABLE 18–4. MONTHLY OPERATING COSTS

System leasing cost	$6,824
Service cost	$1,973
Reagents and supplies	$6,806
Net cost per month	$15,603
Net cost per reportable test result	$0.175

dressed in the original agreement. Some manufacturers actually might guarantee that the price will remain constant over the term of the agreement (**price protection**). Alternatively, they might offer to limit any price increases to a predetermined amount.

FEATURES OF TECHNOLOGY THAT HAVE AN IMPACT ON COSTS

Instrumentation manufacturers have responded to the laboratories' needs by adding to analyzers features that help minimize labor time requirements and other features to minimize operating costs. Such features include barcode readers for patient identification, barcoding of reagents, enhanced data management capabilities, uni- and bidirectional interfacing with the host computer, enhanced throughput, and broad test menus.

Formerly, much of the technologist's time was spent loading the test requested for each patient. A laboratory requisition sheet would accompany the sample. When it arrived in the laboratory, the technologist would enter the patient identifier into the analyzer along with the tests requested. Many hospital and laboratory computers now have the capability of generating a barcode upon order entry. Barcode information includes the patient identifier as well as tests requested. The barcode is placed on the sample and read by the analyzer, obviating the need for the technician to input this information into the analyzer.

Result reporting is also less labor intensive by this system. The technologist can review test results, and the interfacing will allow the technologist then to release the results directly into the computer—no manual entry needed. Obviously, labor time is minimized, as is the risk of reporting errors.

Expanded test menus now found on routine chemistry analyzers offer significant cost-saving potential. Traditionally, the laboratory has had at least one analyzer for routine chemistry, another for STAT routine chemistry tests, another for therapeutic drug testing, and one for drugs of abuse. Each of these workstations incurred a capital cost, a service contract cost, and costs associated with routine maintenance and calibration. In many instances a technologist or a technician was assigned to each of these workstations.

Large test menus have enabled laboratories to reduce the number of workstations, thereby reducing costs associated with maintaining each separate workstation. For example, many routine analyzers have the capability of placing over 35 methods on the analyzer at once. Such methods can include routine chemistries, STATS, electrolytes, therapeutic drugs, drugs of abuse, specific proteins, and thyroid tests. Some of these systems are considered open systems. This means that in addition to using the manufacturer's test methods, the laboratory can adapt the test methods of other vendors. This increases price competition in the marketplace and further enhances the laboratory's ability to consolidate.

The expanding test menus now found on automated analyzers also offer additional cost-saving potential. Many tests currently being sent out to the reference laboratory might now be more economical to process in-house. For example, thyroid testing can now be performed on routine chemistry analyzers or on an immunology analyzer. Previously, many laboratories sent this test to a reference laboratory rather than devoting a technologist to perform this test by using the manual RIA technique.

The rapid increase in the use of certain tests, coupled with the recent automation of such tests, also enables the laboratory to reduce costs by using automated instrumentation in-house to perform the test. Prostate-specific antigen (PSA) is one such test.

Increasing volume of this test has enabled the laboratory to spread the capital and service costs and the cost of running controls over more tests, thereby reducing the cost per patient result. As the test menus of such analyzers continue to expand, the laboratory will be able to spread the **fixed costs** over more tests, thereby further reducing the cost per test and enabling the laboratory to process even more tests cost effectively in-house.

Some companies have prepackaged reagents with barcode identification. The prepackaging or use of dry technologies has minimized labor time for reagent preparation. The barcoding of the reagents allows for the identification by the computer of reagents by lot numbers and allows the analyzer to notify the technologist of the amount of reagent still available. When the reagent is about to be used up, the technologist is notified and simply places the new package on the system. If the same lot number is used, there is no downtime and reagent waste is minimized, further reducing costs.

The data management software enables the automatic flagging of sample analyte concentrations that are outside the linear range. The sample will be automatically diluted to bring it into linear range. This saves time and eliminates sample handling and manual dilution errors.

The new analyzers allow on-board quality control, which includes the automatic downloading of data into quality control files. Out-of-range quality control results are flagged. This compares with the previous work of recording quality control data and plotting quality control results manually. Obviously, less time is spent by using the software available on most of the new analyzers currently available.

Computer software programs also allow for the automatic start-up and daily maintenance routines, thereby eliminating the manual task of performing these required tasks.

Similar labor savings are now achievable as a result of changes in hematology analyzers. Before the introduction of the fully automated counting analyzers, the hematology department was responsible for manual platelet counts and manual differentials on patient samples. With the new counting systems, the analyzer now counts platelets electronically and offers a three-part or five-part differential. Depending on the population pool of patient samples, the automated differential has cut the technologist's manual worktime. The technologist reviews only the abnormal differentials flagged by the counting system.

In addition to the automated differentials, some systems save additional labor time by offering "hands-off" efficiency with automixing, autofeed, autosampling, and barcoding for easy patient identification. The use of trays for convenient loading, along with closed-tube autosampling with cap-piercing tubes that are thoroughly mixed as the trays are moved along the system also insures high-speed operation with unattended processing. The new systems deliver more information at a much faster pace.

In the microbiology laboratory, cost savings can be realized by using bacteriology systems that provide fully automated microbial identification or susceptibility tests. Such systems can also be interfaced with either the laboratory information systems or patient care systems.

Systems such as the Vitek use miniaturized test kits in the form of plastic cards of 30 test wells, each containing substrates for microbial identification testing. Test kits are available for automated identification of commonly occurring gram-negative and gram-positive organisms and yeasts. Test kits that accept a direct inoculation of urine are available in two configurations. These cards provide a bacterial count and identification of the organisms frequently found in urinary tract infections. Test kits are available for testing fastidious organisms and anaerobes, utilizing substrates that react with preformed enzymes, but these must be read manually. The results are entered into the database, and the identification is made by the computer.

The advantage of a fully automated **walk-away system** lies in the elimination of tedious multistep identification procedures using conventional media and the labor involved in manual inoculation of nonautomated single-step commercial identification kits. Further labor is saved after the requisite incubation period by elimination of the steps involving reagent addition and interpretation of reactions for identification and the reading and recording of susceptibility tests.

TECHNOLOGY AND THE LABORATORY'S GROWTH POTENTIAL

As we have discussed, the laboratory is under pressure to control costs. We have also discussed how the technology available today can help bring operating and labor costs under control. The technology can also help the laboratory deal with budget problems by enabling the processing of increases in workflow cost effectively. For example, Table 18–4 identifies the monthly costs of processing 89,375 routine chemistry tests per month. The system and service costs are considered fixed costs. That is, as volume changes, the cost of capital acquisition and service remain constant. As volume expands, reagent and supply costs will expand. They are called **variable,** or incremental, **costs.** In our example, monthly expenditures on these variable costs are $6,806. This amounts to $0.076 per test.

Therefore, incremental increases in testing can be processed for $.076 per test. Of course, we have assumed that additional labor will not be required, but for small increases in testing, this is a reasonable assumption. For example, this laboratory, which processes approximately 250 routine chemistry samples per day, should be able to process an additional 25 samples without requiring additional labor.

Using this concept of incremental cost, or **marginal cost analysis,** let us assume that the laboratory is able to convince a nearby nursing home or several doctors or both to send their patients to the hospital for blood work. Let us also assume that on average the laboratory processes on a daily basis 5 days per week an additional 25 chemistry profiles and 25 CBCs. Since these samples are collected for out-patients, the laboratory can charge for this service. Let's be conservative and assume charges of $12 for the CBC and $15 for the chemistry profile. On a daily basis, the laboratory is able to generate $675 in income. This amounts to $175,500 annually.

The incremental cost to process the 20 chemistry profiles is $1.52. Therefore, the annual incremental cost is $9,880. The incremental costs associated with processing an additional 25 CBCs per day are the insignificant additional costs for isotonic and lysing reagent. Therefore, the laboratory will be able to generate a profit of approximately $165,000.

CASE STUDIES: COST SAVINGS VIA WORKSTATION CONSOLIDATION

The first case study describes how **workstation consolidation** and resulting savings were achieved in the chemistry section of a reference laboratory by acquiring a chemistry analyzer with an expanded test menu. The laboratory adopted the Miles TECHNICON AXON system, but other analyzers with similar capabilities were considered.

The second scenario describes workstation consolidation and cost-saving potential for the special chemistry section of the laboratory. Potentially large cost savings can be achieved. As the technology and the test menus are further developed, this potential will be realized. The scenario we describe notes the current savings offered by such a system and identifies future savings as well.

nology to achieve these objectives. The owner believed that workstation consolidation was key to designing a competitive laboratory. One workstation requires less labor input, fewer controls and standards, and fewer contracts than multiple workstations, thus reducing operating costs and minimizing the need to split samples, resulting in improved turnaround time.

This case study describes how these goals were achieved by acquiring a chemistry analyzer that was able to perform the work currently being performed by two analyzers. The rationale for selecting the particular analyzer is also explained, as well as the impact on operational costs and utilization of labor.

CASE STUDY I

IMPROVING OPERATIONAL EFFICIENCY THROUGH WORKSTATION CONSOLIDATION

Pressures placed on today's laboratory to produce more test results, offer broader test menus, and improve turnaround time continue to grow. The difficulty is to meet these challenges at a time when cost containment is also a priority, and when qualified technologists are in short supply. Fortunately, today's technology offers a means of:

- Improving turnaround time.
- Offering a broad test menu in one workstation.
- Improving worker productivity, thereby providing a means for coping with the labor shortage.
- Reducing operating costs.

A private reference laboratory trying to compete in today's market sought tech-

Rationale for Selecting the TECHNICON AXON System

The primary goal was to be able to consolidate workstations. To accomplish this goal, an analyzer that had a large test menu was required. Obviously, the TECHNICON AXON system, with 38 resident chemistries and the ability to select from among over 100 tests, met this goal.

In addition to routine chemistries, the ability to place TDMs, thyroids, drugs of abuse, immunoassays, and urinary chemistries was required to achieve the desired goal of workstation consolidation.

These times require that operating costs be reduced. Disposable cuvets, which are used by competitive systems, significantly add to operating costs. A system, therefore, that utilizes reusable permanent cuvets cleaned on the system was desired. There was a strong preference that cleaning be accomplished without the need for a water purification system, which incurs an additional expense and additional maintenance. For example, some manufacturers require water quality to be 10 to 18 mega ohms. This would require a water purification system.

Operating costs are lower for systems that enable one to employ user-defined test menus. Rather than be limited to reagent availability of only one particular manufacturer, a system that enables the user to purchase reagents from a variety of vendors assures that operating costs are minimized. Such a system has the added benefit of adapting new methods as they become available.

Previously, a technologist was assigned exclusively to the Olympus DEMAND and a technologist was assigned exclusively to the Abbott TDX. Now, the technologist assigned to the Abbott TDX was made available to evaluate other test methods with the goal of expanding the services of the laboratory.

Impact of Workstation Consolidation on Operating Costs

Obviously, the use of one workstation instead of two reduces service and capital costs. This analysis, however, focuses solely on the operational costs experienced when the Olympus DEMAND and Abbott TDX were used versus the costs associated with the TECHNICON AXON System.

The ability of the data management system to monitor reaction curves was deemed to be an important characteristic of the system. Extensive data storage capabilities (i.e., reaction curves, STAT results, and control values) along with graphic displays of patient means, reaction curves, and QC reports were all considered desired characteristics of the data management system.

In selecting an analyzer such as the TECHNICON AXON system with a broad test menu it was important that throughput not be compromised. In this case, a throughput of over 500 tests per hour was more than adequate to provide the laboratory with the means of assuring acceptable turnaround time. In fact, it is anticipated that turnaround time will actually be improved. Previously, many samples required processing at two workstations. This in itself slows down the processing time. In addition, the Abbott TDX workstation previously used to process samples requiring testing for TDMs was not interfaced with the computer. Results were manually entered, thereby requiring more time and labor.

Figure 18–1 shows that operational costs are reduced by over $2,000 per month by utilizing the TECHNICON AXON system.

Impact of Workstation Consolidation on Labor Utilization

Once the decision was made to purchase the TECHNICON AXON system, all the routine chemistries previously performed on the Olympus DEMAND and the TDMs performed on the Abbott TDX were placed on the TECHNICON AXON system. This consolidation of tests is depicted in Figure 18–2.

The reasons for the reduction are twofold. Supply costs associated with the Olympus DEMAND, which uses disposable cuvets, exceeded the cost of supplies on the TECHNICON AXON system by over $.05 per test. Greater savings were achieved by running the TDMs on the TECHNICON AXON system versus the Abbott TDX. This was due to two factors. The laboratory built its reputation on its ability to provide excellent service and rapid turnaround time. Therefore, tests were not batched. As a result, protocol dictated that three controls be run every time a particular test either on a single or multiple samples is

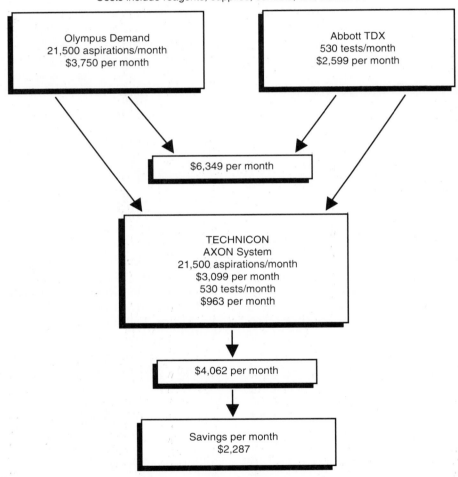

WORKSTATION CONSOLIDATION
Operational Cost Analysis

Costs include reagents, supplies, controls, and standards

Olympus Demand
21,500 aspirations/month
$3,750 per month

Abbott TDX
530 tests/month
$2,599 per month

$6,349 per month

TECHNICON
AXON System
21,500 aspirations/month
$3,099 per month
530 tests/month
$963 per month

$4,062 per month

Savings per month
$2,287

■ **FIGURE 18–1.**

(From Franey RJ, Lehmann C, Leiken A: *Improving Operational Efficiency Through Workstation Consolidation.* Tarrytown, NY, Technicon Instruments Corporation, 1991.)

WORKSTATION CONSOLIDATION
Test Distribution by Workstation

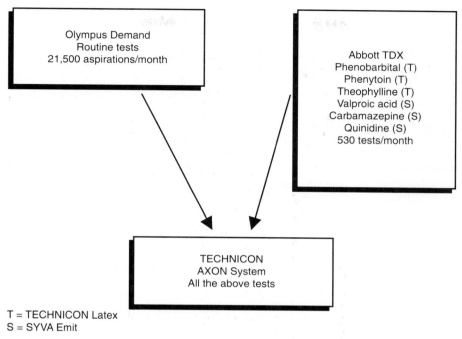

Olympus Demand
Routine tests
21,500 aspirations/month

Abbott TDX
Phenobarbital (T)
Phenytoin (T)
Theophylline (T)
Valproic acid (S)
Carbamazepine (S)
Quinidine (S)
530 tests/month

TECHNICON
AXON System
All the above tests

T = TECHNICON Latex
S = SYVA Emit

■ **FIGURE 18–2.**

(From Franey RJ, Lehmann C, Leiken A: *Improving Operational Efficiency Through Workstation Consolidation.* Tarrytown, NY, Technicon Instruments Corporation, 1991.)

run. The TECHNICON AXON system's superior data management enabled the laboratory to feel confident utilizing fewer controls. More significantly, the fact that it is an open system enabled the laboratory to obtain reagents at less than half the cost of reagents used on the Abbott TDX.

Summary and Conclusion

The need to reduce costs and offer improved and expanded services is apparent. As demonstrated, a means to achieve these goals has been accomplished by consolidating workstations with the TECHNICON AXON system. More work needs to be done and is planned. The open system of the TECHNICON AXON will enable the laboratory to continue to expand its automated test menu without additional workstations and the additional capital and labor costs inherent with multiple workstations.

Labor shortages and the increasing competition warrant that such systems be implemented. Manufacturers are beginning to respond to the needs of the laboratory by offering such systems that are far more user-friendly and reliable than the previous generation of analyzers. The availability of such systems challenges laboratorians to utilize them to improve **operational efficiency** and the services offered.

CASE STUDY II

WORKSTATION CONSOLIDATION IN THE SPECIAL CHEMISTRY/ THERAPEUTIC SECTION

The special chemistry/therapeutic section of a teaching hospital has the volumes and the tests exhibited in Table 18–5. The tests performed are typical of tests performed in these areas. Although other tests are also performed in these areas, these tests were selected because they are either currently available on most immunology analyzers or are in the late stages of development and should be

available in the near future. The second column notes the number of patient results the laboratory produces on a monthly basis. Certain tests that appear in the table are performed in duplicate. These tests are currently being performed using a manual procedure (RIA), and they are run in duplicate to minimize human error. In addition to the duplicate samples, standards, controls, and repeats need to be accounted for. This information appears in the last column of Table 18–5. Therefore, to produce 4,199 patient results, the laboratory has been producing 8,856 test results.

This workload is distributed to four workstations. As can be seen in Figure 18–3, these workstations include an RIA workstation, the Photon ERA, the Amerlite, and the COBAS Fara II. The tests performed at each workstation are noted. Those tests with an asterisk are tests the laboratory is considering moving to an immunology analyzer. (Refer to Chapter 17 on immunology analyzers for tests and analyzers currently available.) As can be seen, the Photon ERA workstation will be eliminated completely, and the Amerlite workstation will be used to process only progesterone.

The workstations identified are labor intensive but experience relatively low reagent and supply costs. Smaller hospitals that process such tests are forced to use more expensive methodologies.

These workstations are staffed five days per week on the day shift. Therapeutic drug tests are also available during the off shifts and the weekends. These workstations are presently staffed by 5.4 medical technologists. Current operating costs, including labor, instrumentation, service, supplies, and reagents, are $30,451 per month.

By processing approximately half the tests currently being processed at the four workstations on the immunology analyzer,

TABLE 18–5. PRESENT MONTHLY TEST VOLUMES

TEST	PATIENT	DUPLICATES	STANDARDS/ CONTROLS/ REPEATS
T3	134	134	96
T4	590	590	213
T3U	453	453	147
HCG	313	313	146
TSH	640	640	235
Fer	232		62
FSH	110	110	89
LH	99	99	87
Prol	90	90	75
Cort	81	81	88
Digox	474		267
Theo	260		214
Tobr	37		41
Gent	380		116
Pheny	205		185
Phenb	101		86
Totals	4199 +	2510 +	2147 = 8856

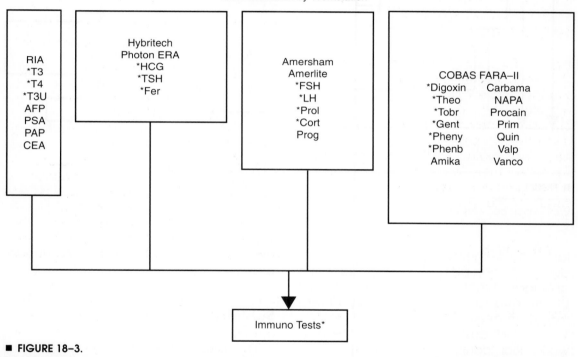

Workstation Consolidation
Test Distribution by Workstation

RIA	
*T3	
*T4	
*T3U	
AFP	
PSA	
PAP	
CEA	

Hybritech
Photon ERA
*HCG
*TSH
*Fer

Amersham
Amerlite
*FSH
*LH
*Prol
*Cort
Prog

COBAS FARA–II
*Digoxin   Carbama
*Theo   NAPA
*Tobr   Procain
*Gent   Prim
*Pheny   Quin
*Phenb   Valp
Amika   Vanco

Immuno Tests*

■ **FIGURE 18–3.**

Workstation consolidation.

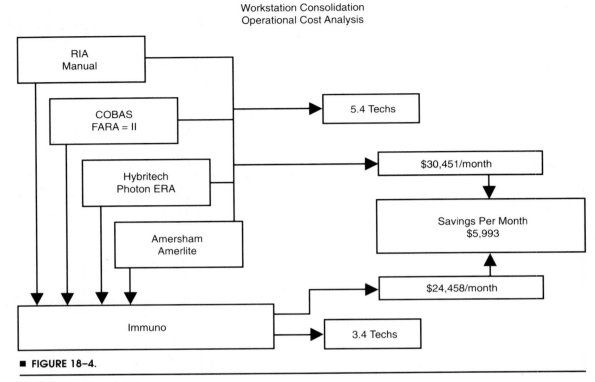

■ **FIGURE 18–4.**

Workstation consolidation.

labor requirements will be substantially reduced. As can be seen in Figure 18–4, it is anticipated that only 3.4 technologists will be needed to process the workload previously processed by 5.4.

When all costs are included, the new workstation configuration will cost $24,458 per month, resulting in a monthly saving of $5,993. As more methods become available on the immunology systems, greater opportunities will exist to consolidate even further. It also might become more economical to perform tests in-house that are currently being sent to a reference laboratory. This not only offers cost savings potential but could provide better turnaround time. Laboratory managers need to assess periodically the appropriateness of performing these ``send-outs'' in the laboratory.

SUMMARY

The technology available today offers many features that can be utilized by the laboratory to help deal with many of the pressures they are facing. Expanding test menus and enhanced computerization enable the laboratory to consolidate workstations, thereby satisfying desires to operate cost effectively as well as provide a broader and better range of services.

The technology also enables the laboratory to process additional work in a cost-effective manner. This provides the opportunity to expand out-patient testing services. As demonstrated, this could be lucrative for the institution and enhance the prestige of the laboratory.

By performing a workflow analysis, as described in Chapter 17, and by understanding the available technologies and the appropriate costs, laboratory managers can organize the laboratory so as to assure the delivery of high-quality, cost-effective services demanded by hospital administrators, physicians, and patients.

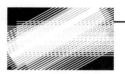

REVIEW QUESTIONS

Choose the best answer to each question.

1. Which is not an advantage of workstation consolidation?

   a. Reduced labor requirements.
   b. Savings on service contracts.
   c. Lower overhead costs.
   d. Reduction in capital costs.

2. If a chemistry department that processed 200 samples per day received an extra 5 samples, which costs would you expect to increase?

   a. The cost of service contracts.
   b. Labor costs.
   c. Reagent costs.
   d. Instrumentation costs.

3. Which of the following is not considered a consumable?

   a. Reagents.
   b. An analyzer.
   c. Sample cups.
   d. Controls.

4. As a result of the use of DRGs to classify Medicare patients and determine a fixed reimbursement

   a. the laboratory cannot bill for tests performed for Medicare in-patients.
   b. the laboratory cannot bill for tests performed for out-patients.
   c. the laboratory cannot bill for any laboratory tests.
   d. None of the above.

A WORD FROM THE MANUFACTURER

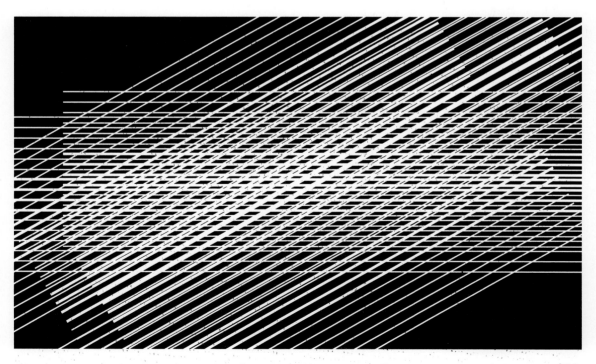

The following is a list of some major companies that manufacture chemistry and hematology analyzers. It does not in any way represent a complete list. The purpose of this section is to provide students with an opportunity to visualize and make comparisons of technology in areas such as throughput, test menu, data management capabilities, maintenance requirements, and so on. The manufacturer's names, addresses, and 800 numbers are listed so that one may write or call for additional information and instrument brochures.

ABBOTT DIAGNOSTICS
Abbott Park, IL 60064
1-800-323-9100

BAXTER HEALTHCARE CORPORATION*
PO Box 25101
Santa Ana, CA 92799-5101
1-800-872-3233

BAXTER DIAGNOSTICS INC.†
Scientific Products Biomedical
1430 Waukegan Road
McGaw Park, IL 60085-6787
1-800-635-4186

BAXTER DIAGNOSTICS INC.‡
PO Box 520672
Miami, FL 33152-0672
1-800-327-2616

BECKMAN INSTRUMENTS
Diagnostic Systems
Brea, CA 92621-6209
1-800-526-3821

BOEHRINGER MANNHEIM CORPORATION
9115 Hague Road
Indianapolis, IN 46250
1-800-428-5030

COULTER CORPORATION
601 Coulter Way
Hialeah, FL 33012-2432
1-800-526-6932

DUPONT DIAGNOSTICS
PO Box 7470
Wilmington, DE 19803
1-800-441-7722

EASTMAN KODAK COMPANY
Clinical Products Division
Rochester, NY 14650
1-800-445-6325

MILES INC.
511 Benedict Ave
Tarrytown, NY 10591-5097
1-800-431-1970

OLYMPUS CORPORATION
4 Nevada Drive
Lake Success, NY 11042-1179
1-800-426-2042

ROCHE DIAGNOSTIC SYSTEMS
1080 U.S. Highway 202
Branchburg, NJ 08876
1-800-526-1247

*Paramax information.
†Hematology information.
‡Stratus immunochemistry information.

ABBOTT TDX FLX

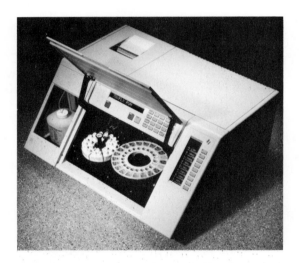

SYSTEM OVERVIEW

Random access analyzer
Closed system
Can perform up to 8 on-board chemistries
Analytic throughput: 40 to 80 samples per hour
Test menu: TDMs, transplant diagnostics, classic chemistries, hormone function, specific proteins, toxicology,
        substance abuse, and fetal management

REAGENTS/SAMPLES

Reagent system: Liquid
Reagent packaging: 100 test kit wedges
On-board reagent inventory
Sample volume: 50 μL
Barcode wand for specimen ID

DATA MANAGEMENT

Interfacing: Unidirectional
Data storage: 200,000 test results
Data reporting: QC Levey-Jennings, Westgard
        Patient demographics
        Multi-tasking

MAINTENANCE

Daily: 5 minutes
Weekly: 30 minutes
Monthly: 1 hour

SPECIAL FEATURES

Barcode wand for data input
Random access
Automated reagent inventory

Printed with permission from Abbott Diagnostics.

ABBOTT CCx CHEMISTRY ANALYZER

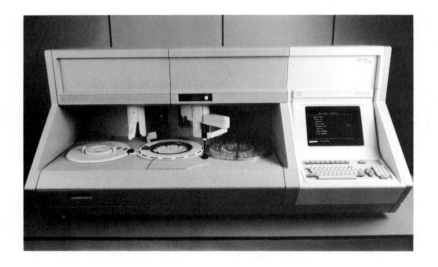

SYSTEM OVERVIEW

Random access analyzer
Open system
Can perform up to 31 on-board chemistries
Analytical throughput: 150–200 based on test requests
Test menu: General chemistries and some special chemistries

REAGENTS/SAMPLES

Reagent system: Liquid
Reagent volume: 25 to 236 μL
Reagent stability: Up to 28 days on-board
Reagent packaging: Reagent cartridges in two sizes
On-board reagent inventory
Primary tube sampling
Sample volume: 1.25 to 25 μL
Sample dilution: Autodilution

DATA MANAGEMENT

Interfacing: Bidirectional
Data storage: 200,000 test results
Touch screen
Data reporting: Color graphic displays include:
          QC reports
          Auto rerun
          Multi-tasking
          Workload analysis
          Calibration summary

MAINTENANCE

Daily: 20 minutes
Weekly: 45 minutes
Monthly: 1 hour

SPECIAL FEATURES

Automated daily maintenance
Liquid level sensing
Auxiliary dispense

Printed with permission from Abbott Diagnostics.

ABBOTT SPECTRUM SERIES II

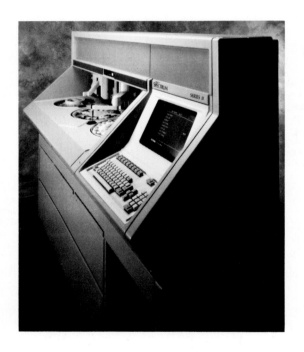

SYSTEM OVERVIEW

Random access analyzer
Open system
Can perform up to 34 on-board chemistries
Analytical throughput: 175 to 200 tests per hour
Test menu: General chemistries, ISEs, and some special chemistries

REAGENTS/SAMPLES

Reagent system: Liquid
Reagent volume: 25 to 236 μL per test
Reagent stability: Up to 28 days on-board
Reagent packaging: Barcoded cartridges
On-board reagent inventory
Direct tube sampling
Sample volume: 1.25 to 25 μL
Sample dilution: Automatically adjusted and reassayed

DATA MANAGEMENT

Interfacing: Bidirectional
Data storage: 200,000 test results
Data reporting: Color graphic displays include:
          QC reports
          Multi-tasking
          Workload analysis
          Auto re-run

MAINTENANCE

Daily: 20 minutes
Weekly: 45 minutes
Monthly: 1 hour

SPECIAL FEATURES

Sample liquid level sensor
Automated daily maintenance
Calibration summary

Printed with permission from Abbott Diagnostics.

ABBOTT SPECTRUM EPx

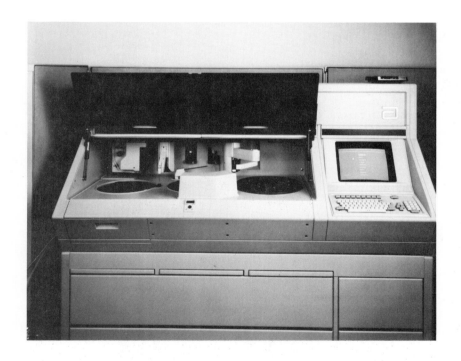

SYSTEM OVERVIEW

Random access analyzer
Open system
Can perform up to 34 on-board chemistries
Analytical throughput: 350 tests per hour
Test menu: General chemistries, ISEs

REAGENTS/SAMPLES

Reagent system: Liquid
Reagent volume: 25 to 236 μL per test
Reagent stability: Up to 28 days on-board
Reagent packaging: Barcoded cartridges in multiple sizes
On-board reagent inventory
Reagent level sensor
Sample bar code with direct tube sampling
Sample volume: 1.25 to 25 μL
Sample dilution: Automatically adjusted and reassayed

DATA MANAGEMENT

Interfacing: Bidirectional
Data storage: 200,000 test results
Data reporting: Color graphic displays include:
                 QC reports (Levey-Jennings graphs)
                 Patient data archive
                 Maintenance logs
                 Patient demographics
                 Touchscreen

MAINTENANCE

Daily: 30 minutes
Weekly: 45 minutes
Monthly: 1 hour

SPECIAL FEATURES

Modem diagnostics
Automatic calibration
Sample liquid sensor
Maintenance tracking

Printed with permission from Abbott Diagnostics.

ABBOTT IMX

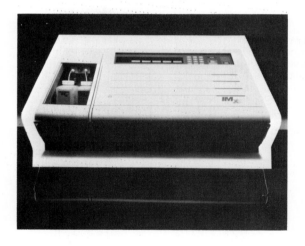

SYSTEM OVERVIEW

Automated immunoassay system
Workflow flexibility
Can perform up to 3 on-board chemistries
Analytical throughput: 48 samples per hour
Test menu: T4, TU, T3, FT_3, FT_4, LH, FSH, prolactin, β-hCG, hCG, CEA, PSA, AFP, Ca 19-9, HTSH, beta-2-micro, SCC, rubella-G, Toxo-G, Toxo-M, CMV-G, CMV-M, theophylline, CK-MB, ferritin, IgE, B_{12}, E_2, havab-B-M and core-M

REAGENTS/SAMPLES

Reagent system: Liquid
Reagent volume: Varies with test
Reagent stability: N/A
On-board reagent liquid sensor
Positions for 24 patients
Sample volume: 150 μL
Sample dilution: Auto calculation of manual dilutions

DATA MANAGEMENT

Interfacing: Bidirectional
Data reporting: Color graphic displays include:
         QC Levey-Jennings, Westgard
         Patient demographics
         Maintenance codes

MAINTENANCE

Daily: 5 minutes
Weekly: 45 minutes
Monthly: 20 minutes

SPECIAL FEATURES

Carousel ID
Barcode ID
LH, PSH, prolactin, random access
Automated reagent inventory
Sample ID
Autodilutions

Printed with permission from the Abbott Diagnostics, a division of Abbott Laboratories.

BAXTER SYSMEX HEMATOLOGY SYSTEMS K-1000

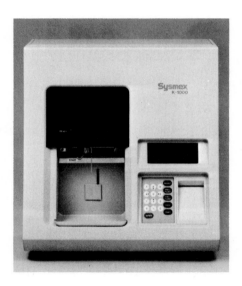

SYSTEM OVERVIEW

24-hr access analyzer
8 CBC parameters plus 10 additional analytical parameters with WBC, RBC, and PLT histograms
Start-up: 10 seconds; from cold start, 5 minutes
Throughput: 80 samples per hour for WB mode; 60 samples per hour for CAP mode
Test menu: WBC, RBC, Hgb, HCT, MCV, MCH, MCHC, PLT, RDW-SD, RDW-CV, PDW, MPV, P-LCR, and Diff
DIFF: Neut (% & #)
       Lymph (% & #)
       Mixed (% & #)

WBC AND RBC FLAGS

Leukocytosis
Left shift
Immature gran
Anisocytosis
Macrocytosis
Anemia

Blasts
Atypical lymphocytes
NRBC
Microcytosis
Hypochromia
Erythrocytosis

REAGENTS/SAMPLES

Reagent volume: 28 mL per cycle
Sample volume:
    Manual mode: 100 μL
    Capillary mode: 40 μL

DATA MANAGEMENT

Interfacing: Bidirectional
Daily and cumulative QC reports
Comprehensive flagging

MAINTENANCE

Daily: 5 minutes
Weekly: 5 minutes
Monthly: 15–20 minutes

Printed with permission from Baxter Diagnostics.

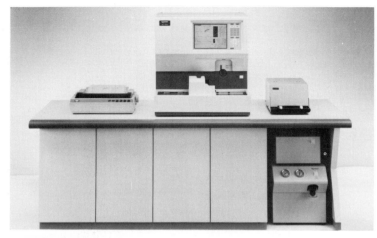

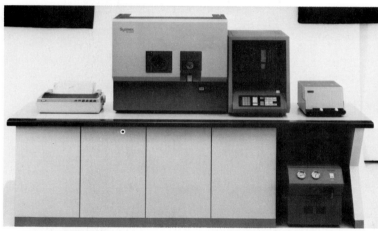

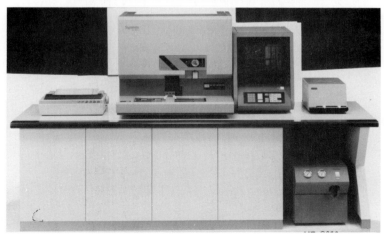

Model NE-1500   Model NE-Alpha
Model NE-5500   Model E-5000
Model NE-8000   Model E-2500

Model R-3000

SYSTEM OVERVIEW

24-hr access analyzer
8 to 23 parameters
Start-up: NE and E systems: 10 seconds, from cold start, 20 minutes, R system: 20 minutes
Throughput:
NE-1500: 90 samples per hour   NE-Alpha: 120 samples per hour
NE-5500: 120 samples per hour   E-5000: 119 samples per hour
NE-8000: 120 samples per hour   E-2500: 119 samples per hour

R-3000: 80 samples per hour

Test menu: WBC, RBC, Hgb, HCT, MCV, MCH, MCHC, PLT, RDW-SD, RDW-CV, PDW, MPV, P-LCR, and Diff
Models NE-1500, NE-5500, and NE-8000: 23 parameters, including 10 WBC differential plus 5 histograms and 1 WBC scattergram

DIFF:	NE-1500	NE-5500	NE-8000	R-1000/3000
Neut	(% & #)	(% & #)	(% & #)	
Lymph	(% & #)	(% & #)	(% & #)	
Mono	(% & #)	(% & #)	(% & #)	
Eos	(% & #)	(% & #)	(% & #)	
Baso	(% & #)	(% & #)	(% & #)	
RBC				#
Retic				% & #

WBC AND RBC FLAGS

Leukocytosis   Blasts
Left shift   Atypical lymphocytes
Immature gran   NRBC
Anisocytosis   Microcytosis
Macrocytosis   Hypochromia
Anemia   Erythrocytosis

REAGENTS/SAMPLES

Reagent volume: Milliliters per cycle
    NE Series: 55 mL; E Series: 36 mL; R Series: 37 mL
Sample volume (all models):
      Closed sample auto: 200 μL
      Manual mode: 125 μL
      Capillary mode: 40 μL
Bar-coded patient ID
Direct tube sampling with cap piercing

DATA MANAGEMENT

Interfacing: Bidirectional
Daily and cumulative QC reports
Comprehensive flagging

MAINTENANCE

	NE Series	E Series	R Series
Daily:	5 minutes	5 minutes	5–10 minutes
Weekly:	10–20 minutes	5–10 minutes	5–10 minutes
Monthly:	10–20 minutes	10–20 minutes	5–10 minutes

Printed with permission from Baxter Diagnostics.

SYSMEX HS-SERIES

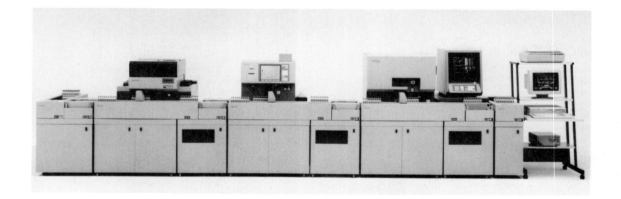

SYSTEM OVERVIEW

Total hematology system HS-330
Automated hematology analyzer, automated reticulocyte analyzer, slide preparation unit and sample transport system
Throughput: HS-330: CBC + WBC Diff, 120 samples per hour; reticulocyte analysis, 80 samples/hr; film preparation, 120 samples per hour
Test menu: WBC, RBC, Hgb, HCT, MCV, MCH, MCHC, PLT, RDW-SD, RDW-CV, RDW, MPV, P-LCR, Diff, Ret% and Ret#
 Diff: Neut (% & #)
  Lymph (% & #)
  Mono (% & #)
  Eos (% & #)
  Baso (% & #)

WBC, RBC, PLT, AND RET FLAGS

Blast	Anisocytosis	Microcytosis
Immature gran	Hypochromasia	Anemia
Left shift	Macrocytosis	Thrombocytopenia
Atypical lymph	Anisochromasia	Thrombocytosis
NRBC	Macrocytosis	

REAGENTS/SAMPLES

Reagent volume: NE-8000 Hematology, 55 mL per cycle
  R-3000 Reticulocyte 37 mL per cycle
Sample volume: NE-8000, 200 µL
  R-3000, 100 µL
  Film preparation, 200 µL
Direct tube sampling
Barcode patient ID

DATA MANAGEMENT

Interfacing: Bidirectional
Daily and cumulative QC reports
Comprehensive flagging

MAINTENANCE

NE System	R System	SPECIAL FEATURES
Daily: 5 minutes	5–10 minutes	Workstation consolidation
Weekly: 10–20 minutes	5–10 minutes	Closed-tube sampling
Monthly: 10–20 minutes	5–10 minutes	Walkaway environment

BAXTER STRATUS INTELLECT

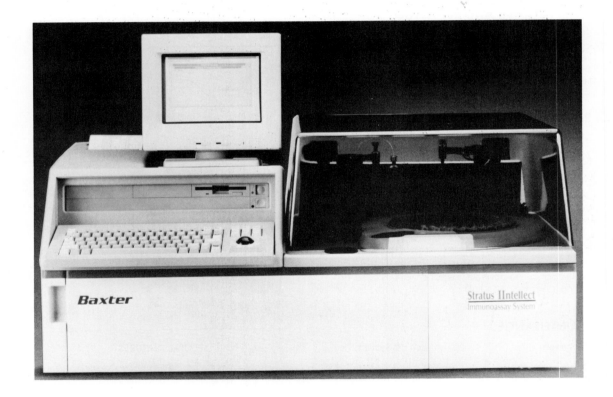

SYSTEM OVERVIEW

Immunoassay batch analyzer
Can perform one on-board chemistries
Analytical throughput: 60 tests per hour
Test menu: Cardiac enzymes, reproductive hormones, allergy tests, cardiac glycosides, antiarrhythmics, antiasthmatics, antiepileptics, antibiotics, tumor markers and infectious disease

REAGENTS/SAMPLE

Reagent system: Solid phase
Reagent volume: 120 tests per kit
Reagent stability: 2 weeks curve stability
Positions for 30 samples
Sample volume: 200 μL
Sample dilution: Serial dilutions for any assay up to 1:1000

DATA MANAGEMENT

Interfacing: RS232 limited bidirectional
Data storage: 240 megabytes.
Data reporting: Color graphics displays include:
                QC reports
                Assay reports
                Patient summary reports
                Calibration reports

MAINTENANCE

Daily: 5 minutes
Weekly: 10 minutes
Monthly: 5 minutes

SPECIAL FEATURES

Roll bar activation
Sample level sensors
Reagent sensors

Printed with permission from Baxter Diagnostics.

BAXTER PARAMAX 720ZX

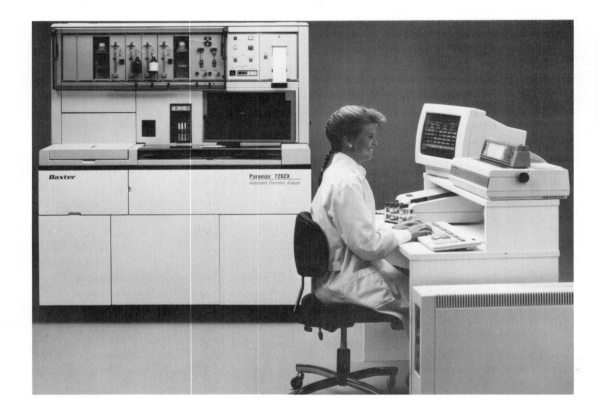

SYSTEM OVERVIEW

24-hour operation
Open system
Can perform up to 52 on-board chemistries, including ISEs
Analytical throughput: Up to 720 tests per hour
Test menu: General chemistries, ISEs, urines, and 10 user-defined

REAGENTS/SAMPLES

Reagent system: Dry tablets
Reagent volume: One tablet
Reagent stability: Up to 90 days on system
Reagent packaging: Barcoded 100 and 300 test packages
On-board reagent inventory
Sample barcode with closed container, direct tube sampling
Sample volume: 2 to 50 μL
Sample dilution: Automatic

DATA MANAGEMENT

Host communications
Touchscreen simplicity/color terminal
15 calculated results
Data storage: 1000 patient records; 10,000 files
Interfacing: Bidirectional
Data reporting: Color graphic displays include:
                        Current statistics and Levey-Jennings charts
                        Range-to-date data summary for QAP
                        Patient demographics

MAINTENANCE

Daily: 5 minutes
Weekly: 15 minutes
Monthly: 30 minutes

SPECIAL FEATURES

No exposure to biohazards
User-defined test menu
Closed container sampling
Positive patient identification
Lithium analysis
Apolipoprotein A1, B
Direct tube sampling (2 to 10 mL)
Dry reagents
Calibration stability 90 days

Printed with permission from Baxter Healthcare Corporation, Paramax Systems Division.

BECKMAN SYNCHRON CX3 CLINICAL CHEMISTRY SYSTEM

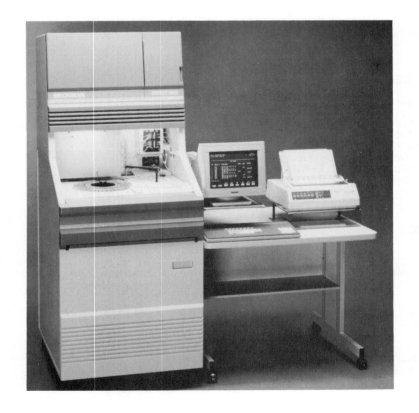

SYSTEM OVERVIEW

24-hour STAT and random access analyzer
Performs up to 8 on-board chemistries
STAT results in less than 1 minute
Analytical throughput of up to 600 tests, or 75 samples per hour
Test menu: Na, KCl and CO_2 by ISE plus glucose, BUN, creatinine and calcium (total protein may be substituted for calcium)

REAGENTS/SAMPLES

Reagent system: Liquid with no preparation required
Reagent volume: 0.22 to 1.25 mL
Reagent stability: Up to 30 days or expiration date on system
Reagent packaging: Bulk packaging for high-volume efficiency
On-board reagent inventory tracking with audible "low-volume" alarm
Sample types: Serum, plasma, urine, CSF
Sample volume: 10 to 62 µL; 144 µL for all 8 tests
Sample barcode with direct tube sampling option
Sample dilution: Automatic overrange detection and correction for glucose

DATA MANAGEMENT

9 user programmable chemistry panels
4 user selectable calculations, such as osmolality and anion gap
Data storage: Holds up to 6,400 patient results
User programmable reference ranges and reporting units
Unidirectional and bidirectional interface options
On-board QC program: Daily QC log
　　　　　　　　　　Daily and monthly cumulative summary statistics
　　　　　　　　　　Levey-Jennings charts

MAINTENANCE

Daily: 5 minutes
Weekly: 10 minutes
Monthly: 20 minutes

SPECIAL FEATURES

Handles 65% of the typical laboratory's workload
True STAT testing and no workflow interruption
Self-checking instrument diagnostics
Extended ISE calibration stability

BECKMAN SYNCHRON CX5 CLINICAL CHEMISTRY SYSTEM

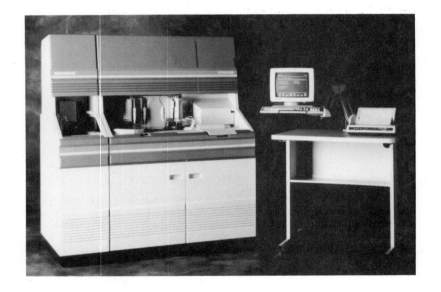

SYSTEM OVERVIEW

24-hour random access analyzer
Open system—100 channels
28 on-board chemistries, including ISEs
Over 60 Beckman chemistries
Analytical throughput: Up to 525 tests per hour
Test menu: General chemistries, ISEs, DAUs, TDMs, thyroids, specific proteins, and esoterics

REAGENTS/SAMPLES

Reagent system: Liquid
Reagent volume: 200 to 327 μL for photometrics
Reagent stability: Up to 42 days on system for photometrics; up to expiration date for ISEs
Reagent packaging: 20–300 tests per cartridge for photometrics; up to 2000 tests per container for STAT side
On-board reagent inventory tracking
Direct tube sampling
Sampling volume: 3 to 25 μL for photometrics; 62 μL for all 4 electrolytes
Sample dilution: Automatic overrange detection and correction

DATA MANAGEMENT

Sample status
Data storage: Holds up to 7,200 test results
Interfacing: Bidirectional
Data reporting: Chartable and laboratory reports
Option of packaging with Cerner PathTrac laboratory information system

MAINTENANCE

Daily: 5 minutes
Weekly: 10 minutes
Biweekly: 5 minutes
Monthly: 30 minutes

SPECIAL FEATURES

Electrolyte profile in <1 minute
Semipermanent glass reaction cuvets
On-board refrigerated reagent storage
Plasma profile capability

Printed with permission from Beckman Instruments, Inc.

BECKMAN SYNCHRON CX7 CLINICAL CHEMISTRY SYSTEM

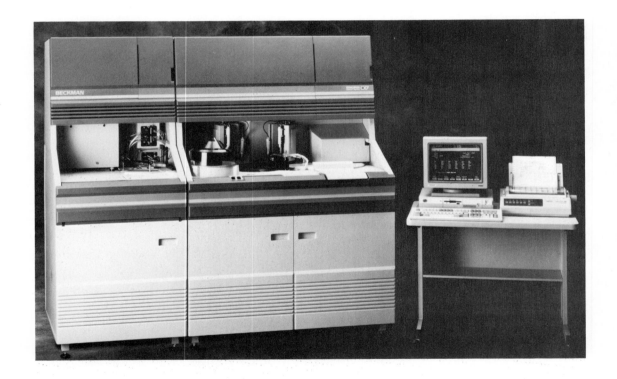

SYSTEM OVERVIEW

24-hour random access analyzer
Open system—100 channels
32 on-board chemistries, including ISEs
Over 60 Beckman chemistries
Analytical throughput: Up to 825 tests per hour
Test menu: General chemistries, DAUs, ISEs, TDMs, thyroids, specific proteins, and esoterics

REAGENTS/SAMPLES

Reagent system: Liquid
Reagent volume: 200 to 327 μL for photometrics
Reagent stability: Up to 42 days on system for photometrics; up to expiration date for ISEs
Reagent packaging: 20–300 tests per cartridge for photometrics; up to 3000 tests per container for STAT side
On-board reagent inventory tracking
Sample barcode with direct tube sampling
Sample volume: 3 to 25 μL for photometrics; 62 μL for all 4 electrolytes
Sample dilution: Automatic overrange detection and correction. Dilution factor entry for prediluted samples

DATA MANAGEMENT

Query host
Sample status
Up to 40 calculations (osmolality, anion gap, and user-defined)
Data storage: Holds up to 10,000 test results
Interfacing: Bidirectional and query host
Data reporting: Color graphic displays include:
    Sample ID reports
    Single patient summary monitors
    QC reports
Supports barcode printer
Option of packaging with Cerner PathTrac laboratory information system, MedPlus barcode printer, and Beckman Spinchron centrifuge with PTS 2000 rotor

MAINTENANCE

Daily: 5 minutes
Weekly: 10 minutes
Biweekly: 30 minutes
Monthly: 30 minutes

SPECIAL FEATURES

Chem 7 profile in <1 minute
Semipermanent glass reaction cuvets
On-board refrigerated reagent storage
Plasma profile capability

Printed with permission from Beckman Instruments, Inc.

BOEHRINGER MANNHEIM/HITACHI 747 SYSTEM

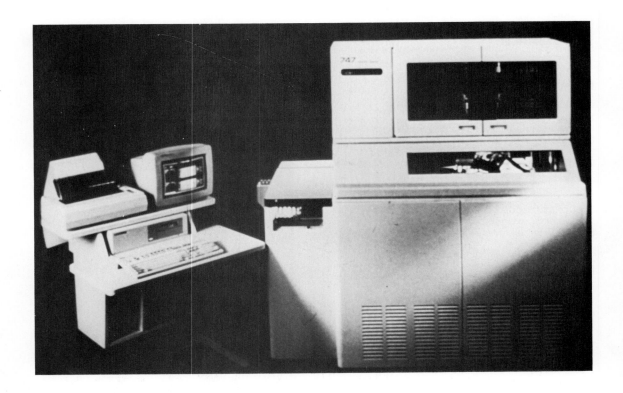

SYSTEM OVERVIEW

Random access analyzer
Open system
Can perform up to 35 on-board chemistries, including ISEs (Na, K and Cl)
Analytical throughput:
747-200 (one ISE unit): 5700 tests per hour, up to 600 samples per hour; 300 samples per hour with ISE max
747-200 (two ISE units): 6600 tests per hour, up to 600 samples per hour max, including ISEs
747-100: 3300 tests per hour, up to 600 samples per hour; 300 samples per hour with ISE max

REAGENTS/SAMPLES

Reagent system: Liquid
Reagent volume: 50–350 µL
Reagent stability: Average working stability: 3 weeks
Reagent packaging: Bottle sizes are 300 and 600 mL
Reagent inventory tracking with low-level alarms
Sample barcode with direct tube sampling
Sample volume: 1–20 µL; average 6–7 µL
Sample dilution: Automatic reassay with reduced sample volume
Insta-Link reagent loading system: No tubes or straws
Refrigerated reagent dispense lines: Minimized frequency and amount of priming

DATA MANAGEMENT

Interfacing: Bidirectional
Data storage: 10K routine, 10K reruns, 400 STAT, for Class 1 (serum) and Class 2 (urine, cerebrospinal fluid)
Data reporting: Color graphic displays include:
    QC reports
    Help windows
    Edit print program
    Sample tracking
    Calculated tests (i.e., BUN/creat)
Data reporting: 8 user-defined calculated tests
50 ABS reading vs. time plotted and printable

SPECIAL FEATURES

Small footprint—inner/outer ring of cuvets
``Stoplight'' (not spotlight) maintenance log
747-200: 300-sample capacity ⎫
747-100: 150 sample capacity ⎭ with STAT interrupt
Optional 2nd ISE only for 747-200 (see throughput)
``Abnormal descent detection'' for all mechanical components
Liquid-level sensing for short sampling
Auto reruns handled as STATs
Operation monitor—unique sample tracking display
AIM—Automated *I*ntegrated *M*aintenance—variable automated maintenance functions similar to macros

MAINTENANCE

	Analyzer Time	Tech Time
Daily:	20 minutes	2 minutes
Weekly:	75 minutes	8 minutes
Monthly:	75 minutes	10 minutes

Printed with permission from the Boehringer Mannheim Corporation.

BOEHRINGER MANNHEIM/HITACHI 911 SYSTEM

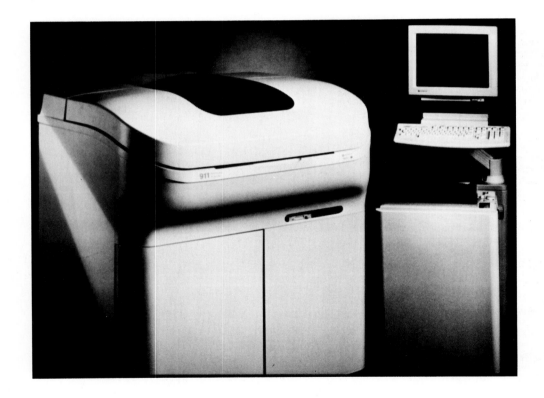

SYSTEM OVERVIEW

24-hour random access analyzer
14 STAT assays under 5 minutes
All routine functions automated:
    Automatic calibration, maintenance, dilution, and rerun
68 programmable channels
Throughput up to 720 tests per hour
Test menu: General chemistries, ISEs, immunoassays, DAUs, TDMs, urine and CSF assays, thyroids, and special chemistries

REAGENTS/SAMPLES

Reagent system: Liquid with on-board refrigeration
Reagent barcoding to allow on-board inventory tracking, automatic bottle changeover, and automatic calibration
Up to 4 reagent additions with variable reaction times
Reagent volume: 50–350 μL
Reagent packaging: 20, 50 and 100 mL
Automatic on-line sample predilution
Immediate STAT sample priority
Refrigerated, covered sample tray for calibrators/QC
Automatic barcode discrimination with direct tube sampling
Low level detection for samples and reagents

DATA MANAGEMENT

Interfacing: Bidirectional with host query and result buffering
Reaction curve monitor
Selectable patient report formats
Data reports: Requisition list
              Maintenance report
              Individual and cumulative QC
              Calibration trace

SPECIAL FEATURES

Automatic calibration tracking and initiation
Automatic Wake-Up feature
Selectable STAT reception mode
Real-time result monitoring

MAINTENANCE

Daily: 2 minutes
Weekly: 5 minutes
Monthly: 25 minutes

BOEHRINGER MANNHEIM ES 300

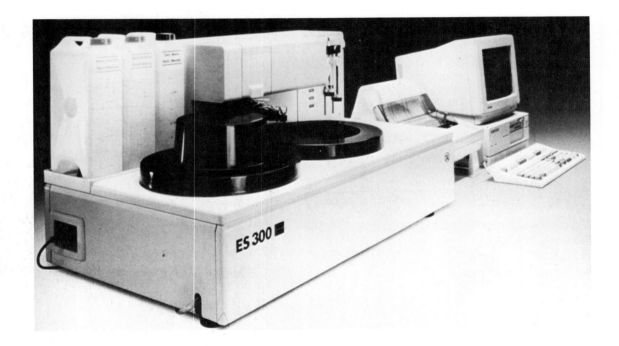

SYSTEM OVERVIEW

Automated immunoassay system
Multichannel, test-selective operation
Can perform up to 12 on-board assays
Analytical throughput: 100 tests per hour
Test menu: T_4, TSH, FT_4, T_3, TU, TBG, progesterone, estradiol, LH, FSH, prolactin, HCG, ferritin, IgE, AFP, cortisol
           and insulin

REAGENTS/SAMPLES

Reagent system: Liquid
Reagent volume: 1000 μL
Reagent stability: Average 2 weeks refrigerated
Liquid level detection for samples and reagents
Positions for 150 patients
Sample volume: 5–200 μL
Sample dilution: Automatic result calculation of manual dilutions

DATA MANAGEMENT

Menu driven software
Interfacing: Bidirectional
Data storage: Holds up to 300 patient files
Data reporting: Color graphic displays include:
     QC reports
     Workload processing
     Calibration curves
Patient-chartable reports

SPECIAL FEATURES

Automated on-line cleaning
3-way alert lights
Trace of run function troubleshooting aid
Run optimization by overlapping sequences
On-line help

MAINTENANCE

Daily: None
Weekly: None
Monthly: 10 minutes

Printed with permission from the Boehringer Mannheim Corporation.

COULTER MAXM HEMATOLOGY SYSTEM

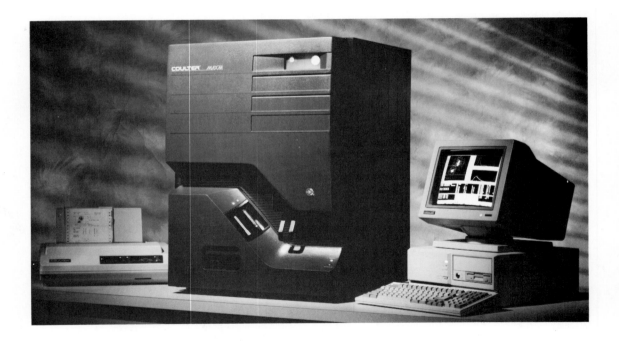

SYSTEM OVERVIEW

24-hour access analyzer
CBC plus 5-part differential
Start-up 60 seconds from standby, 5 minutes from cold start
Throughput: 75 samples per hour
Test menu: WBC, RBC, Hgb, HCT, MCV, MCH, MCHC, RCDW, PLT, MPV
        Diff: Lymph (% & #)
             Mono (% & #)
             Neut (% & #)
             Eos (% & #)
             Baso (% & #)

WBC AND RBC FLAGS

Anisocytosis
Hypochromasia
Macrocytosis
Band 1/band 2

Anisochromasia
Microcytosis
Blasts
Atypical lymphocytes

RBC flags (aniso, poik, hypo,
   macro, micro)
Platelets (clumps and giant)

REAGENTS/SAMPLES

Reagent volume: 45.0 mL Isoton IV, 1.06 mL hype IV diff, 0.60 mL erythrolyse, 0.133 stabilise per cycle
Sample volume: 185 µL primary tube mode
                  125 µL secondary sample mode
                    50 µL predilute mode
Direct tube sampling
Barcode sample ID

DATA MANAGEMENT

Interfacing: Bidirectional
Daily and cumulative QC data (15 files)
Comprehensive flagging
1000 patient result storage
Database query
Multitasking

MAINTENANCE

Daily: None
Weekly: None
Monthly: 10–15 minutes

SPECIAL FEATURES

Autoloader (optional)
Automatic calibration
System monitoring
Closed vial sampling–multiple tube size
Predilute feature
Differential results on WBC counts to 100 cells/µL

Printed with permission from Coulter Corporation.

COULTER STKS HEMATOLOGY SYSTEM

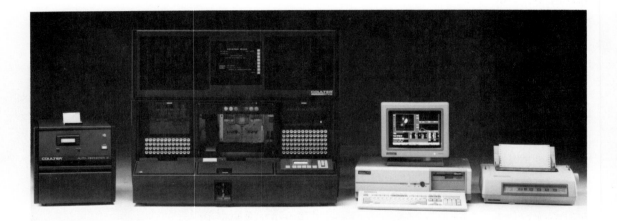

SYSTEM OVERVIEW

COULTER STKS HEMATOLOGY SYSTEM

24-hour access analyzer
CBC plus 5-part differential
Start-up 20 seconds from standby, 1 minute 15 seconds from cold start
Throughput: 109 samples per hour CBC and Diff; 138 per hour CBC only
Test menu: WBC, RBC, Hgb, HCT, MCV, MCH, MCHC, CHCM, RDW, PLT
     Diff: Neut (% & #)
            Lymph (% & #)
            Mono (% & #)
            Eos (% & #)
            Baso (% & #)

WBC AND RBC FLAGS

Anisocytosis	Anisochromasia	RBC flags (aniso, poik, hypo,
Hypochromasia	Microcytosis	macro, micro)
Macrocytosis	Blasts	Platelets (clumps and giant)
Band 1/band 2	Atypical lymphocytes	

REAGENTS/SAMPLES

Reagent volume: 56.3 mL Isoton IV, 1.1 mL hype 111 diff, 1.1 mL erythrolyse, 0.2 mL stabilise per cycle
Sample volume: 250 μL primary tube mode
               150 μL secondary sample mode
Direct tube sampling
Barcode patient ID

DATA MANAGEMENT

Interfacing: Bidirectional
Daily and cumulative QC data (15 files)
Database query
Comprehensive flagging
1000 patient results storage
Multitasking

MAINTENANCE

Daily: None
Weekly: None
Monthly: 10–15 minutes

SPECIAL FEATURES

144-tube STKS cassette
Automatic calibration
System monitoring
Closed-vial sampling
Differential results on WBC counts to 100 cells/μL

Printed with permission from Coulter Corporation.

DU PONT ACA IV ANALYZER

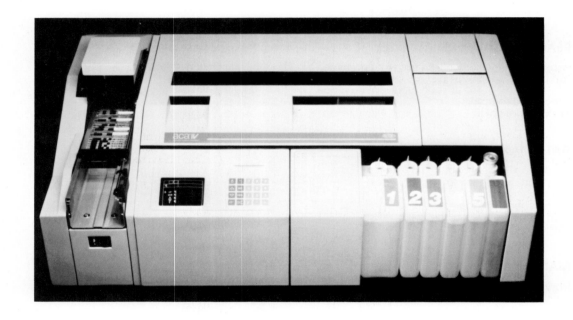

SYSTEM OVERVIEW

Random access bench-top analyzer
Closed system
Can perform up to 85 on-board chemistries
Analytical throughput: 45 tests per hour
Test menu: TDMs, DAUs, toxicology, specialty tests, general chemistries, electrolytes, endocrinology

REAGENTS/SAMPLES

Reagent system: Tablet/liquid
Reagent volume: 1 pack per test
Reagent stability: 4 to 12 months
Reagent packaging: Individual barcoded packages
Samples are placed in covered cups and loaded with any sequence of test packs (barcoded sample cup ID)
Sample volume: 20 to 440 μL
Sample dilution: Manual

DATA MANAGEMENT

Interfacing: Unidirectional
Data storage: 60 test results, patient IDs
Data reporting: Monochromatic CRT, thermal printer, load list printout

MAINTENANCE

Daily: 5–10 minutes
Weekly: 8–10 minutes
Monthly: 30–40 minutes

SPECIAL FEATURES

Random access capability
Broad test menu (85 tests)
No start-up or shut-down required
Automated calibration
Calibration frequency 6 weeks to 6 months

DU PONT DIMENSION CLINICAL CHEMISTRY SYSTEM

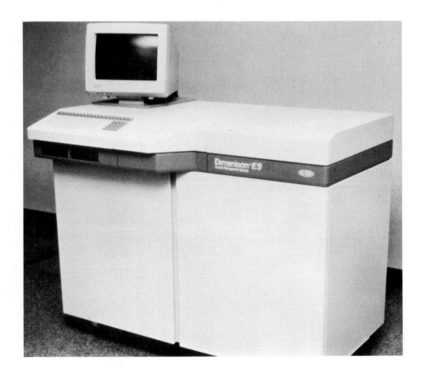

SYSTEM OVERVIEW

24-hour random access analyzer
Closed system
Can perform up to 42 on-board chemistries, including ISEs
Analytical throughput: Up to 400 tests per hour
Test menu: General chemistries, ISEs, TU, T_4, TDMs, and C-reactive protein

REAGENTS/SAMPLES

Reagent system: Liquid, tablets
Reagent volume: 5 to 40 tests per each cartridge well set
Reagent stability: Up to 30 days
Reagent packaging: 15 to 240 tests per cartridge
On-board reagent inventory
Sample entry by sample wheel or barcode ID of primary tube sampling, interchangeably
Sample volume: 2 to 60 μL per test, 5 to 15 μL average
Automatic sample dilution

DATA MANAGEMENT

Interfacing: Bidirectional
External query mode
Data storage: 2000 patient results, 10,000 QC results
Data reporting: Color graphic displays include:
        Present supply of reagent and cuvets
        QC reports
        Levey-Jennings plots
        Previous test results
        Calibration data, plots
        Sample/test-specific histograms
        Method correlation program

MAINTENANCE

Daily: 3–5 minutes
Weekly: 10 minutes
Monthly: 30–40 minutes

SPECIAL FEATURES

Automatic reagent preparation
Blow-molded cuvet system, reduces biohazards and
   costs of cleaning
Programmed calculations (i.e., BUN/crea)
Calibration frequency 2–3 months
Method kinetics display

KODAK EKTACHEM 700XR

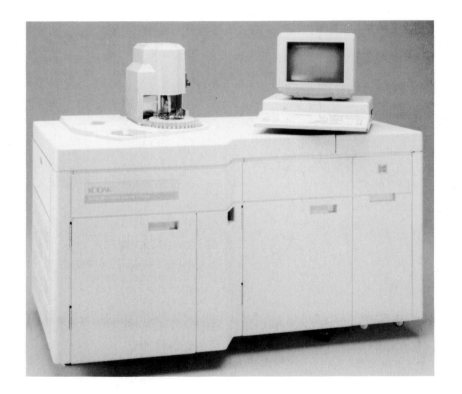

SYSTEM OVERVIEW

24-hour random access analyzer
Closed system
Can perform up to 42 colorimetric, rate and ISEs tests per sample
Analytical throughput: 540 and up to 750 tests per hour by adding the high-volume profiling accessory
Test menu: General chemistries, ISEs, some TDMs, and several urine and CSF chemistries available

REAGENTS/SAMPLES

Reagent system: Dry slides
Reagent volume: One slide per test
Reagent stability: 12 to 18 months (shelf); 2 to 4 weeks on analyzer
Reagent packaging: Barcoded 50-test cartridges (lower-volume tests available in 18-slide cartridges
On-board reagent inventory with continuous monitoring
Sample barcode with direct tube sampling
Sample volume: 10 to 11 μL per test

DATA MANAGEMENT

Touchscreen simplicity
Result integration from other laboratory analyzers
Cap workload recording and calculations
Automatic calculations (i.e., chol/HDL)
Data storage: 5,000 sample results
Interfacing: Bidirectional
Data reporting: Color graphic displays include Levey-Jennings charts

MAINTENANCE

Daily: 5 minutes
Weekly: 10–15 minutes
Monthly: 15 minutes

SPECIAL FEATURES

180-day calibration
No reagent preparation
QC once a day
Specimen liquid level sensor
Minimal interferences (bilirubin, hemolysis, icterus)

Printed with permission from Eastman Kodak Company.

KODAK EKTACHEM 500

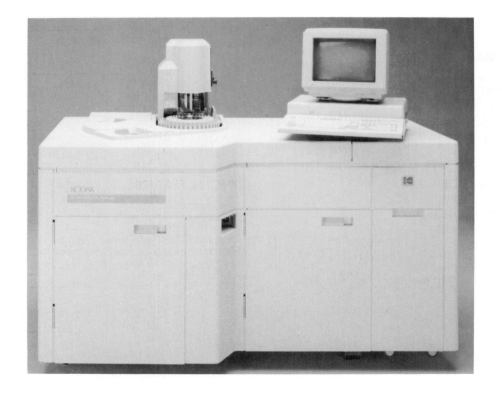

SYSTEM OVERVIEW

24-hour random access analyzer
Closed system
Can perform up to 42 colorimetric, rate and ISE tests per sample
Analytical throughput: Up to 300 tests per hour
Test menu: General chemistries, ISEs, some TDMs and several urine and CSF tests

REAGENTS/SAMPLES

Reagent system: Dry slides
Reagent volume: 1 slide per test
Reagent stability: 12–18 months (shelf), 2–4 weeks on analyzer
Reagent packaging: Barcoded 50-test cartridges (lower-volume tests available in 18 test cartridges)
On-board reagent inventory with continuous monitoring
Sample barcode with direct tube sampling
Sample volume: 10 to 11 μL

DATA MANAGEMENT

Touchscreen simplicity
Result integration from other laboratory analyzers
Cap workload recording and calculations
Automatic calculations (i.e., chol/HDL)
Data storage: 5,000 sample results
Interfacing: Bidirectional
Data reporting: Color graphic displays include Levey-Jennings charts

MAINTENANCE

Daily: 5 minutes
Weekly: 10–15 minutes
Monthly: 15 minutes

SPECIAL FEATURES

180-day calibration
No reagent preparation
QC once a day
Specimen liquid level sensor
Minimal interference (bilirubin, hemolysis, icterus)

KODAK EKTACHEM E250

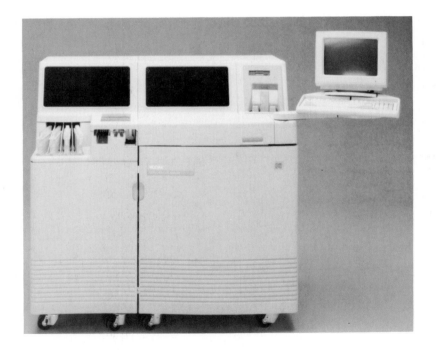

SYSTEM OVERVIEW

24-hour random access analyzer
Closed system
Can perform up to 42 colorimetric, rate, and ISE tests per sample
Analytical throughput: Up to 250 tests per hour
Test menu: General chemistries, ISEs, some TDMs, and several urine and CSF chemistries, some immunoassays (1994)

REAGENTS/SAMPLES

Reagent system: Dry slides
Reagent volume: 1 slide per test
Reagent stability: 12–18 months (shelf), 2–4 weeks on analyzer
Reagent packaging: Barcoded 50-test cartridges (lower-volume tests available)
On-board reagent inventory with continuous monitoring
Sample barcode with direct tube sampling
Sample volume: 10 to 11 μL
Sample dilution: Manual factor input by operator, or automatic dilution for urine chemistries and on-demand dilution for out-of-range

DATA MANAGEMENT

Touchscreen simplicity
Result integration from other laboratory analyzers
Cap workload recording and calculations
Automatic calculations (i.e., LDL/VLDL)
Data storage: 5,000 sample results
Interfacing: Uni- or bidirectional
Data reporting: Color graphic displays include Levey-Jennings charts

MAINTENANCE

Daily: 5 minutes
Weekly: 10–15 minutes
Monthly: 15 minutes

SPECIAL FEATURES

180-day calibration
No reagent preparation
QC once a day
Multiple lots of chemistry stored on analyzer
Specimen liquid level sensor
Minimal interferences (bilirubin, hemolysis, icterus)

Printed with permission from Eastman Kodak Company.

TECHNICON AXON SYSTEM

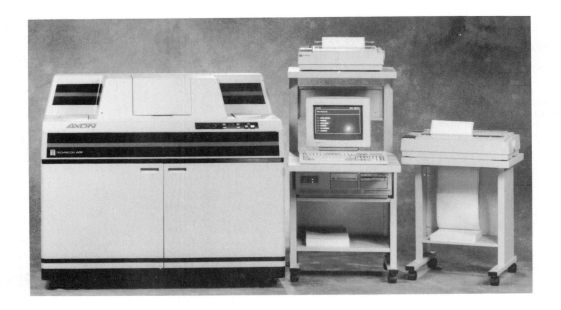

SYSTEM OVERVIEW

24-hour random access analyzer
Open system
38 resident chemistries (36 colorimetric and two ISEs for sodium and potassium)
Analytical throughput: 480 colorimetric tests per hour and up to 576 with ISEs
Test menu: General chemistries, ISEs, urine chemistries with user-defined TDMs, thyroids, DAUs, and
    immunoassays

REAGENTS/SAMPLES

Reagent system: Liquid, with on-board refrigeration
Reagent volume: 10 μL to 400 μL, with most requiring 300–350 μL per test
Reagent stability: Up to 30 days
Reagent packaging: Barcoded 50- to 90-mL sizes
On-board reagent inventory and refrigeration
72-position sample wheel with dedicated STAT and control positions
Sample volume: 3 to 47 μL, generally less than 25 μL
Sample dilution: 5 predefined dilution factors, 5, 10, 20, 50, and 80
STAT dwell time: 9.5 minutes

DATA MANAGEMENT

Menu-driven software
Reaction curve monitor: Real-time display, 65 absorbance readings plotted, ABS vs. time
Data storage: Latest 2000 reaction curves stored; 972 samples, 100 STATS and 80 controls per day for 40 days
Interfacing: 2-way host communications (bidirectional)
Data reporting: Color graphic displays include:
        QC scattergrams and histograms, Westgard
        Histograms of patient means
        Reaction curves
        Test correlation graphs
        Multipoint calibration curves
        Correlation program

MAINTENANCE

Daily: None
Weekly: 10 minutes
Monthly: 20 minutes

SPECIAL FEATURES

Liquid level sensors warn when sample or reagent is
    low
Direct tube sampling
Color-coded reagent cassettes and trays
Permanent Pyrex cuvets

Printed with permission from Miles Inc. Diagnostic Division.

TECHNICON CHEM 1+ SYSTEM

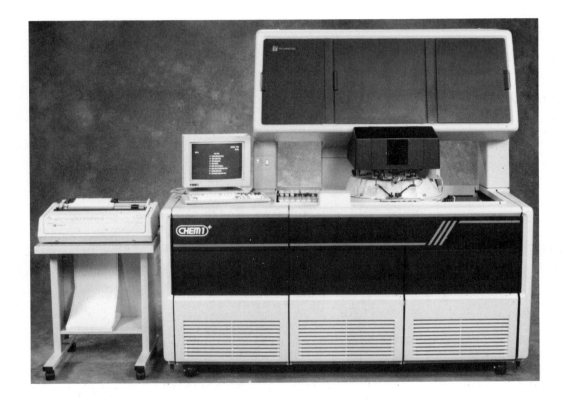

SYSTEM OVERVIEW

24-hour random access analyzer
Proprietary reagent with 10 open channels
35 resident chemistries (including 3 ISEs: Na, K, CO_2)
Analytical throughput: 720 photometric tests per hour and with a maximum of 1800 tests when ideal mix of ISEs
Test menu: General chemistries, ISEs, thyroids, immunoassays, DAUs, and user-defined methods
30+ days' calibration

REAGENTS/SAMPLES

Reagent system: Liquid (capsule chemistry technology)
Reagent volume: 14 μL photometric, 140 μL ISEs
Reagent stability: 30+ days for most reagents
Reagent packaging: Barcoded cassettes of various sizes
On-board inventory and refrigeration
272-sample capacity
Sample volume: 1 μL photometric and 10 μL per ISE
Sample barcode reader

DATA MANAGEMENT

Menu driven
Three levels of on-line content-sensitive help
Data storage: Holds all demographics and up to 43 results for 2,250 patients. Allows to define up to 3 ratios, 32 profiles, 195 sex and age reference ranges and 64 flagging ranges
Interfacing: 2-way host communications (bidirectional)
Data reporting: Color graphic displays include:
     Full-file management, 2,250 records
     Scattergrams for QC and patient means
     Reaction and multipoint calibration curves

MAINTENANCE

Daily: 5 minutes
Weekly: 30 minutes
Monthly: 1 hour

SPECIAL FEATURES

Direct tube sampling
Immunoassay capability
Micro reagents

Printed with permission from Miles Inc. Diagnostic Division.

TECHNICON DAX SYSTEMS

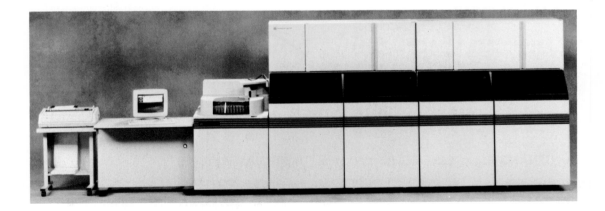

SYSTEM OVERVIEW

24-hour random access analyzer
Open system
Can perform up to 32 colorimetric and 2 ISE tests per sample
Analytical throughput: DAX 96 and 72 can analyze 300 samples per hour; DAX 48 can process 150 samples per hour; and DAX 24 can process 100 samples per hour
Test menu: General chemistries, ISEs, urine chemistries, user-defined TDMs and DAUs, thyroids, and immunoassays

REAGENTS/SAMPLES

Reagent system: Liquid
Reagent volume: 50 to 400 μL
Reagent stability: Up to 30 days
Reagent packaging: 250 to 2000 mL cassettes
On-board reagent inventory
Racks are barcoded and color-coded for STATs, patients, calibrators, and controls
Sample barcode with direct tube sampling from 5-, 7-, or 10-mL Vacutainer tubes
Sample volume: 2 to 30 μL
Sample dilution: 1:2, 1:4, and 1:8

DATA MANAGEMENT

Touchscreen simplicity
ICON-driven software with mouse interaction
Result valildation screen helps
Data storage: Holds up to 5000 patient files
Interfacing: 2-way host communications (bidirectional)
Data reporting: Color graphic displays include:
        QC scattergrams and histograms
        Multipoint calibration curves
        Delta check capability
        File management

MAINTENANCE

Daily: 15 minutes
Weekly: 30 minutes
Monthly: 1 hour

SPECIAL FEATURES

Short sample and clot detector with flushing
Sampler monitor displays position of all samples on sampler, as well as status
Direct tube sampling
Automatic start-up/shut-down
Automatic reruns and dilutions
STAT interrupt

Printed with permission from Miles Inc. Diagnostic Division.

TECHNICON RA-2000 SYSTEM

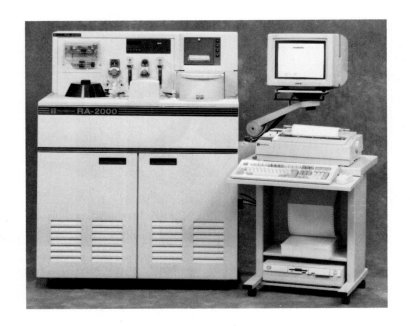

SYSTEM OVERVIEW

24-hour random access analyzer
Open system
26 resident chemistries (26 colorimetric or 23 colorimetric plus 3 ISEs)
Analytical throughput: 240 tests per hour, 720 per hour with ISEs
Test menu: General chemistries, ISEs, colorimetric Na and K, TDMs, T_4, T-UP, specific proteins, DAUs, user-defined methods

REAGENTS/SAMPLES

Reagent system: Liquid
Reagent volume: 5 to 450 μL per test
Reagent stability: Up to 7 days
Reagent packaging: 40 mL reagent boats
On-board refrigeration
30-position sample tray with positive barcode
Sample volume: 1.5 to 30 μL
Sample reruns and dilutions

DATA MANAGEMENT

ICON-driven software with mouse interaction
Optional touchscreen
Data storage: 2000 patient records, up to 70 test results per patient
Interfacing: 2-way host communications (bidirectional)
Data reporting: color graphic displays include:
   Result review and edit with panic and delta flags
   Daily and cumulative quality control
   Patient reports

MAINTENANCE

Daily: <5 minutes
Weekly: 20 minutes
Monthly: N/A

SPECIAL FEATURES

Direct tube sampling
Automatic cuvet washing
255 TECHNICON and user-defined methods can be
   stored in memory

Printed with permission from Miles Diagnostics Inc.

TECHNICON IMMUNO-1 SYSTEM

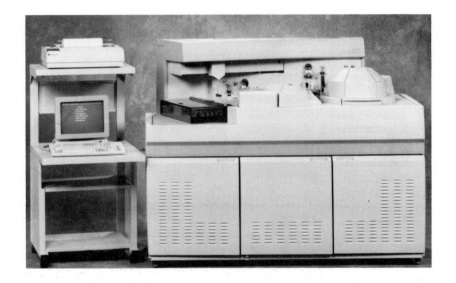

SYSTEM OVERVIEW

24-hour random access analyzer
Closed system
22 resident chemistries
Analytical throughput: Up to 120 tests per hour; time to first result as few as 7 minutes
Test menu: T_3, T_4, T_3U, FSH, LH, TSH, ferritin, prolactin, hCG, pheno, tobra, digox, theoph, genta, phenytoin, cortisol

REAGENTS/SAMPLES

Reagent system: Liquid
Reagent volume: 65–150 µL
Reagent stability: Up to 30 days
Barcoded 100–200 test cassettes
Reagent inventory: Self-monitored on-board
78 samples on-board with continuous sample loading
Sample volume: 2–50 µL
STAT capability

DATA MANAGEMENT

Menu-driven software
Calibration curve: 6-point curves with curve editing
Data storage: 1000 patients with 24 tests per patient
Interfacing: 2-way host communications (1st q93) (bidirectional)
Data reporting: User-defined QC limits
                  Levey-Jennings graphs
                  Cumulative QC means

MAINTENANCE

Daily: None
Weekly: 15 minutes
Monthly: 15 minutes

SPECIAL FEATURES

Ultrasensitive TSH
Similar to a chemistry analyzer
Both homogenous (latex agglutination) and
    heterogeneous (magnetic particle kinetic enzyme
    immunoassay) assays
Reusable reaction cuvet tray washed on-board

Printed with permission from Miles Diagnostics Inc.

TECHNICON H-2 SYSTEM

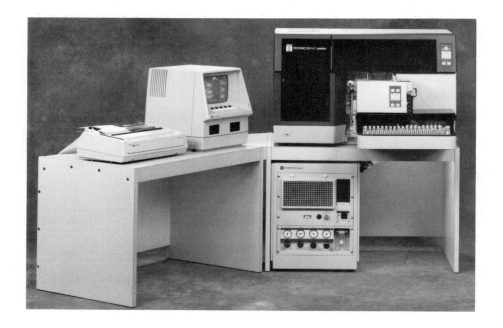

SYSTEM OVERVIEW

TECHNICON H-2 SYSTEM

24-hour access analyzer
CBC plus 6-part differential
Start-up: 40 seconds from standby, 2 minutes 40 seconds from cold start
Throughput: 102 samples per hour
Test menu: WBC, RBC, Hgb, HCT, MCV, MCH, MCHC, CHCM, RDW, PLT, MPV, HDW, RDW
  Diff: Neut (percent absolute)
        Lymph (% and abs. no.)
        Eos (% and abs. no.)
        Monos (% and abs. no.)
        Basos (% and abs. no.)
        Large unstained cells (% and abs. no.)

WBC AND RBC FLAGS

Anisocytosis
Anisochromasia
Hypochromasia
Hyperchromasia
Macrocytosis

Microcytosis
Blasts
Left shift
Atypical lymphocytes
Immature granulocytes

REAGENT/SAMPLE

Reagent volume: 2.9 mL/cycle
Sample volume: 125 µL open tube and 145 µL closed tube sample

DATA MANAGEMENT

Internal computer and parameter self-checks with diagnosis
Patient moving averages
Daily and cumulative QC data
Statistical tables
System error flags
Audio alerts
Interfacing: Bidirectional

MAINTENANCE

Daily: 10 minutes
Weekly: N/A
Monthly: 20 minutes every 3 months

SPECIAL FEATURES

Optional Labfacts data management software
Optional manual barcode reader

Printed with permission from Miles Diagnostics Inc.

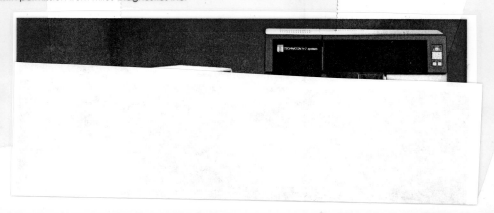

TECHNICON H-1E SYSTEM

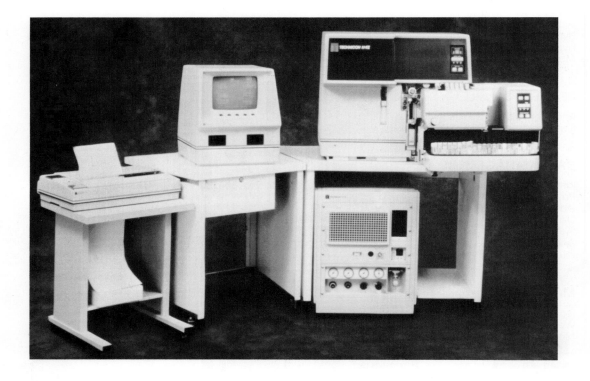

SYSTEM OVERVIEW

24-hour access analyzer
CBC plus 6-part differential
Start-up: 40 seconds from standby, 2 minutes 40 seconds from cold start
Throughput: 80 samples per hour in CBC mode or 60 samples per hour for CBC plus WBC and differential
Test menu: WBC, RBC, Hgb, HCT, MCV, MCH, MCHC, CHCM, RDW, PLT, MPV, HDW, PDW
  Diff: Absolute # and percentage of the following:
    Neut, lymph, mono, eos, baso, large unstained cells, plus lobularity index, and mean peroxidase index

TECHNICON H-1E SYSTEM

WBC AND RBC FLAGS

WBC Flags: Left shift, atypical lymphocytes, blasts, and others (including immature granulocytes)
RBC Flags: RBC size, aniso, micro, macro, Hgb content, variation in Hgb concentration, hypo- and hyperchromia

REAGENTS/SAMPLES

Reagent volume: 2.9 mL per cycle
Reagents packaged to provide approximately 900 assays
Sample volume: 125 µL open tube and 145 µL closed tube sampler

DATA MANAGEMENT

Internal computer and parameter self-checks with diagnosis
Patient moving averages
Daily and cumulative QC data
Statistical tables
System error flags
Audio alerts
Interfacing: Bidirectional

MAINTENANCE

Daily: 10 minutes
Weekly: N/A
Monthly: 20 minutes every 3 months

SPECIAL FEATURES

Optional manual barcode reader
Optional Labfacts data management software

Printed with permission from Miles Diagnostics Inc.

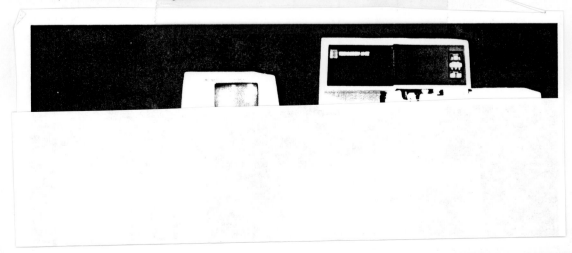

OLYMPUS REPLY

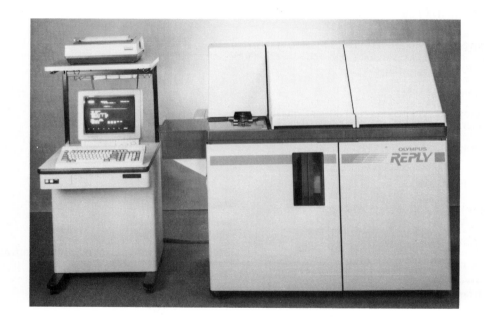

SYSTEM OVERVIEW

24-hour random access analyzer
Open system
Can perform up to 32 colorimetric and 3 ISEs per sample
Analytical throughput: 400 photometric, 600 with ISE unit
Test menu: General chemistries, ISEs, urine chemistries, TDMs, DAUs, thyroids, specific proteins

REAGENTS/SAMPLES

Reagent system: Liquid
Reagent volume: 25 to 300 µL, average of 70 µL per test
Reagent stability: Up to 30 days
Reagent packaging: 18 or 50 mL bottles
On-board reagent inventory
Sample holders are color coded for QC, STATs and controls
Sample barcoded with direct tube sampling
Sample volume: 3 to 50 µL
Sample dilution: Automatic repeat, dilute, or condense

DATA MANAGEMENT

Data management system
5 report formats
Reaction curve monitoring
Datas storage: Stores up to 4000 patient files
Interfacing: Bidirectional
Data reporting: Color graphic displays:
            QC charts
            Data edit functions
            User-defined calculated tests
            Correlation correction

MAINTENANCE

Daily: 5 minutes
Weekly: 15 minutes
Monthly: 45 minutes

SPECIAL FEATURES

Reagent volume detector
198 test menu (user-defined)
Direct tube sampling
Automatic ISE cleaning cycle

Printed with permission from Olympus Corporation, Clinical Instruments Division.

OLYMPUS 5000 SERIES

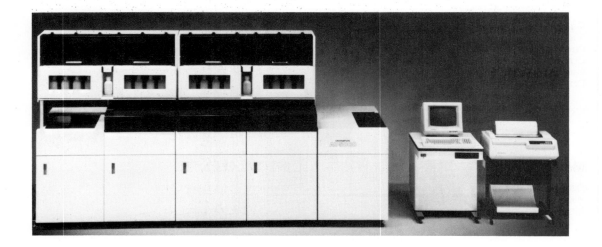

SYSTEM OVERVIEW

Random access analyzer
Open systems
Can perform up to 24 (5021), 16 (5121), 24 (5031), 12 (5131), 24 (5061) on-board chemistries
Analytical throughput: Model 5021, 100 samples per hour
Model 5121, 150 samples per hour
Model 5031, 150 samples per hour
Model 5131, 300 samples per hour
Model 5061, 300 samples per hour
Test menu: General chemistries, DAUs, thyroids, ISEs, and special chemistries

REAGENTS/SAMPLES

Reagent system: Liquid
Reagent volume: 50 to 500 μL
Reagent stability: 7 to 60 days
Reagent packaging: Package sizes are keyed to each system
On-board reagent inventory
Sample barcode with direct tube sampling
Sample volume: 3 to 15 μL

DATA MANAGEMENT

Interfacing: Bidirectional
Data storage: Holds up to 4200 patient files
Data reporting: Color graphic displays include:
QC reports
Data edit functions
Repeat run menu
User-defined calculated tests
Correlation correction

MAINTENANCE

Daily: 15 minutes
Weekly: 1 hour
Monthly: 1 hour

SPECIAL FEATURES

Sample level detector
Secondary STAT printer
Test-dedicated reagent valves

Printed with permission from Olympus Corporation, Clinical Instruments Division.

ROCHE COBAS MIRA PLUS

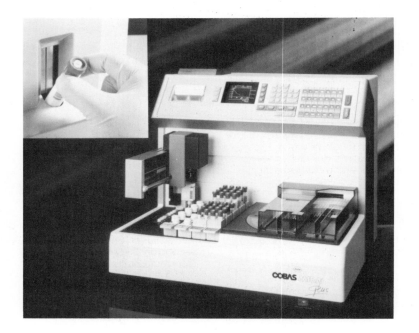

SYSTEM OVERVIEW

24-hour random access analyzer
Open system
60 on-board chemistry reagents
Analytical throughput: Up to 204 tests per hour with ISEs
Test menu: General chemistries, special chemistries, DAUs, TDMs, and specific proteins

REAGENTS/SAMPLES

Reagent system: Liquid
Reagent volume: 100–600 μL
Reagent stability: Reagent-specific
Reagent packaging: Vials with various sizes
Sample entry by sample cups; primary or secondary tube sampling with optional barcode capability and closed-tube safety
Sample volume: 2 to 95 μL
Pre- or postdilution of samples

DATA MANAGEMENT

Interfacing: Bidirectional
Data storage: >4000 patient test results
Data reporting: Daily and monthly QC results
                 Levey-Jennings plotting
                 Plotting calculations using up to 4 tests
                 End-point or linear regression analysis
                 Linear search for enzymes
                 6 nonlinear calculation models
                 104 programmable test channels
                 Software maintenance feature

MAINTENANCE

Daily: 5–10 minutes
Weekly: 1–2 minutes
Monthly: 5–15 minutes

SPECIAL FEATURES

Reagent and sample level detection
Ready-to-use color-coded liquid TDM, DAT, and thyroid reagents
TDMs, STATS in 5 minutes
Automated cuvet handling (optional)

Printed with permission from Roche Diagnostic Systems.

ROCHE COBAS FARA II

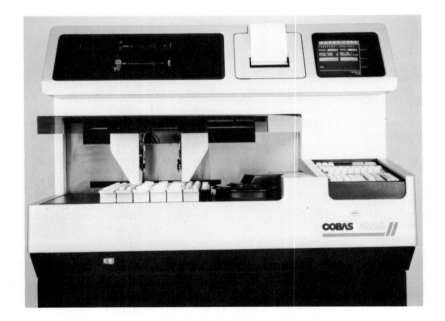

SYSTEM OVERVIEW

24-hour random access analyzer
Open system
90 resident chemistry reagents
Analytical throughput: Up to 400 tests per hour
Test menu: General chemistries, special chemistries, DAUs, specific proteins, ISEs, immunoassays, and TDMs

REAGENTS/SAMPLES

Reagent system: Liquid
Reagent volume: Up to 370 μL
Reagent stability: Test-specific
Reagent packaging: Vials with various sizes
Sample entry: Racks (computer entry)
Sample volume: 2–95 μL
Preprogrammed predilution

DATA MANAGEMENT

Interfacing: Bidirectional
Data storage: >4000 patient test results
Data reporting: Sample and reagent absorbance check
Recalculations of results from raw data
Ratio calculations utilizing up to 4 tests
End-point or linear regression analysis
Linear search for enzymes
6 nonlinear calculation models

MAINTENANCE

Daily: 2–5 minutes
Weekly: 2–5 minutes
Monthly: 5–15 minutes

SPECIAL FEATURES

TDMs, STATS in 5 minutes
Reagent and sample level detection
Ready-to-use color-coded liquid TDM, DAT, and
  thyroid reagents

Printed with permission from Roche Diagnostic Systems.

ROCHE COBAS INTEGRA

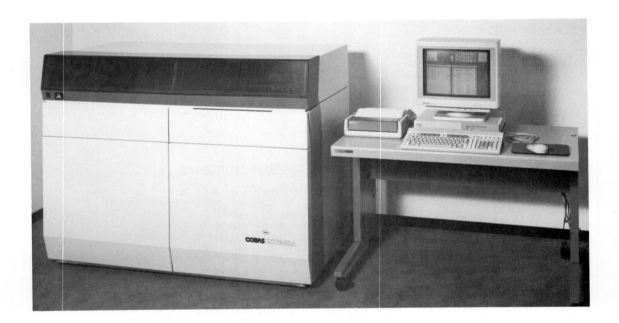

SYSTEM OVERVIEW

24-hour random access analyzer
Closed system
72 resident chemistries, including ISEs
Analytical throughput: 750 tests per hour
Test menu: General chemistries, ISEs, urine chemistries, CSF chemistries, TDMs, thyroids, DAUs, immunoassays,
             and special proteins

REAGENTS/SAMPLES

Reagent system: Liquid
Reagent volume: 100 to 250 µL
Reagent stability: Minimum 30 days (test-specific)
Reagent packaging: 50 to 1000 tests per barcoded cassette
On-board inventory and refrigeration
Sample entry by direct tube sampling with barcode (closed tube)
Sample volume: 2 to 50 µL per test with average below 10 µL
Automatic sample dilution and concentration
STAT dwelltime: 7 minutes with next test run integration

DATA MANAGEMENT

Interfacing: Bidirectional
Query function
Data storage: 200+ megabytes
Data reporting: Color graphic displays include:
                 QC reports
                 Levey-Jennings, Westgard rules
                 Calculated ratios
                 Calibration review
                 Sample tracking
                 Preset supply of reagents and cuvets
                 Test-specific histograms
                 Previous test results
                 Patient-monitoring line graphics

MAINTENANCE

Daily: 5 minutes
Weekly: 5 minutes
Monthly: 10–30 minutes

SPECIAL FEATURES

Reagent on-board reconstruction
Multiworkstation analyzer
68 test cassettes, on-board reagent capacity
One-reagent cassette design
Large test menu
``Load and forget'' one-time loading of reagents
Object-oriented, driven software
Self-start program

Printed with permission from Roche Diagnostic Systems.

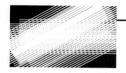

GLOSSARY

Absorbance. Optical density of a substance; $A = 2 - \log \%$ transmittance; $A = abc$, where a is the absorptivity of the substance of interest, b is the light path, and c is the concentration of the substance of interest.

Absorption. Light that will not pass through a solution. It is the process by which energy in the form of electromagnetic radiation is transferred to a substance when the radiation interacts with the substance.

Accuracy. The ability of a method to produce a result close to the true result.

Acridine orange. A fluorochrome that binds to nucleic acid. Its primary use is in highlighting bacteria in blood cultures.

Alpha-particle. A type of radiation, consisting of helium atoms minus their orbiting electrons, that is emitted by radioactive elements.

Alternating current. An electrical circuit in which the flow of electrons is bidirectional, first moving in one direction and then in the other.

Amperometry. The branch of electrochemistry that utilizes information gained from applying a fixed potential to an electrochemical cell and then measuring current produced because of an oxidation or reduction reaction.

Ampholytes. Low molecular weight (300 to 1000 daltons) amphoteric polyaminocarboxylic acids used in isoelectric focusing electrophoresis to create stable pH zones.

Analytical. All functions performed at an instrument to produce a test result.

Analytical sensitivity. The lowest concentration that can be reported with a particular analytical method.

Analytical specificity. Ability of an assay to produce accurate results in the presence of possible interferences.

Analytical throughput. The maximum number of tests or samples an instrument can perform in 1 hour.

Atomic absorption. A spectrophotometric method to determine the concentration of elements in a solution by vaporizing them in a flame and measuring their absorption of characteristic wavelengths.

Autodilution. Dilutes samples automatically when assays are out of linear range.

Automatic indexing. A feature on a densitometer that automatically advances the electrophoresis strip, which contains multiple sample channels, from one channel to the next.

Bandpass (bandwidth). The range of wavelengths between which the peak absorption is half the transmittance. This range represents the distribution of wavelengths that pass through the exit slit of the monochromator. This term corresponds to the slit width of the spectrophotometer.

Barcode. A series of lines and spaces that vary in width to represent alphanumeric symbols. A barcode reader hits the code with a laser beam and interprets the light reflected into a computer-readable form.

Batch analyzer. An instrument designed to perform the same test or a group of tests on multiple patient samples during each analytical run.

Batch systems. Analyzers that perform large numbers of single tests.

Beer's law. An equation that shows the linear relationship existing between absorption and the concentration of the absorbing species. The law states that the absorbance of a homogeneous sample of an absorbing substance is directly proportional to the concentration of the absorbing substance; $A = abc$, where A = Absorbance, a = absorption coefficient, b = distance the light travels through the sample, c = concentration.

Beta particle. A type of radiation, composed of electrons, that is emitted by radioactive elements.

Bias. Observed result minus assigned value.

Bidirectional interface. Allows two-way communication via computer linkage between the laboratory information system (LIS) and any on-line instrument.

Birefringence. The difference between the two indices of refraction seen to exist among some crystalline materials.

Calibration. Prescribed steps performed to establish testing parameters and instrument conditions that provide precise and accurate results.

Calibration verification. The assay of calibration materials to confirm that a test system has remained stable throughout the reportable range.

Capacitor. An electrical circuit element with the ability to store an electrical charge.

Capillary zone electrophoresis. Also referred to as capillary electrophoresis (CE) or high performance capillary electrophoresis (HPCE), this analytic technique combines high performance liquid chromatography and conventional electrophoresis in a single system.

Capital acquisition. The purchase or lease/rental of clinical laboratory instrumentation.

Cathode. The negatively charged pole that attracts more cationic proteins.

Cathode ray tube. A screen or monitor upon which computer data are displayed in the form of numbers, letters, and symbols that allow for communication between the user and the computer.

Cell potential. The measure of potential by a voltmeter in an electrochemical cell, which reflects the difference in electron energy between the two half-cells.

Centrifugal analyzer. A batch analyzer utilizing centrifugation to mix reagent(s) and sample(s) in a self-contained rotary cuvet assembly.

Chemiluminescence. A chemical reaction that produces light.

Chemiluminescent reaction. A chemical reaction in which an unstable product is formed; when it reverts to its ground energy state, it releases energy in the form of visible light.

Chloride electrode. An ion-selective electrode (ISE) constructed of either a liquid membrane or a solid-state crystal of silver chloride/silver sulfite, and responding to chloride ion.

Chloridometer. A device for performing coulometric analysis for the determination of chloride concentration.

Chopper. A component that interrupts an electrical current or light beam, converting it from direct current to alternating current through mechanical or electrical means.

Clinical decision concentration. The concentration at which a caregiver may act if the result is less than or greater than.

Clinical Laboratory Improvement Act (CLIA). A federal law that sets out regulations for the performance of laboratory testing.

Clinical sensitivity. The percent of patients with a disease who have a positive test result.

Clinical specificity. The percent of patients who do not have a disease and do not have a positive result.

Closed reagent system. User can purchase reagents only from instrument manufacturer.

Closed tube sampling. Designed to allow sampling of patient specimen without opening tubes, resulting in cost savings and reduced biohazardous risks for operator.

Coefficient of variation (CV). A statistic that describes the variability of results for a specimen assayed repeatedly, relative to the mean.

Coincidence correction. Electronic circuitry that corrects for the possibility that two cells will pass through an aperture at one time.

"Coincidence" error. An error in analyzers using the electronic impedance principle in which two or more cells simultaneously enter the aperture separating the internal and external electrodes, resulting in one pulse.

Colligative properties. The four physical properties of a solution—boiling point, freezing point, vapor pressure, and osmotic pressure—that are related to the number of particles in solution and can, in turn, be measured to determine the osmolality of a solution.

Colorimeter. A device for estimating the percentage of a colored substance in a solution.

Columns. The component in gas and liquid chromatography systems that houses the stationary phase. Typically, columns are coiled and are contained in an oven.

Competitive immunoassay. An antigen-antibody reaction in which labeled antigen and unlabeled antigen compete for limited antibody sites. The amount of bound labeled antigen is indirectly proportional to the concentration of the analyte.

Conductivity analyzers. A method used in cell counting based on the electrical conductivity difference between particles in a suspension and the diluent as measured between two electrodes.

Consumables. Disposable supplies used to produce test results.

Cost per reportable. All direct costs related to producing a patient test result.

Coulometry. An analytical technique similar to amperometry. The main difference is that the current needed to convert a substance completely is measured and used to determine the concentration.

Current. The flow of electrons through a substance such as a solution or a wire; measured in coulombs of charge per second (i.e., amperes).

Cuvet (cuvette). The receptacle in which the sample is placed, allowing light bands exiting the monochromator to pass through before striking the detector. There is a wide variety of cuvets. The choice depends on the analysis and the sample volume.

Data management. The data management features that can be found on a particular analyzer (e.g., Q.C. programs).

Database. A method for computerized storage of data that allows for quick and easy access of the information as well as simple insertion and deletion of data.

Dedicated instrument. An instrument that is dedicated to perform one or two tests.

Delimiting. A feature in automated electrophoretic systems that allows for deletion, or suppression of fractions, and adjustment of the scanned baselines or slopes.

Delta checking. A procedure that compares a patient's previous result with the current result for a particular analyte.

Densitometer. A modified spectrophotometer that determines the intensity of each band of an electrophoretogram.

Detector. A device designed to convert the energy of incident radiation into an electric output, a useful measure of the radiation that is incident on the device.

Diagnostic programs. Software programs designed to assess instrument function and to report malfunctions to operator.

Dichroic mirror. A mirror that splits a beam of energy and directs specific portions of it in two different directions.

Diffraction grating device. A monochromatic wavelength selector (monochromator) that consists of a series of parallel grooves, equally spaced, allowing a light beam that strikes it to be dispersed into several linear spectra.

Diode. A solid state device (or electron tube) having only two active elements or electrodes that allow current flow in only one direction.

Direct costs. Only those costs incurred as a direct result of producing a test result. Indirect costs such as administrative costs would not be included in this calculation.

Direct current. An electrical current in which the electrons flow in only one direction.

Double antibody separation. The separation of the antigen-antibody complex from the free is accomplished by adding a second antibody (antigammaglobulin) to form a larger precipitating complex.

Double hydrodynamic focusing system. A patented measurement process of the Cobas Argos 5 Diff analyzer that uses two successive measurements on each cell: electronic resistance and optical absorbance.

Downtime. Time during which instrument is not capable of producing patient results that can be reported.

DRG (Diagnosis Related Group). A prospective payment system used by Medicare to classify all hospitalized patients into one of 468 diagnosis-related groups. The hospital receives a fixed payment per DRG to cover operating costs.

Drift. A slow, unidirectional change in the output of an instrument in a system that occurs over several days or weeks, representative of long-term stability. Drift occurs because of temperature changes and/or aging of the light source and electronic components, or both.

Efficiency. A mathematical concept that is determined by calculation of the height equivalent of a theoretical plate. The number generated is representative of the ability of the column to give good separation.

Electrical impedance. A principle for cell counting based on cells acting as insulators momentarily increasing the resistance in an electrical path between two electrodes.

Electrochemistry. The study of chemical reactions occurring because of the flow or presence of electrons between two dissimilar substances.

Electrode. An electrochemical interface or half-cell that can be used with another interface to make useful measurements.

Electron (chemical) ionization. Ionization of sample molecules resulting from striking them with a beam of light.

Electronic transition. A change in the orbital position of an electron or an atom or molecule, such as a change from ground state to excited state.

Electro-osmotic flow. A bulk flow of fluid resulting from excess of positively charged ions in the direction toward the cathode that enhances the separation of the charged ions.

Emission wavelength. The light re-emitted by a substance after having absorbed light energy of a shorter wavelength.

Emitter. One of the elements of a transistor; comparable to the cathode of the electron tube.

Endosmosis (electroendosmosis). The slowing, retardation, or reversal of protein migration when the support medium becomes negatively charged because of the absorption of hydroxyl ions from the buffer.

Enzyme electrode. An indicator electrode utilizing an immobilized enzyme as one of the layers of the membrane. This electrode can be made to respond to nonionic analytes if the enzyme converts the analyte to a reactant that can be sensed by the basic electrode.

Enzyme multiplied immunoassay technique (EMIT). A homogeneous enzyme immunoassay in which an enzyme-labeled drug competes with a free drug in the sample for antibody-binding sites. When the enzyme-labeled drug is bound, the enzyme activity is blocked. The free enzyme-labeled drug is allowed to react with its substrates. The enzyme activity is directly proportional to the concentration of the drug in the sample.

Excitation wavelength. The wavelength of the incident light that is absorbed by the molecule, causing it to be raised to a higher energy level.

Expert systems. A type of information system programmed to solve problems, such as interpretation of test results and/or diagnosis by established criteria.

Filter. A device that selectively passes certain wavelengths of light and will absorb others. A glass (Wratten) filter has one or two layers of colored glass.

Fingerprint. The ridge patterns of the fingers that have become a pillar of modern criminal identification.

Fixed costs. Costs that do not vary as test volume increases. Examples are rental payment, interest on debt, depreciation of plant and equipment, and wages of a skeleton staff that would be employed as long as the hospital stayed in business even if it produced nothing.

Fixed profile system. A sequential system that performs a specific number of tests at one time.

Flame ionization detector (FID). A detector used in chromatographic systems, based on the principle that organic compounds are ionized in a flame; electrons are released and migrate to a detector, producing an electrical current that is amplified and measured.

Flame photometry. A photometric method to determine the concentration of an element in a flame-vaporized sample by measuring the intensity of its emission spectra.

Flow cell. A type of sample holder that is designed as a flow-through cuvet. Sample is introduced via tubing.

Flow cytometer. An instrument that uses light scatter methodology for making multiple measurements of individual cells in a flowing fluid.

Fluorescence. That property of some substances that allows them to absorb light energy at one wavelength and re-emit some of it at a longer wavelength; the immediate emission (10^{-8} sec) of light after it has absorbed radiation.

Fluorescent polarization. When fluorescent molecules are excited with polarized light, they emit partially polarized light whose intensity is indirectly related to the degree of rotation of the molecules. Free molecules have a higher rate of rotation and emit lower intensity light than do bound molecules, which have a low rate of rotation and therefore emit a higher intensity of light.

Fluorochrome. A molecule, used to tag an antigen or an antibody, that is capable of absorbing light and re-emitting it as fluorescence.

Fractional precipitation separation. Antigen-antibody complex can be precipitated by neutral salts, such as ammonium sulfite and ammonium sulfate, and organic solvents, such as ethanol.

Function verification. Those activities that usually involve the checking of system operation.

Gain. The amount of amplification of input voltage to output voltage.

Gamma ray. A form of high-energy electromagnetic radiation emitted by radioactive elements.

Gas chromatography. A chromatographic system in which the mobile phase is a gas.

Gas-sensing electrode. A modified indicator electrode fashioned with a membrane, like Teflon, semipermeable to a gas, and placed around the base of an electrode such as a glass electrode.

Glass electrode. An electrode specially designed with a thin piece of glass as the membrane. The glass can be formulated so that it is sensitive to H^+ or Na^{2+} ions.

Gradient elution. A chromatographic technique in which various solvents are introduced into the mobile phase as the compound elutes through the system. This technique causes changes in polarity of the mobile phase and promotes improved separation.

Hardware. The physical components containing all the electronics necessary for the operation of a computer system.

Hemogram. A group of hematologic direct analyses, usually including hemoglobin, erythrocyte count, and leukocyte count.

Heterogeneous immunoassay. Immunoassay reaction in which a separation step is required to separate the bound label physically from the free label before measurement can be performed.

High performance liquid chromatography (HPLC). A modified liquid chromatography system that utilizes narrow, rigid columns with chemicals containing different function groups that are bonded to a silica column to alter polarity.

High resolution protein electrophoresis. An electrophoresis technique that employs a specialized agarose gel (low content of sulfate and carboxyl groups) under high voltage to achieve greater specificity in protein separation.

Histogram. A computer-generated, single-dimensional display of cellular analyses, such as volume. Analysis or measured values are shown on the X-axis, and the concentration is shown on the Y-axis.

Hollow cathode lamp. A lamp containing an inert gas and a metal cathode that emits wavelengths characteristic of the cathode.

Homogeneous immunoassay. Immunoassay reaction in which no separation step is required by using labeled reagent whose activity is modulated by the binding reaction.

Hospital Information System (HIS). The computer system that stores the data and programs utilized in administrative hospital operations (billing, admitting, medical records) and allows operators access to laboratory data from the Laboratory Information System.

Host computer. A facility's primary computer in which all data are collected and stored.

"Hot line." An emergency, 24-hour, manufacturer-staffed, troubleshooting phone line.

Hydrodynamic focusing. A process in which a stream of isotonic sheath fluid is used to arrange cells in single file and channel them through a counting chamber with an orifice only slightly larger than a leukocyte.

Immunoprecipitation. Certain serum proteins can form insoluble immunocomplexes in the presence of their specific antibody.

Impedance. Opposition to the flow of alternating current, which is a result of the combined effect of resistance and reactance; an application of this principle is used in cell-sorting instrumentation.

Indicator electrode. The electrochemical half-cell with a potential that varies in response to some analyte.

Inductively coupled plasma. A photometric method to determine the concentrations of elements in an electrically heated argon gas ''plasma'' source by measuring the intensity of their emission spectra.

Instrument maintenance. A two component process: first, preventive maintenance per se, and second, troubleshooting and repair.

Integrated circuit. A major electrical device containing several electrical components such as to allow the device to perform multiple electronic functions.

Interface. The electrical connection that allows for communication (passage of data) between multiple computer systems (e.g., the LIS and automated instrumentation).

Interference. The effect of a substance within the sample matrix on the analyte being analyzed.

Internal standard. A known concentration of a substance (element or compound) added to a sample to correct for certain characteristics of a procedure, e.g., flame instability.

Ion-selective electrode (ISE). An indicator electrode used in potentiometry that responds to a specific ion in the sample.

Isoelectric focusing electrophoresis (IFE). A high resolution electrophoresis technique in which proteins migrate through a pH gradient, with the aid of ampholytes, to their respective isoelectric points (pIs).

Junction potential. A potential arising at the interface between the inner electrode fluid of the reference electrode and the sample.

Laboratory Information System (LIS). A computer system within the laboratory that stores patient information and results. The LIS may be interfaced (or linked) to analytical instruments for reporting of results and to a Hospital Information System for retrieval of laboratory results throughout the hospital.

Laser. An acronym for *l*ight *a*mplification by *s*timulated *e*mission *r*adiation; this beam of light is very intense, highly collimated, and often used in nephelometers.

Lease. A contract that allows for the renting of instrumentation for a specified time under specified terms.

Levy-Jennings charts. A quality control procedure that plots consecutive control results over time on a graph.

Light scatter. The interaction of light directed on particles suspended in solution, resulting in the bending of light, at various angles, away from its original path.

Line spectra. Discontinuous emission of essentially monochromatic light.

Linearity. The extent to which a range over a response (e.g., absorbance) is directly proportional to the concentration; also, the relationship between two variables that yields a straight line when plotted on a graph.

Liquid membrane electrode. A porous polymer membrane indicator electrode in which a nonpolar liquid is soaked. A hydrophobic ion-exchanger or neutral carrier ionophore that selectively reacts with the ion of interest is dissolved into the nonpolar liquid.

Lobularity index. A ratio of polymorphonuclear nuclei (PMN) to mononuclear nuclei (MN), indicating the degree of nuclear segmentation.

Local Area Network (LAN). A connection of multiple computers within a localized area that allows for data and hardware and software components to be shared at more than one user terminal.

Luminometer. An instrument designed to measure a flash of light. It consists of a light-tight, temperature-regulated chamber and a sensitive light detector that is capable of measuring light in nanoseconds.

Manual systems. Laboratory tests that are performed manually.

Marginal cost analysis. The additional cost incurred as output expands. It is cost associated with producing an additional patient test result.

Matrix-plot. A high resolution charge produced by the Cobas Argos 5 Diff analyzer in which collected signals from successive measurements of electronic resistance and optical absorbance are computerized and categorized.

0.5 McFarland turbidity standard. A turbidity standard equivalent to 1.5×10^8 cells/ml.

Microparticle-enhanced nephelometric immunoassay. A technique that utilizes submicron-sized particles as carriers of antibodies, so that the reaction of the coated antibody with the antigen will result in a suspended particle large enough to scatter light and thus be detected by a nephelometer.

Microspectrophotometer. An analytical instrument, combining microscopy with spectrophotometry, that provides absorption spectra from trace quantities of evidence being observed microscopically.

Minimal inhibitory concentration (MIC). The minimum concentration of antimicrobial agent needed to yield a 99 percent reduction in colony-forming units (microbial colonies) of a microbial suspension.

Mobile phase. The solvent used in a chromatographic system that serves as the carrier of the compound through a column, i.e., through the stationary phase.

Modem. A specialized communication device that allows for multiple computers to exchange data over telephone lines.

Moderate and high complexity tests. CLIA has defined the complexity of clinical laboratory tests and classified them according to the difficulty in performing and interpreting the test. CLIA has determined who may perform these types of testing based on training, education, and experience.

NCCLS (National Committee for Clinical Laboratory Standards). A nonprofit educational organization composed of laboratory professionals in industry, academia, and laboratorians. The committee produces protocols for operation of clinical laboratories.

Nephelometer. An instrument that measures light scattered at a 90° angle from the primary beam.

Nephelometry. The technique of employing a specially designed spectrophotometer to detect light scatter, produced by particles suspended in solution, at an angle different from that of the incident light source.

Neutron activation analysis. The technique of bombarding specimens with neutrons and measuring the resultant gamma ray radioactivity.

Noise. Random fluctuations in a system that occur abruptly, representative of short-term stability.

Noncompetitive immunoassay. Immunoassay reaction in which the antibody is labeled.

Normal phase. A chromatographic separation with a nonpolar mobile phase and a polar stationary phase.

Normal reference range. The range of values for a particular analyte, obtained from patients thought to be healthy. It is used to help determine whether a result from a patient may be abnormal compared with healthy patients. This range, however, does not define health. Some healthy patients may have results outside this range and patients with disease may have results within this range.

On-board stability. The life span of a reagent once placed on an instrument.

On-site testing. Laboratory testing performed in the same location and at the same time that the patient is seen by the physician.

Open system. Reagents and consumable supplies can be purchased from any available vendor.

Operational efficiency. Making the fullest utilization of available inputs. Alternatively, minimizing the use of inputs to produce the desired level of test results.

Optical density (absorbance). Microbes in solution refract and deflect light from passing through a solution. By using a device such as a colorimeter or spectrophotometer, turbidity can be expressed in units of absorbance.

Panic value. A result that may indicate that a patient's life is in jeopardy and an immediate response may be required by a physician.

Parallel analysis. A comparison of results for select analytes between different analyzers and/or methodologies.

pCO_2 electrode. A gas electrode that responds selectively to CO_2 gas; the outer membrane is separated from a pH glass electrode by a bicarbonate buffer solution.

PCR (polymerase chain reaction). Procedure by which hundreds of thousands of copies of a specific sequence of DNA are synthesized.

Peak height ratio. The peak height of the analyte of interest divided by the peak height of the internal standard.

Peak resolution (R_s). The extent to which two peaks are separated in a chromatographic system; calculated by

$$R_s = \frac{2(t_B - t_A)}{W_A W_B}$$

Performance verification. Activities designed to test and ensure that an instrument is working correctly and is properly calibrated.

pH electrode. An electrode system utilizing a glass membrane placed around an internal Ag/AgCl reference electrode.

Phosphorescence. The delayed release (10^{-2} to 100 sec) of absorbed radiation.

pO$_2$ electrode. An electrode composed of a small platinum cathode and an Ag/AgCl anode placed in a supporting electrolyte (typically a phosphate buffer) and enclosed by a gas-permeable membrane. The potential at the cathode is adjusted so that oxygen is reduced.

POL (physician office laboratory). A small laboratory that relies on smaller instrumentation.

Polarized light. Light that travels in a single plane.

Polarography. A voltammetric technique in which a working electrode has a continually renewable surface, such as the dropping mercury electrode.

Polymer enhancement. Nonionic hydrophilic polymers, such as polyethylene glycol (PEG) and dextran, are used to improve the speed and sensitivity of nephelometric reactions.

Postanalytical. All functions performed after analyzer results to get test results back to physician.

Postanalytical variation. Changes in patient results after analysis. This may be due to inaccurate calculations or to transcribing incorrect results.

Potassium electrode. An ISE utilizing the antibiotic valinomycin as the ionophore in the membrane, and responding to potassium ion.

Potential. The ability to do electrochemical work.

Potentiometry. An analytic technique making use of the information gained from determining a potential difference (volts) between two interfaces (e.g., electrodes) measured at equilibrium and with no current.

Preanalytical. All functions performed prior to instrumentation.

Preanalytical variation. Changes in patients' results due to inappropriate specimen handling, test ordering, or specimen collection.

Precipitate-impregnated membrane. An indicator electrode constructed of a polymer into which a precipitate containing the ion of interest is introduced.

Precision. The ability of a method to repeat a result over numerous analyses. Good precision indicates that the results are reproducible, thus having a low standard deviation and coefficient of variation.

Preventive maintenance. Scheduled inspection (of instruments or equipment) resulting in minor adjustment or repair to delay or avoid major repair and emergency or premature replacement.

Price protection. An agreement whereby the vendor agrees to limit price increases by an agreed upon amount during the term of the agreement.

Proficiency testing. The testing of specimens whose concentrations are unknown to the participating laboratory. Results are returned to the specimen provider, and the results are graded by comparing with results from all laboratories or reference laboratories. They are evaluated using criteria determined by either CLIA or the proficiency provider.

Pyrolysis. The decomposition of organic substances by heat.

Quadripole mass filter. A mass analyzer that separates ions based on their movement through a field. The quadripole, four rods in a rectangular configuration, uses radio frequency in an electronic field.

Quality assurance. A process that assures clinically useful results by monitoring procedures that affect the handling of patient samples, patient orders, patient reports, and other factors affecting the quality of patient results.

Quality control. A process that assures an accurate result of an analytical method.

Quality control checks. Performance tests run daily, weekly, or monthly to verify photometric linearity and wavelength accuracy, and to determine whether stray light is entering the system.

Radioimmunoassay (RIA). Immunoassay reaction in which the labeling molecule is a radioisotope such as ^{125}I.

Random access analyzers. Analyzers that process different tests simultaneously and discretely.

Reference electrode. An electrode that has a known, constant half-cell potential and against which the relative potential of the working or indicator electrode is measured.

Reference method. A method whose accuracy and precision is understood, which is used to validate methods used on a day-to-day basis. These procedures are usually very time consuming and are not appropriate for routine analyses.

Reference range. The range of values for a given analyte in a defined population. Usually used to guide the physician in detecting abnormal results. Reference range may depend on the population's age and sex.

Refraction. The bending of incident light after it passes from one medium to another of different density. Light scatter at right angles is strongly influenced by this phenomenon.

Reportable range. The lowest and highest concentrations that can be reported without dilution or other treatment of the specimen.

Resistance. The opposition of a substance to current flow; measured in ohms.

Resolution. In spectrophotometry, this term can be substituted for bandwidth.

Retardation factor (R_f). The distance a compound travels, on a thin layer plate, from the point of application to the distance the mobile phase (solvent) travels within the same time period.

Retention time (T_R). The time it takes for a retained compound to elute from a chromatographic system.

Retention volume (V_R). The volume it takes for a retained compound to elute from a chromatographic system.

Reverse phase chromatography. A chromatographic separation accomplished with a polar mobile phase and a nonpolar stationary phase.

RFLP (restriction fragment length polymorphism). Variation in DNA sequence that can be detected as a change in the length of the DNA fragments produced by a restriction enzyme.

Robotic system. A mechanized device designed to perform repetitive tasks with a high degree of precision and accuracy.

Run. An interval within which the accuracy and precision of a testing system are expected to be stable, but it cannot be greater than 24 hours. For some methods, a run may be every time patients, calibrators, and controls are assayed, whereas other methods may define a run as once each day, or once each shift.

Sample splitting. The sharing of a sample between multiple workstations.

Sandwich (2-site) immunoassay. Immunoassay reaction in which the molecule is first incubated with an antibody immobilized on a solid phase and then with a second labeled antibody directed at the second antigenic site on the molecule. Excess labeled antibody is removed by washing the solid phase, and the concentration of the analyte is directly proportional to the amount of bound label on the solid phase.

Satellite testing. Testing performed in locations other than the main laboratory site, such as a critical care unit.

Saturated calomel electrode (SCE). A practical reference electrode containing an inert wire (e.g., platinum) in contact with elemental mercury, mercurous chloride (calomel), and a saturated solution of potassium chloride.

Scanning. The collection of data (e.g., absorbance) over an entire wavelength range. This feature on a spectrophotometer allows one to determine the maximal absorbance wavelength of an absorbing solution.

Scanning electron microscope. An instrument that focuses a beam of electrons on a specimen and produces a highly magnified image upon a TV tube.

Scatter measurements. A methodology for analyzing cell characteristics that uses a focused beam of light which is interrupted (scattered) when cells are encountered in a flowing fluid.

Scatterplots. A display of data points or cells classified by two or more measurable characteristics. This is used to identify the presence of abnormalities in subpopulations, primarily from conductivity.

Semiconductor. A material with a resistivity between that of conductors and insulators; a solid state electrical device, called a diode, made of silicon (or germanium) ``doped'' crystal.

Sequential batch systems. Automated system that automatically adds samples and reagents to an analytical stream for a particular test.

Service contract. Contracts in which the vendor agrees to supply maintenance and repair of instrumentation. The contract could cover response time and hours and days (i.e., including weekends) during which the services will be provided.

Silver-silver chloride electrode (Ag/AgCl). A popular reference electrode constructed of a silver wire, or platinum wire coated with silver, for which some of the silver is converted to silver chloride by electrolysis in hydrochloric acid.

Sodium electrode. A membrane electrode in which sodium from the sample reacts with ion-exchange sites selective for this ion on the outer membrane surface. These membranes have been made of glass or liquid.

Software. The programmed instructions that operate the computer system.

Solid phase separation. Antigen or antibody can be immobilized onto a solid phase surface, such as polymer beads, plastic tubes, glass fiber, filter paper, or magnetized particles. Separation of the bound from the free label can be achieved by centrifugation, decantation, simple washing, or the application of a magnetic field.

Solid state circuit. Electrical circuits that use semiconductor diodes and transistors instead of vacuum tubes.

Solid state membrane electrode. A type of indicator electrode in which the active portion of the membrane is actually a solid crystal or salt pellet of the ion of interest.

"Sort logic." A computerized logic that is applied to a cell-sorter instrument in which cells are identified electronically as they pass a laser beam; this results in certain cells being charged and redirected for further analyses.

Specification sheets (spec sheets). A manufacturer's list of performance and special features provided by a particular instrument.

Spectrogram. A graph or photograph of a spectrum.

Spectrophotometer. An instrument that measures the amount of monochromatic light passing through a solution by means of an adjustable monochromator such as a prism or a diffraction grating.

Standard deviation (SD). A statistic that describes how results vary about the mean when a specimen is assayed repetitively.

Standard deviation index (SDI). A measure that describes the number of standard deviations away from the mean that a result is.

STAT systems. Systems that are dedicated to performing only STAT tests.

Stationary phase. The separating material that remains in a fixed position (liquid or solid).

Stray radiant energy (stray light). Light (wavelengths), other than that exiting from the sample, which strikes the detector. Usually this is room light that has entered the instrument.

Susceptibility testing. Determining an antibiotic's capability of killing or suppressing the growth of microorganisms.

Sweep flow technology. A modification in the Coulter STKS analyzer that improves platelet count accuracy by preventing red cell recirculation.

Target range. The range of results that are considered acceptable by the proficiency agency. Some of these target ranges are defined by CLIA.

Target value. The concentration of an analyte from a proficiency sample. This concentration is assumed to be the true concentration. The target value is based on the mean of all participants, or the mean established by reference methods.

Terminal. The point at which the user may interact with the computer by entering or retrieving data. Usually consists of a monitor and a keyboard along with any other specialized input/output devices (modems, barcode scanners).

Test menu. The number of available chemistry tests available for a particular instrument.

Test profile. A group of tests designed to provide information about a specific organ function or disease process.

Thermal conductivity detector (TCD). A detector used in gas chromatography systems that utilizes the principle of changes in heat conductivity (heat conduction) of a carrier gas caused by mixture of the sample. An increase in temperature decreases the resistance and causes a current flow.

Thermocouple. A thermoelectric device consisting of two dissimilar metals joined so that a potential difference generated between the points of contact is a measure of the temperature difference between the points.

Thin-layer chromatography (TLC). A chromatographic system in which flat beds or planar supports are used as the stationary phase.

Transducer. A device that changes physical energy, such as pressure, light, and heat, into electrical energy.

Transformer. A device containing a primary and a secondary coil, linked by magnetic lines of force, used to transfer and increase or decrease electrical energy from one circuit to another.

Transistor. A solid state, three-electrode semiconductor device that functionally replaced the vacuum tube.

Troubleshooting. The process by which apparently unsatisfactory instrument performance is traced down to root causes, which permits the correct solution to be applied to identified problems.

Turbidimetry. The measurement of a decrease in percent transmittance of an incident beam of light as it passes through a solution containing suspended particles.

Turbidity. Cell (microbial) suspensions appear turbid because each cell scatters light. The amount of turbidity is proportional to the quantity of microbes present.

Turnaround time. Typically refers to time required to produce a test result once a sample arrives in the laboratory.

Two-dimensional (2D) electrophoresis. An electrophoretic process that applies a two-stage approach to separation of proteins. Separation is accomplished first based on charge and then upon molecular mass.

Variable costs. Costs that change as output (i.e., test volume) fluctuates.

VCS. An acronym for volume (V), conductivity (C), and laser light scatter (S) describing the technology used in multiple measurements for leukocyte differentials in the Coulter STKS.

Voltammetry. An analytical technique similar to amperometry in which the potential is varied in some way and the current-potential relationship is monitored.

Waivered tests. Tests that, according to CLIA, are either cleared by the FDA for home use, employ simple and accurate methodologies that have a negligible likelihood of erroneous results, or pose no reasonable risk of harm to the patient if performed incorrectly.

"Walkaway" systems. Laboratory systems that allow the operator to walk away from the systems after they have been loaded with patient samples and test requests are entered.

Wheatstone bridge. An electrical configuration using four resistors that act in pairs to compare some unknown parameter to a known parameter according to Ohm's law.

Wick flow. The upward movement of buffer through both immersed ends of a membrane to replace lost moisture. This phenomenon can reduce separation and compression of the final band patterns.

Workflow analysis. The monitoring of all functions from the time a test is requested to results reported.

Working electrode. The electrode that consumes or produces electrons, which can be measured as current and related to the amount of analyte.

Workload. Quantity of work accomplished by an instrument, a laboratorian, or an entire laboratory staff in a defined time.

Workstation consolidation. Reducing the number of laboratory instruments needed to meet testing demands.

X-ray diffraction. The technique of directing x-radiation at a crystal and studying the reflection patterns that are produced.

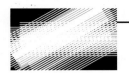

ANSWERS

Chapter 1

1.	c	7.	c
2.	a	8.	c
3.	c	9.	c
4.	b	10.	b
5.	d	11.	b
6.	d		

Chapter 2

1.	a and d	4.	b and c
2.	a	5.	c and d
3.	b		

Chapter 3

1.	a	5.	c
2.	d	6.	c
3.	c	7.	b
4.	d	8.	b

Chapter 4

1.	c	9.	a
2.	d	10.	b
3.	d	11.	b
4.	b	12.	a
5.	b	13.	d
6.	a	14.	a
7.	b	15.	e
8.	d	16.	d

Chapter 5

1.	b	4.	b
2.	d	5.	c
3.	d	6.	b

Chapter 6

1.	c	4.	c
2.	d	5.	d
3.	d	6.	b

Chapter 7

1.	b	5.	a
2.	d	6.	d
3.	a	7.	a
4.	d	8.	d

Chapter 8

1.	b	5.	a
2.	d	6.	d
3.	e	7.	b
4.	c		

Chapter 9

1.	d	7.	a
2.	b	8.	b
3.	c	9.	c
4.	b	10.	a
5.	a	11.	c
6.	b	12.	d

Chapter 10

1.	a	4.	c
2.	b	5.	d
3.	c		

Chapter 11

1.	d	6.	a, c, d
2.	a, b, d	7.	b, c, d
3.	b, c	8.	a, c
4.	a, b, c	9.	a, b, c, d
5.	b	10.	a, b, c, d

Chapter 12

1.	d	4.	c
2.	c and d	5.	b
3.	e		

Chapter 13

1.	a, c, e	4.	c
2.	b, c, e	5.	c
3.	b	6.	a, b

Chapter 14

1.	b	4.	b
2.	a	5.	b
3.	b		

Chapter 15

1.	b	5.	All
2.	a	6.	d
3.	f	7.	d
4.	e		

Chapter 16

1.	a	4.	b
2.	b	5.	d
3.	d		

Chapter 17

1.	c	5.	b
2.	a	6.	b
3.	c	7.	b
4.	d		

Chapter 18

1.	c	3.	b
2.	c	4.	a

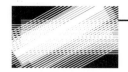

INDEX

Note: Page numbers in *italics* refer to illustrations; page numbers followed by t refer to tables.